ADVANCES IN NEUROLOGY
VOLUME 24

Advances in Neurology

INTERNATIONAL ADVISORY BOARD

Advances in Neurology
Volume 24

The Extrapyramidal System and its Disorders

*VIth International Symposium
on Parkinson's Disease,* 6th, Québec, Québec, 1978

Editors

Louis J. Poirier, M.D., Ph.D.
*Professeur de Neurologie Expérimentale
Université Laval
Directeur, Centre de Neurobiologie
Hôpital de l'Enfant-Jésus
Québec, P.Q., Canada*

Theodore L. Sourkes, Ph.D.
*Professor of Psychiatry
Director, Laboratory of Neurochemistry
McGill University
Montréal, P.Q., Canada*

Paul J. Bédard, M.D., Ph.D.
*Professeur Agrégé
Université Laval
Centre de Neurobiologie,
Hôpital de l'Enfant-Jésus
Québec, P.Q., Canada*

Raven Press ■ New York

Raven Press, 1140 Avenue of the Americas, New York, New York 10036

Made in the United States of America

Library of Congress Cataloging in Publication Data

International Symposium on Parkinson's Disease, 6th,
    Québec, Québec, 1978.
    The extrapyramidal system and its disorders.

    (Advances in Neurology; v. 24)
    Includes index.
    1. Parkinsonism—Congresses. 2.   Extrapyramidal
tracts—Diseases—Congresses. 3.   Extrapyramidal tracts
—Congresses. 4.   Neurotransmitters—Congresses.
I.   Poirier, Louis Joseph, 1918– II.   Sourkes,
Theodore L. III.   Bédard, Paul J. IV.   Title.
V.   Series. [DNLM: 1.   Basal ganglia diseases—
Congresses. 2.   Extrapyramidal tracts—Congresses.
3.   Parkinson disease—Congresses. W3 IN921BK 6th
1978e / WL400 I61 1978e]
RC321.A276   vol. 24 [RC382]   616.8'08s   79–2461
ISBN 0–89004–369–8   [616.8'3]

Advances in Neurology Series

Preface

Over approximately the last two decades, neurobiology has profited by the development of refined methodologies and techniques. This new technology has lent itself particularly well to the study of the extrapyramidal system and related nervous structures so that neuroscientists have been encouraged to give more consideration to understanding this system and its clinical disorders. These efforts have resulted in important breakthroughs that greatly contribute not only to a better knowledge of the nervous mechanisms involved in extrapyramidal disorders but also to a more rational and efficient management of the underlying disturbances in patients. In this area, advances in basic and clinical science have clearly gone hand in hand.

The topics presented in this volume were selected on the basis of their originality and their reflection of the present state of knowledge of the extrapyramidal system and its disorders. They represent a concise summary of the contributions of approximately 120 scientists who reported at the VIth International Symposium on Parkinson's Disease, held in Quebec, September 24–27, 1978.

Within the spectrum of research delineated in this book, fine morphology and neuroanatomy are coupled with histochemistry and neurochemistry; neurochemical pathways have been morphologically identified and, correspondingly, neuromodulators can be topographically located in discrete areas of the brain. Increasingly precise knowledge of neurochemical topography has guided the neuropharmacologists and the electrophysiologists in their enlightening findings in reference to the control of motor activity and its disturbances. All this evidence, together with hints concerning the possible agents involved in the production of extrapyramidal disorders has, in turn, led to improved therapeutic procedures. In perusing this volume, therefore, the reader will recognize how the interaction between the various disciplines and approaches has resulted in greater knowledge of the control of motor activity and its disturbances, and how basic research has helped alter clinical experience.

This volume will be of interest to clinical neurologists and to neuroscientists.

The Editors

Acknowledgment

The VIth International Symposium on Parkinson's Disease was sponsored by:

Le Conseil de Recherche en Santé du Québec (Quebec Health Research Council)
The Medical Research Council of Canada
The Parkinson Foundation of Canada
The American Parkinson Disease Association
The World Federation of Neurology

Bibliography of Proceedings of the International Symposia on Parkinson's Disease

1. Elliot, H., and Nashold, B. Jr., editors (1960): *The Shaking Palsy (Parkinson's Disease)*, 160 pp. McGill University Press, Montreal. (Montreal, October 10, 1959.)
2. Nashold, B. Jr., and Huber, W. E., editors (1966): The Second Symposium on Parkinson's Disease. *J. Neurosurg*, 24 (Part 2) (Suppl.): 117–248. (Washington, D.C., November 18–20, 1963.)
3. Gillingham, F. J., and Donaldson, I. M. L., editors (1969): *Third Symposium on Parkinson's Disease*, 302 pp. E. & S. Livingstone, Edinburgh. (Edinburgh, May 20–22, 1968.)
4. Siegfried, Editor (1972): *Volume 1: Lead of Statement*, 219 pp., *Volume 2: Selected Communications on Topic*, 375 pp. Hans Huber Publishers, Bern, Stuttgart, Vienna. Fourth Symposium on Parkinson's Disease. (Zurich, September 22–24, 1972.)
5. Birkmayer, W., and Hornykiewicz, O., editors (1976): *Advances in Parkinsonism: Biochemistry, Physiology, Treatment*, 627 pp. Editiones Roche, Basle. (Vienna, September 17–20, 1975.)
6. Poirier, L. J., Sourkes, T. L., and Bédard, P. J., editors (1979): *The Extrapyramidal System and Its Disorders, Advances in Neurology Volume 24*, 552 pp. Raven Press, New York. VIth International Symposium on Parkinson's Disease. (Québec, September 24–27, 1978.)

Contents

x

Neurochemistry and Neuropharmacology of the Extrapyramidal System

Therapy of Parkinson's Disease and Management of Side Effects

Contributors

Y. Agid
Clinique de Neurologie et Neuropsychologie
Hôpital de la Salpétrière
75634 Paris, France

L. F. Agnati
Department of Histology
Karolinska Institutet
S-104 01 Stockholm, Sweden

H. Allain
Laboratoire de Pharmacologie
Faculté de Médecine
Rennes 35000, France

M. Grabowska-Andén
Department of Pharmacology
University of Göteborg
S-400 33 Göteborg, Sweden

N. -E. Andén
Department of Pharmacology
University of Göteborg
S-400 33 Göteborg, Sweden

F. Andermann
Departments of Neurology and Neurosurgery
Montréal Neurological Institute
Montréal, Québec, H3A 2B4 Canada

K. Andersson
Department of Histology
Karolinska Institutet
S-104 01 Stockholm, Sweden

A. Barbeau
Department of Neurobiology
Clinical Research Institute of Montréal
Montréal, Québec, H2W 1R7 Canada

H. Barden
Departments of Anatomy, Pathology (Division
of Neuropathology), and Neurology
Columbia University
College of Physicians and Surgeons
and New York State Psychiatric Institute
New York, New York 10032

M. Barden
Department of Physiology
Faculty of Medicine
Laval University
Quebéc, P.Q., G1K 7P4 Canada

R. E. Barrett
Neurological Institute
New York, New York 10032

G. Bartholini
Research Department
Synthélabo-L.E.R.S.
75013 Paris, France

N. Bathien
Service de Neurologie
Centre Hospitalier Sainte-Anne
75014 Paris, France

A. F. Battista
Department of Neurosurgery
Neurochemistry Laboratories
New York University Medical Center
New York, New York 10016

P. Bawa
Playfair Neuroscience Unit
University of Toronto
Toronto, Ontario, M5T 2S8 Canada

D. W. Baxter
Division of Neurology
Department of Medicine
Montréal General Hospital
Montréal, Québec, H3G 1A4 Canada

P. J. Bédard
Laboratoires de Neurobiologie
Pavillon Notre-Dame
Québec, P.Q., G1J 5B3, Canada

C. Bertrand
Division of Neurosurgery
Hôpital Notre-Dame
Montréal, P.Q., H2L 1M4 Canada

W. Birkmayer
Evangelisches Krankenhaus
A-1090 Vienna, Austria

G. A. Bishop
Department of Anatomy
Michigan State University
East Lansing, Michigan 48824

J. R. Boissier
Centre de Recherches Roussel-Uclaf
Romainville, 93230 France

A. -M. Bonnet
Clinique de Neurologie et Neuropsychologie
Hôpital de la Salpétrière
75634 Paris, France

J. D. Brown
Departments of Physiology and Clinical Neuro-
*   logical Sciences*
University of Western Ontario
London, Ontario, N6A 5C1 Canada

I. C. Bruce
Playfair Neuroscience Unit
University of Toronto
Toronto, Ontario, M5T 2S8 Canada

L. L. Butcher
Department of Psychology
University of California
Los Angeles, California 90024

D. Calne
Laboratory of Neurophysiology
National Institute of Mental Health and Ex-
*   perimental Therapeutics Branch*
National Institute of Neurological and Commu-
*   nicative Disorders and Stroke*
Bethesda, Maryland 20014

A. Carlsson
University of Göteborg
Department of Geriatric and Long-Term Care
*   Medicine*
Vasa Hospital
S-411 33 Göteborg, Sweden

P. M. Carvey
Department of Neurological Sciences
Rush University
Chicago, Illinois 60612

I. Casson
New York University School of Medicine
New York, New York 10016

T. N. Chase
Experimental Therapeutics Branch
National Institute of Neurological and Commu-
*   nicative Disorders and Stroke*
Bethesda, Maryland 20013

A. Cheramy
Groupe NB, INSERM U 114
Collège de France
75231 Paris, France

T. Chida
Department of Neurology
Juntendo Medical School
Hongo, Bunkyo-ku, Tokyo, Japan 113

J. Constantinidis
University Psychiatric Clinic
Geneva, Switzerland

J. D. Cooke
Departments of Physiology and Clinical Neuro-
*   logical Sciences*
University of Western Ontario
London, Ontario, N6A 5C1 Canada

J. Dankova
Laboratoires de Neurobiologie
Pavillon Notre-Dame
Québec, P.Q., G1J 5B3 Canada

L. Davidson
Department of Psychopharmacology
Clarke Institute of Psychiatry
Toronto, Ontario, M5T 1R8 Canada

A. Debono
University Department of Neurology
Institute of Psychiatry and King's College Hos-
*   pital*
Medical School
Denmark Hill, London SE5, United Kingdom

M. R. Delong
Departments of Physiology and Neurology
The Johns Hopkins University School of
*   Medicine*
Baltimore, Maryland 21205

J. M. Deniau
Laboratoire de Physiologie des Centres Nerveux
75230 Paris, France

S. G. Diamond
Reed Neurological Research Center
University of California at Los Angeles School
*   of Medicine*
Los Angeles, CA 90024

T. Dipaolo
Department of Physiology
Faculty of Medicine
Laval University
Québec, P.Q., G1K 7P4 Canada

J. Van den Driessche
Laboratoire de Pharmacologie
Faculté de Médecine
Rennes 35000, France

R. Durso
New York University School of Medicine
New York, New York 10016

R. C. Duvoisin
Mount Sinai School of Medicine
New York, New York 10029

J. Emile
Departments of Immunology and Neurology
Centre Hospitalier Universitaire
49036 Angers, France

C. Euvrard
Centre de Recherches Roussel-Uclaf
Romainville 93230, France

E. Evarts
Laboratory of Neurophysiology
National Institute of Mental Health and Experimental Therapeutics Branch
National Institute of Neurological and Communicative Disorders and Stroke
Bethesda, Maryland 20014

S. Fahn
Neurological Institute
New York, New York 10032

J. Féger
Laboratoire de Physiologie des Centres Nerveux
75230 Paris, France

S. H. Foo
New York University, School of Medicine
New York, New York 10016

F. Fuxe
Department of Histology
Karolinska Institutet
S-104 01 Stockholm, Sweden

A. P. Georgopoulos
Departments of Physiology and Neurology
The Johns Hopkins University School of Medicine
Baltimore, Maryland 21205

J. Glowinski
Groupe NB, INSERM U 114
Collège de France
75231 Paris, France

M. Goldstein
Department of Psychiatry
Neurochemistry Laboratories
New York University Medical Center
New York, New York 10016

M. Gonce
Department of Neurobiology
Clinical Research Institute of Montréal
Montréal, Québec, Canada

G. K. Hodge
Department of Psychology
University of California
Los Angeles, California 90024

A. K. Granérus
University of Göteborg
Department of Geriatric and Long-Term Care Medicine
Vasa Hospital
S-411 33 Göteborg, Sweden

S. Gravel
Laboratoires de Neurobiologie
Pavillon Notre-Dame
Québec, P.Q., G1J 5B3 Canada

I. Grofova
Anatomical Institute
University of Oslo
Oslo 1, Norway

J. H. Growdon
Tufts-New England Medical Center
Boston, Massachusetts 02111

C. Hammond
Laboratoire de Physiologie des Centres Nerveux
75230 Paris, France

R. Hassler
Department of Neurobiology
Max-Planck-Institut für Hirnforschung
D-6000 Frankfurt/M. 71, Germany

T. Hirai
Department of Neurosurgery
Gunma University School of Medicine
Gunma, Japan

A. Hitri
Department of Neurological Sciences
Rush University
Chicago, Illinois 60612

T. Hökfelt
Department of Histology
Karolinska Institutet
S-104 01 Stockholm, Sweden

O. Hornykiewicz
Institute of Biochemical Pharmacology
University of Vienna
A-1090 Vienna, Austria

K. Hoyte
Department of Psychiatry
Montréal General Hospital
Montréal, Québec, H3G 1A4 Canada

D. Hurez
Departments of Immunology and Neurology
Centre Hospitalier Universitaire
49036 Angers, France

R. Iizuka
Department of Psychiatry
School of Medicine
Tokyo, 113 Japan

S. Imai
Department of Neurosurgery
Gunma University School of Medicine
Gunma, Japan

S. Inagaki
Department of Anatomy
Fujita-Gakuen University School of Medicine
Toyoake, Aichi 470–11 Japan

V. T. Innanen
Kinsmen Laboratory of Neurological Research
Department of Psychiatry
University of British Columbia
Vancouver, B.C., V6T 1W5 Canada

P. Jenner
University Department of Neurology
Institute of Psychiatry and King's College
  Hospital
Medical School
Denmark Hill, London SE5, United Kingdom

A. J. Joffroy
Centre de Recherche en Sciences Neurologiques
Département de Physiologie
Université de Montréal
Montréal, Québec, H3C 3T8 Canada

T. Kato
Laboratory of Cell Physiology
Department of Life Chemistry
Graduate School at Nagatsuta
Tokyo Institute of Technology
Yokohama 227, Japan

M. Khayali
New York University School of Medicine
New York, New York 10016

M. E. Kiely
Department of Psychiatry
Montréal General Hospital
Montréal, Québec, H3G 1A4 Canada

J. -K. Kim
Department of Physiology
Catholic Medical College
Seoul, Korea

S. T. Kitai
Department of Anatomy
Michigan State University
East Lansing, Michigan 48824

H. L. Klawans
Department of Neurological Sciences
Rush University
Chicago, Illinois 60612

J. D. Kocsis
Department of Anatomy
Michigan State University
East Lansing, Michigan 48824

T. Kondo
Department of Neurology
Juntendo Medical School
Hongo, Bunkyo-ku
Tokyo, 113 Japan

Y. Kondo
Department of Anatomy
Fujita-Gakuen University School of Medicine
Toyoake, Aichi 470–11 Japan

M. Kupersmith
New York University School of Medicine
New York, New York 10016

H. C. Kwan
Department of Physiology
University of Toronto
Toronto, Ontario, M4B 1K7 Canada

H. Laaksonen
Department of Neurology
University of Turku
Turku, Finland

R. Labrecque
Department of Neurobiology
Clinical Research Institute of Montréal
Montréal, P.Q., Canada

F. Labrie
Department of Physiology
Faculty of Medicine
Laval University
Québec, P.Q., G1K 7P4 Canada

S. Lal
Department of Psychiatry
Montréal General Hospital
Montréal, Québec H3G 1A4 Canada

Y. Lamarre
Centre de Recherche en Sciences Neurologiques
Département de Physiologie
Université de Montréal
Montréal, P.Q., H3C 3T8 Canada

P. Langelier
Laboratoires de Neurobiologie
Pavillon Notre-Dame
Québec, P.Q., G1J 5B3 Canada

R. A. Levine
Department of Pharmacology
The George Washington University Medical
   Center
Washington, D.C. 20037

J. Y. Lew
Department of Psychiatry
Neurochemistry Laboratories
New York University Medical Center
New York, New York 10016

F. Lhermitte
Clinique de Neurologie et Neuropsychologie
Hôpital de la Salpétrière
75634 Paris, France

A. N. Lieberman
New York University School of Medicine
New York, New York 10016

K. G. Lloyd
Research Department
Synthélabo-L.E.R.S.
75621 Paris, France

W. Lovenberg
Section on Biochemical Pharmacology
National Heart, Lung and Blood Institute
National Institutes of Health
Bethesda, Maryland 20014

R. Marchand
Laboratoires de Neurobiologie
Pavillon Notre-Dame
Québec, P.Q., G1J 5B3 Canada

C. H. Markham
Reed Neurological Research Center
University of California at Los Angeles School
   of Medicine
Los Angeles, California 90024

C. D. Marsden
University Department of Neurology
Institute of Psychiatry and King's College
   Hospital
Medical School
Denmark Hill, London SE5, United Kingdom

J. Martin
School of Public Health
The Johns Hopkins School of Medicine
Baltimore, Maryland 21205

S. N. Martinez
Division of Neurosurgery
Hôpital Notre-Dame
Montréal, P.Q., H2L 1M4 Canada

E. G. McGeer
Kinsmen Laboratory of Neurological Research
Department of Psychiatry
University of British Columbia
Vancouver, B.C., V6T 1W5 Canada

P. L. McGeer
Kinsmen Laboratory of Neurological Research
Department of Psychiatry
University of British Columbia
Vancouver, B.C., V6T 1W5 Canada

K. Missala
Department of Psychiatry
McGill University
Montréal, Québec, H3A 1A1 Canada

P. Molina-Negro
Division of Neurosurgery
Hôpital Notre-Dame
Montréal, P.Q., H2L 1M4 Canada

J. T. Murphy
Department of Physiology
University of Toronto
Toronto, Ontario, M4B 1K7 Canada

I. Nagatsu
Department of Anatomy
Fujita-Gakuen University School of Medicine
Toyoake, Aichi 470–11 Japan

T. Nagatsu
Laboratory of Cell Physiology
Department of Life Chemistry
Graduate School at Nagatsuta
Tokyo Institute of Technology
Yokohama 227 Japan

H. Nakajima
Department of Neurosurgery
Gunma University School of Medicine
Gunma, Japan

S. Nakamura
Department of Neurosurgery
Neurochemistry Laboratories
New York University Medical Center
New York, New York 10016

H. Narabayashi
Department of Neurology
Juntendo Medical School
Hongo, Bunkyo-ku, Tokyo 113 Japan

P. A. Nausieda
Department of Neurological Sciences
Rush University
Chicago, Illinois 60612

A. Nieoullon
Institut de Neurophysiologie et
  Psychophysiologie du C.N.R.S.
Département de Neurophysiologie Générale
13274 Marseille, France

C. Nitsch
Department of Neurobiology
Max-Planck-Institut für Hirnforschung
D-6000 Frankfurt/M. 71
German Federal Republic

C. Ohye
Department of Neurosurgery
Gunma University School of Medicine
Gunma, Japan

A. Olivier
Departments of Neurology and Neurosurgery
Montréal Neurological Institute
Montréal, P.Q., H3A 2B4 Canada

K. -S. Paik
Department of Physiology
Brain Research Institute
Yonsei University
Seoul, Korea

A. Parent
Laboratoires de Neurobiologie
Pavillon Notre-Dame
Québec, P.Q., G1J 5B3 Canada

J. D. Parkes
University Department of Neurology
Institute of Psychiatry and King's College
  Hospital
Medical School
Denmark Hill, London SE5, United Kingdom

M. Pérez de la Mora
Department of Histology
Karolinska Institutet
S-104 01 Stockholm, Sweden

L. J. Poirier
Laboratoires de Neurobiologie
Pavillon Notre-Dame
Québec, P.Q., G1J 5B3 Canada

L. Possani
Departamento de Biologia Experimental
UNAM
México 20, D.F.

A. Pouplard
Departments of Immunology and Neurology
Centre Hospitalier Universitaire
49036 Angers, France

F. Pouplard
Departments of Immunology and Neurology
Centre Hospitalier Universitaire
49036 Angers, France

R. J. Preston
Department of Anatomy
Michigan State University
East Lansing, Michigan 48824

P. Price
University Department of Neurology
Institute of Psychiatry and King's College
Hospital
Medical School
Denmark Hill, London SE5, United Kingdom

W. D. Rausch
L. Boltzmann Institute of Clinical Neurobiology
Lainz-Hospital
A-1130 Vienna, Austria

M. W. Repeck
Department of Physiology
University of Toronto
Toronto, Ontario, M4B 1K7 Canada

J. L. Ribadeau-Dumas (deceased)
Service de Neurologie
Centre Hospitalier Bretonneau
F-37000 Tours, France

P. Riederer
L. Boltzmann Institute of Clinical Neurobiology
Lainz-Hospital
A-1130, Vienna, Austria

U. K. Rinne
Department of Neurology
University of Turku
SF-20520 Turku 52, Finland

E. Rinvik
Anatomical Institute
University of Oslo
Oslo 1, Norway

D. S. Robinson
Section on Biochemical Pharmacology
National Heart, Lung and Blood Institute
National Institutes of Health
Bethesda, Maryland 20014

P. Rondot
Service de Neurologie
Centre Hospitalier Sainte-Anne
75014 Paris, France

M. Roy
Department of Neurobiology
Clinical Research Institute of Montréal
Montréal, Québec, H2W 1R7 Canada

O. Sabouraud
Service de Neurologie
Hôpital Pontchaillou
rue Henri Guilloux
Rennes 35000, France

M. Budininkas-Schoenebeck
Departments of Anatomy, Pathology (Division
of Neuropathology), and Neurology
Columbia University College of Physicians and
Surgeons
and New York State Psychiatric Institute
New York, New York 10032

R. Schwarcz
Department of Histology
Karolinska Institutet
S-104 01 Stockholm, Sweden

B. T. Shahani
Department of Clinical Neurophysiology
Massachusetts General Hospital and Harvard
Medical School
Boston, Massachusetts 02114

T. Shibazaki
Department of Neurosurgery
Gunma University School of Medicine
3–39–22 Showa-Machi Maebashi
Gunma, Japan

J. -L. Signoret
Clinique de Neurologie et Neuropsychologie
Hôpital de la Salpétrière
75634 Paris, France

V. Sonninen
Department of Neurology
University of Turku
SF-20520 Turku, 52 Finland

T. L. Sourkes
Department of Psychiatry
McGill University
Montreal, P.Q., H3A 1A1 Canada

A. Svanborg
University of Göteborg
Department of Geriatric and Long-Term Care
Medicine
Vasa Hospital
S-411 33 Göteborg, Sweden

C. A. Tamminga
Adult Psychiatry Branch
National Institute of Mental Health
Bethesda, Maryland 20014

R. Tapia
Departamento de Biologia Experimental
UNAM
México 20, D.F. México

T. Tartaro
New York University School of Medicine
New York, New York 10016

W. G. Tatton
Playfair Neuroscience Unit
University of Toronto
Toronto, Ontario, M5T 2S8 Canada

V. M. Tennyson
Department of Pathology (Division of
Neuropathology)
Columbia University College of Physicians and
Surgeons
New York, New York 10032

H. Teräväinen
Laboratory of Neurophysiology
National Institute of Mental Health and Ex-
perimental Therapeutics Branch
National Institute of Neurological and Commu-
nicative Disorders and Stroke
Bethesda, Maryland 20014

R. Tissot
University Psychiatric Clinic
Geneva, Switzerland

S. Toma
Service de Neurologie
Centre Hospitalier Sainte-Anne
75014 Paris, France

A. Villeneuve
Department of Psychiatry
Faculty of Medicine
Laval University
Québec, P.Q., G1K 7P4 Canada

W. J. Weiner
Department of Neurological Sciences
Rush University
Chicago, Illinois 60612

A. C. Williams
Experimental Therapeutics Branch
IRP, National Institute of Neurological
and Communicative Disorders and Stroke
National Institutes of Health
Bethesda, Maryland 20014

P. Worms
Research Department
Synthélabo-L.E.R.S.
75013 Paris, France

R. R. Young
Harvard Medical School
Department of Neurology
Massachusetts General Hospital
Boston, Massachusetts 02114

M. Ziegler
Service de Neurologie
Centre Hospitalier Sainte-Anne
75014 Paris, France

Advances in Neurology, Vol. 24, edited by
L. J. Poirier, T. L. Sourkes, and P. J. Bédard.
Raven Press, New York © 1979.

The Extrapyramidal and Limbic Systems Relationship at the Globus Pallidus Level: A Comparative Histochemical Study in the Rat, Cat, and Monkey

*A. Parent, *S. Gravel, and **A. Olivier

*Laboratoires de Neurobiologie et Département d'Anatomie, Faculté de Médecine, Université Laval, Québec, G1K 7P4, Canada; **Department of Neurology and Neurosurgery, Montréal Neurological Institute, Montréal, H3A 2B4, Canada

The mammalian globus pallidus, the main output device of the extrapyramidal system, is intimately surrounded by forebrain structures related to the limbic system. Among these structures are the lateral hypothalamic area and the so-called basal nucleus of Meynert, composed of large-sized neurons scattered within the substantia innominata. Topographically, the lateral hypothalamic area borders the ventromedial aspect of the medial pallidal segment in primates or its acknowledged equivalent—the entopeduncular nucleus—in rats and cats, whereas the substantia innominata and basal nucleus are found immediately beneath the globus pallidus in the three groups. In addition to the fact that these limbic and extrapyramidal structures lie in close proximity to each other, some recent neuroanatomical studies in cats (15) and in rats (9) suggest that the entopeduncular nucleus neurons themselves project toward the habenula, an important limbic system relay station. Although the existence of such a pallidohabenular pathway has been confirmed in rats (8), results from more recent anatomical and physiological studies suggest that, in squirrel monkeys and in cats at least, most of the neurons of the pallidal area that project to the habenula are part of limbic structures intimately surrounding the pallidal complex rather than being typical pallidal neurons (5,8,18).

In view of the divergence between some of the above-mentioned findings, which appears to reflect significant species variations, we thought it useful to undertake a comparative study of the topographical organization of the peripallidal limbic structures—especially the basal nucleus of Meynert—in the rat, cat, and rhesus monkey *(Macaca mulatta).* In the present account, the neurons of the peripallidal limbic nuclei have been identified on the basis of, first, their high acetylcholinesterase (AChE) content (see refs. 10,13,16,19) and of, second, their morphological characteristics, which differ markedly from those of the globus pallidus.

In the present investigation, the new pharmacohistochemical procedure was used, which involves pretreatment of the animals with diisopropylfluorophosphate (DFP). Such a method permits optimal visualization of AChE neuronal somata and proximal processes without strong background staining (see ref. 1). The brains of all DFP-treated animals were processed for AChE according to the Karnovsky-Roots histochemical method (12). Numerous brains of untreated rats, cats, and rhesus monkeys, either stained for AChE according to the Gomori-Koelle (6) or the Karnovsky-Roots histochemical procedures, or according to the Nissl method, were also available for this study.

RESULTS

The Rat (Figs. 1–6)

Although the existence of a substantia innominata–basal nucleus complex has not always been recognized as such in rodents (7), a large population of voluminous and strongly stained AChE neurons is nevertheless present beneath the rostral pole of the globus pallidus of the rat (Fig. 1A). Rostrally, this cellular aggregate merges with the morphologically similar and strongly stained AChE neurons of the nucleus of the diagonal band of Broca and of the medial septal nucleus. At the level of the anterior commissure, numerous neurons of this cell group, lying in an area that appears to be equivalent to the substantia innominata found in other mammals (3), form a typical S-shaped cell column that reaches dorsally the medial border of the globus pallidus (Fig. 1A). At this level, the AChE neurons appear as a tight neuronal net that completely surrounds the medial aspect of the globus pallidus. These intensely stained AChE neurons, as well as those of the substantia innominata below, are large (40–50 μm in diameter), multipolar, and possess numerous thick AChE-containing processes. They thus differ markedly from the much smaller (20–30 μm) triangular or fusiform globus pallidus cells that are only weakly to moderately stained for AChE.

FIG. 1. Semischematic drawings of transverse half-sections through the forebrain of the rat illustrating the distribution of strongly stained AChE neurons *(full circles)* and weakly reactive cells *(empty circles)* within and around the pallidal complex. The drawings are placed in a rostrocaudal order from **A** to **C.** The lightly shaded areas in the caudatoputamen and in the olfactory tubercle indicate a weak background AChE staining.

FIGS. 2–4. Transverse sections through the rostral (Fig. 2), the middle (Fig. 3), and the caudal (Fig. 4) portions of the pallidal complex of a DFP-treated rat, showing the distribution of the strongly stained AChE neurons.

FIGS. 5–6. High-power views depicting some of the large-sized and strongly stained AChE neurons that occur among the small and pale cells of the entopeduncular nucleus (Fig. 5) and of the globus pallidus (Fig. 6) of a DFP-treated rat.
AC, anterior commissure; CC, corpus callosum; CP, caudatoputamen; E, entopeduncular nucleus; FX, fornix; H, hypothalamus; IC, internal capsule; OC, optic chiasma; OT, optic tract; OTB, olfactory bulb; P, globus pallidus; PA, preoptic area; THAL, thalamus.

A few voluminous and strongly stained AChE neurons are also found within the bed nucleus of the anterior commissure (Fig. 1A). These neurons are closely packed and appear to form a nearly complete ring around the anterior commissure.

As we proceed further caudally, the number of intensely stained AChE neurons

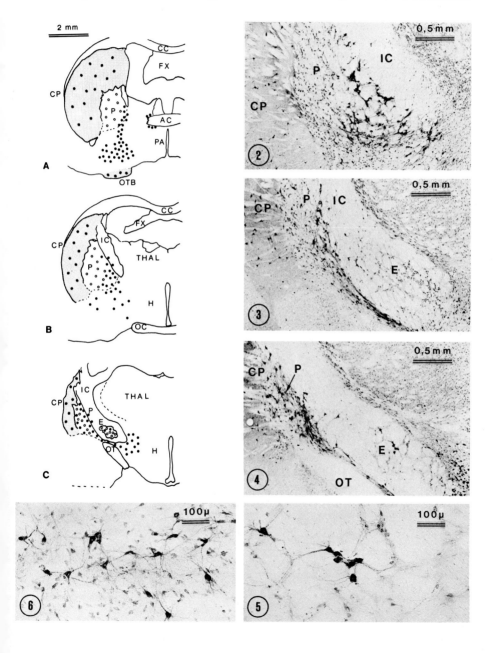

decreases strikingly beneath the globus pallidus (Fig. 1B), whereas progressively more neurons of this type are found within the globus pallidus itself (Fig. 2). At the level of the middle third of the globus pallidus (Fig. 3), the strongly positive AChE neurons present within the globus pallidus are continuous, with a rather thick cell band of similar neurons located along the dorsal edge of the optic tract.

At the level of the caudal third of the globus pallidus, the intensely stained AChE neurons present within the globus pallidus are even more numerous (Fig. 1C). They are much more uniformly distributed throughout the whole structure (Fig. 4). Their long and radiating AChE-containing processes are intimately intermingled with the weakly stained pallidal neurons (Fig. 6). Numerous strongly positive AChE neurons are also found within the lateral hypothalamic area (Figs. 1C,4). The latter cell group is directly continuous with the AChE neuronal population of the globus pallidus through the thin cell band of strongly stained AChE neurons located along the optic tract (Figs. 1C,4).

Even in animals that have not been treated with DFP, some strongly positive AChE neurons can be visualized—although in much less detail—in the lateral hypothalamic area and in the caudal portion of the globus pallidus of the rat, as also noted by Jacobowitz and Palkovits (10). Moreover, the rostral and caudal poles of the globus pallidus of the rabbit are known to be completely surrounded by large and strongly stained AChE neurons (3). At variance with the above-mentioned findings in the rat, however, these AChE neurons referred to as "interstitial nerve cells" in the rabbit appear to have their dendritic fields strictly confined to the white matter surrounding the globus pallidus (3). Some findings based on retrograde cell changes after cortical ablation in the rabbit suggest that these interstitial nerve cells, in contrast to the typical pallidal neurons, project directly to the motor and premotor cortex (2).

In normal (pharmacologically unmanipulated) rats, the entopeduncular nucleus displays an overall AChE staining that is only weak to moderate in intensity. After DFP treatment, the entopeduncular neurons stand out more clearly. Most consist of medium-sized (20–30 μm) triangular, fusiform, or round cells that stain only weakly for AChE. These neurons thus resemble the typical pale globus pallidus cells, except that some of them, particularly the round cells, are slightly smaller in size (20–25 μm). In addition, a small number of large and strongly stained AChE neurons are also present in the rostral and caudal poles of the entopeduncular nucleus (Fig. 4). These cells are morphologically similar to the large and highly reactive AChE neurons present within and around the globus pallidus. They possess numerous long AChE-containing processes intertwined with the weakly reactive fiber bundles that give to the entopeduncular nucleus its typical reticular appearance (Fig. 5).

The Cat (Figs. 7–12)

As in the rat, numerous intensely reactive AChE neurons are present at the level of the pallidal complex in the cat. The pattern of their topographical distribution around and within the globus pallidus is basically similar to that disclosed in the rat. For instance, neurons of this type are present within the cat substantia innominata, immediately beneath the rostral pole of the globus pallidus (Figs. 7A,8). At this level, the whole substantia innominata displays a weak background AChE staining. Within this structure, the large-sized (40 μm) and strongly stained AChE neurons are clustered into lateral and medial cell groups that are more or less differentiated from one another. The most dorsally located AChE cells of the lateral group invade the medullary laminas that separate the globus pallidus from the putamen. In addition, numerous AChE neurons of the same type are spread along the dorsomedial border of the globus pallidus, partly within the fibers of the internal capsule (Fig. 7A). Ventrally, this cell column merges with the AChE neurons of the medial group of the substantia innominata (Figs. 7A,8).

More caudally, the number of AChE neurons present beneath the globus pallidus decreases markedly, whereas more neurons of this type occur along the lateral and dorsomedial borders of the pallidum (Fig. 7B). The central portion of the globus pallidus, however, still contains numerous typical weakly stained pallidal cells. These neurons have triangular or fusiform cell bodies that are smaller in size (20–30 μm) than those of the strongly stained AChE neurons.

In the caudal third of the globus pallidus, a great number of strongly stained, large AChE neurons are evenly scattered throughout the pallidum, among the small and pale cells. At this level, however, AChE-containing neuronal somata are no longer found beneath the globus pallidus (Figs. 7C,9). The large and multipolar pallidal neurons that contain high amounts of AChE possess numerous long and ramified processes that also stain for the enzyme (Fig. 12).

Large and multipolar AChE neuronal somata are also found in the lateral preopticohypothalamic area of the cat. Unlike those in the rat, however, the hypothalamic AChE neurons in the cat are not continuous with those of the globus pallidus (Fig. 7C).

The entopeduncular nucleus of the cat differs markedly from that of the rat. In non-DFP-treated cats, this structure displays a very intense background AChE staining (Fig. 10). This enzyme staining is as intense as it is in the caudate nucleus and putamen and thus obscures all the cell bodies. After DFP treatment, however, weakly stained AChE neurons can be visualized in the entopeduncular nucleus (Fig. 11). The shape and size of the entopeduncular neurons are similar to those of the small to medium-sized, weakly stained cells of the globus pallidus.

The Rhesus Monkey (Figs. 13–18)

The basal nucleus of Meynert is particularly well developed in primates, including man (7,11). The presence of a strong AChE activity at this level has been already acknowledged by some authors (see refs. 4,14). Indeed, in untreated rhesus monkeys, the whole substantia innominata displays an overall AChE activity that is as intense as that found in the neostriatum (16). After DFP treatment, however, it becomes possible to visualize numerous large multipolar, and intensely reactive AChE neurons, which appear to correspond to those of the basal nucleus.

At the level of the anterior commissure, this AChE neuronal population is composed of two more-or-less continuous cell groups located within the medial

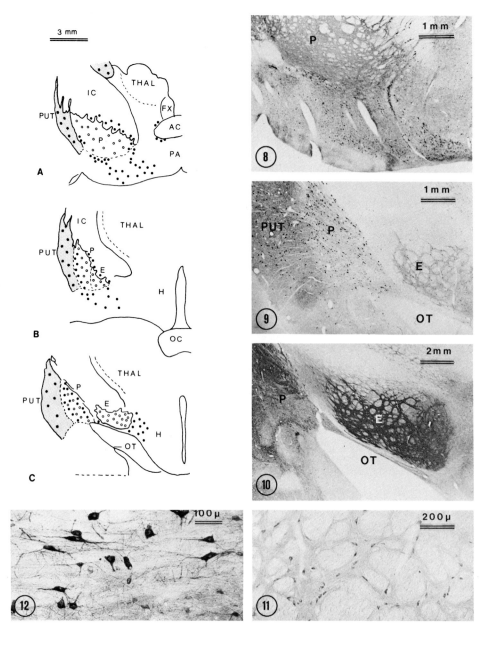

and lateral parts of the substantia innominata, respectively (Figs. 13A,14). The neurons of the medial group have a mean diameter of 40 to 45 μm and display numerous AChE-containing processes. The intensely reactive AChE neurons of the lateral group are slightly smaller (30–35 μm) than those of the medial group and are embedded in a mesh of very fine and granular AChE material.

Both the medial and lateral AChE neuronal groups of the substantia innominata extend rostrocaudally for a considerable distance beneath the lenticular nucleus. At the level of the optic chiasma, the more dorsally located multipolar neurons of the medial group are continuous with morphologically identical neurons situated along the ventromedial aspect of the pallidum and the base of the anterior limb of the internal capsule (Figs. 13B,14,16). The more dorsally located neurons of the lateral group, on the other hand, invade the rostral pole of the internal division of the globus pallidus (Figs. 14,15). More caudally, the intensely stained AChE neurons of the lateral group form two cell plates that invade the internal and external medullary lamina of the lenticular nucleus (Figs. 13C,18). Other large multipolar AChE-containing neurons, more or less continuous with those of the basal nucleus, are present within the lateral preoptic and lateral hypothalamic areas, whereas other similar neurons are scattered among the fibers of the ansa lenticularis in an area that appears to correspond to the so-called nucleus ansae lenticularis (20). As in the rat and the cat, the bed nucleus of the anterior commissure also contains highly reactive neurons with numerous thick AChE-containing processes (Figs. 13A,17).

FIG. 7. Semischematic drawings of transverse half-sections through the forebrain of the cat illustrating the distribution of strongly stained AChE neurons *(full circles)* and weakly reactive cells *(empty circles)* within and around the pallidal complex. The drawings are set out in a rostrocaudal order from A to C. The lightly shaded area in the putamen indicates a weak background AChE staining.

FIG. 8. Transverse section through the rostral pole of the globus pallidus of a DFP-treated cat showing the intensely reactive AChE neurons bordering ventromedially the globus pallidus (see **A** in Fig. 7).

FIG. 9. Transverse section through the middle portion of the pallidal complex of a DFP-treated cat showing the numerous strongly stained AChE neurons present within the globus pallidus itself.

FIG. 10. Transverse section through the entopeduncular nucleus of a normal (pharmacologically unmanipulated) cat. The structure displays a very strong background AChE staining.

FIG. 11. Photomicrograph showing some of the pale neurons that can be visualized within the entopeduncular nucleus of the cat after DFP treatment.

FIG. 12. High-power view illustrating some of the large and strongly stained AChE neurons that occur within the globus pallidus of the cat. DFP-treated animal.
AC, anterior commissure; E, entopeduncular nucleus; FX, fornix; H, hypothalamus; IC, internal capsule; OC, optic chiasma; OT, optic tract; P, globus pallidus; PA, preoptic area; PUT, putamen; THAL, thalamus.

In contrast to what has been found in the rat and cat, however, the abundant and intensely reactive peripallidal cells do not directly invade the globus pallidus itself, except at the level of the rostral pole of the medial division of this structure. Both divisions of the primate globus pallidus are in fact mostly composed of

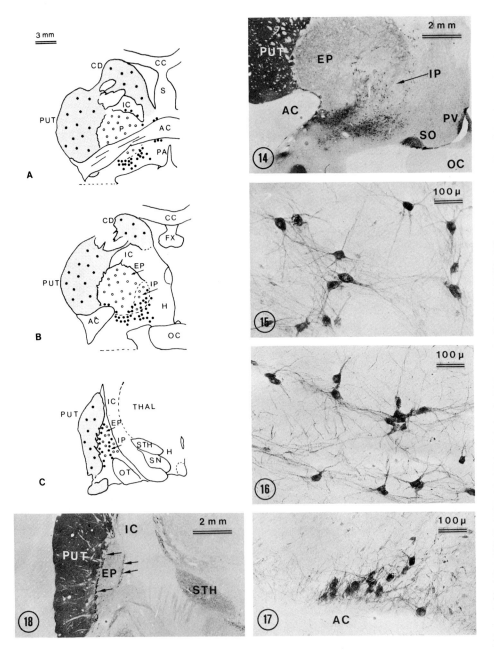

medium-sized (20–25 μm) triangular or fusiform neurons that stain only weakly for AChE. These pallidal neurons in primates thus appear morphologically and histochemically similar to the typical pale cells present in the globus pallidus and entopeduncular nucleus of the rat and the cat.

CONCLUSIONS AND SUMMARY

In the present study, the topographical organization and the morphological characteristics of the intensely stained AChE neurons belonging to various peri-pallidal limbic structures have been investigated in the rat, cat, and rhesus monkey. The main conclusions of this study may be summarized as follows.

In the three species, a well-characterized substantia innominata–basal nucleus complex has been found. It consists of numerous large and heavily stained AChE neurons scattered beneath the rostral half of the globus pallidus. Rostrally, this cellular population merges with the highly reactive cell groups of the nucleus of the diagonal band of Broca and of the medial septum. In the monkey, the substantia innominata–basal nucleus complex prolongs itself caudally for a con-siderable distance beneath the lenticular nucleus and invades only slightly this extrapyramidal structure, particularly at the level of the medullary lamina and within the rostral pole of the internal division of the globus pallidus. In contrast, in the rat and even more strikingly in the cat, the AChE neurons of the substantia innominata do not persist at the basis of the caudal half of the globus pallidus but instead appear to invade massively the globus pallidus itself. Therefore, in both of these species, the globus pallidus is composed of two types of neurons: (a) the small- to medium-sized weakly reactive neurons that are typical of the

---

FIG. 13. Semischematic drawings of transverse half-sections through the forebrain of the rhesus monkey illustrating the distribution of strongly stained AChE neurons *(full circles)* and weakly reactive cells *(empty circles)* within and around the pallidal complex. The drawings are placed in a rostrocaudal order from **A** to **C**. The lightly shaded areas in the putamen and caudate nucleus indicate a weak background AChE staining.

FIG. 14. Low-power view of the lenticular nucleus of a DFP-treated rhesus monkey showing numerous strongly stained AChE neurons of the basal nucleus, some of which invade the rostral pole of the internal segment of the globus pallidus (see **B** in Fig. 13).

FIGS. 15–17. High-power views depicting some large-sized and highly reactive AChE neurons present within the rostral pole of the internal segment of the globus pallidus (Fig. 15), in-between the dorsal border of the globus pallidus and the internal capsule (Fig. 16) (see **A** in Fig. 13), and along the dorsal border of the anterior commissure (Fig. 17) (see **A** in Fig. 13).

FIG. 18. Low-power view of the caudalmost portion of the lenticular nucleus of a DFP-treated rhesus monkey illustrating the strongly stained AChE neurons present within the internal and external medullary lamina *(arrows)* (see **C** in Fig. 13).
AC, anterior commissure; CC, corpus callosum; CD, caudate nucleus; EP, external segment of the globus pallidus; FX, fornix; H, hypothalamus; IC, internal capsule; IP, internal segment of the globus pallidus; OC, optic chiasma; OT, optic tract; P, globus pallidus; PA, preoptic area; PUT, putamen; PV, paraventricular nucleus; S, septum; SN, substantia nigra; SO, supraoptic nucleus; STH, subthalamic nucleus.

globus pallidus and/or entopeduncular nucleus in the three species and (b) the large and strongly stained AChE neurons that are continuous with and morphologically similar to the neurons of the substantia innominata. The morphological and histochemical similarities of the pale cells present in the globus pallidus and entopeduncular nucleus of the rat and cat and in both divisions of the pallidum of primates suggest that these neuronal populations could have arisen, phylogenetically, from a similar forebrain anlage in all three species.

On the other hand, the entopeduncular nucleus of the cat differs from that of the rat in at least two aspects. First, this structure in pharmacologically unmanipulated cats displays a very strong background AChE staining that does not occur—at least with the same intensity—in the rat entopeduncular nucleus nor in the internal division of the primate globus pallidus. The origin and significance of this intense neuropil AChE staining in the feline entopeduncular nucleus remain to be investigated. The striatofugal fibers could contribute substantially to this enzyme activity, however, because lesions of the cat neostriatum have been shown to cause a marked decrease in the background AChE staining of the entopeduncular nucleus (17). Second, the cat entopeduncular nucleus appears to be composed chiefly of pale and small- to medium-sized cells, whereas some large-sized and strongly stained AChE neurons occur in the rostral and caudal poles of the rat entopeduncular nucleus.

In the three species, large-sized and intensely reactive AChE neurons are also present at the level of certain other limbic structures bordering the pallidal complex, particularly the lateral preopticohypothalamic area. The topographical distribution of these neurons and their relationship with those of the substantia innominata–basal nucleus complex appear somewhat similar in the three species.

In conclusion, therefore, there appears to be highly significant species variations, from rodents to primates, in the degree of topographical overlap between limbic and extrapyramidal systems at the level of the globus pallidus. The neurons of the peripallidal limbic structures are much more intimately associated with pallidal neurons—but not as much with entopeduncular neurons—in "lower" mammalian species than in primates.

ACKNOWLEDGMENT

This research was supported by grant MT-5781 of the Medical Research Council of Canada to A. Parent.

REFERENCES

1. Butcher, L. L., Talbot, K., and Bilezikjian, L. (1975): Acetylcholinesterase neurons in dopamine regions of the brain. *J. Neural. Trans.*, 38:127–153.
2. Das, G. D. (1971): Projections of the interstitial nerve cells surrounding the globus pallidus: A study of retrograde changes following cortical ablation in rabbits. *Z. Anat. Entwicklungsgesch.*, 133:135–160.
3. Das, G. D., and Kreutzberg, G. W. (1968): Evaluation of interstitial nerve cells in the central

nervous system: A correlative study using acetylcholinesterase and Golgi techniques. *Ergeb. Anat. Entwicklungsgesch.,* 41:1–58.

4. Divac, I. (1975): Magnocellular nuclei of the basal forebrain project to neocortex, brain stem, and olfactory bulb—Review of some functional correlates. *Brain Res.,* 93:385–398.

5. Filion, M., and Harnois, C. (1978): A comparison of projections of entopeduncular neurons to the thalamus, the midbrain and the habenula in the cat. *J. Comp. Neurol.,* 181:763–780.

6. Gomori, G. (1952): *Microscopic Histochemistry: Principles and Practice.* University of Chicago Press, Chicago.

7. Gorry, J. D. (1963): Studies on the comparative anatomy of the ganglion basale of Meynert. *Acta Anat. (Basel),* 55:51–104.

8. Gravel, S., Boucher, R., Scarabin, J.-M., and Parent, A. (1977): Comparative study of forebrain afferents to the habenula in the cat and the rat as revealed by HRP neuronography. *Neurosci. Abstr.,* 3:198.

9. Herkenham, M., and Nauta, W. J. H. (1977): Afferent connections of the habenular nuclei in the rat. A horseradish peroxidase study, with a note on the fiber-or-passage problem. *J. Comp. Neurol.,* 173:123–146.

10. Jacobowitz, D., and Palkovits, M. (1974): Topographic atlas of catecholamine- and acetylcholinesterase-containing neurons in the rat brain, Part I: Forebrain (telencephalon, diencephalon). *J. Comp. Neurol.,* 157:13–28.

11. Jones, E. G., Burton, H., Saper, C. B., and Swanson, L. W. (1976): Midbrain, diencephalic and cortical relationships of the basal nucleus of Meynert and associated structures in primates. *J. Comp. Neurol.,* 167:385–420.

12. Karnovsky, M. J., and Roots, L. (1964): A "direct-coloring" thiocholine method for cholinesterases. *J. Histochem. Cytochem.,* 12:219–221.

13. Koelle, G. B. (1954): The histochemical localization of cholinesterases in the central nervous system. *J. Comp. Neurol.,* 100:211–228.

14. Mesulam, M.-M., and Van Hoesen, G. W. (1976): Acetylcholinesterase-rich projections from the basal forebrain of the rhesus monkey to neocortex. *Brain Res.,* 109:152–157.

15. Nauta, H. J. W. (1974): Evidence of a pallidohabenular pathway in the cat. *J. Comp. Neurol.,* 156:19–28.

16. Olivier, A., Parent, A., and Poirier, L. J. (1970): Identification of the thalamic nuclei on the basis of their cholinesterase content in the monkey. *J. Anat. (Lond.),* 106:37–50.

17. Olivier, A., Parent, A., Simard, H., and Poirier, L. J. (1970): Cholinesterasic striatopallidal and striatonigral efferents in the cat and the monkey. *Brain Res.,* 18:273–282.

18. Parent, A., and Boucher, R. (1978): Is there a pallidohabenular pathway in monkeys? *Neurosci. Abstr.,* 4:48.

19. Parent, A., Poirier, L. J., Boucher, R., and Butcher, L. L. (1977): Morphological characteristics of acetylcholinesterase-containing neurons in the CNS of DFP-treated monkeys. Part 2: Diencephalic and medial telencephalic structures. *J. Neurol. Sci.,* 32:9–28.

20. Poirier, L. J., Parent, A., Marchand, R., and Butcher, L. L. (1977): Morphological characteristics of the acetylcholinesterase-containing neurons in the CNS of DFP-treated monkeys. Part 1: Extrapyramidal and related structures. *J. Neurol. Sci.,* 31:181–198.

Advances in Neurology, Vol. 24, edited by
L. J. Poirier, T. L. Sourkes, and P. J. Bédard.
Raven Press, New York © 1979.

Cytohistochemical Study of the Primate Basal Ganglia and Substantia Nigra

R. Marchand, L. J. Poirier, and A. Parent

Laboratoires de Neurobiologie, Département d'Anatomie, Faculté de Médecine, Université Laval, Québec, Québec, G1K 7P4, Canada

In a previous study based on the pharmacohistochemical procedure for the demonstration of *de novo* synthesis of acetylcholinesterase (AChE) as applied by Butcher et al. (3) and Kreutzberg et al. (17), we described the distribution of AChE neurons within the extrapyramidal and associated structures (24) in the *Macaca mulatta.* Since this approach permits a better visualization of the cytological characteristics of the AChE-containing neurons of the CNS (2,18,23), it was of particular interest to undertake a detailed study of the types of neurons and of their distribution within the substantia nigra, the globus pallidus, and the neostriatum of the primate brain. In addition, the different types of neurons containing AChE were compared with similar neurons in material prepared according to the Nissl method of staining.

METHODOLOGY

Four monkeys were injected i.m. with bis-(1-methylethyl) phosphofluoridate [diisopropylfluorophosphate (DFP)] at various times prior to being killed. The brains of these animals were blocked in the coronal plane, and the blocks were then frozen and sectioned at 40 μm on a freezing microtome. The sections of the brain were processed for AChE. Transverse sections of normal monkey brains stained with basic fuchsin or cresyl violet and/or fast blue were available for comparison. A more detailed description of the methodology used in this study has been published by Poirier et al. (24).

RESULTS

The Substantia Nigra

In the monkey, the substantia nigra, corresponding to the *locus niger* in man as described by Sommering, is made up of a fibrillar and cellular plate. It extends over the entire extent of the midbrain and lies on the cerebral peduncle on either side of the midline.

In transverse sections of the brainstem stained with basic stains, two areas somewhat irregular but rather well delineated from each other may be identified at different levels of the substantia nigra. The area occupied by more closely packed neurons corresponding to the *pars compacta* is more dorsomedially located, whereas the area containing fewer neurons or *pars reticulata* is more ventrally and ventrolaterally located within the substantia nigra.

The rostralmost part of the substantia nigra is almost entirely covered by the subthalamic nucleus. At this level, it is represented exclusively by the pars reticulata, which is continuous with the pallidum through the neuropil of the comb bundle. At the level of the caudal pole of the mamillary bodies, the pars compacta is represented by a thin band of neurons along the dorsomedial edge of the substantia nigra. It overlies the pars reticulata, which extends more laterally than the pars compacta. More caudally, the neurons of the pars compacta are greater in number and constitute rows of cells which extend into the underlying pars reticulata. These cellular bands constitute rings which envelope zones of the pars reticulata (Figs. 1,2). These annular formations thus subdivide the pars reticulata of this level into three areas: medial, lateral, and intraannular. Caudally to the level of the emergence of the third nerve root fibers, the pars reticulata is progressively replaced by the neurons of the pars compacta. At the more caudal levels, the neurons of the pars compacta are less abundant and are represented by an oblique band of sparsed neurons which is in contiguity with the similar neurons of the more dorsally located nucleus *parabrachialis pigmentosus.* The latter group of neurons occupies the area between the magnocellular division of the red nucleus and the decussation of the superior cerebellar peduncles.

Cytology

In nervous tissue of the monkey brain either stained according to the modified method of Klüver and Barrera (15) or prepared for the demonstration of AChE, five types of neurons may be identified at the level of the substantia nigra.

FIGS. 1–10. Microphotographs of sections through the substantia nigra of the monkey illustrating the distribution and cytological characteristics of different types of neurons. AChE activity (Figs. 1,2,5,6,8,10) from DFP-treated animals, and Nissl stain (Figs. 3,4,7,9) from nontreated animals. **1:** Transverse section through the intermediary level of the substantia nigra illustrating the distribution of AChE activity. × 6.5. **2:** Distribution of the nerve cells at the level of a ring of neurons of the pars compacta which envelops nervous tissue of the pars reticula as illustrated in Fig. 1. The arrow indicates the pyramid-shaped neuron of type C2 illustrated in Fig. 6. Calibration bar = 100 μm. **3,4:** Types C2 (Fig. 3) and C1 (Fig. 4) neurons of the pars compacta. Type C1 cells, which outnumber type C2 neurons, constitute the main nerve cells of the pars compacta. Calibration bar = 50 μm. **5:** AChE activity in types C1 and C2 *(arrow)* neurons. Note more intense enzymatic activity in the cell body and processes of type C2 neurons. Calibration bar = 50 μm. **6:** A C2 neuron of pyramidal shape. Note the axon detaching from its base. Calibration bar = 50 μm. **7,8:** Type R1 neurons in Nissl stain. Calibration bar = 50 μm. **9,10:** Type R2 neurons after Nissl stain (Fig. 10) and in section prepared for the demonstration of AChE (Fig. 11). Calibration bar = 50 μm.

Two types of neuron may be identified in the pars compacta of the substantia nigra. The first type (C1) is the most common neuron of the pars compacta. The medium-sized body (25–45 μm) has an ovoid, triangular, or somewhat elongated shape. In tissue prepared with basic stains, the cytoplasm of these neurons has a peculiar appearance due to the presence of intensely stained striae which alternate with lightly stained bands. Therefore, these neurons have a typical tigroid aspect. The eccentrically situated large nucleus is well delineated,

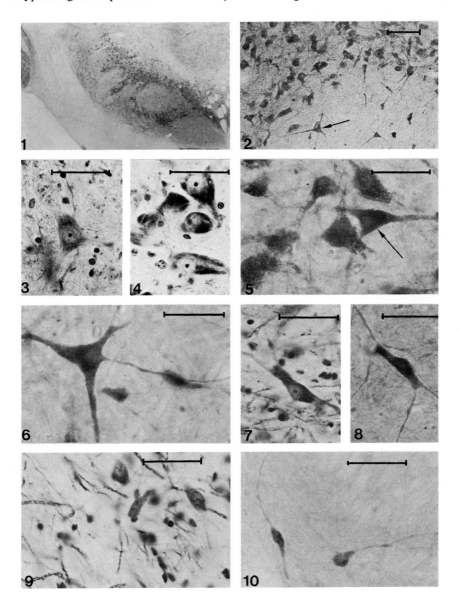

although it is often partially masked by the Nissl substance of the cytoplasm. In this material, the apparently broad dendrites are occasionally stained (Fig. 4).

In cholinesterasic material, the AChE activity of the cytoplasm of the C1 type neurons is moderate. It is not homogeneously distributed, and under such conditions, the cell bodies have a granular appearance. Their dendrites show a lighter AChE activity. The C1 type neurons occupy the more dorsal (lemniscal) and dorsolateral areas of the pars compacta, where the background enzymatic activity is weaker. They display long and broad neurites. The enzymatic activity, however, seems to be restricted to the neurilemma (Figs. 2,5).

Type C2 neurons of the pars compacta are fewer than type C1. In AChE material of the monkey brain, type C2 neurons stand out sharply. As a matter of fact, the pyramidal or triangular cell bodies (40–60 μm) have a moderate-to-intense enzymatic activity which is uniformly distributed in the cytoplasm. The site of the slightly eccentric nucleus corresponds to an area of lighter AChE activity. The enzymatic activity is also important in the long neurites which give rise to few branches (Figs. 5,6).

This type (C2) of neuron is more precisely located either along the ventral edge of the pars compacta or along the internal edge of its annular structures. The processes of these neurons are orientated toward either the pars compacta or the pars reticulata (Fig. 5); occasionally, processes of the same neuron are distributed to both divisions of this structure (Fig. 2, *arrow*). In Nissl material, the C2 type neuron is more difficult to identify. Figure 3 illustrates a neuron that, on the basis of its location within the substantia nigra and of the shape of the cell body, most likely corresponds to a C2 type neuron. The Nissl substance is more or less uniformly distributed throughout the cytoplasm. The eccentrically located nucleus is to a great extent masked by the chromophil substance of the cytoplasm, and the neurites are broad and long.

A third type of neuron (R1) of the substantia nigra is most often located within the medial part of the pars reticularis. In Nissl preparations, this type of cell with an elongated or triangular cell body is intensely stained. It gives rise to long and usually well-stained processes. The nucleus is often masked by the Nissl substance, but occasionally it may be seen, and under such conditions, it has an elongated shape similar to that of the cell body. The nucleus is somewhat eccentrically located. In AChE material, the R1 type neuron has a moderate-to-intense enzymatic activity which is somewhat lighter at the site occupied by the nucleus. The proximal parts of the processes appear relatively thick and have few branches (Figs. 7,8).

The fourth type of neuron (L) of the substantia nigra is of medium size (30–50 μm). These neurons are mainly located within the lateral and ventro-lateral areas of the rostral and intermediate parts of the pars reticulata. They are not present in the caudal part of the substantia nigra. In material prepared with basic fuchsin and fast blue, the L type nerve cells are the commonly found neurons within the fibrous and lateral part of the substantia nigra. The rounded or triangular cell body contains Nissl substance that has a punctiform appearance. The tigroid substance is more abundant midway between the nuclear and cytoplasmic membranes. The nucleus is almost centrally located (Fig. 11). In AChE material, the corresponding areas of the substantia nigra show neurons that have a light-to-moderate enzymatic activity (Fig. 12). The cytoplasm has a fine and granular appearance, and lightly AChE-rich processes originate from each angle of the cell body. This type of neuron is very similar to the neurons of the internal division of the globus pallidus as shown in Figs. 13 and 14. In both Nissl and AChE material, the type "L" neurons, which are more rostrally located in the substantia nigra, and the corresponding neurons of the internal division of the pallidum share the same cytological characteristics (Figs. 11–14).

A fifth type of neuron (R2) is also present in the substantia nigra of the monkey. These neurons have small rounded or somewhat elongated cell bodies and are disseminated over most of the pars compacta and the pars reticulata. The pale nucleus is eccentrically located in the lightly stained cytoplasm (Fig. 9). These neurons and their long processes display moderate and light AChE activity, respectively (Fig. 10).

Neostriatum

In the monkey, the neostriatum is represented by the caudate nucleus, including the nucleus accumbens septi, the putamen, and the bridges of striatal tissue that link the caudate nucleus and the putamen. The latter structures are more abundant at the level of the anterior limb of the internal capsule (Fig. 15). As disclosed in Nissl material, the nervous elements are homogeneously distributed over all the different parts of the neostriatum. The larger neurons, however, have a somewhat more elongated shape at the level of the bridges of striatal tissue. Three types of neurons—small-, medium-, and large-sized—may be disclosed in such material. The larger neurons (type I) have ovoid or bulbous cell bodies with a maximum diameter of 30 to 40 μm. The Nissl substance is mainly situated at both ends of the perikaryon, and the nucleus is eccentrically located (Figs. 16,19). The medium-sized (type II) and small-sized (type III) neurons contain much less Nissl substance. The nucleus is more sharply outlined in the medium-sized neurons, whereas the cytoplasm is scanty in the small-sized ones (Figs. 16,19).

As a consequence of the relatively light cholinesterasic background of the neuropil following DFP treatment (Figs. 16,17), the cell bodies and processes of the AChE-containing neurons of the striatum are easily visualized. Two types of neurons, which represent only a small percentage of the total number of striatal neurons, may be identified within the various areas of the neostriatum. They are evenly distributed, and both show an intense AChE activity. Type I neurons, somewhat more abundant, have fusiform, bulbous cell bodies (Figs. 17,18) with broad and variegated processes which taper and become thinner

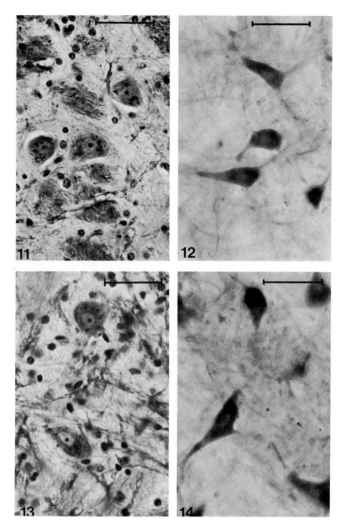

FIGS. 11–14. Microphotographs of sections through the substantia nigra (Figs. 11,12) and the internal division of the globus pallidus (Figs. 13,14) of the brain of the monkey. Calibration bar = 50 μm. **11,12:** Type "L" neurons of the substantia nigra in sections stained with a basic dye (Fig. 11) and prepared to demonstrate AChE (Fig. 12), respectively. **13,14:** Neurons of the pallidum from sections stained with a basic dye (Fig. 13) and prepared to demonstrate AChE (Fig. 14). Note the resemblance between these neurons and the type "L" neurons of the substantia nigra.

away from the cell body. Their AChE activity is somewhat lighter than that of the cell body. Type I neurons located in the bridges of striatal tissue are more elongated (as in Nissl material) (Fig. 17), whereas the processes of those located at the periphery of the caudate or putamen course along the edge of

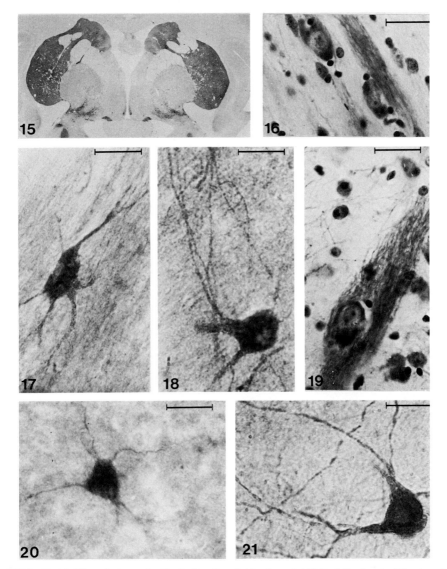

FIGS. 15–21. Microphotographs illustrating the distribution of AChE at the level of the basal ganglia and the cytohistochemical characteristics of individual neurons within these structures in the brains of DFP-treated monkeys. AChE (Figs. 15,17,18,20,21) and basic fuchsin and fast blue (Figs. 16,19) stains. **15:** Transverse section through the intermediate parts of the basal ganglia illustrating the distribution of AChE in the caudate nucleus, the putamen, and both divisions of the pallidum. Note also the intense AChE activity at the level of the nucleus basalis of Meynert and the supraoptic nuclei. × 25. **16:** Nissl- and myelin-stained striatal tissue at the level of the tail of the caudate nucleus. **17,18:** AChE activity of individual type 1 neurons located in the bridges of tissue between the caudate nucleus and the putamen (17) and in the tail of the caudate nucleus along the periphery (closing neuron) (18). Calibration bar = 25 μm. **19:** Nissl- and myelin-stained striatal tissue at the level of the putamen. Calibration bar = 25 μm. **20:** AChE activity of a type II neuron located in the head of the caudate nucleus. Calibration bar = 25 μm. **21:** AChE activity of a neuron of the nucleus ansa lenticularis. The long processes of the neuron spread and ramify into the above-located internal division of the pallidum. Calibration bar = 25 μm.

these structures (Fig. 18). Type I neurons most likely correspond to the large or giant chromatic cells. Type II neurons, somewhat smaller (maximum diameter, 25–30 μm), possibly correspond to the spidery aspiny neurons described by Fox et al. (8). The perikaryon, which contains an eccentrically situated nucleus, is polygonal, and these smooth and smaller processes branch in the vicinity of the cell body (Fig. 20). Numerous other medium- and small-sized neurons are unstained in AChE material. Under these conditions (DFP-treated animal), the strionigral fibers display minimal AChE activity as disclosed at the level of the comb bundle.

Globus Pallidus

Corresponding neurons of the internal division of the pallidum may be observed in material prepared with a Nissl stain and for demonstration of AChE (Figs. 13,14). In Nissl material, the neurons of the two divisions of the pallidum are morphologically similar to type L neurons located in the lateral and ventrolateral part of the substantia nigra (compare Figs. 11 and 13; 12 and 14). The medium-sized round or triangular cell body contains Nissl substance, mainly situated midway between the nuclear and cell membranes, that has a punctiform appearance. The nucleus is almost centrally located (Fig. 13). In AChE material, the cell bodies and processes display moderate and light enzymatic activity, respectively (Fig. 14).

Other large neurons closely related to the globus pallidus constitute the nucleus ansae lenticularis. In AChE material, the cell bodies and processes of these neurons show an intense AChE-activity (Fig. 21). The bulbous and multipolar cell bodies give rise to thick processes which taper and ramify in fine branches ending in the above-located pallidum. Other thinner but intensely stained processes course below the ventral edge of the pallidum and apparently join the ansa lenticularis.

DISCUSSION

On the basis of cytohistochemical characteristics, five types of neurons may be identified in the substantia nigra of the monkey. Such neurons are particularly obvious in DFP-treated animals because of the light AChE activity of the background (2,3,24) in comparison with the intense background AChE activity observed in nontreated monkeys (21) and rats (12,16). Two types of neuron are present in the pars compacta of the substantia nigra. Type C1 has a medium-sized and ovoid cell body which displays a moderate AChE activity. Its processes occasionally show a light enzymatic activity (24). This type of neuron (C1) most likely corresponds to the medium-sized neurons thought by Gulley and Wood (11) to give rise to the nigrostriatal dopaminergic pathways. In this regard, the morphological, statistical, and histopathological studies of the substantia nigra of the rat by Butcher et al. (3) strongly suggest that the C1 type neurons correspond to the dopaminergic neurons of the substantia nigra. In monkeys with ventromedial tegmental lesions, the associated retrograde cellular degeneration apparently involves type C1 neurons (Marchand and Poirier, *unpublished data*), which suggests that the loss of this class of AChE-containing neurons is most likely responsible for the decreased concentration of dopamine in the corresponding striatal tissue (25,26).

Type C2 neurons of the substantia nigra of the monkey have triangular or pyramidal cell bodies and relatively long processes, both of which show an important AChE activity (24). However, this type of neuron, which stands out sharply in tissue from DFP-treated monkeys prepared for the demonstration of AChE, is more difficult to identify in Nissl material.

Type L neurons more especially occupy the lateral and ventrolateral parts of the substantia nigra of the monkey. They are larger and more numerous in the fibrous (lateral) and rostral parts of the substantia nigra. On the basis of their cytological characteristics both in AChE and Nissl material, they are very similar to the neurons of the internal division of the pallidum as first suggested by Mirto (19) in man, later by Olszewski and Baxter (22) in Nissl material, and more recently by Fox et al. (7) and Schwyn and Fox (29) in Golgi and other material of the monkey brain. Olszewski and Baxter (22) have also observed that the substantia nigra pars reticulata and the internal division of the pallidum are continuous at the level of the fields of Sano (28). Schwyn and Fox (29) have also noted that the nervous tissue of the comb bundle, which links the rostral part of the substantia nigra and the pallidum, is very similar to the tissue of these two structures. As suggested by Poirier et al. (24), it is therefore conceivable that the type "L" neurons have the same origin as the pallidal neurons and could correspond to neurons that have migrated more caudally (19), or else they have been isolated from the globus pallidus by the fibers of the internal capsule during the development of the brain. In view of the fact that the neurons of the internal division of the pallidum project to the thalamus (20) and in light of the above data, it appears that the type L neurons of the substantia nigra could give rise to similar projections. As a matter of fact, a nigrothalamic bundle originating in the pars reticulata has been proposed by Faull and Carmen (6) and Carpenter and Peter (5). Gulley and Wood (11) have suggested that the larger neurons of the rostrolateral area of the substantia nigra give rise to the nigrothalamic projection. In this regard, Rinvik (27) has reported that the injection of horseradish peroxidase (HRP) into the dorsal thalamus results in marking of the larger neurons of the pars reticulata of the substantia nigra in the cat.

Types R1 and R2 neurons are less abundant than types C1 and L in the substantia nigra of the monkey. Type R1 neurons, which are intensely stained in Nissl material, are most common in the ventromedial area of the pars reticulata of the substantia nigra. Type R2 neurons, which have small cell bodies, are found in both the pars compacta and the pars reticulata. They most likely correspond to the small neurons described by Ramon y Cajal (4) and Schwyn and Fox (29). Gulley and Wood (11), who observed similar neurons in the rat brain, believe that they are interneurons.

As a consequence of the application of the pharmacohistochemical method (1,3), AChE neurons of the neostriatum, which are obscured by the intense background activity in the pharmacologically unmanipulated animals, may be readily identified in the brain of DFP-treated animals. Under the particular conditions used in this study, medium- and large-sized neurons with intensely stained cell bodies and processes were observed throughout the neostriatum. They represent a small percentage of the neuronal population of the neostriatum. The larger type neurons, apparently identical to the type III neurons in rat brain described by Butcher et al. (3), have cell bodies that have a fusiform or bulbous shape. They most likely correspond either to the large chromatic neurons observed in Nissl preparations, or to the giant or large aspiny neurons described in Golgi preparations of the neostriatum of monkeys (7) and rats (13). In the cat, the large aspiny neurons represent <1% of the striatal neurons (13). The other type of AChE-positive neuron in the neostriatum of the monkey, probably corresponding to the type II AChE neurons of the rat striatum described by Butcher et al. (3), is represented by medium-sized neurons whose perikarya are polygonal. These neurons, which are fewer than the larger neurons, most likely correspond to the "spidery aspiny" neurons described by Fox et al. (8). The large AChE neurons observed in the neostriatal tissue of the DFP-treated monkey could be the source of the acetylcholinesterasic striatopallidal and stria-tonigral fibers (21) as suggested by Fox et al. (9). In view of the fact that the destruction of the neostriatum results in a significant decrease of gamma-amino-butyric acid (GABA) in the corresponding pallidum and substantia nigra (14), it is conceivable that the neostriatal GABAergic neurons are identical to the large AChE-containing neurons of the neostriatum. It must be pointed out, however, that this hypothesis does not receive support from observations by Grofova (10). In injecting HRP into the substantia nigra, this investigator reported no labeling of giant cells in the cat neostriatum, while, at least in one brain, approximately 100 medium-sized neurons were labeled. Therefore, the acetylcholinesterasic and/or GABAergic striatofugal fibers may originate exclusively from medium-sized neurons.

In contradistinction to the caudate nucleus and putamen, where only a small percentage of neurons show an AChE activity, most cell bodies and processes of the neurons of both divisions of the globus pallidus display a light-to-moderate enzymatic activity. Their spindle-shaped or triangular cell bodies and their processes are similar to those shown in Golgi preparations of the pallidum (7). Moreover, these neurons are morphologically similar to the type "L" neurons mainly located in the rostrolateral part of the substantia nigra.

Another group of large bulbous and multipolar neurons interspersed among the fibers of the ansa lenticularis below the pallidum are closely related to the latter structure. This group of large neurons with intensely AChE-stained cell bodies and processes corresponds to nucleus ansae lenticularis. They are most likely related morphologically and functionally to the globus pallidus, as suggested by the fact that their dendrites abundantly ramify within the pallidal tissue.

SUMMARY

On the basis of Nissl material and of the distribution of AChE, five types of neurons may be identified in the substantia nigra of the monkey. Types C1 and C2 are present in the pars compacta. Type C1 neurons, which have medium-sized and ovoid cell bodies, most likely correspond to the dopaminergic neurons. The fewer type C2 neurons have triangular or pyramidal cell bodies and processes which show an important AChE activity. Type L neurons, mainly located in the lateral and ventrolateral parts of the substantia nigra, have rounded or triangular cell bodies. They are very similar to the neurons of the pallidum. Type R1 neurons, which are intensively stained in Nissl material, occupy the ventromedial area of the substantia nigra. Type R2 neurons, with small cell bodies, are diffusely distributed. In AChE material, the perikarya and processes of two types of neurons of the neostriatum, representing a small percentage of all neurons in this structure, are intensely stained.

ACKNOWLEDGMENT

This research was supported by grant MT-732 of the Medical Research Council of Canada. Dr. Marchand holds a postdoctoral fellowship from the Quebec Health Science Council, and Dr. Poirier is the recipient of a Killam commemorative scholarship.

REFERENCES

1. Butcher, L. L., and Hodge, G. K. (1976): Postnatal development of acetylcholinesterase in the caudate-putamen nucleus and substantia nigra of rats. *Brain Res.,* 106:223–240.
2. Butcher, L. L., Marchand, R., Parent, A., and Poirier, L. J. (1977): Morphological characteristics of acetylcholinesterase-containing neurons in the CNS of DFP-treated monkeys. Part III. Brain stem and spinal cord. *J. Neurol. Sci.,* 32:169–185.
3. Butcher, L. L., Talbot, K., and Bilezikjian, L. (1975): Acetylcholinesterase neurons in dopamine-containing regions of the brain. *J. Neural Trans.,* 38:127–153.
4. Cajal, S. Ramon y (1909, 1911): Histologie du système nerveux de l'homme et des vertébrés, 2 vols. Norbert Maloine, Paris.
5. Carpenter, M. B., and Peter, P. (1972): Nigrostriatal and nigrothalamic fibers in the rhesus monkey. *J. Comp. Neurol.,* 144:93–116.
6. Faull, R. L. M., and Carman, J. B. (1968): Ascending projections of the substantia nigra in the rat. *J. Comp. Neurol.,* 132:73–92.
7. Fox, C. A., Andrade, A. N., Luqui, I. J., and Rafols, J. A. (1974): The primate globus pallidus. A Golgi and electron microscopic study. *J. Hirnforsch.,* 15:75–93.
8. Fox, C. A., Andrade, A. N., Schwyn, R. C., and Rafols, J. A. (1971/72): The aspiny neurons and the glia in the primate striatum—A Golgi and electron microscopic study. *J. Hirnforsch.,* 13:341–362.
9. Fox, C. A., Rafols, J. A., and Cowan, W. M. (1975): Computer measurements of axis cylinder diameters of radial fibers and "comb" bundle fibers. *J. Comp. Neurol.,* 159:201–224.

10. Grofova, I. (1975): The identification of striatal and pallidal neurons projecting to substantia nigra—An experimental study by means of retrograde axonal transport of horseradish peroxidase. *Brain Res.,* 91:286–291.
11. Gulley, R. L., and Wood, R. L. (1971): The fine structure of the neurons in the rat substantia nigra. *Tissue Cell,* 3:675–690.
12. Jacobowitz, D. M., and Palkovits, M. (1974): Topographic atlas of catecholamine and acetylcholinesterase-containing neurons in the rat brain, Part I [Forebrain (telencephalon, diencephalon)]. *J. Comp. Neurol.,* 157:13–28.
13. Kemp, J. M., and Powell, T. P. S. (1971): The structure of the caudate nucleus of the cat— Light and electron microscopy. *Phil. Trans. Roy. Soc. (Lond.), B,* 262:383–410.
14. Kim, J. S., Bak, I. J., Hassler, R., and Oakada, Y. (1971): Role of aminobutyric acid (GABA) in the extrapyramidal motor system, Part 2 (Some evidence for the existence of a type of GABA-rich strionigral neurons). *Exp. Brain Res.,* 14:95–104.
15. Klüver, H., and Barrera, E. (1953): A method for the combined staining of cells and fibers in the nervous system. *J. Neuropathol. Exp. Neurol.,* 12:400–403.
16. Koelle, G. B. (1954): The histochemical localization of cholinesterases in the central nervous system. *J. Comp. Neurol.,* 100:211–228.
17. Kreutzberg, G. W., Toth, L., and Kaiya, H. (1975): AChE as marker for dendritic transport and secretion. In: *Advances in Neurology, Vol. 12: Physiology and Pathology of Dendrites,* edited by G. W. Kreutzberg, pp. 269–281. Raven Press, New York.
18. Marchand, R., Parent, A., and Poirier, L. J. (1976): Distribution of acetylcholinesterase within various groups of neurons of the midbrain, pons-medulla and spinal cord of monkeys treated with DFP. *Neurosci. Abstr.,* 2:629.
19. Mirto, D. (1896): Contributo alla fina anatomia della substantia nigra di Sommering e del pedunculo cerebrale dell'unomo. *Riv. Sper. Freniatr.,* 22:197–210.
20. Nauta, W. J. H., and Mehler, W. R. (1966): Projections of the lentiform nucleus in the monkey. *Brain Res.,* 1:3–48.
21. Olivier, A., Parent, A., Simard, H., and Poirier, L. J. (1970): Cholinesterasic striopallidal and striatonigral efferents in the cat and the monkey. *Brain Res.,* 18:273–282.
22. Olszewski, J., and Baxter, D. (1954): *Cytoarchitecture of the Human Brain Stem,* p. 199. J. Lippincott, Philadelphia.
23. Parent, A., Poirier, L. J., Boucher, R., and Butcher, L. L. (1977): Morphological characteristics of acetylcholinesterase-containing neurons in the CNS of DFP-treated monkeys, Part 2 (Diencephalon and medial telencephalic structures). *J. Neurol. Sci.,* 32:9–28.
24. Poirier, L. J., Parent, A., Marchand, R., and Butcher, L. L. (1977): Morphological characteristics of acetylcholinesterase-containing neurons in the CNS of DFP-treated monkeys, Part I (Extrapyramidal and related structures). *J. Neurol. Sci.,* 31:181–198.
25. Poirier, L. J., and Sourkes, T. L. (1964): Influence du locus niger sur la concentration des catécholamines du striatum. *J. Physiol. (Paris),* 56:426–427 (abstr.).
26. Poirier, L. J., and Sourkes, T. L. (1965): Influence of the substantia nigra on the catecholamine content of the striatum. *Brain,* 88:181–192.
27. Rinvik, E. (1975): Demonstration of nigrothalamic connections in the cat by retrograde axonal transport of horseradish peroxidase. *Brain Res.,* 90:313–318.
28. Sano, T. (1910): Beitrag zur vergleichenden Anatomie der Substantia nigra des Corpus luysii und der Zona incerta. *Monatsschr. Psychiatr. Neurol.,* 27:110–127.
29. Schwyn, R. C., and Fox, C. A. (1974): The primate substantia nigra—A Golgi and electron microscopic study. *J. Hirnforsch.,* 15:95–126.

Advances in Neurology, Vol. 24, edited by
L. J. Poirier, T. L. Sourkes, and P. J. Bédard.
Raven Press, New York © 1979.

Effects of Chronic Reserpine Treatment on the Brains of Rabbits and Their Fetuses

*Virginia M. Tennyson, *Mary Budininkas-Schoenebeck, *†John Martin, and **Herbert Barden

*Departments of Anatomy, Pathology (Division of Neuropathology), and Neurology, Columbia University, College of Physicians and Surgeons, and **The New York State Psychiatric Institute, New York, New York 10032*

When brain tissue is treated by the Falck–Hillarp technique (12), the neostriatum exhibits a diffuse and intense greenish-yellow fluorescence due to the presence of high concentrations of dopamine (8) scattered in minute axonal terminals throughout the neuropil (9,13). Dahlström and Fuxe (11) suggested that fluorescent neurons of the substantia nigra, pars compacta, project their axons to the neostriatum. The nigroneostriatal pathway is not fluorescent in the normal adult animal, but its existence has been confirmed using a variety of techniques after the tract has been experimentally lesioned (1,2,7,10,20,25,34). Although the nigroneostriatal pathway does not fluoresce in the adult, it can be visualized directly in the fetus because the early outgrowing axons from the substantia nigra are fluorescent for a short period of time all along their course when they first enter the putamen (14,15,19,21–23,29). In the rabbit, fluorescent neostriatal terminals are found initially only in the ventral putamen, at gestation days 18 to 20; however, by day 28, there are scattered individual terminals and "islands" of linear, punctate, and diffuse fluorescence in both the caudate nucleus and putamen (see reviews of refs. 26,27,30).

Studies of fetal or early postnatal development of substantia nigra neurons and their terminals in the neostriatum have been done in the mouse (14,15), rat (18,19,22,23), rabbit (26,27,29,30), and human (21). Substantia nigra neuroblasts become fluorescent (Fig. 1) as soon as they migrate away from the primitive ependymal zone at gestation day 14 in the rabbit (29). The fluorescent cell bodies have wispy processes, but axons have not grown out from these neuroblasts to any extent.

Since axonal pathways have not been established between the substantia nigra and neostriatum as yet, the early neuroblasts of the substantia nigra cannot be carrying out their mature function of innervating the neostriatum. Therefore,

---

†Present address: School of Public Health, Johns Hopkins School of Medicine, Baltimore, Maryland 21205.

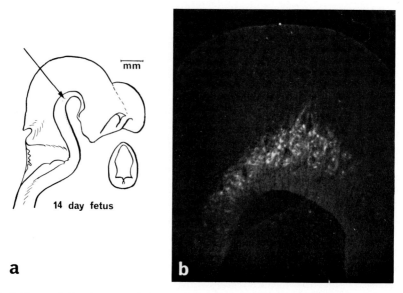

FIG. 1. Stage of development of the midbrain of a fetal rabbit at 14 days' gestation. **a:** A diagram of a transverse section of the midbrain, a parasagittal section of the brain, and the gross appearance of the fetus. The arrow indicates the location of the fluorescent cells in **(b)**. **b.** A fluorescence micrograph showing fluorescent cell bodies and short processes in the mantle layer of the basal plate of the caudal mesencephalon. ×115. (Reproduced from Tennyson et al., ref. 29, with permission.)

dopamine may be present at this early stage to subserve a different function. We wish to test the hypothesis that at early stages, dopamine may play a role in normal development of the nigroneostriatal tract.

A possibility that intrigues us is that dopamine may be released from the cell body and act as a humoral agent to initiate communication between neurons of one region and another. If this is so, it would ultimately lead to the establishment of appropriate neural connections. Dopamine, therefore, may be a link in a feedback mechanism to direct axons to their target. In addition, maintenance of the postsynaptic target may be dependent on presynaptic innervation, or on receiving a catecholaminergic developmental signal at an appropriate time.

If drugs that interfere with catecholamine metabolism are administered at critical periods of development, the proper migration of axons may be altered, and degeneration may occur in target areas. For this study, we used repeated administration of reserpine to pregnant rabbits to deplete dopamine from their fetuses during critical periods of development of substantia nigra neuroblasts and their axons. We have found large compound bodies suggestive of degeneration in the putamen of the reserpine-treated fetus, and in late fetal life there are fewer terminals and less mature neurons than in the normal fetal putamen. In addition, some of the adult rabbits receiving reserpine had lesions or an increase of intraneuronal lipofuscin in their brains. Preliminary reports have appeared on these studies (31–33).

MATERIALS AND METHODS

Pregnant rabbits received repeated subcutaneous injections of reserpine over a period of 9 to 11 days during the middle of gestation or were left untreated as controls. The lowest total dose for the entire period was 0.34 mg, and the highest dose was 6.0 mg. The fetuses were killed on days 22 to 28 of gestation. We studied the brains of some fetuses by fluorescence microscopy using the Falck-Hillarp technique (12). Littermate fetuses were perfused with a glutaraldehyde–paraformaldehyde–acrolein mixture and then postfixed with 2% osmium tetroxide for electron microscopy. For light microscopic study of lesions in the brains of adults, 10 μm sections of the same paraffin-embedded freeze-dried tissue used for the fluorescence microscopy study were stained by the following methods: Harris hematoxylin and eosin (H & E), cresyl violet, Sudan black B (6), periodic acid-Schiff (PAS) (6), and acetic acid carbolfuchsin (3) utilized as an acid-fast stain for lipofuscin (4,5). Lipofuscin, which contains a modified lipid component, can be identified by various staining techniques which include the latter three stains (24,35).

RESULTS AND DISCUSSION

As mentioned, normal neuroblasts of the substantia nigra are fluorescent by day 14 of gestation (Fig. 1b). Their axons have reached the putamen by days 18 to 20, and from days 22 to 28 of gestation widespread individual fluorescent terminals as well as "islands" of linear or diffuse fluorescence develop (27,29). To determine whether the doses of reserpine given to the dam were effective in completely depleting dopamine from axons in the fetal putamen, the brains of some fetuses were examined 4 hr after the last dose of drug on day 22 of gestation. Fluorescence was absent in the fetal putamen even at the lowest dose given to the dam. Thus, the drug crossed the placenta and exerted its effects on the fetus.

To determine the time required for fluorescence to return to the putamen of drug-treated fetuses, fetuses were killed on gestation day 28, 3 days after cessation of reserpine treatment. (The dam had received a total of 5.1 mg of reserpine over a period of 11 days during the middle of gestation.) The substantia nigra of the control fetus had well-developed neurons which exhibited a moderately intense dopamine fluorescence in their cell bodies and dendrites (Fig. 2a) and fluorescent terminals in the neuropil. The neurons of the reserpine-treated fetus often appeared as "ghosts," having only small amounts of fluorescence (Fig. 2c). The putamen of the control fetus had scattered fluorescent terminals and moderately intense fluorescent "islands" of punctate and linear profiles (Fig. 2b). There were very few isolated terminals in the putamen of the reserpine-

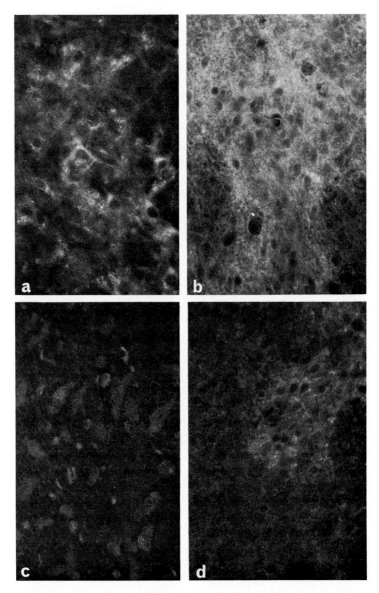

FIG. 2. Fluorescence micrographs of control **(a** and **b)** and reserpine-treated **(c** and **d)** fetuses at day 28 of gestation. (The dam of the reserpine-treated fetus received a total of 5.1 mg of reserpine over a period of 11 days and was killed 3 days later.) **a:** Neuroblasts of the substantia nigra of the control fetus have moderately intense fluorescence in cell bodies and processes. **b:** Axons from these cells form diffuse linear patterns that appear as "islands" of fluorescence in the putamen. **c:** Neuroblasts of the substantia nigra of the reserpine-treated fetus appear as "ghosts" with only small amounts of fluorescence in their cell bodies. **d:** Axons of these cells form only a few small "islands," which have a very low fluorescence. ×320.

treated fetus, and the "islands" were smaller and their fluorescence very weak (Fig. 2d). Even 6 days after cessation of reserpine treatment of another rabbit which received a total of 0.7 mg of reserpine over a period of 8 days, there were only a few fluorescing profiles in the fetal putamen.

How can one explain the presence of the few fluorescent processes 3 to 6 days after cessation of reserpine treatment, and why is the rest of the neuropil nonfluorescent? Did reserpine actually stop the growth of most of the dopamine-containing axons, as postulated by the hypothesis being tested? If this is the case, the few fluorescent axons present in Fig. 2d would represent a new growth of axons that occurred after stopping reserpine treatment. An alternative explanation would be that axons from the substantia nigra are present in the nonfluorescent regions of the putamen, but they have not yet been supplied with dopamine and synthesizing enzymes from the cell bodies in the substantia nigra. We have tried to answer these questions by taking low-magnification electron micrographs of the neuropil of the putamen of control and reserpine-treated fetuses and counting the number of vesicle-containing profiles. Although some characteristics of the dopamine-containing axons have been reported after 5-hydroxydopamine uptake (16,28), dopamine processes and terminals have not yet been conclusively demonstrated. Thus, we counted all profiles that could possibly correspond to the fluorescent images seen in the normal fetus. The profiles counted were vesicle-containing terminals with or without synaptic specializations, axonal growth cones with vesicles, and thin axons with vesicles extending along their length. In the adult rabbit neostriatum, all of these processes except the growth cone, which is not present in mature brain, incorporated 5-hydroxydopamine (28).

We have only preliminary data, but there appears to be a decrease in vesicle-containing profiles in the putamen of reserpine-treated fetuses. The control fetuses had a mean of 49 vesicle-containing processes in an area of 300 sq μm. Three reserpine-treated fetuses from different dams receiving a total of 5.1, 3.1, and 3.0 mg over 11 to 12 days had 33, 43, and 45%, respectively, of control values. We intend to increase the number of animals in this study, and we will label the vesicle-filled profiles with 5-hydroxydopamine or tritiated catecholamines to determine what proportion of the terminals in the putamens of these fetuses are catecholaminergic. We do not know how many axons and terminals at this fetal stage have grown into the putamen from other areas, such as cerebral cortex and thalamus.

Littermate fetuses of those that had been studied by fluorescence microscopy were examined by electron microscopy. There were multiple small and large heterogeneous bodies (Fig. 3) and other evidence of degeneration in processes scattered throughout the neuropil in the putamen of reserpine-treated fetuses. Multivesicular bodies (Fig. 3a) are commonly altered and appear to be one of the early changes that takes place. Some of the degenerative bodies are in processes of uncertain origin, but other processes can be identified by their content of ribosomes and endoplasmic reticulum, as dendrites of neuroblasts in the putamen. Therefore, at least some of the degeneration is taking place in target

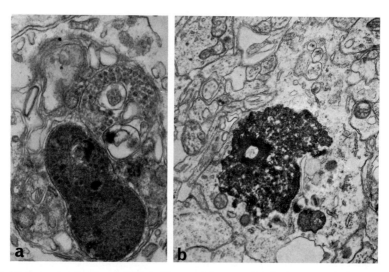

FIG. 3. Electron micrographs showing evidence of degeneration in the neuropil of the putamen of reserpine-treated fetuses. **a:** Early alterations in large and small multivesicular bodies in the putamen of a 22-day fetus. ×27,000. (The dam received a total of 0.56 mg of reserpine over a period of 9 days and was killed 4 hr later.) **b:** Large and small heterogeneous bodies are present in processes in the putamen of a 28-day fetus. ×10,200. (The dam received a total of 3.0 mg of reserpine over a period of 12 days and was killed 3 days later.)

tissue of axons of the substantia nigra. We do not know yet whether the degenerative changes are due to a cytotoxic effect of the drug or whether the alterations represent transsynaptic degeneration due to absence of dopamine terminals or of dopamine itself.

We also noticed that the neuroblasts of reserpine-treated fetuses generally appeared less mature (Fig. 4b) than those of controls (Fig. 4a). There was much less cytoplasm and dendrites were not as obvious in the experimental fetus. This observation is consistent with the findings of Lauder and Krebs (17), who injected parachlorophenylalanine into pregnant rats. These investigators used tritiated thymidine to mark the date of origin of neurons that are targets of serotonergic terminals and examined the animals 1 month after birth. They found that target neurons arose at later times than normal, and thus were less mature for a given age.

Adult Brains

The dam's brain was always examined in these experiments to determine how effective the dose of reserpine was in depleting catecholamines from her neostriatum. In general, the lower doses at least partially depleted the neostriatum, but had less effect on the mesolimbic system. The highest doses depleted both the mesolimbic system and neostriatum.

We made a serendipitous finding when we examined these brains with fluores-

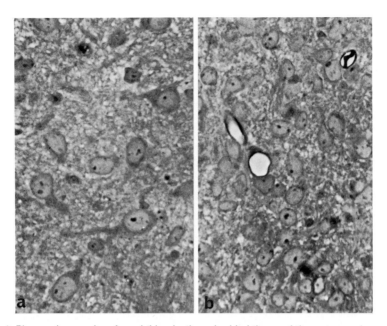

FIG. 4. Phase micrographs of semi-thin plastic-embedded tissue of the putamen from control **(a)** and reserpine-treated **(b)** fetuses at day 28 of gestation. (The dam of the reserpine-treated fetus received a total of 5.1 mg of reserpine over a period of 11 days and was killed 3 days later.) **a:** Neuroblasts from the control fetus are relatively large and have a distinct zone of cytoplasm, large nuclei, and prominent dendrites. **b:** Neuroblasts of the reserpine-treated fetus are closely packed together, and are smaller and have very little cytoplasm or dendritic processes evident. ×470.

cence microscopy. Of 15 pregnant females, 11 had either increases in the number and size of intraneuronal lipofuscin granules, particularly in the prepiriform cortex and often in the dorsal cortex, or else they had areas of autofluorescent tissue that were identified as lesions in the brain. Figure 5a shows the typical appearance of lipofuscin granules in the prepiriform cortex of a normal pregnant rabbit, and Fig. 5b shows the increases in number and size of these granules from a pregnant rabbit receiving 0.56 mg reserpine over a period of 9 days. This rabbit also had a lesion in the lateral cortex. Since it seemed possible that this effect of reserpine was limited to pregnant rabbits, we examined males and virgin females as well. Fluorescence microscopy revealed an autofluorescent lesion (Fig. 6a) in the dorsal cortex of a virgin rabbit given a total of 0.63 mg of reserpine over a period of 10 days. Histologic stains showed many cells, probably phagocytes, forming the periphery of the lesions and necrosis in the center. Stains for lipofuscin demonstrated that many of the cells of the lesions had numerous small spherical granules of lipofuscin (Fig. 6b,c,d). The formation of lipofuscin is believed to proceed primarily by the progressive oxidation of lipid, a major component of the granule. A male rabbit also had a lesion in the dorsal cortex after receiving a total of 0.7 mg of reserpine over a period

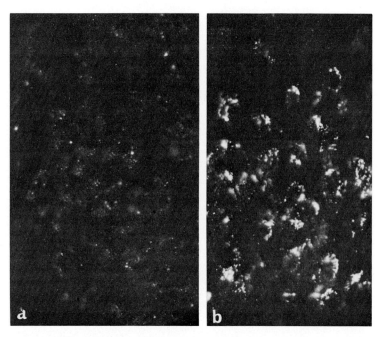

FIG. 5. Fluorescence micrographs of autofluorescent intraneuronal lipofuscin granules in the prepiriform cortex of a control pregnant rabbit (a) and of a pregnant rabbit that had received a total of 0.56 mg of reserpine over a period of 9 days and was killed 6 days later. **a:** Very small granules are present in control neurons. **b:** The granules are markedly increased in size and number in the reserpine-treated rabbit. ×320.

of 8 days. It should be pointed out that all of the reserpine-treated adult rabbits were relatively young, about 7 to 10 months of age. Since reserpine treatment in some of these young adults resulted in increases in intraneuronal lipofuscin, it might represent a premature aging of their brains. In this regard, the brains of reserpine-treated young adults resembled the brain of a healthy untreated old male rabbit in our colony whose age was at least 3 years. There were large numbers of lipofuscin granules throughout his brain.

SUMMARY

Reserpine has been administered during critical periods of development of neuroblasts of the substantia nigra in the rabbit, that is, just before or at the time that normal fetuses first develop dopamine in these neuroblasts until their terminals are well established in the putamen. There are fewer fluorescent processes in the putamen 3 to 6 days after cessation of treatment. Preliminary studies in which the number of vesicle-containing profiles were counted in electron micrographs support the fluorescence microscopy data showing that there are fewer terminals in the reserpine-treated fetus. In addition, there are large

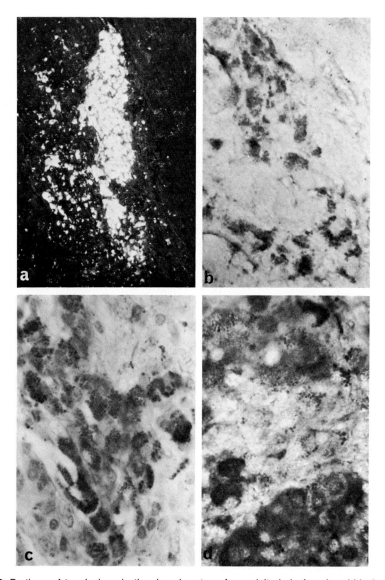

FIG. 6. Portions of two lesions in the dorsal cortex of an adult virgin female rabbit that had received a total of 0.6 mg of reserpine over a period of 10 days. The cells of the lesion appear to be phagocytes. (**a, b,** and **c** are from the same lesion; **d** is from an adjacent lesion.) **a:** Fluorescence micrograph showing autofluorescence in the central necrotic zone and in cells surrounding it. ×120. **b:** Sudan-black-B staining demonstrates numerous small spherical lipofuscin granules in cells. ×340. **c:** Acid-fast staining with Barbeito-Lopez carbolfuchsin shows numerous small, spherical, lipofuscin granules in cells. ×340. **d:** Periodic acid-Schiff staining occurs variously as small spherical lipofuscin granules, diffuse cytoplasmic staining, or as granules on a deeply tinted background. ×340.

heterogeneous bodies in target tissue, which suggests selective degeneration. Reserpine also affects the brains of adult rabbits. A large proportion of adult rabbits receiving repeated reserpine injections showed increases in the number and size of intraneuronal lipofuscin granules and/or lipofuscin granule-containing lesions in their brains.

ACKNOWLEDGMENTS

The authors wish to express their gratitude to Mr. Francisco Aviles for valuable histologic assistance and to Mr. Moshe Rosen for management of the electron microscope. These studies were supported by USPHS grant NS-11870, NSF grant BNS 78–13733, the Cerebral Palsy Research and Educational Foundation, the Clinical Center for Research in Parkinson's and Allied Diseases, and the Muscular Dystrophy Associations of America, New York.

REFERENCES

1. Andén, N.-E., Dahlström, A., Fuxe, K., and Larsson, K. (1965): Further evidence for the presence of nigro-neostriatal dopamine neurons in the rat. *Am. J. Anat.,* 116:329–334.
2. Andén, N.-E., Dahlström, A., Fuxe, K., Larsson, K., Olson, L., and Ungerstedt, U. (1966): Ascending monoamine neurons to the telencephalon and diencephalon. *Acta Physiol. Scand.,* 67:313–326.
3. Barbeito-Lopez, J. (1946): A new staining method for histologic sections: Preliminary report. *Am. J. Clin. Pathol. (Tech. Sect.),* 10:53–56.
4. Barden, H. (1979): Acid fast staining of oxidized neuromelanin and lipofuscin in human brain. *J. Neuropathol. Exp. Neurol.,* 38:(5), *(in press).*
5. Barden, H., Rivers, W., and Aviles, F. (1978): Interference filter microfluorometry and acid fast staining of bleached neuromelanin and lipofuscin age pigments in human brain. *Age,* 1:74 *(abstr.).*
6. Barka, T., and Anderson, P. J. (1963): *Histochemistry, Theory, Practice and Bibliography.* Hoeber, New York.
7. Bédard, P., Larochelle, L., Parent, A., and Poirier, L. J. (1969): The nigrostriatal pathway: A correlative study based on neuroanatomical and neurochemical criteria in the cat and the monkey. *Exp. Neurol.,* 25:365–377.
8. Carlsson, A. (1959): The occurrence, distribution and physiological role of catecholamines in the nervous system. *Pharmacol. Rev.,* 11:490–493.
9. Carlsson, A., Falck, B., and Hillarp, N. Å. (1962): Cellular localization of brain monoamines. *Acta Physiol. Scand.,* 56 (Suppl. 196):1–28.
10. Carpenter, M. B., and Peter, P. (1972): Nigrostriatal and nigrothalamic fibers in the rhesus monkey. *J. Comp. Neurol.,* 144:93–116.
11. Dahlström, A., and Fuxe, F. (1964): Evidence for the existence of monoamine-containing neurons in the central nervous system. I. Demonstration of monoamines in the cell bodies of brain stem neurons. *Acta Physiol. Scand.,* 62 (Suppl. 232):1–55.
12. Falck, B., Hillarp, N.-Å., Thieme, G., and Torp, A. (1962): Fluorescence of catecholamines and related compounds condenses with formaldehyde. *J. Histochem. Cytochem.,* 10:348–354.
13. Fuxe, K., Hökfelt, T., and Nilsson, O. (1965): A fluorescence and electron microscopic study on certain brain regions rich in monoamine terminals. *Am. J. Anat.,* 117:33–46.
14. Golden, G. S. (1972): Embryologic demonstration of a nigro-striatal projection in the mouse. *Brain Res.,* 44:278–282.
15. Golden, G. S. (1973): Prenatal development of the biogenic amine systems of the mouse brain. *Dev. Biol.,* 33:300–311.
16. Hökfelt, T. (1968): *In vitro* studies on central and peripheral monoamine neurons at the ultrastructural level. *Z. Zellforsch. Mikrosk. Anat.,* 91:1–74.

17. Lauder, J. M., and Krebs, H. (1978): Serotonin and early neurogenesis. In: *Maturation of Neurotransmission.* Satellite Symposium, 6th Meeting of the International Society of Neurochemistry, St.-Vincent, pp. 171–180. S. Karger, Basel.
18. Loizou, L. A. (1972): The postnatal ontogeny of monoamine-containing neurons in the central nervous system of the albino rat. *Brain Res.,* 40:395–418.
19. Maeda, T., and Dresse, A. (1968): Possibilités d'étude du trajet des fibres cérébrales monoaminergiques chez le rat nouveau-né. *C.R. Soc. Biol. (Belge),* 162:1626–1629.
20. Moore, R. Y., Bhatnager, R. K., and Heller, A. (1971): Anatomical and chemical studies of a nigro-neostriatal projection in the cat. *Brain Res.,* 30:119–135.
21. Nobin, A. and Björklund, A. (1973): Topography of the monoamine neuron systems in the human brain as revealed in fetuses. *Acta Physiol. Scand.,* Suppl. 388:3–40.
22. Olson, L., Boreus, L. O., and Seiger, Å. (1973): Histochemical demonstration and mapping of 5-hydroxytryptamine- and catecholamine-containing neuron systems in the human fetal brain. *Z. Anat. Entwicklungsgesch.,* 139:259–282.
23. Olson, L., Seiger, Å., and Fuxe, K. (1972): Heterogeneity of striatal and limbic dopamine innervation: Highly fluorescent islands in developing and adult rats. *Brain Res.,* 44:283–288.
24. Pearse, A. G. E. (1972): *Histochemistry, Theoretical and Applied, 3rd ed., Vol. 2.* Williams & Wilkins, Baltimore.
25. Szabo, J. (1971): A silver impregnation study of nigrostriate projections in the cat. *Anat. Rec.,* 169:441 (abstr.).
26. Tennyson, V. M. (1976): Development of the substantia nigra, pars compacta, and neostriatum. In: *Progress in Neuropathology, Vol. 3,* edited by H. M. Zimmerman, pp. 359–381, Grune & Stratton, New York.
27. Tennyson, V. M., Barrett, R. E., Cohen, G., Côté, L., Heikkila, R., and Mytilineou, C. (1972): The developing neostriatum of the rabbit: Correlation of fluorescence histochemistry, electron microscopy, endogenous dopamine levels, and H³-dopamine uptake. *Brain Res.,* 46:251–285.
28. Tennyson, V. M., Heikkila, R., Mytilineou, C., Côté, L., and Cohen, G. (1972): 5-Hydroxydopamine "tagged" boutons in rabbit neostriatum: Interrelationship between vesicles and axonal membrane. *Brain Res.,* 82:341–348.
29. Tennyson, V. M., Mytilineou, C., Barrett, R. E. (1973): Fluorescence and electron microscopic studies of the early development of the substantia nigra and area ventralis tegmenti in the fetal rabbit. *J. Comp. Neurol.,* 149:233–257.
30. Tennyson, V. M., Mytilineou, C., Heikkila, R., Barrett, R. E., and Côté, L. (1975): Dopamine-containing neurons of the substantia nigra and their terminals in the neostriatum. In: *UCLA Forum in Medical Sciences, Brain Mechanisms in Mental Retardation,* edited by M. A. B. Brazier and N. Buchwald. Academic Press, New York.
31. Tennyson, V. M., Schoenebeck, M., Martin, J. (1977): Reserpine and/or α-methyl-*p*-tyrosine induced lesions in brains of pregnant rabbits and their fetuses. 7th Annual Meeting of the Society of Neuroscience, Anaheim, California, Abstr. Vol. III, p. 121.
32. Tennyson, V. M., Schoenebeck, M., Martin, J. (1978): Fluorescence and electron microscopic studies of the fetal neostriatum after administration of reserpine to the dam. *Anat. Rec.* 190:557–558.
33. Tennyson, V. M., Schoenebeck, M., Martin, J. (1979): Degeneration of targets deprived of catecholaminergic innervation. *Can. J. Neurol. Sci. (in press).*
34. Ungerstedt, U. (1971): Stereotaxic mapping of the monoamine pathways in the rat brain. *Acta Physiol. Scand.* [Suppl. 367]:1–48.
35. Wolman, M. (1975): Biological peroxidation of lipids and membranes. *Israel J. Med. Sci.,* 11 (Suppl):1–248.

Advances in Neurology, Vol. 24, edited by
L. J. Poirier, T. L. Sourkes, and P. J. Bédard.
Raven Press, New York © 1979.

Glutamic Acid as a Possible Neurotransmitter of Neo- and Allocortical Projections to the Fundus Striati

Cordula Nitsch, R. Hassler, *J.-K. Kim, and **K.-S. Paik

Department of Neurobiology, Max-Planck-Institut für Hirnforschung, D-6000 Frankfurt/ M. 71, German Federal Republic

The basomedial extension of the caudatum and putamen, the fundus striati, or nucleus accumbens septi (for terminology see refs. 1,5), receives as an integral part of the striatum (20) a projection from the neocortex (2,8), but it also receives fiber terminals from the hippocampal formation. Most of the latter fibers do not arise in the cornu ammonis proper, but in the subiculum (15,19). Therefore, the term *hippocampus* as defined by Stephan (17) and including the cornu ammonis, the area dentata, and the subiculum should be used.

Several lines of investigation suggest that L-glutamic acid (Glu), a neuroexcitatory amino acid, could be the transmitter of the corticostriatal fibers (4,10,11,16) and of the hippocampal efferents as well (14,18). In these reports, however, afferents to the fundus striati were not considered. In the present work, the possibility that the fundus striati receives Glu-ergic terminals from neo- and allocortical areas will be discussed. The degenerations that occur in the fundus striati after hippocampal deafferentation will be described.

EFFECT OF FRONTAL CORTEX ABLATION ON REGIONAL Glu CONTENT

Male Wistar rats were anesthetized with phenobarbital, and large unilateral or bilateral ablations of the frontal cortex (in rats the frontal cortex is primarily involved in motor functioning) were performed exactly as described by Kim et al. (10). After a survival period of 20 days, the animals were decapitated, regional brain areas dissected out, and the Glu content estimated using an enzymatic assay procedure (14).

In the caudate nucleus, the Glu content decreased significantly to 83% of its control value both after unilateral (compared to the contralateral side, as

---

* Present address: Department of Physiology, Catholic Medical College, Seoul, Korea.
** Present address: Department of Physiology, Brain Research Institute, Yonsei University, Seoul, Korea.

shown in Fig. 1a) and after bilateral removal of the frontal cortex (compared to the Glu content in naive control rats, as shown in Fig. 1b). This result further substantiates the role of Glu in the corticostriatal fiber system. In addition, the fact that the percentage of decrease is identical for both unilateral and bilateral lesions indicates that the fibers from the frontal motor cortex in rats project preferentially to the ipsilateral striatum.

In the fundus striati, the Glu concentration decreased significantly in animals with unilateral lesions (calculated by the *t*-test for paired values of the ipsilateral and contralateral samples; Fig. 1a). After bilateral ablation of the frontal cortex the fall in the Glu level was not significant when compared to that in naive controls (Fig. 1b). In the hippocampus, which does not receive projections from the motor and premotor cortex (see Stephan, ref. 17), no differences in Glu content were observed after either type of operation. Hence, the fact that the lesion had an effect, although a rather small one, may indicate that the fundus striati also receives some Glu-containing synapses from the frontal motor cortex, in the same way as the other parts of the striatum.

EFFECT OF EXTIRPATION OF THE HIPPOCAMPUS ON REGIONAL Glu CONTENT

In male Wistar rats, the hippocampus was completely extirpated on both sides by suction through a small hole in the parietal bone (for details on the surgical technique and the behavioral effects of these lesions see ref. 9). Rats with an identical lesion of the parietal cortex alone served as sham-operated controls.

Whereas Glu content remained unchanged in the caudate nucleus 20 days after hippocampus extirpation, it decreased to 86% in the fundus striati (Fig. 2). This decrease was significant when experimental animals were compared with the sham-operated animals and the naive controls. In the septum, a major target structure of hippocampal efferents, Glu content fell even further to 75% (Fig. 2). Considering that in the caudate, a brain region devoid of limbic inputs (12,17), the Glu level is not affected by the hippocampus extirpation, it is reasonable to suggest that the hippocampal projection to the fundus striati contains the excitatory transmitter candidate, Glu.

ELECTRON MICROSCOPIC EVALUATION OF DEGENERATIONS IN THE FUNDUS STRIATI AFTER EXTIRPATION OF THE HIPPOCAMPUS

Rabbits in which the hippocampus had been removed unilaterally (13) were perfused transaortically with an aldehyde fixative 2, 4, and 6 days postoperatively. Regional brain areas were dissected out, postfixed in OsO_4 and embedded in Epon 812. From each tissue block, 1-μm thick sections were stained with toluidine blue and checked under the light microscope to control the exact position for final trimming. Ultrathin sections were stained with uranyl acetate and lead nitrate and viewed in a Siemens Elmiskop 1A.

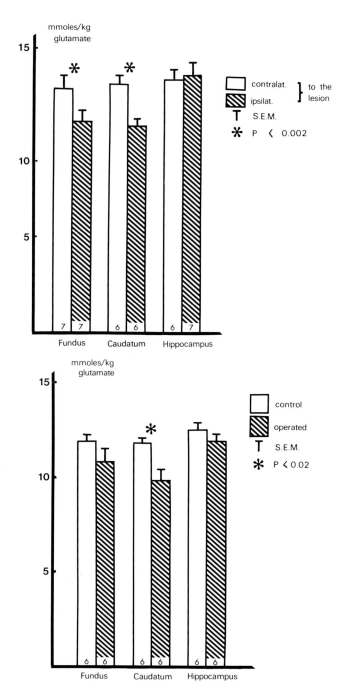

FIG. 1. Glutamate levels in the fundus striati, the head of the caudate nucleus, and the hippocampus 20 days after frontal cortex ablation. **a:** After unilateral operation: Comparison between glutamate levels ipsilateral and contralateral to the lesion. **b:** After bilateral operation: Comparison between glutamate levels in naive controls and lesioned animals.

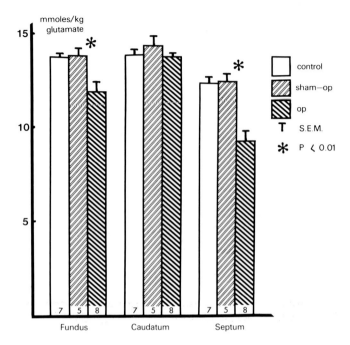

FIG. 2. Glutamate levels in the fundus striati, the head of the caudate nucleus, and the septum in naive controls and 20 days after sham operation or hippocampus extirpation, respectively.

After hippocampus extirpation through the parietal cortex, several types of synapses exhibit signs of degeneration, such as shrinkage of the bouton with darkening of its matrix, clumping of the vesicles, and engulfment and later digestion of the bouton remnants by reactive astroglia. In order to describe these morphological changes in more detail, nine types of striatal synapses have been distinguished according to the classification system for cat striatum proposed by Hassler and Chung (6; see also R. Hassler, *this volume*).

The synapses that are most commonly degenerated possess the features of type VII synapses (Fig. 3a). These are axosomatic or axodendritic synapses on the large efferent nerve cells of the striatum which contain densely packed, small, round vesicles. Type VII synapses have been reported to degenerate after ablation of somatosensory and premotor areas (2,7) as well as after parafascicular-center median lesions (3). Since we did not find such degenerating terminals in sham-operated animals with lesions of the parietal cortex, it may be assumed that some of them represent terminals of the hippocampal projection.

Degenerating type III synapses were observed, not as frequently, but consistently (Fig. 3b). They appear as slender boutons with densely packed, round vesicles which make narrow asymmetric contacts with spines of the small spiny interneurons of the striatum. As is the case with the type VII boutons, the type III boutons degenerate after cortical lesions (7), but in the fundus striati, some of them may be terminals of the hippocampal efferents.

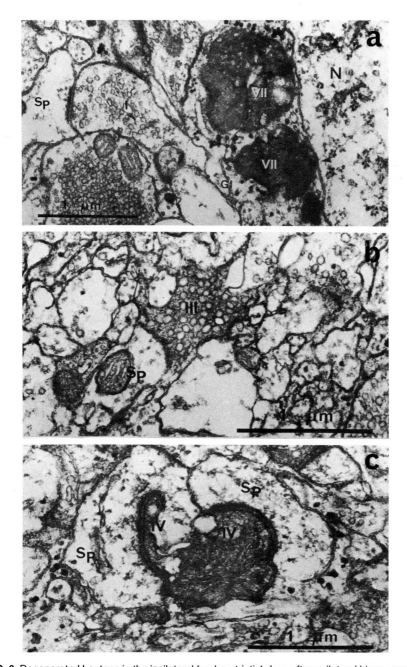

FIG. 3. Degenerated boutons in the ipsilateral fundus striati 4 days after unilateral hippocampus extirpation. **a:** Directly adjacent to the soma of a large neuron (N), degenerated masses (VII) in which a vesicular structure can still be recognized are engulfed by reactive astroglial processes (Gl). A type I bouton (I) contacting a spine (Sp) is not affected by the lesion. **b:** A shrunken type III bouton (III) surrounded by heavily altered neuropil has an asymmetric contact with a spine (Sp). Many vesicles are well preserved in the dark matrix. **c:** A degenerated bouton (IV) exhibiting a heavily electron-dense matrix contacts two neighboring spines (Sp). The strongly asymmetric, curved, and divided synaptic junction permits classification of this bouton as type IV.

The third type of bouton undergoing degeneration after hippocampus extirpation exhibited the characteristics of a type IV synapse (Fig. 3c), i.e., a divided, mostly curved, strongly asymmetric contact with one or several neighboring spines. In the fundus striati, these boutons are considered to derive exclusively from the thalamic parafascicular nucleus (3). In some of our preparations, careful checking of serial frontal sections revealed that superficial areas extending from the dorsomedial to dorsolateral part of the thalamus had either been injured or else showed some glial reaction. Thus, further and more restricted experiments with lesions are required to determine whether some of the type IV boutons also originate from the allocortex.

All other types of synapses present in the fundus striati do not degenerate after hippocampus extirpation; namely, the type I synapses, the terminals of the nigral projection, are well preserved (Fig. 3a).

CONCLUSIONS

The present investigation shows that after hippocampus extirpation, numerous boutons degenerate in the basomedial part of the caudate and putamen corresponding to the fundus striati. Previously, it had been demonstrated that terminal degeneration occurs there after somatomotor cortex ablation (2). The Glu level in the fundus striati decreased after lesion of either the hippocampal or the motor input, whereas in the caudate it decreased only after cortical ablation. Thus, the caudate and putamen receive only neocortical afferents, which are probably Glu-ergic in nature. In contrast, the fundus striati possesses Glu-ergic input from both the motor cortex and the hippocampus, indicating its role as a limbic part of the striatum. Whether and to what extent the limbic striatum is the brain site responsible for some of the psychiatric disorders occurring in Parkinson's disease must await further investigation.

REFERENCES

1. Brockhaus, H. (1942): Zur feineren Antomie des Septum und des Striatum. *J. Psychol. Neurol. (Leipzig.),* 51:1–56.
2. Chung, J. W., and Hassler, R. (1976): Experimental degeneration of different types of synapses in the fundus striati of the cat. In: *Aktuelle Probleme der Neuropathologie, Vol. 3,* edited by K. Jellinger, pp. 48–54. Facultas Verlag, Wien.
3. Chung, J. W., Hassler, R., and Wagner, A. (1976): Degenerated boutons in the fundus striati (nucleus accumbens septi) after lesions of the parafascicular nucleus in the cat. *Cell Tissue Res.,* 172:1–14.
4. Divac, I., Fonnum, F., and Storm-Mathisen, J. (1977): High affinity uptake of glutamate in terminals of corticostriatal axons. *Nature (Lond.),* 266:377–378.
5. Hassler, R. (1978): Striatal control of locomotion, intentional actions and integrating and perceptive activity. *J. Neurol. Sci.,* 36:187–224.
6. Hassler, R., and Chung, J. W. (1976): The discrimination of nine different types of synaptic boutons in the fundus striati (nucleus accumbens septi). *Cell Tissue Res.,* 168:489–505.
7. Hassler, R., Chung, J. W., Rinne, U., and Wagner, A. (1978): Selective degeneration of two out of nine types of synapses in cat caudate nucleus after cortical lesions. *Exp. Brain Res.,* 31:67–80.

8. Kemp, J. M., and Powell, T. S. P. (1970): The cortico-striate projection in the monkey. *Brain,* 93:525–546.
9. Kim, C., Kim, C. C., Kim, J. K., Kim, M. S., Chang, H. K., Kim, J. Y., and Lee, I. G. (1971): Fear response and aggressive behavior of hippocampectomized house rats. *Brain Res.,* 9:237–251.
10. Kim, J. S., Hassler, R., Haug, P., and Paik, K.-S. (1977): Effect of frontal cortex ablation on striatal glutamic acid level in rat. *Brain Res.,* 132:370–374.
11. McGeer, P. L., McGeer, E. G., Scherer, U., and Singh, K. (1977): A glutamatergic corticostriatal path? *Brain Res.,* 128:369–373.
12. Nauta, W. J. H., and Domesick, V. B. (1977): Cross roads of limbic and striatal circuitry: Hypothalamo-nigral connections. In: *Limbic Mechanisms,* edited by K. E. Livingston and O. Hornykiewicz, pp. 75–93. Plenum Press, New York.
13. Nitsch, C., Kim, J.-K., and Shimada, C. (1979): The commissural fibers in rabbit hippocampus: Synapses and their transmitter. *Prog. Brain Res., (in press).*
14. Nitsch, C., Kim, J.-K., Shimada, C., and Okada, Y. (1979): Effect of hippocampus extirpation on glutamate levels in target structures of hippocampal efferents. *Neurosci. Lett.,* 11:295–299.
15. Rosene, D. L., and Van Hoesen, G. W. (1977): Hippocampal efferents reach widespread areas of cerebral cortex and amygdala in the rhesus monkey. *Science,* 198:315–317.
16. Spencer, H. J. (1976): Antagonism of cortical excitation of striatal neurons by glutamic acid diethylester: Evidence for glutamic acid as an excitatory transmitter in the rat striatum. *Brain Res.,* 102:91–101.
17. Stephan, H. (1975): *Handbuch der mikroskopischen Anatomie des Menschen, Vol. 4, Nervensystem, Part 9, Allocortex,* pp. 494–602. Springer-Verlag, Berlin.
18. Storm-Mathisen, J., and Opsahl, M. W. (1978): Aspartate and/or glutamate may be transmitters in hippocampal efferents to septum and hypothalamus. *Neurosci. Lett.,* 9:65–70.
19. Swanson, L. W., and Cowan, W. M. (1975): Hippocampo-hypothalamic connections: Origin in subicular cortex, not Ammon's horn. *Science,* 189:303–304.
20. Swanson, L. W., and Cowan, W. M. (1975): A note on the connections and development of the nucleus accumbens. *Brain Res.,* 92:324–330.

Advances in Neurology, Vol. 24, edited by
L. J. Poirier, T. L. Sourkes, and P. J. Bédard.
Raven Press, New York © 1979.

Striatal Projection Neurons: Morphological and Electrophysiological Studies

S. T. Kitai, R. J. Preston, G. A. Bishop, and J. D. Kocsis

Department of Anatomy, Michigan State University, East Lansing, Michigan 48824

Although anatomical studies (20–22,24) indicate that fibers from the striatum project to the substantia nigra, the cells of origin of these fibers have not yet been clearly established. Cytoarchitectonic studies reveal the presence of large and small cells in the caudate nucleus (2,17) which through Golgi and electron microscopic analysis can be further divided into at least six types of neurons (1,5–7,11,18). The most numerous type is a medium-sized spiny neuron. Some investigators have considered this medium spiny neuron to be an intrinsic element (6,11). Recently, however, retrograde transport of horseradish peroxidase (HRP) from the substantia nigra has been observed to occur in many medium-sized caudate neurons (4,10,23). In some caudate areas, as many as 30 to 50% of the cells were found to take up HRP (4). These percentages conflict with the suggestion from Golgi studies that minority elements, the giant and medium aspiny neurons that together appear to comprise <5% of caudate neurons (11), form the caudate nucleus output (7). Still, neither Bunney and Aghajanian (4) nor Grofová (10) could demonstrate conclusively that the striatal projection originated from medium spiny neurons. Recent Golgi studies (5,18; J. A. Rafols, C. A. Fox, *personal communication*) have shown, however, that this neuron's axon does extend beyond the neuron's dendritic arborization, and in addition, they have established that the axon is myelinated (J. A. Rafols, C. A. Fox, *personal communication*). They still did not determine if the axon projected out of the striatum.

The purpose of the present study was (a) to activate striatal projection neurons antidromically by stimulation of the substantia nigra, (b) to characterize the projection neurons' extrinsic responses, (c) to assess their membrane characteristics, and (d) to describe their morphological properties.

MATERIALS AND METHODS

Rats and cats were used. Cats were anesthetized with either sodium pentobarbital (35 mg/kg) or a combination of sodium thiamylal (20 mg/kg) and α-chloralose (60 mg/kg). Male Long-Evans hooded rats were anesthetized with urethane (1.2 g/kg). The surgical preparations and the recording and electrical stimulation procedures have been described elsewhere for the cat (13,15,16,19) and for the rat (3). The substantia nigra (SN), the anterior sigmoid gyrus (Cx), and the centromedian parafascicular complex (CMP) of the intralaminar thalamus were stimulated with current pulses of 0.05 to 0.1 msec duration. Intracellular recording electrodes were filled with 2 M K-citrate or 2 M KCl and had direct current (DC) resistance of 30 to 60 MΩ. Some electrodes were filled with an HRP solution, which was introduced into the impaled neuron by electrophoresis in order to permit later morphological identification and analysis. The procedure for HRP injection and histological processing has been described elsewhere (12).

RESULTS

Antidromic Activation of the Striatal Neurons

Stimulation of the SN often induced antidromic spike potentials in cat caudate (Cd) nucleus neurons. The antidromic nature of these spikes was established by their all-or-none appearance and constant latency at threshold (Fig. 1A) and by collision of the SN-induced antidromic spike with a preceding spontane-

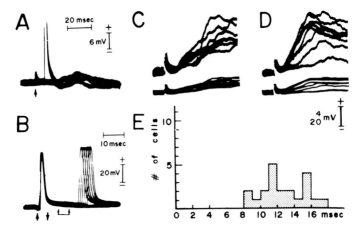

FIG. 1. Antidromic and orthodromic responses of Cd neurons. **A:** All-or-none constant latency action potential elicited by SN stimulation. **B:** Superimposed records of responses to paired stimuli in a test for collision between an intracellularly evoked spike (conditioning) and an SN-evoked spike (test). Upward and downward arrows indicate onset and offset of depolarizing pulse. First small upward *arrow* indicates the point at which SN stimulation failed to induce an action potential, and the second upward small *arrow* indicates SN stimulation corresponding to longest latency potential. **C:** Excitatory postsynaptic potentials evoked by SN stimulation. Variation of stimulus intensity elicits graded amplitude, but constant latency responses. Bottom traces show low-gain DC records. **D:** Centromedian-parafascicular-complex-induced EPSPs recorded from the same neuron as in **C.** Bottom traces are low-gain DC. Ten milliseconds per calibration in **B** applies also to **C** and **D.** High gain 4 mV and low gain 20 mV in **D** also applies to **C. E:** Latency histogram for antidromic action potentials evoked by SN stimulation.

ous or intracellularly induced spike (Fig. 1B). The latency of antidromic spikes ranged from 8 to 20 msec (Fig. 1E). These latencies, which are similar to those reported in previous studies (9,14), suggest conduction velocities for Cd projection neurons falling mainly in the range of 1 to 2 m/sec, and are consistent with estimates (1,8) of small Cd efferent fiber diameter (mean 0.2–0.7 μm). It should be noted that some impaled Cd neurons could not be antidromically activated by SN stimulation and yet had orthodromic response properties and morphological properties identical to those of antidromically activated neurons (detailed below). This probably results from a low security for antidromic invasion of the projection neuron. The cause of this blockage, whether extrinsic (e.g., inhibition at axonal or initial segment sites), intrinsic (e.g., low safety factor for antidromic propagation at axon collateral branch points), or both, is not yet known.

Synaptic Responses

In the cat, the antidromically activated Cd neurons also responded orthodromically to SN, Cx, and CMP stimulation. In all cases, the initial orthodromic response was an excitatory postsynaptic potential (EPSP) with latencies of 3 to 20, 3 to 12, and 4 to 12 msec, respectively. The monosynaptic nature of these EPSPs was shown by absence of a latency change (i.e., no temporal facilitation), despite an increase in either intensity or frequency of stimulation (Fig. 1C,D). Often, EPSPs were followed by a hyperpolarizing potential having a duration of 100 msec or more. Similarly, SN stimulation in the rat evoked monosynaptic EPSPs in striatal projection neurons with latencies of 1.3 to 5.7 msec. These EPSPs were followed by hyperpolarization lasting approximately 100 msec and by rebound depolarization.

Membrane Electrical Constants

Cat caudate neurons were found to have an input resistance of 12 to 24 MΩ. This value was obtained from the relation between the amplitude of intracellularly injected current and the plateau level of the resultant membrane voltage response. In addition, the time course of these membrane responses to weak hyper- and depolarizing injection currents yielded membrane time-constant estimates with a mean value of 11.3 msec. Figure 2 shows these membrane responses for a neuron that responded antidromically (as well as orthodromically) to SN stimuli. The 20-MΩ input resistance and 12.5-msec time-constant values for this neuron fall within the range of values obtained from neurons that could not be antidromically activated. This would be expected since, as noted earlier, caudate neurons are particularly susceptible to antidromic blockade, and in addition, all membrane measurements were probably taken from the same morphological type of neuron (i.e., in our laboratory, for a sample of >70 intracellularly recorded and identified cells, only the medium spiny neuron was impaled).

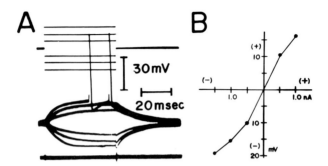

FIG. 2. Input resistance (Ro) determination for a cat Cd neuron. **A:** Membrane responses to hyper- and depolarizing currents of 0.5, 1.0, and 1.5 nA. Bottom trace of the record is extracellular control. **B:** The current voltage relation (Ro = 20 MΩ for the linear portion of the curve).

From the obtained input resistance together with an estimate of the medium spiny neuron membrane area, membrane resistance was calculated to be nearly 8,000 $\Omega \cdot cm^2$, a value higher than those reported for other CNS neurons. This high resistance would facilitate somatopetal spread of synaptic currents from distal dendritic sites. Such currents would originate at postsynaptic sites on spines that have been found (5,6,11) to occur with an extremely high and relatively uniform density along the entire length of this neuron's dendrites.

Morphological Characteristics of Striatal Projection Neurons

Intracellular injections of HRP were made into both antidromically and nonantidromically activated cat Cd neurons. All of the recovered neurons were found to have similar somatodendritic morphology. Both the somata, which ranged from 13 to 22 μm in size, and the proximal dendrites were found to be spine free. The secondary and tertiary dendrites, however, were densely covered with both sessile and pedunculated spines. Such somatodendritic features, which distinguish this neuron from all other Cd elements, identify these recovered neurons with the medium spiny neurons of Kemp and Powell (11) and Fox et al. (6) or the spiny I neurons of DiFiglia et al. (5). The axon arose from the soma and gave rise to several fine collaterals, each of which bifurcated repeatedly to form a fine plexus within the dendritic domain of the parent cell. The parent axon followed a tortuous course and could be followed within the caudate nucleus to a point near the internal capsule. Figure 3A is a drawing reconstructing a cat Cd projection neuron that responded antidromically and synaptically to SN stimulation.

In the rat, the parent axon of the striatal projection neuron was seen to leave the striatum and enter the globus pallidus. Some axons were traced further to a point near the entopeduncular nucleus, but the precise area of termination of these fibers has not yet been established. Figure 3B is a reconstruction of a

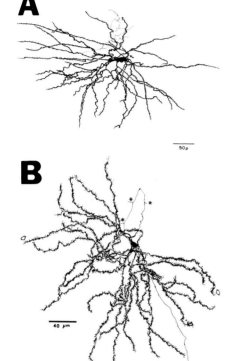

50µ

40 µm

FIG. 3. Striatal projection neurons reconstructed with the aid of a drawing tube. **A:** Caudate projection neuron in the cat. *Arrow* indicates the axon. **B:** Striatal projection neuron in the rat. *Arrows* indicate the fine terminal portion of the dendrites. *Asterisks* indicate the points of axon collateral origin.

striatal projection neuron whose axon was traced into the globus pallidus. These striatal projection neurons had spherical or elliptical somata ranging in size from 14 to 24 µm. Four to nine primary dendrites arose from the soma, divided into secondary and tertiary branches, and terminated after extending for distances of 200 to 250 µm. As in the cat, the soma and primary dendrites of the rat projection neuron were spine free, while the secondary and tertiary dendrites were heavily covered with pedunculated and sessile spines. The axon arose either directly from the soma or from a primary dendrite and gave rise to several collaterals which branched extensively to form a fine axonal plexus within and occasionally beyond the dendritic domain of the parent cell. This anatomical identification of the projection neuron in the rat striatum demonstrates conclusively that the medium spiny neuron, which comprises the majority of the striatal elements, is one type of projection neuron.

In summary, the striatal projection neuron receives convergent monosynaptic excitatory inputs from the cerebral cortex, the intralaminar thalamus, and the substantia nigra. Combined electrophysiological and anatomical studies clearly demonstrate that the medium spiny neuron is a striatal projection neuron in both the cat and the rat.

ACKNOWLEDGMENTS

This study was supported by USPHS grants NS-00405 and NS-14866. The authors express their gratitude to Dr. A. C. Bonduki and H. Chang for their helpful comments, criticisms, and technical assistance throughout the study.

REFERENCES

1. Adinolfi, A. M., and Pappas, G. D. (1968): The fine structure of the caudate nucleus of the cat. *J. Comp. Neurol.*, 113:167–184.
2. Bielschowsky, M. (1919): Einige Bemerkungen zur normalen und pathologischen Histologie des Schweif- und Linsenkerns. *J. Psychol. Neurol.*, 25:1–11.
3. Bishop, G. A., Preston, R. J., and Kitai, S. T. (1979): Medium spiny neuron projection from the rat striatum: An intracellular horseradish peroxidase study. *Brain Res. (in press).*
4. Bunney, B. S., and Aghajanian, G. K. (1976): The precise localization of nigral afferents in the rat as determined by a retrograde tracing technique. *Brain Res.*, 117:423–435.
5. DiFiglia, M., Pasik, P., and Pasik, T. (1976): A Golgi study of neuronal types in the neostriatum of monkeys. *Brain Res.*, 114:245–256.
6. Fox, C. A., Andrade, A. N., Hillman, D. E., and Schwyn, R. C. (1971–1972): The spiny neurons in the primate striatum. A Golgi and electron microscopic study. *J. Hirnforsch.*, 13:181–201.
7. Fox, C. A., Andrade, A. N., Schwyn, R. C., and Rafols, J. A. (1971–1972): The aspiny neurons and the glia in the primate striatum: A Golgi and electron microscopic study. *J. Hirnforsch.*, 13:341–362.
8. Fox, C. A., Rafols, J. A., and Cowan, W. M. (1975): Computer measurements of axis cylinder diameters of radialfibers and "Comb" bundle fibers. *J. Comp. Neurol.*, 159:201–224.
9. Fuller, D. R., Hull, C. D., and Buchwald, N. A. (1975): Intracellular responses of caudate output neurons to orthodromic stimulation. *Brain Res.*, 96:337–341.
10. Grofová, I. (1975): The identification of striatal and pallidal neurons projecting to substantia nigra. An experimental study by means of retrograde axonal transport of horseradish peroxidase. *Brain Res.*, 91:286–291.
11. Kemp, J. M., and Powell, T. P. S. (1971): The structure of the caudate nucleus of the cat. Light and electron microscopy. *Philos. Trans. R. Soc. Lond. [Biol. Sci.]*, 262:383–401.
12. Kitai, S. T., Kocsis, J. D., Preston, R. J., and Sugimori, M. (1976): Monosynaptic inputs to caudate neurons identified by intracellular injection of horseradish peroxidase. *Brain Res.*, 109:601–606.
13. Kitai, S. T., Sugimori, M., and Kocsis, J. D. (1976): Excitatory nature of dopamine in the nigro-caudate pathway. *Exp. Brain Res.*, 21:351–362.
14. Kitai, S. T., Wagner, A., Precht, W., and Ohno, T. (1975): Nigro-caudate and caudato-nigral relationship: An electrophysiological study. *Brain Res.*, 85:44–48.
15. Kocsis, J. D., and Kitai, S. T. (1977): Dual excitatory inputs to caudate spiny neurons from substantia nigra stimulation. *Brain Res.*, 138:271–283.
16. Kocsis, J. D., Sugimori, M., and Kitai, S. T. (1977): Convergence of excitatory synaptic inputs to caudate spiny neurons. *Brain Res.*, 124:403–413.
17. Namba, M. (1957): Cytoarchitecktonische Untersuchungen am Striatum. *J. Hirnforsch.*, 3:24–48.
18. Pasik, P., Pasik, T., and DiFiglia, M. (1976): Quantitative aspects of neuronal organization in the neostriatum of the macaque monkey. In: *Research Publications: Association for Research in Nervous and Mental Disease, Vol. 55, The Basal Ganglia,* pp. 57–90. Raven Press, New York.
19. Sugimori, M., Preston, R. J., and Kitai, S. T. (1978): Response properties and electrical constants of caudate nucleus neurons in the cat. *J. Neurophysiol.*, 41:1662–1675.
20. Szabo, J. (1962): Topical distribution of striatal efferents in the monkey. *Exp. Neurol.*, 5:21–36.
21. Szabo, J. (1967): The efferent projections of the putamen in the monkey. *Exp. Neurol.*, 19:463–476.

22. Szabo, J. (1970): Projections from the body of the caudate nucleus in the rhesus monkey. *Exp. Neurol.,* 27:1–15.
23. Szabo, J. (1979): Striato-nigral and nigral-striatal connection. An anatomical study. *Appl. Neurophysiol., (in press).*
24. Voneida, T. J. (1960): An experimental study of the course and destination of fibers arising in the head of caudate nucleus in the cat and monkey. *J. Comp. Neurol.,* 115:75–87.

Advances in Neurology, Vol. 24, edited by
L. J. Poirier, T. L. Sourkes, and P. J. Bédard.
Raven Press, New York © 1979.

A Study of the Afferent Connections to the Subthalamic Nucleus in the Monkey and the Cat Using the HRP Technique

*E. Rinvik, *I. Grofová, **C. Hammond, **J. Féger, and **J. M. Deniau

*Anatomical Institute, University of Oslo, Oslo 1, Norway; and **Laboratoire de Physiologie des Centres Nerveux, 75230 Paris, France

In spite of the well-known clinicopathologic correlation of hemiballismus with lesions of the subthalamic nucleus (STH), remarkably little is known about the details of STH fiber connections. In fact, until very recently the only well-established connection of STH seemed to consist of a heavy input from the external segment of the globus pallidus (GPe) and projections from the STH back to the internal pallidal segment (GPi) (5,6).

In an electrophysiological study, Ohye et al. (31) concluded that the monkey's striatum exerts a direct, monosynaptic effect on neurons of the STH. Since this observation is at variance with the few known anatomical data, it was deemed necessary to reexamine the sources of afferents to the monkey's STH by means of the technique of retrograde transport of horseradish peroxidase (HRP). To our knowledge, these findings have not been previously reported.

MATERIALS AND METHODS

Following stimulation of the striatum, physiological recordings were made in the STH of eight adult monkeys *(Macaca cynomolgus)*. These experiments were followed by unilateral or bilateral pressure injections in the STH of 0.1 to 0.2 μl of a 25% solution of HRP (Serva). The animals were kept alive for 2 to 4 days. The first five animals were perfused with a mixture of 0.4% formaldehyde and 1.25% glutaraldehyde in a 0.1 M phosphate buffer. The brains were dissected out and postfixed overnight before being transferred to a buffered 30% sucrose solution. The whole brain was cut on the freezing microtome into 50-μm thick coronal sections. Every fifth section was treated with 3,3-diaminobenzidine (DAB) according to the method of Graham and Karnovsky (15). The last four animals were perfused with a mixture of 1% paraformaldehyde and 1.25% glutaraldehyde. Serial sections from the brains of these animals were treated with benzidine dihydrochloride (BDHC) according to the method of Mesulam (25). Alternating sections were also treated with DAB. The sections that were treated with DAB were counterstained with cresyl violet, whereas the sections treated with BDHC were counterstained with neutral red.

The exact location and number of labeled cells were determined using a pantograph, and the borders of cell groups were superimposed on the plots by means of a camera lucida. The location of the cannula tip and the extent of the reaction product at the injection site were carefully mapped in each case.

For the purpose of the present investigation, the brains of two monkeys could not be used. The HRP was injected bilaterally into the STH in one animal (M 12015, Fig. 1).

In addition to injecting the monkeys with HRP, unilateral iontophoretic ejections of HRP were made in five cats. A micropipette with a tip between 20 and 50 μm in diameter was filled with a 5% solution of HRP in 0.1 M KCl, and a constant current of 5 μA was passed through the brain for 20 min. Following a survival time of 2–4 days, the animals were perfused with saline followed by a mixture of 1% paraformaldehyde and 1.25% glutaraldehyde in a 0.1 M phosphate buffer. Finally, the animals were perfused with a 10% solution of sucrose in a phosphate buffer. The brains were dissected out and immediately cut on the freezing microtome into 50-μm thick coronal sections, and every fifth section was treated according to the method of Mesulam (25).

In one cat, a large electrolytic lesion was made through the pars compacta and the pars reticulata of the substantia nigra (SN). A lateral stereotaxic approach was used in order to minimize the damage to structures other than the SN. Following a survival time of 4 days, the animal was perfused and the brain processed for the electron-microscopic examination of the STH, as previously described (34).

RESULTS

The Use of the Brown Versus the Blue Reaction Procedures for the Demonstration of HRP

While treating alternating sections with DAB and with BDHC, it has become apparent that, in our hands, the latter procedure is more sensitive than the former. This is obvious at the injection site, where the spreading of the injected HRP appears much larger in the BDHC-treated section than in the neighboring DAB-treated section. Furthermore, the number of labeled cells and the intensity of the labeling is greater in the section treated with BDHC than in the section treated with DAB. Moreover, the use of BDHC enables us to distinguish between the exogenously administered HRP, visualized as dark-bluish granules, and the endogenously occurring oxidizing substances in the soma of cells in some particular brainstem nuclei of the monkey, such as the locus ceruleus and the SN (25,26). These brown-yellowish granules can only with very great difficulty be distinguished from exogenously administered HRP in the DAB-treated material.

For these reasons, the brains of the last series of operated monkeys and of all cats were treated with BDHC. This should be kept in mind when comparing the injection sites in various animals (Figs. 1,2) and when judging the distribution of labeled cells in various nuclei indicated in Table 1.

Distribution of Labeled Cells Following HRP Injections in the Monkey's STH

In four monkeys (M 12015 L and R, M 12017, M 12018), the injection cannula was located well within the STH, and the injected HRP was mainly confined to the nucleus. In two other monkeys (M 12327, M 12329), only the tip of the cannula had penetrated the dorsal border of STH, but the injected HRP was highly concentrated within a large part of the nucleus. There was always some spreading of HRP to neighboring structures, and this was more pronounced for the BDHC- than for the DAB-treated material (Figs. 1,2). In these six animals, the external segment of the GPe is repeatedly the central nervous structure showing the largest number of labeled cells (Fig. 3). We have, moreover, been able to confirm the topographical organization of the pallidosub-thalamic projection described earlier in the monkey (7). In addition to the GPe, several other nuclei constantly show a substantial number of labeled cells in these cases, namely the SN, the locus ceruleus including the peribrachial nuclei (LC) (Fig. 4), the dorsal nucleus of the raphe (DR) (Fig. 5a,b), the nucleus pedunculopontinus (PP) (Fig. 5a), the hypothalamus, and the central nucleus of the amygdala. In these nuclei, however, the number of labeled cells is lower than in the GPe (see Table 1). In the SN, the largest number of labeled cells is seen in the pars compacta (SNC), but a considerable number of labeled cells are also seen in the pars reticulata (SNR), as well as in the paranigral cell groups (PN), including the ventral tegmental area of Tsai.

A variable and small number of labeled cells is also seen in the cerebral cortex, especially the frontal cortex, including the motor cortex and the opercular cortex of the insula. A few labeled cells are occasionally seen in the GPi (see Table 1 and Fig. 2). Similarly, a few labeled cells are seen in the bed nucleus of the stria terminalis (BSt) in most cases, but their number is quite negligible. Except for a few labeled cells that lie at the border between the BSt and the ventralmost part of the caudate nucleus, we have never seen in this material labeled cells in the striatum. In cases with a unilateral injection of HRP into the STH, we have never seen labeled cells in the contralateral STH.

Injections of HRP Dorsolateral to the Caudal STH (M 12325) and Dorsal to the Rostral STH (M 12330)

In these two cases, the tip of the cannula was outside of the STH, but some HRP diffused within the dorsolateral part of the nucleus. In both cases, however, there is not a single labeled cell in the GPe. In animal M 12330 in which the HRP was injected within the pallido- and cerebellothalamic projections, a large

M-12015

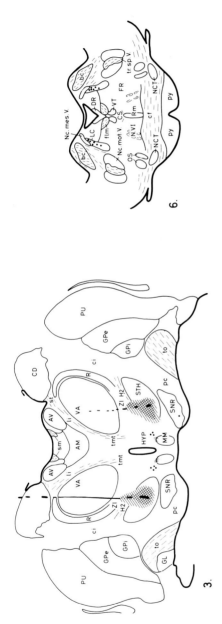

FIG. 1. Distribution of labeled cells in monkey M 12015, which was treated with DAB (see text). Each *dot* represents one labeled cell in the particular section shown.

Abbreviations Used in All Figures

AHL	area hypothalamica lateralis	Nc.mes.V	nucleus mesencephalicus nervi trigemini
AM	nucleus anterior medialis thalami	Nc.mot.V	nucleus motorius nervi trigemini
AMYG	amygdala	NCT	nucleus corporis trapezoidei
AV	nucleus anterior ventralis thalami	N.II	nucleus lemnisci lateralis
bc	brachium conjunctivum	NR	nucleus ruber
BST	bed nucleus of stria terminalis	NRT	nucleus reticularis tegmenti
Ca	commissura anterior	OS	oliva superior
CD	nucleus caudatus	PB	nucleus parabrachialis
ch	chiasma opticum	pc	pedunculus cerebri
ci	capsula interna	PN	paranigral cell groups
CL	nucleus centralis lateralis	PO	nucleus posterior thalami
CM	centrum medianum	PP	nucleus pedunculopontinus
CS	nucleus centralis superior	PU	putamen
ct	corpus trapezoideum	Pulv.	pulvinar
CU	nucleus cuneiformis	PV	nucleus paraventricularis hypothalami
DR	nucleus dorsalis raphe	py	pyramis
EN	nucleus entopeduncularis	R	nucleus reticularis thalami
f	fornix	Rm	nucleus raphe magnus
FF	Forel's field	RR	nucleus retrorubralis
flm	fasciculus longitudinalis medialis	Sep	septum
fr	fasciculus retroflexus	SGC	substantia grisea centralis
FR	formatio reticularis	SI	substantia innominata
GL	corpus geniculatum laterale	sm	stria medullaris
GM	corpus geniculatum mediale	SNC	substantia nigra compacta
GP	globus pallidus	SNR	substantia nigra reticulata
GPe	globus pallidus externus	st	stria terminalis
GPi	globus pallidus internus	STH	nucleus subthalamicus
HYP	hypothalamus	tmt	tractus mammilothalamicus
IP	nucleus interpeduncularis	to	tractus opticus
LD	nucleus lateralis dorsalis thalami	tr.sp.V	tractus spinalis nervi trigemini
Li	lamina medullaris interna	VA	nucleus ventralis anterior thalami
lm	lemniscus medialis	VL	nucleus ventralis lateralis thalami
LP	nucleus lateralis posterior thalami	VPL	nucleus ventralis posterior lateralis
MD	nucleus medialis dorsalis thalami	VPM	nucleus ventralis posterior medialis
MM	nucleus mammilaris medialis	VT	nucleus ventralis tegmenti Gudden
N.III	nervus oculomotorius	VTA	area ventralis tegmenti
N.VI	nervus abducens	ZI	zona incerta
Nc.III	nucleus oculomotorius		

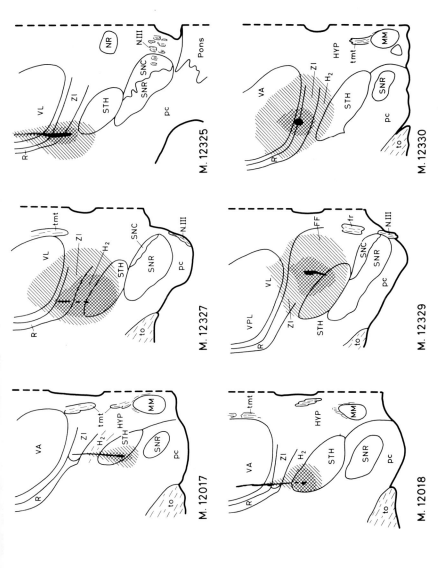

FIG. 2. Drawings showing the site and maximal spreading of injected HRP in six monkeys. Animals M 12017 and M 12018 were treated with DAB, the others with BDHC (see text). *Solid black* indicates the cannula track and *double hatchings* the highest concentration of HRP in the section.

TABLE 1. *Distribution of labeled cells in monkeys with HRP injections*

Case & procedure	GPe	SNC/SNR	PN	DR	LC + PB	HYP	AMYG	PP	GPi	Cerebellar nuclei
HRP injection in the STH										
M 12015 L DAB	++++	++/+	+	+		+	+	+	0	
M 12015 R DAB	++++	++/+	+	++		+	+	+	±	
M 12017 DAB	++++	++/+	+	+		+	+	++	+	
M 12018 DAB	++++	++/+	+	+		++	++	++	±	
M 12327 BDHC	++++	++/+	++	++	+++	++	++	++	0	+
M 12329 BDHC	++	++/+	+	++	++	+		+	+	+++
HRP injection outside the STH										
M 12330 BDHC	0	0/±	0	0	+	+	0	+	++	+++
M 12325 BDHC	0	±/0	±	0	±	±	0	0	0	

Distribution of labeled cells in various nuclei in monkeys with HRP injections in the STH and outside of the STH. In each animal, all labeled cells were counted on every fifth section throughout the entire nucleus in question. ++++, more than 400 labeled cells; +++, 200–400 labeled cells; ++, 50–200 labeled cells; +, 10–50 labeled cells; ±, <10 labeled cells.

AMYG, amygdala; BDHC, benzidine dihydrochloride; DAB, 3,3-diaminobenzidine; DR, nucleus dorsalis raphe; GPe, globus pallidus externus; GPi, globus pallidus internus; HRP, horseradish peroxidase; HYP, hypothalamus; LC, locus ceruleus; PB, nucleus parabrachialis; PN, paranigral cell groups; PP, nucleus pedunculopontinus; SNC, substantia nigra compacta; SNR, substantia nigra reticulata; STH, nucleus subthalamicus.

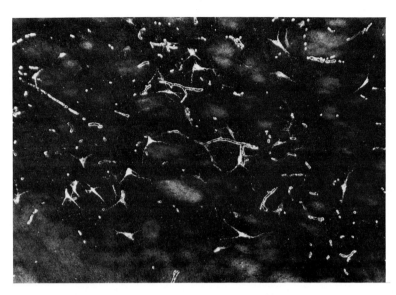

FIG. 3. Dark-field photomicrograph showing labeled cells in GPe in case 12017. DAB-treated section. ×65.

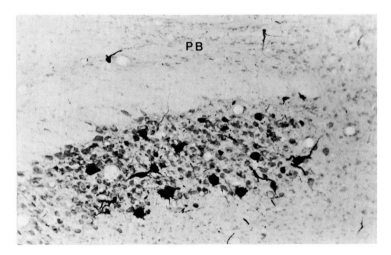

FIG. 4. Labeled cells in the LC and the PB of monkey M 12327. ×75.

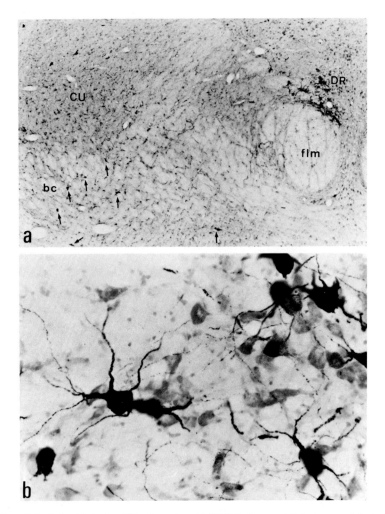

FIG. 5. a: Labeled cells in the DR of monkey M 12327. *Arrows* point at some labeled cells in the PP. ×27. **b:** Details from the DR shown in **a.** ×240.

number of cells of the GPi and the cerebellar nuclei are labeled. In case M 12325, the HRP was injected caudal to the pallidothalamic pathway, and no cells are labeled in the GPi of this animal.

In these two animals no cells are labeled in the DR or in the amygdala, but some cells are labeled in the LC, their number being quite a bit lower than that in the LCs of animals in which the tip of the injecting cannula had encroached on the borders of the STH [compare, for example, case M 12327 (Fig. 2 and Table 1)].

Very few labeled cells are seen in the SNC and the SNR and in the paranigral cell groups. The number of labeled nigral cells is much lower than in the SN of monkeys in which the tip of the injecting cannula was inside the edge of the STH. In the hypothalamus, the number of labeled cells is negligible.

Iontophoretic Ejection of HRP in Cats

Horseradish peroxidase was successfully ejected within various parts of the STH in five cats. The distribution of labeled cells in one of these animals is shown in Fig. 6. Since the amount of ejected HRP was small, the number of labeled cells is of course lower than in monkeys injected with HRP. The distribution of labeled cells, however, closely corresponds with that seen in monkeys in which the tip of the injecting cannula had been placed within the borders of the STH. The only striking difference in our investigation appears to be a higher number of labeled cells in the BSt in cats. In addition, we have never seen labeled cells in the cat's motor cortex following HRP ejections in the STH. Labeled cells, however, are repeatedly seen in the proreus gyrus, i.e., the frontal granular cortex.

In two cats, the HRP was ejected in the ventralmost part of STH lying on the cerebral peduncle. In these cases, labeled cells are seen only in the ventral part of the striatum. No labeled cells are seen in the entopeduncular nucleus (the feline homolog of the GPi).

Electron-microscopic Observations

In one cat with a large electrolytic lesion of the SNC and the SNR, boutons in varying stages of a dark type of degeneration are seen in the ipsilateral STH (Fig. 9). No such boutons are seen in the contralateral STH.

DISCUSSION

In their physiological study in the monkey, Ohye et al. (31) suggested that the striatum exerts a direct monosynaptic effect on the STH. The present investigation, however, does not appear to support this suggestion since no labeled cells were found in the striatum of monkeys following the injection of HRP within the STH, with the exception of a few labeled cells at the border between the BSt and the ventralmost part of the caudate nucleus. In two cats, however, with HRP ejected along the ventral border of the STH, labeled cells were seen in the ventral striatum. We believe that these cells belong to striatonigral fibers, since fibers arising in the ventral striatum course partly through the ventral STH on their way to the SN. We cannot, of course, exclude the possibility that these fibers may give off collaterals to the STH on their way to the SN, and this could explain the physiological observations made by Ohye et al. (31). An electron-microscopic study might help to solve this problem. In any event,

C - 12424

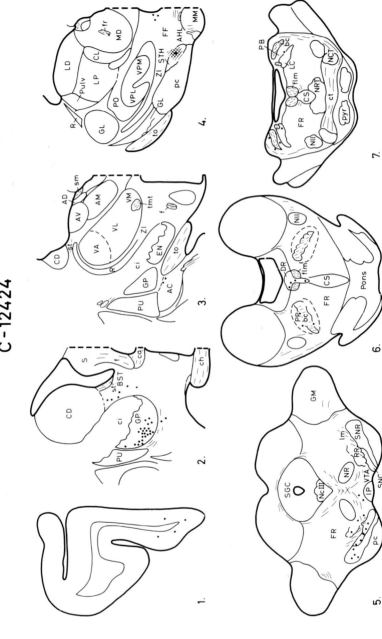

FIG. 6. Distribution of labeled cells in cat C 12424, which had an iontophoretic ejection of HRP in the STH. The brain sections were treated with BDHC.

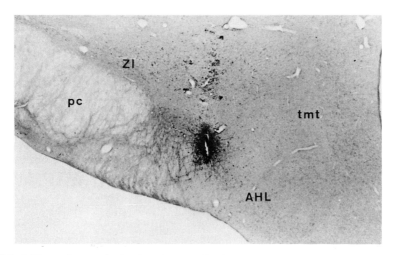

FIG. 7. Photomicrograph showing ejected HRP in the medial STH of cat C 12473. ×6.

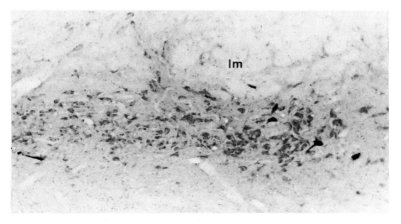

FIG. 8. Labeled cells in the SNC of cat C 12424 (see Fig. 6). ×95.

our observations in monkeys and cats suggest that the dorsal four-fifths of the STH does not receive afferents from the striatum.

It thus appears from our investigation that the striatum can influence the STH only indirectly. Quantitatively, it appears indisputable that the GPe is the main mediator of a striatal influence on cells in the STH, since the largest number of labeled cells following HRP injection/ejection in the STH is invariably found in the GPe. This finding thus is in agreement with the well-established documentation in the literature of a prominent pallidosubthalamic projection (7,16,20,28,30). Whether or not the GPi also contributes to the pallidosub-thalamic projection has been a more controversial issue. On the basis of silver

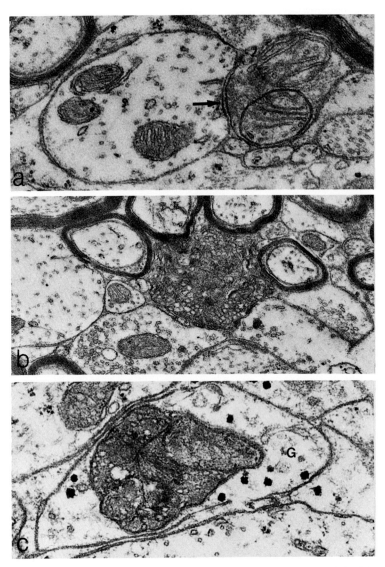

FIG. 9. a, b, c: Electron micrographs of degenerating boutons in the cat's STH following a lesion of the SN. *Arrow* points at synaptic specialization. G, glial process containing glycogen. **a:** ×64,500, **b:** ×33,000, **c:** ×48,450.

impregnation studies, Carpenter et al. (7) tentatively suggested the existence of a minor contingent of STH afferents from the GPi in the monkey. In an autoradiographic study in the cat, Nauta (28) could not from his material either confirm or deny the existence of a projection from the entopeduncular nucleus to the STH. In an autoradiographic study in the monkey, Kim et al. (20) conclude that the GPi probably does not project on the STH. This conclusion is in accordance with the observations made in the present study. Labeled cells were seen in the GPi only in monkeys in which a considerable concentration of HRP was deposited at the level of rostral H2 where the pallido*thalamic* fibers are known to course (21,30). The conclusions drawn from the study of our monkey material is supported by the total absence of labeled cells in the entopeduncular nucleus following iontophoretically ejected HRP within the cat's STH. The observations made by Kim et al. (20) and those reported here thus emphasize that the connections between the pallidum and the STH are not totally reciprocal. Nauta and Cole (29) in a recent autoradiographic study in the cat and the monkey, however, described a prominent subthalamic projection reaching both pallidal segments and not only to the GPi as generally stated in the literature (see 5,6 for references).

In their study, Nauta and Cole (29) also report the existence of a massive projection from the STH onto the SN, confirming previous observations made in the rat (19). These findings together with our observations of a substantial labeling of SN cells following HRP injections/ejections in monkeys and cats thus indicate that there exists a reciprocal connection between the two nuclei. A nigrosubthalamic projection has not been previously reported in the literature (5,6). Admittedly, our observations could be explained by an uptake of HRP by nigrostriatal fibers which are known to course along the dorsal border of the STH and even to travel through the medial part of the nucleus (8,9,27,36). Although our monkeys with HRP injected dorsally to the STH [cases M 12330, M 12325 (Fig. 2, Table 1)] display a few labeled cells in the SN, the number of such cells is substantially lower than in those animals in which the tip of the injection cannula entered the STH [compare cases M 12325 and M 12327 (Fig. 2, Table 1)]. However, even our cases with iontophoretically ejected HRP within the cat's STH do not exclude the possibility that nigrostriatal fibers coursing through the STH—and not nigrosubthalamic fibers themselves—have taken up the marker. However, the electron-microscopic demonstration of boutons in various stages of degeneration following electrolytic lesion of the SN (Fig. 9) appears to confirm the existence of a nigrosubthalamic projection. It is interesting that cells in both the SNC and the SNR, as well as the PN, are labeled following injections/ejections of HRP in the STH. The fact that the largest number of labeled cells is seen in the SNC appears at first glance to be difficult to reconcile with the reports in the literature to the effect that there are virtually no catecholaminergic nerve terminals in the STH (14,22). In this regard, however, it should be recalled that not all SNC cells are necessarily dopaminergic, as indirectly suggested in some reports (11,12,23).

The possible existence of a ceruleosubthalamic projection as suggested in the present study also appears to be in conflict with the reports pointing to the absence of catecholaminergic nerve terminals in the STH. However, it is worth mentioning that Jones and Moore (17) state that not all cells in the cat's LC show histochemical fluorescence for catecholamines. On the other hand, it could be argued that the labeled cells in the LC—and in the DR—in our material are the result of an uptake of injected HRP by ascending fibers originating in the LC and DR and coursing in the vicinity of the STH (1–4,10,18,24, 33,35). It is remarkable, however, that in two monkeys with HRP injected along the dorsal border of the STH (case M 12330) or dorsolaterally to the nucleus (case M 12325), not a single labeled cell was seen in the DR. In the LC, a few cells were labeled in these cases, but the number was quite a bit lower than that seen in two cases where the tip of the injection cannula entered the STH [cases M 12327 and M 12329 (Fig. 2 and Table 1)]. Furthermore, labeled cells are repeatedly seen in the ipsilateral DR and LC following iontophoretically ejected HRP within the cat's STH, suggesting that the cells in these nuclei have axons that either travel through the STH or actually terminate there, or, of course, do both. Electron-microscopic studies are currently in progress in order to help settle this question.

Concerning the PP nucleus, nothing is known about its efferent projections, at least to our knowledge. The observations made in the cat as well as in the monkey in the present study clearly suggest that cells in the PP project onto the STH. In this regard, it is interesting that Nauta (28) and Nauta and Cole (29) in autoradiographic investigations describe a modest projection from the STH to the PP in the cat and the monkey. This projection appears quantitatively less important than the input to the PP from the GPi (28–30).

Our material does not permit a complete assessment of the corticosubthalamic projection (32). In our monkey material, we have seen a few labeled cells in the precentral gyrus, but their number varies from case to case without apparent relationship to the injected HRP. It is not possible from our material to decide whether these cells belong to corticosubthalamic neurons or to other corticofugal cells. The only cortical region in the monkey that repeatedly displays a few labeled cells when the HRP is injected within STH is the opercular insula. However, in the monkey, a prominent, somatotopically organized projection to the lateral half of the STH from the precentral gyrus has been seen using the autoradiographic technique (K. Akert, *personal communication*). In our cat material, however, we have never seen a labeled cell in the primary motor cortical area following HRP ejections in the STH. In these cases, only a small number of labeled cells are seen in the proreus gyrus.

In a recent investigation, it was shown that the pallidosubthalamic projection may be GABA-ergic (13). The present study has disclosed several other possible sources of afferents to the STH. Investigations of putative transmitter substance in some of these pathways are currently being carried out.

REFERENCES

1. Azmitia, E. C., and Segal, M. (1978): An autoradiographic analysis of the differential ascending projections of the dorsal and median raphe nuclei in the rat. *J. Comp. Neurol.,* 179:641–668.
2. Bobillier, P., Petitjean, F., Salvert, D., Ligier, M., and Seguin, S. (1975): Differential projections

of the nucleus raphe dorsalis and nucleus raphe centralis as revealed by autoradiography. *Brain Res.,* 85:205–210.

3. Bobillier, P., Seguin, S., Petitjean, F., Salvert, D., Touret, M., and Jouvet, M. (1976): The raphe nuclei of the cat brain stem: A topographical atlas of their efferent projections as revealed by autoradiography. *Brain Res.,* 113:449–486.

4. Bowden, D. M., German, D. C., and Poynter, W. D. (1978): An autoradiographic, semistereotaxic mapping of major projections from locus coeruleus and adjacent nuclei in *Macaca mulatta. Brain Res.,* 145:257–276.

5. Carpenter, M. B. (1976): Anatomy of the basal ganglia and related nuclei: A review. In: *Advances in Neurology, Vol. 14,* edited by R. Eldridge and S. Fahn, pp. 7–48. Raven Press, New York.

6. Carpenter, M. B. (1976): Anatomical organization of the corpus striatum and related nuclei. In: *The Basal Ganglia,* edited by M. D. Yahr, pp. 1–36. Raven Press, New York.

7. Carpenter, M. B., Fraser, R. A. R., and Shriver, J. E. (1968): The organization of pallidosubthalamic fibers in the monkey. *Brain Res.,* 11:522–539.

8. Carpenter, M. B., Nakano, K., and Kim, R. (1976): Nigrothalamic projections in the monkey demonstrated by autoradiographic technics. *J. Comp. Neurol.,* 165:401–416.

9. Carpenter, M. B., and Peter, P. (1972): Nigrostriatal and nigrothalamic fibers in the rhesus monkey. *J. Comp. Neurol.,* 144:93–116.

10. Conrad, L. C. A., Leonard, C. M., and Pfaff, D. W. (1974): Connections of the median and dorsal raphe nuclei in the rat: An autoradiographic and degeneration study. *J. Comp. Neurol.,* 156:179–206.

11. Feltz, P., and De Champlain, J. (1972): Persistence of caudate unitary responses to nigral stimulation after destruction and functional impairment of the striatal dopaminergic terminals. *Brain Res.,* 43:595–600.

12. Fibiger, H. C., Pudritz, R. E., McGeer, P. L., and McGeer, E. G. (1972): Axonal transport in nigro-striatal and nigro-thalamic neurons: Effects of medial forebrain bundle lesions and 6-hydroxy-dopamine. *J. Neurochem.,* 19:1697–1708.

13. Fonnum, F., Grofová, I., and Rinvik, E. (1978): Origin and distribution of glutamate decarboxylase in the nucleus subthalamicus of the cat. *Brain Res.,* 153:370–374.

14. Fuxe, K. (1965): Distribution of monoamine nerve terminals in the central nervous system. *Acta Physiol. Scand.,* 64 (Suppl. 247):36–85.

15. Graham, R. C., and Karnovsky, M. J. (1966): Glomerular permeability. Ultrastructural cytochemical studies using peroxidase as protein tracers. *J. Exp. Med.,* 124:1123–1134.

16. Grofová, I. (1969): Experimental demonstration of a topical arrangement of the pallidosubthalamic fibers in the cat. *Psychiatr. Neurol. Neurochir.,* 72:53–59.

17. Jones, B. E., and Moore, R. Y. (1977): Catecholamine-containing neurons of the nucleus locus coeruleus in the cat. *J. Comp. Neurol.,* 157:43–52.

18. Jones, B. E., and Moore, R. Y. (1977): Ascending projections of the locus coeruleus in the rat. II. Autoradiographic study. *Brain Res.,* 127:23–53.

19. Kanazawa, I., Marshall, G. R., and Kelly, J. S. (1976): Afferents to the rat substantia nigra studied with horseradish peroxidase with special reference to fibers from the subthalamic nucleus. *Brain Res.,* 115:485–491.

20. Kim, R., Nakano, K., Jayaraman, A., and Carpenter, M. B. (1976): Projections of the globus pallidus and adjacent structures: An autoradiographic study in the monkey. *J. Comp. Neurol.,* 169:263–290.

21. Kuo, J.-S., and Carpenter, M. B. (1973): Organization of pallidothalamic projections in the rhesus monkey. *J. Comp. Neurol.,* 151:201–236.

22. Lindvall, O., Björklund, A., Nobin, A., and Stenevi, U. (1974): The adrenergic innervation of the rat thalamus as revealed by the glyoxylic acid fluorescence method. *J. Comp. Neurol.,* 154:317–348.

23. Ljungdahl, Å., Hökfelt, T., Goldstein, M., and Park, D. (1975): Retrograde peroxidase tracing of neurons combined with transmitter histochemistry. *Brain Res.,* 84:313–319.

24. McBride, R. L., and Sutin, J. (1976): Projections of the locus coeruleus and adjacent pontine tegmentum in the cat. *J. Comp. Neurol.,* 165:265–284.

25. Mesulam, M.-M. (1976): The blue reaction product in horseradish peroxidase neurohistochemistry: Incubation parameters and visibility. *J. Histochem. Cytochem.,* 24:1273–1280.

26. Mesulam, M.-M., and Rosene, D. L. (1977): Differential sensitivity between blue and brown reaction procedures for HRP neurohistochemistry. *Neurosci. Lett.,* 5:7–14.

27. Moore, R. Y., Bhatnagar, R., and Heller, A. (1971): Anatomical and chemical studies of a nigro-neostriatal projection in the cat. *Brain Res.,* 30:110–135.
28. Nauta, H. J. W. (1974): Efferent projections of the caudate nucleus, pallidal complex, and subthalamic nucleus in the cat. (Thesis.) Case Western Reserve University, Cleveland, Ohio.
29. Nauta, H. J. W., and Cole, M. (1978): Efferent projections of the subthalamic nucleus: An autoradiographic study in monkey and cat. *J. Comp. Neurol.,* 180:1–16.
30. Nauta, W. J. H., and Mehler, W. R. (1966): Projections of the lentiform nucleus in the monkey. *Brain Res.,* 1:3–42.
31. Ohye, C., LeGuyader, C., and Feger, J. (1976): Responses of subthalamic and pallidal neurons to striatal stimulation: An extracellular study on awake monkeys. *Brain Res.,* 111:241–252.
32. Petras, J. M. (1965): Some fiber connections of the precentral and postcentral cortex with basal ganglia, thalamus and subthalamus. *Trans. Am. Neurol. Assoc.,* 91:274–275.
33. Pickel, V. M., Segal, M., and Bloom, F. E. (1974): A radioautographic study of the efferent pathways of the nucleus locus coeruleus. *J. Comp. Neurol.,* 155:15–42.
34. Rinvik, E., and Grofová, I. (1974): Light and electron microscopical studies of the normal nuclei ventralis lateralis and ventralis anterior thalami in the cat. *Anat. Embryol.,* 146:57–93.
35. Shimizu, N., Ohnishi, S., Tohyama, M., and Maeda, T. (1974): Demonstration by degeneration silver method of the ascending projection from the locus coeruleus. *Exp. Brain Res.,* 21:181–192.
36. Usunoff, K. G., Hassler, R., Romansky, K., Usunova, R. P., and Wagner, A. (1976): The nigrostriatal projection in the cat. Part I. Silver impregnation study. *J. Neurol. Sci.,* 28:265–288.

Advances in Neurology, Vol. 24, edited by
L. J. Poirier, T. L. Sourkes, and P. J. Bédard.
Raven Press, New York © 1979.

Selective Bilateral Lesions of Pars Compacta of the Substantia Nigra: Effects on Motor Processes and Ingestive Behaviors

Larry L. Butcher and *Gordon K. Hodge

Department of Psychology and Brain Research Institute, University of California, Los Angeles, California 90024

The value of animal models of human neurologic disorders is directly related to how accurately the experimentally induced neuropathology and its consequences mimic the human disorder. Although loss of neuronal somata in the substantia nigra as an important correlate of human parkinsonism was suggested over 40 years ago in the brilliant studies of Hassler (8), only recently have animal models based on nigral involvement been used extensively to facilitate our understanding of basic neuropathologic mechanisms in Parkinson's disease (for review see ref. 11). Prominent among these models has been the circling rodent. Pioneered by Andén and his associates (2), this model was produced originally by unilaterally destroying various areas of the forebrain electrolytically. Such animals turned toward the side of the ablation (2), and this circling was correlated with a loss of dopamine in the substantia nigra and caudate-putamen complex (3). Furthermore, loss of neuronal somata in pars compacta of the substantia nigra was seen (3). These observations, among others, gave rise to the hypothesis that rodents circle toward the side of the body containing the less efficacious nigro-striatal "dopamine" system, a conjecture consistent with the findings that intrastriatal infusion of dopamine elicits circling contralateral to the side of injection and that this circling can be blocked by chlorpromazine (14).

A major advance in thinking about animal models of parkinsonism based on nigro–striatal dopamine involvement was put forth by Ungerstedt (12,13) in a series of landmark experiments based on the use of 6-hydroxydopamine. Similar to electrolytic lesions, unilateral 6-hydroxydopamine ablations in the mesencephalon were correlated with drug-elicited turning toward the side of neuropathology (12). Perhaps more intriguing, however, was Ungerstedt's (13) observation that bilateral infusion of 6-hydroxydopamine into various areas in the mesencephalon, diencephalon, and telencephalon produced hypokinesia,

---

* Present address: Department of Psychology; University of New Mexico, Albuquerque, New Mexico 87131.

aphagia, and adipsia. These motor and ingestive deficits were attributed by Ungerstedt (12,13) to damage to the nigro-striatal dopamine system.

All of these studies have contributed substantially to our understanding of the functions of the substantia nigra and neuroanatomically interconnected structures. The question can be raised, however, whether or not the manipulations described above were confined exclusively to the structures and systems given prominence in the published works *(vide infra)*. If not, then perhaps other neural systems contributed to the observed behavioral deficits (e.g., see ref. 15). In the present report we attempt to clarify the role of pars compacta of the substantia nigra in motor and consummatory activity by making lesions confined virtually exclusively to that structure and observing the subsequent behavior.

WHAT THE WHITE KNIGHT TELLS US ABOUT ABLATION PROCEDURES

In a passage from *Through the Looking Glass,* Lewis Carroll (6) has pointed out the necessity of careful thinking in using words to describe actual events. The White Knight, attempting to cheer Alice, proposes to sing her a song:

> ". . . . The name of the song is called *'Haddocks' Eyes'.* "
>
> "Oh, that's the name of the song, is it?" Alice said, trying to feel interested.
>
> "No, you don't understand," the Knight said, looking a little vexed. "That's what the name is *called.* The name really is *'The Aged Aged Man'.* "
>
> "Then I ought to have said 'That's what the *song* is called'?" Alice corrected herself.
>
> "No, you oughtn't: that's quite another thing! The *song* is called *'Ways and Means':* but that's only what it's *called,* you know!"
>
> "Well, what *is* the song, then?" said Alice, who was by this time completely bewildered.
>
> "I was coming to that," the Knight said.

In the dialogue between Alice and the White Knight it is important to appreciate the differences among *the song itself, the name of the song, what the song is called,* and *what the name of the song is called.* Similar difficulties confront us in attempting to assess the nature of lesions in studies on the functions of the nigro-striatal dopamine system. In many of these experiments, given that the authors present the relevant histology or histochemistry, the name of the lesion and the lesion itself do not represent the same thing; this we call the "White Knight syndrome." In the carefully done study of Hökfelt and Ungerstedt (9), for example, a large nonselective lesion of 1 mm in diameter is displayed (Fig. 7) after injection of 8 $\mu g/4$ μl 6-hydroxydopamine into the ventral mesencephalon. Varying degrees of nonselective damage in other locations of the midbrain are shown in other figures of their report (e.g., Figs. 5,8), even though the same dose of 6-hydroxydopamine was used and the infusion cannula was situated in approximately the same place. In the behavioral studies of Ungerstedt (12,13), however, comparisons between the histopathologic profile of each rat and its subsequent behavior were not made, and all of these ablations would presumably be described as lesions of the nigro-striatal dopamine system. But the correlation between the name of the lesion and the actual lesion would clearly vary from animal to animal, and this is a problem that we have encountered also. In the present report, therefore, we have attempted to make sufficiently precise lesions of pars compacta of the substantia nigra such that the name of the ablation and the actual damage are virtually the same entity.

EXPERIMENTAL PROCEDURES

Adult female rats were used. Unilateral or bilateral radio-frequency lesions were made in pars compacta of the substantia nigra (group PC, Fig. 2; compare with Fig. 1), the location of A9 dopamine-containing cell bodies projecting prominently to the caudate–putamen complex (10). The electrode was oriented

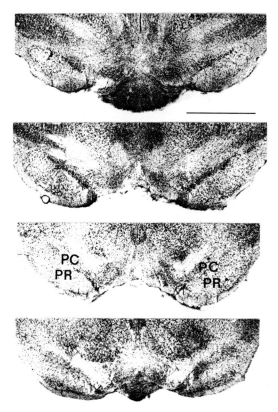

FIG. 1. Ventral mesencephalon of an unoperated, control rat. Sections are arranged rostrocaudally. PC, pars compacta, substantia nigra; PR, pars reticulata, substantia nigra. Thionin stain, scale = 2 mm.

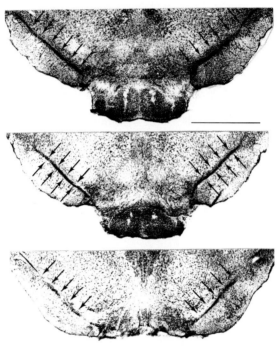

FIG. 2. Bilateral radio-frequency lesions in pars compacta of the substantia nigra. All sections are from a single rat in group PC. Sections arranged rostrocaudally. Arrows point to residual gliosis in pars compacta. Thionin stain, scale = 2 mm.

45° from the horizontal to take advantage of the position and elongated shape of pars compacta. Since the lesion probe was essentially parallel to pars compacta neuronal somata, the ensuing thermal ablation was almost entirely confined to that nigral subdivision (Fig. 2).

Sham-operated controls consisted of rats that were surgically manipulated in the same way that experimental groups were treated except that no electrical current was passed.

For comparison purposes radio-frequency lesions were made that involved (a) substantial or complete loss of pars compacta somata in addition to medial lemniscus damage (group PC–ML), (b) extensive but subtotal portions of pars compacta with moderate extracompacta damage (group SPC), (c) minimal to moderate subtotal portions of pars compacta with moderate extracompacta damage, including portions of the medial lemniscus (group SPC–ML), and (d) extensive portions of the median raphe area and adjacent reticular formation (group MR, Fig. 3).

In addition, unilateral and bilateral nigral lesions were attempted with 8 μg/ 4 μl (Fig. 4) and 4 μg/2 μl 6-hydroxydopamine (groups 6-OHDA-8 and 6-OHDA-4, respectively). In group 6-OHDA-4 the animals were pretreated with 25 mg/kg desipramine. According to Agid et al. (1), use of 8 μg/4 μl 6-hydroxy-

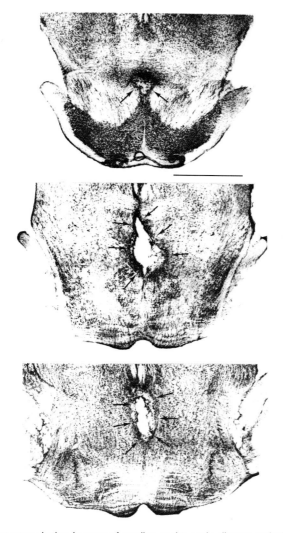

FIG. 3. Radio-frequency lesion in area of median raphe and adjacent reticular formation. All sections are from a single rat in group MR, and are arranged rostrocaudally. Arrows point to cavitation. Thionin stain, scale = 2 mm.

dopamine, because this dose produces significant nonselective damage, does not constitute proper usage of the cytotoxin, a viewpoint with which we agree. Yet virtually all researchers engaged in behavioral studies have used this dose or greater (e.g., 12,13); accordingly, we have tested this dose in the present experiments. When used properly, 6-hydroxydopamine apparently must be intra-cerebrally infused in doses not exceeding 4 μg/2 μl (1); to increase selectivity desipramine pretreatment is recommended (4). We have followed this protocol also.

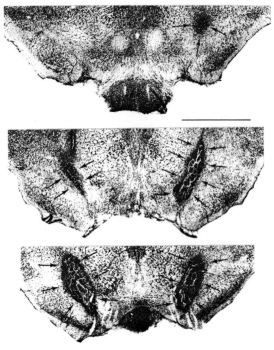

FIG. 4. Histopathology after bilateral intramesencephalic infusion of 8 μg/4 μl 6-hydroxydopamine. All sections are from a single rat in group 6-OHDA-8 and are arranged rostrocaudally. Arrows point to massive gliosis. Thionin stain, scale = 2 mm.

Bilaterally lesioned animals were used in behavioral studies. Although histologic and histochemical evaluations of these animals were performed at the termination of behavioral testing, additional histologic and histochemical studies were conducted on animals with unilateral ablations. Brains were processed for monoamines according to the glyoxylic acid procedure of de la Torre and Surgeon (7). Thionin staining was done also.

Baseline food and water intakes, body weights, and spontaneous locomotor activity were recorded for a period of at least 7 days preceding surgery. Postoperative behavioral measures were continued daily for a minimum of 2 weeks; additional observations for most animals were made during the fifth and eighth postoperative weeks. For some rats, ingestive and locomotor behaviors, as well as body weights, were measured daily for 25 weeks. Behaviors of rats recorded on a discontinuous basis did not differ from measures taken daily on rats with comparable treatments.

HISTOLOGIC AND HISTOCHEMICAL EVALUATIONS

The most complete and selective lesions of pars compacta were those in group PC animals (Fig. 2, compare with Fig. 1). Occasionally a few cell bodies remained in pars compacta at caudo-medial levels and in pars lateralis. Lesions restricted almost exclusively to pars compacta (Fig. 2) produced severe but not complete loss of histochemically assessed dopamine in the caudate–putamen complex, whereas dopamine content in nucleus accumbens and the olfactory tubercle was unaffected or only slightly decreased, at least as assessed histochemically. Catecholamine fibers and terminals in the septum and amygdala showed only slight, if any, decrements in fluorescence. Slight to moderate loss of dopamine was observed, however, in the interstitial nucleus of the stria terminalis.

Fluorescence decrements in the striata of rats sustaining ablations similar to those of experimental groups PC–ML, 6-OHDA-4, 6-OHDA-8, SPC, and SPC–ML were positively correlated with the degree of pars compacta involvement, which ranged from minimal to virtually complete. Little or no loss of telencephalic catecholamine fluorescence was seen after lesions in group MR (Fig. 3) except when those ablations infringed upon known catecholamine systems originating in and/or traversing the pons and midbrain.

Ablations made with 6-hydroxydopamine were of variable size and shape (Fig. 4). In combinations with desipramine, 4 μg/2 μl 6-hydroxydopamine produced moderate nonselective damage accompanied by extensive degeneration of compacta somata. With 8 μg/4 μl 6-hydroxydopamine, however, a prominent nonselective component to its action was frequently seen (Fig. 4). When nonselective necrosis in groups 6-OHDA-4 and 6-OHDA-8 invaded the ventromedial mesencephalic tegmentum (e.g., Fig. 4), then extensive loss of fluorescence was noted in nucleus accumbens, the olfactory tubercle, septum, interstitial nucleus of the stria terminalis, and the amygdala, as well as in the caudate–putamen complex. In all lesion groups, there was a tendency for glial scarring and lesion size to diminish with the passage of time.

BEHAVIORAL EVALUATIONS

Animals with lesions restricted principally to pars compacta (group PC, Fig. 2) were chronically hyperactive, sometimes as long as 23 weeks postoperatively (Fig. 5). The photocell activity levels were more than twice as high as those of controls. The intensity and duration of hyperactivity were correlated with degree of selective destruction of pars compacta. Animals in group PC were somewhat more active and remained so for longer durations (Fig. 5) than animals with less discrete compacta lesions involving the medial lemniscus as well (group PC–ML). Both groups PC and PC–ML were significantly more active than groups SPC and SPC–ML, which sustained partial damage to pars compacta; group SPC and SPC–ML rats were hyperactive only during the first 3–4 days postsurgically (Fig. 5).

Animals with lesions of areas that included the median raphe became hyperactive immediately upon recovery from surgery. Like rats in groups PC and PC–ML, animals in group MR remained hyperactive throughout the course of the experiments (Fig. 5). Qualitatively, they differed from compacta-ablated rats (group PC and PC–ML) in that animals with raphe lesions tended to wander

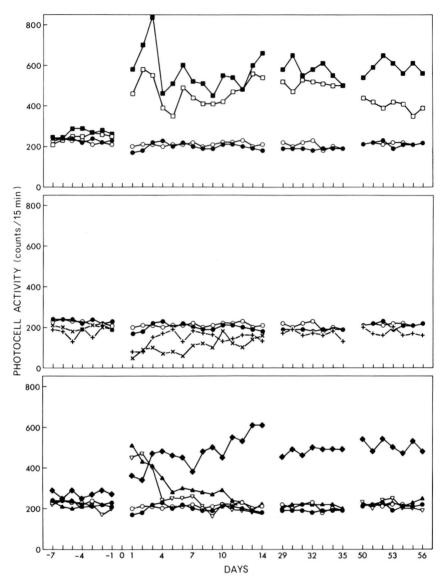

FIG. 5. Effects of bilateral brainstem lesions on spontaneous locomotor activity. Nonoperated controls *(open circles)*, sham-operated controls *(closed circles)*, group PC *(closed squares)*, group PC–ML *(open squares)*, group 6-OHDA-4 (+), group 6-OHDA-8 (×), group SPC *(closed triangles)*, group SPC–ML *(inverted, open triangles)*, and group MR *(closed diamonds)*. Surgery was performed on day 0. Activity from the preceding 7 days and subsequent 56 days is shown. Control data are displayed in all panels to facilitate comparisons. Significance level for all statistical comparisons: $P < 0.05$. Rats in groups PC, PC–ML, and MR were significantly more active than control groups throughout the postoperative period. Animals that were transiently hyperactive were significantly different from controls on postoperative days 1–3 for group SPC-ML and days 1–4 for group SPC. Group 6-OHDA-4 rats were significantly less active than control groups on days 1–2 after surgery. Animals in group 6-OHDA-8 were significantly hypoactive on days 1–6 after surgery. No other comparisons were statistically significant.

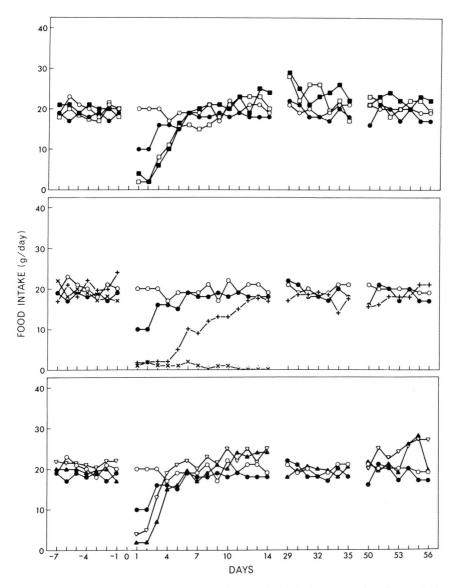

FIG. 6. Effects of bilateral mesencephalic lesions on 24-hr food consumption. For symbols, figure format, and significance level see legend of Fig. 5. On postoperative days 1 and 2, all lesioned groups consumed significantly less food than nonoperated rats. Furthermore, all lesioned groups ate less than sham-lesioned controls on these days. On postoperative day 3, only the two 6-OHDA groups ate less than both control groups, the SPC–ML group did not differ significantly from either control group, and all other rats ate significantly less than nonoperated but not sham-operated controls. On postoperative days 4 and 5, only the 6-OHDA-4 and 6-OHDA-8 animals differed from controls. From postoperative days 6–14, the duration of their testing period, the 6-OHDA-8 group differed significantly from the control groups. No other comparisons were statistically significant.

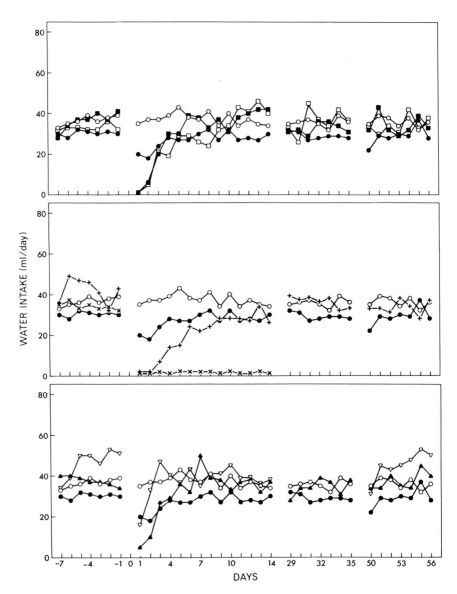

FIG. 7. Effects of bilateral mesencephalic lesions on 24-hr water consumption. For symbols, figure format, and significance level see legend of Fig. 5. On postoperative day 1, all groups drank significantly less water than nonoperated rats; moreover, all lesioned groups with the exception of group SPC-ML differed significantly from sham-operated animals. On postoperative day 2, all groups except SPC–ML differed from nonoperated but not from sham-operated animals. From postoperative days 3–56 none of the radio-frequency lesioned rats differed from either nonoperated or sham-operated controls. From postoperative days 3–5, the 6-OHDA-4 group drank significantly less than nonoperated rats. From postsurgical days 3–14, the duration of their testing period, the 6-OHDA-8 group drank significantly less than either control group. No other comparisons were statistically significant.

about more in their home cages rather than engaging in the continuous gnawing and manipulatory behaviors characteristic of compacta-ablated rats.

Despite the fact that animals with radio-frequency lesions of the pars compacta (group PC) often sustained virtually complete destruction of compacta cell bodies without appreciable damage to the medial lemniscus or pars reticulata, water and food intakes of these animals, as well as in rats with radio-frequency lesions encompassing other loci (groups PC–ML, SPC, SPC–ML), were reduced only briefly during the immediate postoperative period (Figs. 6 and 7), and body weights were unaffected. Indeed, these brief decrements in consummatory behaviors did not appear well correlated with extent of compacta damage, since food intakes were reduced to approximately the same degree in groups PC, PC–ML, SPC, and SPC–ML (Fig. 6), even though compacta damage varied greatly among these animals. Similarly, water consumption decrements were approximately the same in groups PC, PC–ML, and SPC (Fig. 7), and group SPC–ML did not differ from sham-operated controls (Fig. 7).

Although we did not quantify food and water consumption in group MR rats, they showed no weight losses, and their body weights did not differ from other experimental groups sustaining radio-frequency lesions. We conclude, therefore, that ablations in the median raphe area did not adversely affect food and water consumption.

Rats receiving 4 μg/2 μl 6-hydroxydopamine in combination with desipramine pretreatment displayed only slight to moderate locomotor impairments (Figs. 5–7), but food intakes remained significantly lower than sham-lesioned rats through postoperative day 5 (Fig. 6). Water consumption was decreased on postsurgical days 1–5 (Fig. 7).

The only animals in the current experimental series that became aphagic and adipsic with accompanying weight decrements were those treated with 8 μg/4 μl 6-hydroxydopamine without desipramine pretreatment (Figs. 6 and 7). As detailed elsewhere in this report, damage inflicted was typically pervasive and nonselective, but there were occasional exceptions where gliosis was minimal. Photocell activities were lower than controls on days 1–6 after surgical procedures (Fig. 5), and the general behavior displayed by these rats was characterized by poverty of movement. Their vertebral columns were frequently arched, and they were often hyperresponsive to touch.

CONCLUSIONS

Neither aphagia nor adipsia was found as a consequence of virtually complete or partial destruction of pars compacta of the substantia nigra, a finding that indicates the need for reevaluation of theories addressing the significance of nigral dopamine alone in the control of ingestive behaviors. Pars compacta does appear, however, to exert a modulating influence on locomotor activity such that absence of this influence is accompanied by chronic hyperkinesia. Under physiologic conditions it is possible that compacta neurons provide an activational set-point for their various target cells (5). Whatever functions the striatum has, therefore, might be potentiated or diminished by alterations in nigro-striatal activity, but the pathway itself would not mediate specific behaviors.

ACKNOWLEDGMENT

This research was supported by USPHS Grant NS-10928 to L.L.B.

REFERENCES

1. Agid, Y., Javoy, F., Glowinski, J., Bouvet, D., and Sotelo, C. (1973): Injection of 6-hydroxydopamine into the substantia nigra of the rat. II. Diffusion and specificity. *Brain Res.,* 58:291–325.
2. Andén, N.-E., Dahlström, A., Fuxe, K., and Larsson, K. (1966): Functional role of the nigro-neostriatal dopamine neurons. *Acta Pharmacol. Toxicol.,* 24:263–274.
3. Andén, N.-E., Dahlström, A., Fuxe, K., Larsson, K., Olson, L., and Ungerstedt, U. (1966): Ascending monoamine neurons to the telencephalon and diencephalon. *Acta Physiol. Scand.,* 67:313–326.
4. Breese, G. R., Smith, R. D., Cooper, B. R., Hollister, A. S., Kraemer, G., and McKinney, W. T. (1975): Use of neurocytotoxic compounds in neuropsychopharmacology. In: *Chemical Tools in Catecholamine Research, Vol. 1,* edited by G. Jonsson, T. Malmfors, and C. Sachs, pp. 335–342. North Holland Publishing Co., Amsterdam.
5. Butcher, L. L., and Talbot, K. (1978): Acetylcholinesterase in rat nigro-neostriatal neurons: experimental verification and evidence for cholinergic–dopaminergic interactions in the substantia nigra and caudate–putamen complex. In: *Cholinergic–Monoaminergic Interactions in the Brain,* edited by L. L. Butcher, pp. 25–95. Academic Press, New York.
6. Carroll, L. (1871): Through the Looking Glass. In: *The Annotated Alice* (1960), introduction and notes by M. Gardner, p. 306. Bramhall House, New York.
7. de la Torre, J. C., and Surgeon, J. W. (1976): A methodological approach to rapid and sensitive monoamine histofluorescence using a modified glyoxylic acid technique: The SPG method. *Histochemistry,* 49:81–93.
8. Hassler, R. (1938): Zur Pathologie der Paralysis agitans und des postenzephalitischen Parkinsonismus. *J. f. Psych. Neurol.,* 48:387–476.
9. Hökfelt, T., and Ungerstedt, U. (1973): Specificity of 6-hydroxydopamine induced degeneration of central monoamine neurones: an electron and fluorescence microscopic study with special reference to intracerebral injection on the nigro-striatal dopamine system. *Brain Res.,* 60:269–297.
10. Lindvall, O., and Björklund, A. (1974): The organization of the ascending catecholamine neuron systems in the rat brain as revealed by the glyoxylic acid fluorescence method. *Acta Physiol. Scand. (Suppl.),* 412:1–48.
11. Marsden, C. D., Duvoisin, R. C., Jenner, P., Parkes, J. D., Pycock, C., and Tarsy, D. (1975): Relationship between animal models and clinical parkinsonism. In: *Advances in Neurology, Vol. 9: Dopaminergic Mechanisms,* edited by D. B. Calne, T. N. Chase, and A. Barbeau, pp. 165–175. Raven Press, New York.
12. Ungerstedt, U. (1971): Postsynaptic supersensitivity after 6-hydroxydopamine induced degeneration of the nigro-striatal dopamine system. *Acta Physiol. Scand. (Suppl.),* 367:69–93.
13. Ungerstedt, U. (1971): Adipsia and aphagia after 6-hydroxydopamine induced degeneration of the nigro-striatal dopamine system. *Acta Physiol. Scand. (Suppl.),* 367:95–122.
14. Ungerstedt, U., Butcher, L. L., Butcher, S. G., Andén, N.-E., and Fuxe, K. (1969): Direct chemical stimulation of dopaminergic mechanisms in the neostriatum of the rat. *Brain Res.,* 14:461–471.
15. Zeigler, H. P., and Karten, H. J. (1974): Central trigeminal structures and the lateral hypothalamic syndrome in the rat. *Science,* 186:636–638.

Advances in Neurology, Vol. 24, edited by
L. J. Poirier, T. L. Sourkes, and P. J. Bédard.
Raven Press, New York © 1979.

Experimental Study of Spontaneous Postural Tremor Induced by a More Successful Tremor-Producing Procedure in the Monkey

Chihiro Ohye, Shuji Imai, Hideo Nakajima, Toru Shibazaki, and Tatsuo Hirai

Department of Neurosurgery, Gunma University School of Medicine, Maebashi, Japan

Lesions involving the midbrain ventromedial tegmental area may produce spontaneous sustained tremor like that of Parkinson's disease in man as well as in monkey (5,6,16,17,20). However, production of the experimental tremor by midbrain lesions might be a difficult task [for example, Gybels (4) produced it in 30% of the operated monkeys] because the usual stereotaxic method is not sufficiently accurate to reach a specific deep subcortical target in the monkey (15).

To overcome the inaccuracy of stereotaxy in monkeys, we have developed a method involving radiological control (2). The principle of this method is to visualize the ventricular system in reference to the deep-seated subcortical structures as in stereotaxy applied to the human brain (19).

Thus, we have succeeded in producing spontaneous tremor in most of the operated monkeys (20 of 26). Six have died in the immediate postoperative period. Neurophysiological studies have been conducted on these monkeys to elucidate the neural mechanism of tremor.

PRODUCTION OF SPONTANEOUS TREMOR

A total of 26 small Java monkeys *(Macaca irus,* body wt = 1–3 kg) were used in this study.

The first 9 were operated using only neurophysiological controls. They were lightly anesthetized with pentobarbital (20 mg/kg) and the head fixed in the usual stereotaxic apparatus. Referring to the stereotaxic atlas of the monkey brain by Atlas and Ingram (1), a pair of coagulating needles (diameter = 1.5 mm, distance =2 mm, effective length = 2 mm) of Leksell's stereotaxic apparatus for human brain (8) were introduced stereotaxically to the lower border of the red nucleus. During the intracerebral descent of the needle, the electrical background activity of the deep subcortical structures was recorded continuously by a concentric bipolar needle electrode (outer diameter = 0.6 mm, interpolar distance = 200 to 300 μ, tip = 10 to 20 μ, electrical resistance about 100 k Ω). Each of the subcortical structures showed characteristic electrical activity as in the human (3,12). For example, the lower border of the thalamus and the red nucleus were reliable landmarks in our vertical approach. Moreover, several points in and around the red nucleus were stimulated electrically (100 Hz, 5 V, for 1–2 sec) by the same electrode to induce and record motor responses. Stimulation of the third cranial nerve resulted in pupillary constriction, various types of ocular movement and palpebral opening. Finally, the needle electrode was replaced by a thermo-controlled needle for coagulation and a lesion was placed at the lower border of the red nucleus (65°C, 15–20 sec). The theoretical size of the lesion was estimated to be 2 × 2 × 1.5 mm³. All these procedures were performed under sterile conditions.

By this stereotaxic method, determination of the exact target point on the first attempt is uncertain on account of the large individual variations in stereo-taxy. As a matter of fact, we were often forced to change the trajectory of the needle without finding the proper point to be coagulated.

Therefore, in another series of experiments, monkeys were operated under radiological control. The details of the radiological procedure have already been presented elsewhere (14). In brief, after taking simple craniograms to verify the exact fixation of the head, stereotaxic ventricular puncture was made, refer-ring to the position of limbus sphenoidalis. The anterior horn of the lateral ventricle was found about 10 mm above the limbus sphenoidalis, and about 4 mm lateral to the midline in our monkeys. About 0.3 ml of radiopaque substance (Conray[1]) was injected to visualize the third ventricle (Fig. 1). The midbrain ventromedial tegmental area was roughly estimated in relation to the anterior and posterior commissures and to the distance of the intercommissural line. A pair of coagulating needles were introduced at this point which is situated a few millimeters anterior to the posterior commissure, several millimeters below the intercommissural line, and 1.0–2.0 mm lateral to the midline. Vertical as well as oblique approaches were used to reach the target. Again, the background activity was recorded during lowering the needle and the responses to electrical stimulation of the third cranial nerve were recorded as in the first series. After establishing the precise target point, a final radiograph was taken to ascertain the position of the needle tip and the lesion was placed at this point (Fig. 1).

NEUROLOGICAL OBSERVATIONS

Immediately after coagulation, ipsilateral third nerve palsy, dilated pupil, loss of light reaction and ptosis could be seen even while the monkey was still in the stereotaxic apparatus. All but four monkeys initially showed these

---

[1] Methylglucamine salt of 5-acetamide = 2,4,6 = triiode N = methyl isothalamic acid, produced by Dai-ichi Seiyaku Co., Ltd., Tokyo, Japan.

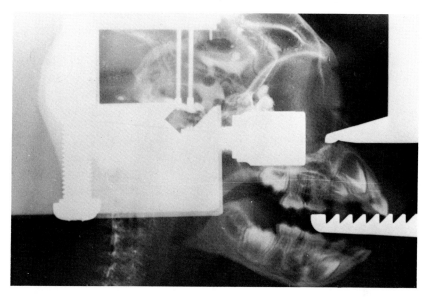

FIG. 1. Radiographic lateral view of the third ventricle and site of coagulation. The lesion was placed between the tips (2 mm in length and distance) of two vertical electrodes. The posterior electrode is anterior to the posterior commissure in this lateral view. Laterality, 1.5 mm from the midline.

signs that lasted about 1 month. These signs gradually decreased to some extent.

After recovery from general anesthesia, all monkeys but 3 showed torticollis, with the occiput directed to the contralateral side. The degree of torticollis differed from case to case; some animals exhibited rotation of the neck of almost 90°, others only slight turning or tilting. In 3 animals, these immediate effects were so strong that they could not stand up and body axial turning on the floor toward the contralateral side resulted. Forced circling toward the contra-lateral side was observed in all other cases. The direction of circling was generally contrary to that of torticollis, but occasionally ipsilateral turning occurred. At the same time, all animals showed a characteristic posture of the contralateral upper limb. The shoulder was adducted, the elbow flexed at about 90°, the wrist extended or slightly flexed with all digits naturally extended. The monkey was generally reluctant to use this limb except under emergency while climbing on the bar after being excited or threatened. On passive flexion or extension of the wrist and elbow joints, some resistance was noticed, especially in the biceps brachii and forearm extensor muscles as illustrated on the EMG (Fig. 2B). The lower limb did not show such abnormal posture but it also was obviously hypokinetic and paretic. These disturbances also tended to improve to a consider-able extent within 1 or 2 months; however, the flexed posture of the contralateral upper limb remained almost unchanged.

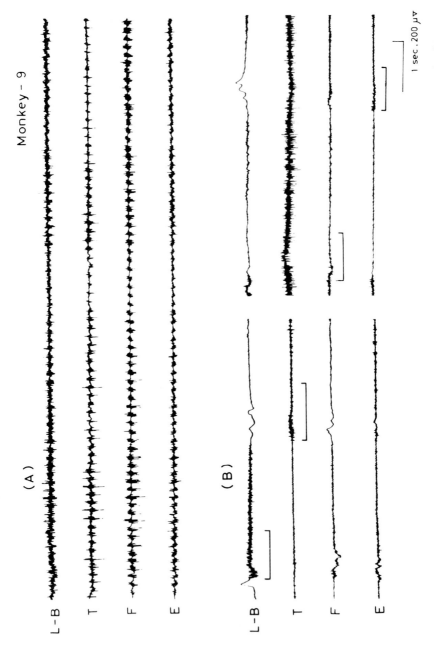

FIG. 2. A: EMG recordings from the left (L) upper limb by surface plate electrodes to show the spontaneous sustained tremor. **B:** Rigidity is assessed by passive stretch *(horizontal bars)* of the muscles. B, biceps brachii; T, triceps brachii; F, forearm flexor; E, forearm extensor muscle. Note the tonic discharge especially in biceps when stretched.

Table I   Several features of tremor (7 cases)

NO.	lesion side	tremor side	delay	frequency (Hz)	site neck	site upper limb	site lower limb	character postural	character intentional
1	R	R	10 D	5	−	+	−	+	+ +
		L	3 w	5	−	+	−	+ +	−
2	L	R	5 w	7	−	+	−	+ +	−
3	R	L	2 w	7−8	−	+	−	+ +	−
5	L	R	4 w	9−10	−	+	+	+	−
6	L	R	3 w	6	−	+	−	+ +	−
7	R	L	8 w	9−10	−	+	+	+	−
9	R	L	3 w	6	+	+	+	+	+

In the course of recovery from these immediate disturbances, spontaneous tremor appeared in the contralateral extremities in all 20 cases which survived. In one case there was tremor of the ipsilateral upper limb as well. The precise moment of onset of tremor was difficult to determine because it usually developed gradually, beginning at the distal part of the contralateral extremity and gradually affecting the proximal part within several days. The delay of onset of tremor ranged from 2 to 8 weeks, its mean value being 4 weeks. The upper limb was involved in all 20 cases while the lower limb trembled concomitantly in 9 cases. The frequency of tremor differed in individual cases; most of them showed 5–7 Hz while in 2 cases it was more rapid (9–10 Hz). The characteristics of tremor were rather constant in a given case but sometimes changed depending on the posture of the limb affected. For example, when the animal was resting, the tremor was observed only in the distal part of the limb, in a manner quite similar to parkinsonian pill-rolling tremor. However, when excited, the tremor became very intense, of a coarse and flapping type involving the whole limb, neck, and shoulder. In the forearm, alternative pronation–supination or flexion–extension were often observed. EMG analysis revealed that the grouping discharges were reciprocal between antagonists (Fig. 2A). In any case, once tremor appeared, it persisted almost unchanged until the animal was sacrificed up to a maximum of 2 years after the operation. Several features of the tremor in the first seven cases are given in Table 1.

NEUROPHYSIOLOGICAL STUDY ON THE RHYTHMIC ACTIVITY IN THE SPINAL CORD

In the monkeys in which the spontaneous tremor was sufficiently marked and sustained, extracellular recordings from various parts of the deep subcortical

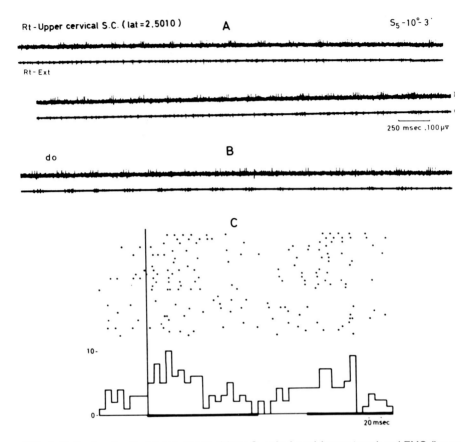

Rt - Upper cervical S.C. (lat = 2.5010)   **A** $S_5 - 10°·3'$

Rt - Ext

250 msec .100 μv

do   **B**

C

10 -

0 -

20 msec

FIG. 3. Multiunit spike discharges recorded from C_1 spinal cord (upper trace) and EMG (lower trace) from the ipsilateral forearm extensor muscle (Rt-Ext). **A:** Rhythmic spinal discharges not accompanied by peripheral tremor. Note the positive spikes. **B:** The same rhythmic discharges in the spinal cord are synchronized with the peripheral tremor. **C:** Time relationship between the spike discharges in the spinal cord *(dots and histogram)* and the EMG *(thick bar on abscissa)* from the ipsilateral forearm extensor muscle. Each grouping discharge of tremor EMG is aligned at its starting point *(horizontal bar)*.

structures were performed in an attempt to elucidate the neural mechanism of tremor. For this purpose, a special extension was devised, consisting of a metal plate fixed on the skull and placed exactly parallel to the stereotaxic apparatus. The head of the monkey was mounted on the stereotaxic frame with the help of this plate, thus making it possible to reach the deep subcortical structures while the animal was awake and trembling. Preliminary results of the recording from the cerebellum and brainstem have been already reported (10,13). To date, only ipsilateral cerebellar neurons have been involved passively during the tremor, especially two groups of neurons lying deep in the ipsilateral lobulus paramedianus and receiving afferent impulses from the mechanical stimulus of the tremor.

To test the hypothesis that the rhythmic activity responsible for production of tremor originates in the central nervous system and descends in the spinal cord (7,11), an attempt was made to find rhythmic discharges in the upper cervical cord of 2 animals. Under local anesthesia, a laminectomy was performed at the C_1 and C_2 level to expose spinal cord; the head of monkey was fixed on the stereotaxic apparatus as described above.

With the aid of a glass micropipette or a metal (tungsten or Elgiloy) electrode, systematic trackings were made searching for rhythmic discharges related to the tremor monitored by EMG. In the awake trembling monkey, stable extracellular recording from the spinal cord was rather difficult but several unitary or multiunitary rhythmic spike discharges were found. For each rhythmic unit, time relation between the spike and the corresponding EMG discharge was analyzed as shown in Fig. 3. Up to now, we have identified five units which were considered to discharge before the EMG bursts, suggesting the existence of descending tremor-driving activities. Such rhythmic discharges were found always deep in the ipsilateral ventral quadrant of the spinal cord, 1–2 mm lateral to the midline. In fact, responses to natural *upper limb* stimulation were encountered in the dorsal part of the cord before reaching the responsive target. This represented a good landmark to determine the proper laterality. One of the recorded points was marked by ferrocyanide using an Elgiloy electrode. Histological examination revealed that the marked point was located at the lateral edge of the ventral horn around Rexed's area VII at the C_1 level (Fig. 4). As this monkey had no tremor of the neck and the spike discharges

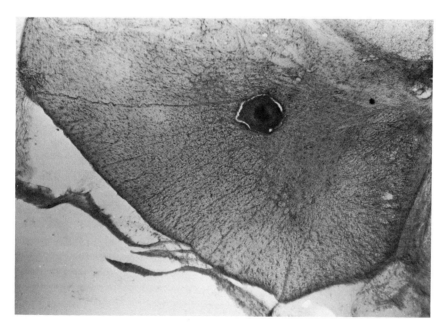

FIG. 4. Right ventral quadrant of the C_1 spinal cord illustrating a point from which rhythmic discharges were recorded. The point is marked by ferrocyanide using Elgiloy electrode.

were positive at C_1, it seems that the fiber activity most likely corresponds to nervous impulses in the descending pathway mediating the tremor.

SUMMARY AND COMMENT

A stereotaxic method to produce experimental spontaneous tremor in the monkey is described. With the aid of radiological and neurophysiological control methods, a spontaneous sustained tremor could be produced in a high percentage of the operated animals. Although histological study has not been included in this paper, the restricted lesions more or less occupied the area between rostral part of the red nucleus and the substantia nigra (9). This is a slightly different area from that described by Poirier et al. (18). The detailed pathological study of the lesions in our series will be presented elsewhere.

Now that the first requirement, i.e., constant production of experimental tremor, is established, the way is open to identify the neural mechanisms of tremor. As a first step toward this end, a neurophysiological study was carried out to localize descending rhythmic discharges in the spinal cord. Such activity was found at the end of the ventral quadrant of the cervical cord ipsilateral to the tremor. At present, it is not yet quite clear which pathway is responsible for this activity. However, it might be correct to assume that the corticospinal tract is not necessarily involved as a tremor-mediating pathway.

REFERENCES

1. Atlas, D., and Ingram, W. R. (1937): Topography of the brain stem of the rhesus monkey with special reference to the diencephalon. *J. Comp. Neurol.*, 66:263–289.
2. Feger, J., Ohye, Ch., Gallouin, F., and Albe-Fessard, D. (1975): A stereotaxic technique for stimulation and recording in non-anesthetized monkeys: application to the determination of connections between caudate nucleus and substantia nigra. In: *Advances in Neurology, Vol. 10,* edited by B. S. Meldrum and C. D. Marsden, pp. 35–45. Raven Press, New York.
3. Fukamachi, A., Ohye, Ch., Saito, Y., and Narabayashi, H. (1977): Estimation of the neural noise within the human thalamus. *Acta Neurochir. (Suppl.),* 24:121–136.
4. Gybels, J. M. (1963): *The Neural Mechanism of Parkinsonian Tremor.* Presses Académiques Européennes, Bruxelles.
5. Holmes, G. (1904): On certain tremors in organic cerebral lesions. *Brain,* 27:327–375.
6. Kremer, M., Russell, W. R., and Smyth, G. E. (1947): A mid-brain syndrome following head injury. *J. Neurol. Neurosurg. Psychiatry,* 10:49–60.
7. Lamarre, Y. (1975): Tremorigenic mechanisms in primates. In: *Advances in Neurology, Vol. 10,* edited by B. S. Meldrum and C. D. Marsden, pp. 23–34. Raven Press, New York.
8. Leksell, L. (1971): *Stereotaxis and Radiosurgery. An Operative System.* Charles C Thomas, Springfield, Ill.
9. Ohye, Ch. (1978): Pathophysiology of extrapyramidal disorders in primate models. *Adv. Neurol. Sci.,* 23:765–767 *(Japanese).*
10. Ohye, Ch., and Albe-Fessard, D. (1978): Rhythmic discharges related to tremor in humans and monkeys. In: *Abnormal Neuronal Discharges,* edited by N. Chalazonitis, p. 37–48. Raven Press, New York.
11. Ohye, Ch., Bouchard, R., Larochelle, L., Bédard, P., Boucher, R., Raphy, B., and Poirier, L. J. (1970): Effect of dorsal rhizotomy on postural tremor in the monkey. *Exp. Brain Res.,* 10:140–150.
12. Ohye, Ch., Fukamachi, A., Miyazaki, M., Isobe, I., Nakajima, H., and Shibazaki, T. (1977):

Physiologically controlled selective thalamotomy for the treatment of abnormal movement by Leksell's open system. *Acta Neurochir.,* 37:93–104.

13. Ohye, Ch., Miyazaki, M., Isobe, I., and Shibazaki, T. (1977): Constantly produced spontaneous sustained tremor and its relation to neural activity of the cerebellum in monkey. *Proc. IUPS (Paris),* 13:562.

14. Ohye, Ch., and Narishige, E. (1977): A new stereotaxic approach to the deep subcortical structures in the awake monkey. *Clin. Physiol.,* 7:170–176 *(Japanese).*

15. Percheron, G., and Lacourly, N. (1973): L'imprécision de la stéréotaxie thalamique utilisant les coordonnées crâniennes de Horsley-Clarke chez le macaque. *Exp. Brain Res.,* 18:355–373.

16. Peterson, E. W., Magoun, H. W., McCulloch, W. S., and Lindsely, D. B. (1949): Production of postural tremor. *J. Neurophysiol.,* 12:371–384.

17. Poirier, L. J. (1960): Experimental and histological study of midbrain dyskinesias. *J. Neurophysiol.,* 23:534–551.

18. Poirier, L. J., Bouvier, G., Bédard, P., Boucher, R., Larochelle, L., Olivier, A., and Singh, P. (1969): Essai sur les circuits neuronaux impliqués dans le tremblement postural et l'hypokinésie. *Rev. Neurol.,* 120:12–40.

19. Talairach, J., de Ajuriaguerra, J., and David, M. (1952): Etudes stéréotaxiques des structures encéphaliques profondes chez l'homme. *Presse Méd.,* 28:605–609.

20. Ward, Jr., A. A., McCulloch, W. S., and Magoun, H. W. (1948): Production of an alternating tremor at rest in monkeys. *J. Neurophysiol.,* 11:317–330.

Advances in Neurology, Vol. 24, edited by
L. J. Poirier, T. L. Sourkes, and P. J. Bédard.
Raven Press, New York © 1979.

Electronmicroscopic Differentiation of the Extrinsic and Intrinsic Types of Nerve Cells and Synapses in the Striatum and Their Putative Transmitters

R. Hassler

*Neurobiology Department, Max-Planck-Institut für Hirnforschung,
Frankfurt/Main, Germany*

The three main parts of the striatum—the putamen, caudate nucleus, and so-called limbic striatum or nucleus accumbens septi—have very similar, if not the same myelo- and cytoarchitecture (51). Each is made up of a few large cells and numerous small nerve cells that have always been regarded as interneurons. Recently it was found that each of the three main parts of the striatum contains the same nine types of synapses with only a few differences (10,24,25). Furthermore, since architectonic (5,41) and fine structural methods have demonstrated that the nucleus accumbens septi has the same features as the caudate nucleus and the putamen, Brockhaus suggested that a more accurate description would be the "fundus striati." The finer differentiations made by Brockhaus, as well as the nerve cell ratio determined by Namba, though entirely justified and realistic, may be disregarded initially for practical physiological or pharmacological reasons.

Since the time of Nothnagel (42), Ramon (47), Cajal (6), and Déjerine (11), the striatum has been regarded as a forebrain structure characterized by a large number (more than 90%) of Golgi type II small neurons, or interneurons having only intrinsic connections, a few (1%) giant projecting neurons, a few (5%) large neurons with undetermined projections, and a few dwarf neurogliaform cells (1%). The time-tested concept of the striatum as an integrative brain center, based on clinico-anatomical findings (2,50,55,56), Golgi material, and neurophysiological and experimental evidence (1,34) has been recently discarded by Grofová (19), Di Figlia et al. (13), and Pasik et al. (44), mainly on the basis of studies involving the use of horseradish peroxidase (HRP) and Golgi methods. The value of the Golgi method is limited because it cannot be used experimentally or quantitatively, and the HRP method must also be questioned on account of its endogenous labeling of distinct types of nerve cells without localized HRP injection and the difficulties of restricting the uptake of HRP to a specific and uniform neuronal system. The papers of Kitai et al. (32,33) seemed to confirm that the "spiny" striatal cells are not interneurons, since only those neurons from which antidromic spikes had been recorded during stimulation of the nigra can be labeled afterwards by HRP iontophoresis into the caudate nucleus. However, in these studies HRP labeling was not done by the typical retrograde method, but rather by direct labeling of more than one single "spiny" neuron, which does not allow identification of the single neuron from which the antidromic spike had been recorded before.

The earlier concept of the striatum as a regulatory center has been also supported by the fact that most studies suggest that no signs of retrograde degeneration in the striatum follow extensive lesions in the substantia nigra. Therefore, retrograde nerve cell degeneration in the striatum had to be investigated electron-microscopically. The experimental technique for identifying the intrinsic and extrinsic nerve cells and synapses consists of isolating a vertical column of striatal tissue by introducing a stainless steel tube (5 mm in diameter), and leaving the tissue cylinder isolated from all afferent and efferent connections *in situ* (Fig. 1). The effect of "columnar isolation" in the caudate nucleus and limbic striatum (or fundus striati) were studied after survival periods of 2, 14, and 28 days, respectively.

EXTRINSIC AND INTRINSIC TYPE OF STRIATAL NERVE CELLS

The ultrastructural differentiation of the various cell types was based on the distinction between "aspiny" and "spiny" neurons (16,17,46). The striatal giant neurons (7), which are rich in intracellular organelles [Mori's type II large cells (40)], are "aspiny" in the sense that the soma and stem dendrites bear

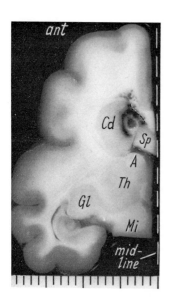

FIG. 1. Unstained horizontal section of cat's brain showing a columnar isolation of caudate nucleus tissue after 2 weeks' survival time following punching with a 5-mm metal tube. The shrunken tissue cylinder is demarcated by small hemorrhages.

many axosomatic synapses, whereas the "spiny" neurons almost completely lack axosomatic contacts. In these neurons the vast majority of the synaptic terminals contact the spines of the dendrites. The few "aspiny" neurons, identifiable by the intact axosomatic contacts (Fig. 2), undergo severe electron-dense degeneration after 28 days of columnar isolation of the striatal tissue (Fig. 2). The cytoplasm is extremely shrunken; the perinuclear space is filled with proliferated and very dense small mitochondria that are intermingled with some lysosomes and elongated tubes of the Golgi apparatus. The peripheral and the perinu-

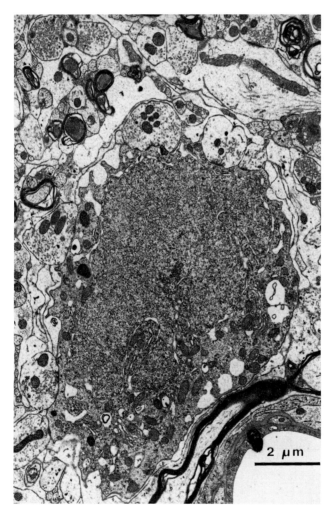

FIG. 2. Dark degeneration of a giant aspiny striatal neuron in contact with many well preserved axosomatic boutons. Four weeks survival time after mechanical isolation from all afferent and efferent connections.

clear zone of the perikaryon are filled with proliferated and very electron-dense endoplasmic reticulum with enlarged cisterns and numerous proliferated ribosomes and polysomes. Two days after the experimental procedure, the endoplasmic reticulum has considerably proliferated and the number of enlarged lysosomes and lipofuscin bodies have increased. After 2 days, as after 4 weeks, the cell membrane is indented by astrocytic vacuoles or by synaptic boutons with well-preserved synaptic vesicles. In Fig. 2, the nucleus, that is deeply indented by fingerlike processes of the proliferated endoplasmic reticulum, is strongly electron-dense but shows only moderate shrinkage. The picture is the same 2 days and 4 weeks after the intervention. During the 2- to 28-day period, the number of darkly degenerated nerve cells in proportion to the other nerve cells is always less than 2%. According to the law of the neuron theory, the dark degeneration of the giant neurons represents retrograde degeneration. These neurons are extrinsic projection cells.

Most of the smaller nerve cells that are "spiny" neurons because they lack axosomatic synapses, show only important swellings of the cytoplasm and the nucleus 2 days as well as 2 and 4 weeks after columnar isolation (Fig. 3). The smooth nuclear membrane shows multiple indentations produced by fingerlike outgrowths of the proliferated endoplasmic reticulum. The number of lysosomes and mitochondria is slightly increased (Fig. 3). Because the small neurons do not show signs of dark degeneration or irreversible disintegration of organelles, one must assume that these neurons and their processes do not extend outside the isolated tissue cylinder. If the rare dwarf cells of the striatum (18) could be differentiated at all on the basis of chromatin agglomeration on the membrane of the extraordinarily small nuclei, it must be concluded that they do not undergo alterations except for cytoplasmic swelling. Like dwarf cells, the spiny neurons belong to the Golgi type II neurons and are functionally interneurons. The spiny neurons represent the intrinsic striatal nerve cells.

Another group of large or medium-sized nerve cells, that usually have axosomatic synaptic contacts show a moderate but still more severe type of alteration than the small spiny neurons. Even 2 days after the isolation of the tissue, the size of the cell but not the nucleus is slightly reduced. Also, the rough endoplasmic reticulum has moderately proliferated and the number of ribosomes, polysomes, and lysosomes or lipofuscin bodies is increased (Fig. 4); the cytoplasm is only slightly darker than normal, in contrast to the dark degeneration of the cells shown in Fig. 2. The nucleus with its large prominent nucleolus shows more and deeper infoldings caused by the rough-surfaced endoplasmic reticulum. The cytoplasmic matrix shows more floccular profiles than normal and some sharply bordered cytoplasmic clearings (Fig. 4). This type of alteration may be called "penumbral alteration." It occurs in 2–4% of all striatal large-sized aspiny neurons that contain few cytoplasmic organelles. They were classified electronmicroscopically as "large nerve cells type I" by Mori (40).

We view this alteration as representing a reversible retrograde reaction to a minor neuronal damage, which does not result in dark degeneration and necrosis.

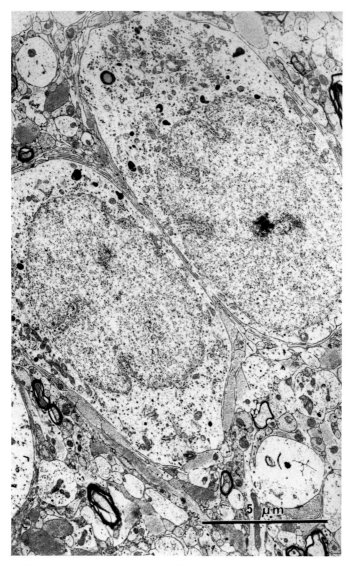

FIG. 3. Two adjacent spiny neurons (note lack of axosomatic boutons) 4 weeks after columnar isolation of striatal tissue. Moderate increase of organelles in the swollen cytoplasm and nuclear membrane indentations may be observed.

The neurons seem to survive the damage caused to the short peripheral parts of their axons, which presumably terminate in the pallidum. The penumbral alteration of the large type I striatal cells (40) indicates that they undergo a slight retrograde alteration, because their terminals have been severed close to the striatum and separated from their perikarya. These aspiny neurons which

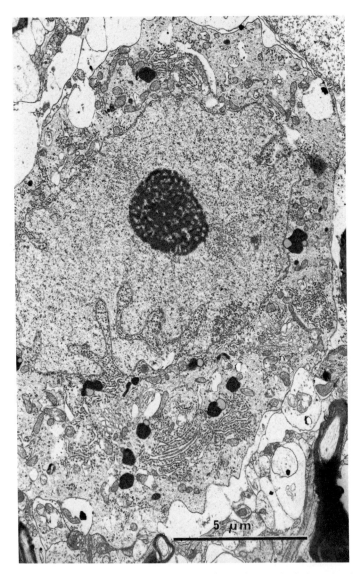

FIG. 4. Aspiny large neuron type I of Mori 2 days after columnar isolation of striatal tissue from the cerebral surrounding areas. Cytoplasm contains cytoplasmic clearing proliferated floccular material and endoplasmic reticulum without electron-dense degeneration, as well as many lysosomes and lipofuscin bodies. The nuclear membrane is indented at several points by proliferated endoplasmic reticulum, although the nucleoplasm is not degenerated.

undergo penumbral alteration are extrinsic nerve cells and presumably project to the pallidum.

EXTRINSIC AND INTRINSIC TYPES OF STRIATAL SYNAPSES

Of the nine different types of synapses we have distinguished in the cat striatum, all three types of axospinous synapses undergo dark degeneration two days after the tissue cylinder has been isolated from all afferent and efferent connections. In Fig. 5, a presynaptic bouton of a caudate type IV synapse is shown to have undergone a dark degeneration; synaptic vesicles can no longer be recognized although the large spine that engulfs the bouton does not show any alteration except for swelling and increased number of floccular elements. The axodendritic type VII bouton (10) that contacts the larger clear dendrite is severely altered. The axoplasm is extremely dark and the synaptic vesicles fuse. A dark microglia process is sandwiched between the degenerated bouton and the large, swollen, although not degenerated, dendrite. The bouton type VIII is much less altered, although the shrunken and darkened small vesicles are aggregated so that large areas of dendroplasm are free of vesicles. In contrast,

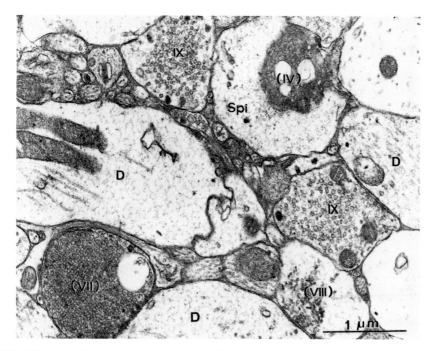

FIG. 5. Electron micrograph of caudate tissue 2 days after columnar isolation from the surrounding cerebral structures. Severely degenerated boutons of axospinous type IV and axodendritic type VII. Type VIII dendrodendritic bouton with aggregated small vesicles. Well-preserved synaptic vesicles in axodendritic type IX (intrinsic) boutons. [After Hassler (25).]

the axodendritic boutons type IX contain well-preserved clear large vesicles of approximately 60 nm diameter and a few dense core vesicles in the periphery.

In the isolated caudate tissue cylinder (Fig. 1), a type VI bouton has lost many of the flattened vesicles, and in others, the membranes are disintegrating and confluent with the darkened axoplasm. The type V (axon-collateral) bouton with pleomorphic vesicles is altered only moderately, if at all, and contains disintegrating vesicles (Fig. 6). The type VIII dendrodendritic bouton has undergone slight alteration although most of the small vesicles have disappeared. The large round vesicle boutons (type IX) contact a dendrite that contains a large number of microtubules (probably a stem dendrite of a type I large cell of Mori). They are intact and even contain some dense core vesicles (Fig. 7).

From these pictures and a large number of other isolation experiments, it becomes clear that the axospinous boutons type I, III, and IV undergo an irreversible dark degeneration in the isolated striatal tissue cylinder after 2 days.

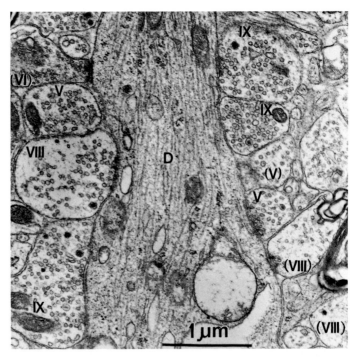

FIG. 6. Mechanically isolated caudate tissue 2 days after punching shows completely preserved large round vesicle boutons type IX contacting a longitudinal-sectioned dendrite (D), in which the microtubules are closer together. The bouton type (VI) containing elongated vesicles has undergone dissolution of most synaptic vesicles which fuse with the darkened axoplasm in the center of bouton. In two type (V) boutons, the pleomorphic vesicles are more or less preserved. The type (VIII) bouton can still be recognized, although it has lost most synaptic vesicles.

These types of boutons are extrinsic, i.e., their cell of origin is outside the striatal tissue cylinder.

The same is true for the axodendritic or axosomatic synapses of types VI and VII. In the experimental material it was not possible to identify intact or degenerated boutons type II *(en passage),* which is understandable since this type is very rare and the boutons have lost the typical synaptic *en passage* contact. The type IX (large round vesicle axodendritic or axosomatic bouton) is completely preserved in almost all samples, or shows only a small decrease of synaptic vesicles. The type V boutons that are regarded as belonging to axon-collaterals of striatal projection cells because they are pleomorphic like the strionigral boutons are either preserved or only moderately altered as seen in Fig. 6. The various ways in which the same type of boutons react to the interruption of all afferent connections could be related to their different origins, i.e., whether they arise from the giant striatal nerve cells that undergo dark degeneration, or from the large striatal nerve cells that undergo only a penumbral alteration. As to the type VIII bouton, it is remarkable that they never undergo dark degeneration in isolated striatal tissue cylinders, but frequently show a

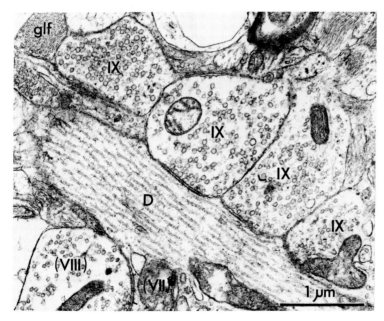

FIG. 7. Caudate tissue 2 weeks after columnar isolation from the surrounding cerebral structures. The three type IX axodendritic boutons contacting the longitudinally cut dendrite (D) contain unchanged large round vesicles and synaptic contacts like the fourth type IX bouton. The small vesicles in the clear dendroplasm of type VIII bouton are only slightly altered, whereas the type VII bouton *(bottom)* had undergone a dark degeneration. The bouton compartment *(upper left)* is filled with glia fibers.

light alteration with rarefaction of the synaptic vesicles which fuse together. In the fundus striati, they are usually well preserved and may even be entirely intact. The origin of these presumably dendrodendritic synapses could be the abundantly branched dendrites of dwarf cells, which have longer processes in the caudate than in the fundus striati.

THE TRANSMITTERS OF THE DIFFERENT TYPES OF SYNAPSES

In the great majority of synapses, synaptic transmission involves chemical transmitters, that differ according to the neuronal system involved. The question should be asked whether each of the nine types of synapses distinguished in the three main parts of the striatum has a different and well-defined transmitter. Since 1959 and the work of Bertler and Rosengren (4) as well as Carlsson (8) dopamine (DA) has been known to be one transmitter in the striatum. One year later, Ehringer and Hornykiewicz (14) and then Hornykiewicz (27) demonstrated that in human Parkinson syndromes, the concentration of DA in the striatum (and also in the substantia nigra) is much reduced. Following experimental interruption of the nigrostriatal fibers in rat, cat, and monkey, DA concentration in the striatum is strongly decreased. It is generally established that DA is the transmitter of the nigrostriatal pathway. From the work of Bak et al. (3) and Chung and Hassler (9), it is known that the terminal boutons of the nigrostriatal fibers are type I (axospinous) and type II (axodendritic *en passage*). Therefore, it can be concluded that DA is stored as a transmitter in these two types of striatal boutons.

Since Fahn and Côté (15) it has been known that the substantia nigra of monkeys has the highest concentration of γ-aminobutyric acid (GABA). Okada et al. (43) demonstrated an equally high GABA content in the substantia nigra and an only slightly lower GABA content in the pallidum, also in rat, rabbit, cat, and baboon [see Hassler (23)]. After interruption of nigrostriatal fibers, GABA concentration drops to 30–40% (30). GABA is probably a transmitter of strionigral neurons. Recent immunohistochemical investigations indicate that the peptide substance P is a concurrent transmitter of the strionigral neurons, mainly of the neurons whose fibers terminate in the rostral nigra reticulata. The terminal boutons of these nigrostriatal fibers are of the pleomorphic type (20,21,30). The same pleomorphic type of boutons exist in the striatum. They store GABA or substance P in the nigra as well as in the striatum without a morphologic distinction so far between GABA-ergic and substance P-ergic boutons.

It has been assumed for a long time that the thalamostriatal fibers originate in the nerve cells of the center median parafascicular complex (22,37,52). These terminals are axospinous type IV boutons, or axosomatic and axodendritic type VII boutons (10). The transmitter substance of these neurons is probably acetylcholine (23,29,48,53).

Webster (54), using the rat, and Kemp and Powell (28), using the monkey, have established that corticostriate connections originate from almost all cortical areas and reach different parts of the striatum. The transmitter of these cortico-striate neurons whose endings are either type III or type VII boutons (25), seems to be glutamate. This is supported by the results of Spencer (49), who found that cortical excitation of striatal neurons is antagonized by glutamic acid diethylester, and Kim et al. (31), who found a drop of striatalglutamic acid level after frontal cortex ablation. In addition, Divac et al. (12) and McGeer et al. (35,36) reported a high affinity uptake of glutamate in terminals of cortico-striatal axons.

The intrinsic synapses type IX of the striatum, which does not degenerate after complete interruption of all extrinsic afferents, seem to have acetylcholine (ACh) as the transmitter, in view of the fact that the caudate nucleus at least has a cholinergic mechanism (38,45). The active transmitters in type VI and type VIII synapses are not known so far.

THE CAUDATE NIGRAL MESHED REVERBERATING NEURONAL CIRCUIT

In the light of this detailed study of distinct synaptic contacts and their transmitters, in the neuronal circuit, we will attempt to give our view of the switching arrangements between the caudate nucleus, the anterior part of nigra compacta, and the other inputs to the caudate nucleus, taking into account the excitatory or inhibitory nature of their transmitters.

The nerve cells of nigra compacta anterior (Ni.a), which are under the inhibitory control of the GABA-ergic caudatal projection cells, give rise to the dopaminergic feedback fibers (Fig. 8, black), which in turn, reach the interneuronal pool of the caudate nucleus. Other inputs from the center median neurons (possibly cholinergic) (green) and from the frontal, prefrontal, and perhaps premotor cortical areas (red), which are glutamatergic, also converge on this interneuronal apparatus. As in most other highly integrating structures, the majority of the nerve cells are interneurons (greater than 90% in the caudate nucleus). More than two-thirds of the synaptic contacts occur on these interneurons. They are excited by the glutamic acid transmitter of the cortical afferents, inhibited by the DA of the substantia nigra synapses (39), and perhaps moderated by the ACh of the center median afferents (green). In the caudate nucleus, the center median afferents predominate over the other two inputs of the interneurons. A great amount of evidence has been accumulated suggesting that the interneurons act through intrinsic synapses by ACh on the giant or large output neurons. This action is in competition with other synaptic contacts originating directly from (a) the nigra-neurons (black) through the *en passage* synaptic contacts with DA as transmitter, (b) the glutamatergic cortical neurons (red) through the type VII contacts, and (c) the cholinergic neurons of the center median nucleus (green), also acting through type VII contacts.

An even greater number of synapses converge on the few giant and large

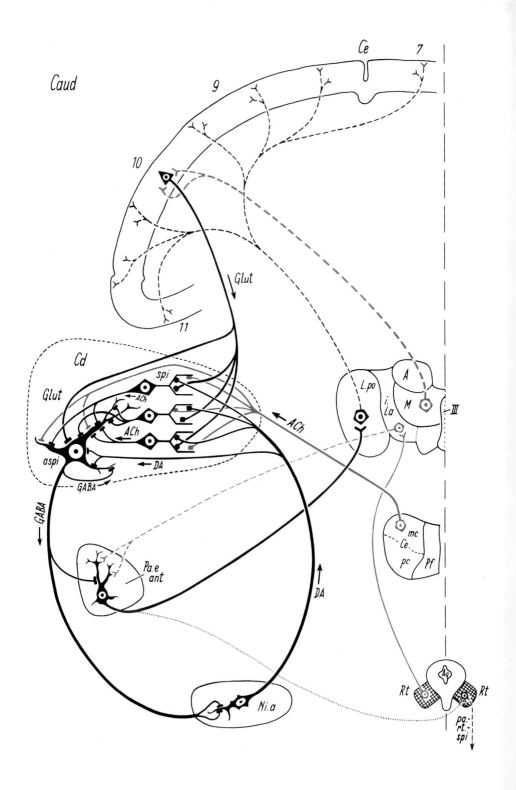

projecting neurons of the caudate nucleus. The mode of action of the three different transmitters (there are at least three) on the large and giant neurons are still unknown, although some of them seem to act in the opposite direction than they do on the striatal interneurons. The efferent fibers of the projecting cells, as well as the intracaudatal axon-collaterals, are either GABA-ergic or substance P-ergic. An inhibitory influence is exerted on the pallidum externum cells as well as the nigra compacta anterior cells. In contrast to the feedback circuit of the putamen, that of the caudate has only a minimal descending influence, if any at all, on the reticulospinal neurons.

In view of the fact that the nigra anterior also has a predominantly ascending action on the caudate nucleus, the main output of this circuit acts on the rostral pole of the lateral thalamic nuclei (L.po. or VA). Recent electrophysiological studies indicate that this nucleus has a nonspecific activating influence on many cortical areas (Fig. 8, red).

It is important to realize that the caudatonigral circuit is not a simple one, but a complicated meshed circuit interacting with at least two other afferent systems at the level of the interneuronal apparatus. The functional significance of this meshed circuit is discussed elsewhere (23a).

SUMMARY

In order to analyze the neuronal organization and the synaptic transmission of the three different parts of the striatum (putamen, caudate, and the so-called limbic striatum), experiments have been made in which a vertical column of striatal tissue was isolated from all afferent and efferent connections by inserting a stainless steel tube measuring 5 mm in diameter. Two, fourteen, or twenty-eight days after such isolation of tissue columns, all "aspiny" giant nerve cells (representing less than 2% of neurons) were darkly degenerated. Three to six percent of the larger spiny cells underwent penumbral alteration characterized by moderate proliferation of the endoplasmic reticulum, polysomes and lysosomes, and cytoplasmic incorporation of floccular profiles, as well as sharply bordered clearings without an irreversible shrinking of cytoplasmic organelles. More than 90% of all nerve cells, including the dwarf cells of Cajal, show only a cytoplasmic swelling without any sign of dark degeneration. According to the neuron theory, the latter small "spiny" neurons cannot have lost any important parts of their neuronal constituents. Therefore, they should be re-

----

FIG. 8. Meshed caudatonigral feedback circuit. *Black:* Afferent dopaminergic (DA) nigra neurons (only Ni. a). The spiny (cholinergic) interneurons with dendritic spine tree on which converge nigral and cholinergic (ACh) centrothalamo *(green)* -caudatal afferents, and glutamatergic cortico–caudate *(red)* afferents. *Black* also represents the interneuronal pool with its cholinergic (ACh) synaptic contacts to the aspiny projection cells. The latter neurons terminate as GABA-ergic synapses on the dendrites of nigra cells and on the dendrites of cells of pallidum externum anterius *(red)*. The thalamocortical semispecific pathway projects [through nucleus lateropolaris (L. po)] to most prefrontal and premotor areas including parietal area 7. Each of the three inputs, known so far, have an emergency break synapse on the large projecting neurons.

garded as intrinsic neurons. The dark degeneration of the "aspiny" giant nerve cells is a retrograde one, due to the loss of the most important parts of the axon. They are the cells with long extrinsic projections presumably to the substantia nigra. The undergoing penumbral alterations of the long "aspiny" large neurons are tentatively explained as a consequence of the reaction to the interruption of their longer axonal processes at the level of the adjacent pallidum. The dopaminergic synapses type I and the type II *("en passage")* are darkly degenerated because they lose their perikaryon outside of the striatum, as do the glutamatergic types III and VII, and the probably cholinergic types IV and VII. All of these are extrinsic types of synapses. The type IX synapses with large round vesicles seem to be intrinsic because they are completely preserved in the isolated tissue; they originate from the intrinsic "spiny" neurons and are probably cholinergic. The pleomorphic type V synapses are in most instances intact, and are regarded as GABA-ergic synapse from axon collaterals. The type VIII dendro-dendritic synapse is better preserved in the isolated fundus striati than in the caudate. It may be speculated that type VIII synapse is the dendritic terminal of the intrinsic dwarf cells.

REFERENCES

1. Akert, K., and Andersson, B. (1951): Experimenteller Beitrag zur Physiologie des Nucleus caudatus. *Acta Physiol. Scand.,* 22:281–298.
2. Anton, G. (1896): Über die Beteiligung der grossen basalen Gehirnganglien bei Bewegungsstörungen und insbesondere bei Chorea. *Jb. Psychiat.,* 14:141–181.
3. Bak, I. J., Choi, W. B., Hassler, R., Usunoff, K. G., and Wagner, A. (1975): Fine structural synaptic organization of the corpus striatum and substantia nigra in rat and cat. In: *Advances in Neurology; Vol. 9: Dopaminergic Mechanisms,* edited by D. B. Calne, T. N. Chase, and A. Barbeau, pp. 25–41. Raven Press, New York.
4. Bertler, A., and Rosengren, E. (1959): On the distribution in brain of monoamines and of enzymes responsible for their formation. *Experientia,* 15:382–385.
5. Brockhaus, H. (1942): Zur feineren Anatomie des Septum und des Striatum. *J. Psychol. Neurol.,* 51:1–56.
6. Cajal, S. R. (1894): Algunas contribuciones al conocimiento de los ganglios del encéfalo: v. Cuerpo estriado. *Anat. Soc. espan. Historia natural,* 2 agosto.
7. Cajal, S. R. (1911): *Histologie du Système Nerveux Central, Vol. II.* Maloine, Paris.
8. Carlsson, A. (1959): The occurrence distribution and physiological role of catecholamines in the nervous system. *Pharmacol. Rev.,* 11:490–493.
9. Chung, J. W., Hassler, R., and Wagner, A. (1976): Degenerated boutons in the fundus striati (nucleus accumbens septi) after lesion of the parafascicular nucleus in the cat. *Cell Tissue Res.,* 172:1–14.
10. Chung, J. W., Hassler, R., and Wagner, A. (1977): Degeneration of two of nine types of synapses in the putamen after center median coagulation in the cat. *Exp. Brain Res.,* 28:345–361.
11. Dèjèrine, J. (1901): *Anatomie des Centres Nerveux, Vol. 2.* Rueff, Paris.
12. Divac, I., Fonnum, F., and Storm-Mathisen, J. (1977): High affinity uptake of glutamate in terminals of corticostriatal axons. *Nature (Lond),* 266:377–378.
13. Di Figlia, M., Pasik, P., and Pasik, T. (1976): A Golgi study of neuronal types in the neostriatum of monkeys. *Brain Res.,* 114:245–356.
14. Ehringer, H., and Hornykiewicz, O. (1960): Verteilung von Noradrenalin und Dopamin (3-Hydroxytyramin) im Gehirn des Menschen und ihr Verhalten bei Erkrankungen des extrapyramidalen Systems. *Klin. Wochenschr.,* 38:1236–1239.

15. Fahn, S., and Côté, L. J. (1968): Regional distribution of γ-aminobutyric acid (GABA) in brain of the Rhesus monkey. *J. Neurochem.,* 15:209–213.
16. Fox, C. A., Andrade, A. N., Hillman, D. E., and Schwyn, R. C. (1971): The spiny neurons in the primate striatum: A Golgi and electron microscopic study. *J. Hirnforsch.* 13:181–201.
17. Fox, C. A., Andrade, A. N., Schwyn, R. C., and Rafols, J. A. (1971/72): The aspiny neurons and the glia in the primate striatum: a Golgi and electron microscopic study. *J. Hirnforsch.,* 13:341–362.
18. Fox, C. A., Lu Qui, I. J., and Rafols, J. A. (1975): Further observations on Ramon y Cajal's "dwarf" or "neuroglioform" neurons and the oligodendroglia in the primate striatum. *J. Hirnforsch.,* 15:517–527.
19. Grofová, I. (1975): The identification of striatal and pallidal neurons projecting to substantia nigra. An experimental study by means of retrograde axonal transport of horseradish peroxidase. *Brain Res.,* 91:286–291.
20. Grofová, I., and Rinvik, E. (1970): An experimental electron microscopic study on the striato-nigral projection. *Exp. Brain Res.,* 11:249–262.
21. Hajdu, R., Hassler, R. and Bak, I. J. (1973): Electron microscopic study of the substantia nigra and the strio-nigral projection in the rat. *Z. Zellforsch. Mikrosk. Anat.,* 146:207–221.
22. Hassler, R. (1949): Über die afferente Leitung und Steuerung des striären Systems. *Nervenarzt,* 20:537–541.
23. Hassler, R. (1974): Fiber connections within the extra-pyramidal system. *Confin. Neurol.,* 36:237–255.
23a. Hassler, R. (1978): Striatal control of locomotion, intentional actions and of integrating and perceptive activity. *J. Neurol. Sci.,* 36:187–224.
24. Hassler, R., and Chung, J. W. (1976): The discrimination of nine different types of synaptic boutons in the fundus striati (nucleus accumbens septi). *Cell Tissue Res.,* 168:489–505.
25. Hassler, R., Chung, J. W., Rinne, U., and Wagner, A. (1978): Selective degeneration of two out of the nine types of synapses in cat caudate nucleus after cortical lesions. *Exp. Brain Res.,* 31:67–80.
26. Hassler, R., Chung, J. W., Wagner, A., and Rinne, U. (1977): Experimental demonstration of intrinsic synapses in cat's caudate nucleus. *Neurosci. Lett.,* 5:117–121.
27. Hornykiewicz, O. (1963): Die topische Lokalisation und das Verhalten von Noradrenalin und Dopamin (3-Hydroxytypamin) in der Substantia nigra des normalen und Parkinson-kranken Menschen. *Wien. Klin. Wochenschr.,* 75:309–312.
28. Kemp, J. M., and Powell, T. S. P. (1970): The cortico-striate projection in the monkey. *Brain,* 93:525–546.
29. Kim, J. S. (1978): Transmitters for the afferent and efferent systems of the neostriatum and their possible interactions. In: *Advances in Biochemical Psychopharmacology Vol. 19,* edited by P. J. Roberts, G. N. Woodruff, and L. L. Iverson, pp. 217–233. Raven Press, New York.
30. Kim, J. S., Bak, I. S., Hassler, R., and Okada, Y. (1971): Role of γ-aminobutyric acid (GABA) in the extrapyramidal motor system. 2. Some evidence for the existence of a type of GABA-rich strio-nigral neurons. *Exp. Brain Res.,* 14:95–104.
31. Kim, J. S., Hassler, R., Haug, P., and Paik, K. S. (1977): Effect of frontal cortex ablation on striatal glutamic acid level in rat. *Brain Res.,* 132:370–374.
32. Kitai, S. T., Kocsis, J. D., Preston, R. J., and Sugimori, M. (1976): Monosynaptic inputs to caudate neurons identified by intracellular injection of horseradish peroxydase. *Brain Res.,* 109:601–606.
33. Kitai, S. T., Sugimori, M., and Kocsis, J. D. (1976): Excitatory nature of dopamine in the nigro-caudate pathway. *Exp. Brain Res.,* 21:351–362.
34. Laursen, A. M. (1963): Corpus striatum. *Acta Physiol. Scand., (Suppl. 211),* 59:1–106.
35. McGeer, E. G., and McGeer, P. L. (1977): A glutamatergic cortico-striatal path? *Proc. Int. Soc. Neurochem. (Kbh),* 6:229.
36. McGeer, P. L., McGeer, E. G., Scherer, U., and Singh, K. (1977): A glutamatergic cortico-striatal path? *Brain Res.,* 128:369–373.
37. McLardy, T. (1948): Projection of the centromedian nucleus of the human thalamus. *Brain,* 71:290–303.
38. McLennan, H., and York, D. H. (1966): Cholinergic mechanisms in the caudate nucleus. *J. Physiol.,* 187:163–175.
39. McLennan, H., and York, D. H. (1967): The action of dopamine on neurones of the caudate nucleus. *J. Physiol,* 189:393–402.

40. Mori, S. (1966): Some observations on the fine structure of the corpus striatum of the rat brain. *Z. Zellforsch. Mikrosk. Anat.,* 70:461–488.
41. Namba, M. (1957): Cytoarchitektonische Untersuchungen am Striatum. *J. Hirnforsch.,* 3:24–48.
42. Nothnagel, H. (1873): Experimentelle Untersuchungen über die Funktion des Gehirns. *Virchows Arch. Path. Anat.* 57:184–214.
43. Okada, Y., Nitsch-Hassler, C., Kim, J. S., Bak, I. J. and Hassler, R. (1971): The role of γ-aminobutyric acid (GABA) in the extrapyramidal motor system. 1. Regional distribution of GABA in rabbit, rat and guinea pig brain. *Exp. Brain Res.,* 13:514–518.
44. Pasik, P., Pasik, T., and DiFiglia, M. (1976): Quantitative aspects of neuronal organization in the neurostriatum of the macaque monkey. *Res. Publ. Assoc. Res. Nerv. Ment. Dis.,* 55:57–90.
45. Portig, P. J., and Vogt, M. (1969): Release into the cerebral ventricles of substances with possible transmitter function in the caudate nucleus. *J. Physiol.,* 204:687–715.
46. Rafols, J. A., and Fox, C. A. (1971/72): Further observations on the spiny neurons and synaptic endings in the striatum of the monkey. *J. Hirnforsch.,* 13:299–308.
47. Ramon Cajal, P. (1889): Trabajos de la seccion de tecnica anatomica de la Facultad de medicina de Zaragoza.
48. Simke, J. P., and Saelens, J. K. (1977): Evidence for a cholinergic fiber tract connecting the thalamus with the head of the striatum of the rat. *Brain Res.* 126:487–495.
49. Spencer, H. J. (1976): Antagonism of cortical excitation of striatal neurons by glutamic acid diethyl ester: evidence for glutamic acid as an excitatory transmitter in the rat striatum. *Brain Res.,* 102:91–101.
50. Vogt, C. (1911): Quelques considérations générales á propos du syndrome du corps strié. *J. Psychol. Neurol.,* 18:479–488.
51. Vogt, C., Vogt, O. (1919): Erster Versuch einer pathologisch-anatomischen Einteilungstriärer Motilitätsstörungen nebst Bemerkungen über seine allgemeine wissenschaftliche Bedeutung. *J. Psychol. Neurol.* 24:1–19.
52. Vogt, C., and Vogt, O. (1941): Thalamusstudien I–IV. *J. Psychol. Neurol.,* 50:32–153.
53. Wagner, A., Hassler, R., and Kim, J. S.: Striatal cholinergic enzyme activities following discrete centro-median nucleus lesion in cat thalamus. *5th Int. Meeting of the Int. Soc. Neurochemists (Abstr. 59),* Barcelona.
54. Webster, K. E. (1961): Cortico-striate interrelations in the albino rat. *J. Anat.,* 95:532–544.
55. Wilson, S. A. K. (1912): Progressive lenticular degeneration: a familial nervous disease associated with cirrhosis of the liver. *Brain,* 34:295–509.
56. Wilson, S. A. K. (1914): An experimental research into the anatomy and physiology of the corpus striatum. *Brain,* 36:427–492.

Advances in Neurology, Vol. 24, edited by
L. J. Poirier, T. L. Sourkes, and P. J. Bédard.
Raven Press, New York © 1979.

Experimental Tremor in Monkey: Activity of Thalamic and Precentral Cortical Neurons in the Absence of Peripheral Feedback

Yves Lamarre and Alfred J. Joffroy

Centre de Recherche en Sciences Neurologiques, Départment de Physiologie, Université de Montréal, Montréal, Québec, Canada; and Service de Neurochirurgie et Laboratoire de Neurochirurgie Expérimentale, Université Libre de Bruxelles, Bruxelles, Belgique

Studies on experimental disorders in animals can contribute to our understanding of the physiopathology of abnormal movements in the human. For several years, we have tried to elucidate the mechanisms responsible for the postural Parkinson-like tremor produced in the monkey by certain lesions of the central nervous system (CNS) (23). Neurons firing in phase with the tremor have been found in the contralateral sensorimotor cortex (5) and in the ventrolateral thalamus (VL) (14), which may be the site of tremorogenesis. However, as was stressed by Cordeau et al. (5), in this type of study one is confronted with a problem of cause and effect. The rhythmic pattern of neuronal activity could be the result of the tremor rather than its cause.

One way to suppress all rhythmic afferent input to the CNS from the trembling limbs is curarization. But, in the curarized unanesthetized preparation, posture as well as movement is lost and the animal is totally flaccid and shows a marked tendency to sleep (8). It is well known that in the normal animal VL units begin to discharge in rhythmic bursts as the state of vigilance is reduced (11,15) but this is not accompanied by tremor. In the present study, a second approach was used in order to avoid peripheral feedback: deafferentation of the trembling limb by section of the dorsal roots. Early observations in the parkinsonian patient (25) and in the monkey with experimental tremor (21) have shown that deafferentation does not prevent the occurrence of postural tremor in the affected limb. Chronic deafferentation thus provides the opportunity of recording episodes of tremor and other movements simultaneously with central unit activity without peripheral feedback from the limb under study.

This chapter presents results on microelectrode recordings made in the thalamus and in the precentral cortex in the deafferented or paralyzed unanesthetized monkey. Some data have been obtained after intravenous administration of harmaline. This substance is able to enhance or provoke tremor in the monkey with midbrain or cerebellar lesions, but has no such effect in the normal animal (24).

METHODS

Lesions were placed by electrocoagulation in the ventromedial portion of the pons and midbrain tegmentum of adult monkeys *(Macaca mulatta)* under aseptic conditions and general anesthesia. Eleven monkeys were selected and showed, in the days following the operation, a sustained postural tremor involving one or two limbs. The tremor appeared either spontaneously or after administration of harmaline. A certain degree of hypokinesia in the affected limb(s) was usual but no other major motor impairment was observed. A chamber for microelectrode insertion was attached to the skull using a method described elsewhere (17). The main feature of this method is that the chamber is also used to fasten the animal's head. The recording situation allows easy observation and recording of tremor and other movements. The same technique was used for recording in the monkey paralyzed with gallamine triethiodide. In this case, the animals were intubated for artificial ventilation and placed on a table. Three to five recording sessions were usually carried out in each animal during a period of 6 to 20 days. In two animals, the dorsal roots C_2–T_4 on the side of tremor were cut intradurally during a second operation.

The unit recordings were carried out with steel microelectrodes of 1-to 2-μ tip diameter. Electrodes were connected through a cathode follower input to a capacity coupled amplifier (bandpass: 30 Hz to 10 KHz). Other recordings included a precentral EEG derived from an epidural vitallium bone screw, electromyograms (EMG) recorded from pairs of stainless steel, noninsulated short needles, and limb displacement from a transducer attached to the trembling limb. The signals were monitored on an oscilloscope, recorded on moving film and were also fed in parallel to a magnetic tape recorder. Data were converted into digital form and processed by means of a PDP9 computer. Auto- and cross-correlations were performed to demonstrate rhythmicity and phase relationships. The effect of intravenous injections of harmaline on neuronal activity was tested on several occasions.

At the end of some microelectrode tracks a lesion was made by passing a 10-μA DC current through the tip of the electrode for 10 sec. After the last recording session, the animal was killed by an overdose of intravenous pentobarbital and perfused with 10% formaldehyde solution in 0.9% saline. The head was placed in a standard stereotaxic apparatus and a block of brain including the thalamus and midbrain was cut between two frontal planes. This block was fixed in 10% neutral formalin, after which serial frontal sections were stained according to the Klüver–Barrera technique. The extent of the pons and midbrain lesions was verified. The microelectrode tracks were reconstructed with reference to the atlas of Olszewski (22) for identification of thalamic nuclei. Detailed histological examination was made in order to identify nucleus ventralis lateralis (VL) and nucleus ventralis posterolateralis, pars oralis (VPL$_o$) from neighboring thalamic nuclei. Due to the imprecise boundaries between certain thalamic nuclei, definitive localization of each cell was not always possible.

RESULTS

Thalamic Recordings

From a total of 51 microelectrode tracks identified on histological sections, 505 thalamic neurons were recorded, 208 after paralysis with gallamine. Various observations were made concerning the relationships of unity activity with the state of vigilance (as judged from the EEG), passive movements, and other natural peripheral stimuli. The aim of this part of the study was to find thalamic neurons discharging rhythmically at a frequency comparable to the frequency of the tremor recorded in the same animal before curarization.

The majority of neurons recorded in the anterior part of the thalamus (VL_o, VA) (see Fig. 3B) had the same general characteristics of spontaneous activity as were described in the normal monkey (11,15): either a sustained firing at a mean discharge rate of up to 30/sec, or bursts of spikes occurring at about 5/sec, often contemporary with slow waves on the EEG (Figs. 1 and 2). As mentioned earlier, paralyzed animals have a tendency to sleep and this was reflected in both the EEG (slow waves) and the increase in bursting activity recorded from thalamic neurons. About 40% of the neurons recorded in VL_o showed a response to peripheral stimuli of the contralateral limbs (mainly quick pressure on tissues or passive movements of joints). In more posterior areas (Fig. 3B, shaded area), most cells showed continuous bursting unrelated to the state of vigilance and were unresponsive to any type of peripheral stimulation. Such cells have not been encountered in the normal paralyzed monkey (11). They were situated mainly in front and above the specific relay nuclei (in VPL_o and in posterior VL_o and VL_c). They were found in a zone extending rostrocaudally for about 4 to 5 mm and involving mainly the midportion of the lateral

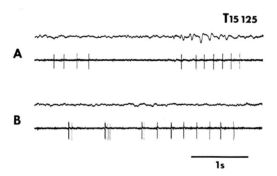

FIG. 1. Spontaneous activity of a thalamic unit (VL_c) recorded in a curarized, unanesthetized monkey on the same side as a midbrain tegmental lesion that had provoked a contralateral postural tremor in the arm. In **A** and **B**, the upper trace is the motor cortex EEG and the lower trace is the unit discharge during periods of spontaneous bursting. **A:** bursting occurs at a frequency of about 6.5/sec during the occurrence of an EEG spindle. **B:** in the absence of cortical slow waves, bursting occurs at a lower frequency of 4.5/sec.

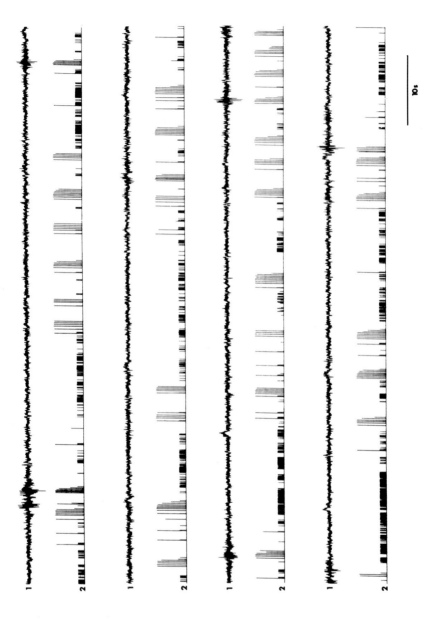

10s

FIG. 2. Ongoing activity of the same cell shown in Fig. 1. **Line 1:** motor cortex EEG. **Line 2:** unit discharge display obtained by feeding an ink-writing polygraph with a standard pulse triggered by each spike. Due to the high firing rate within the bursts, the deflection of the pen exceeds the standard pulse height during episodes of bursting. Periods of bursting activity alternate with periods of tonic activity. The four sets of records are continuous and the total time of recording is 5.5 min.

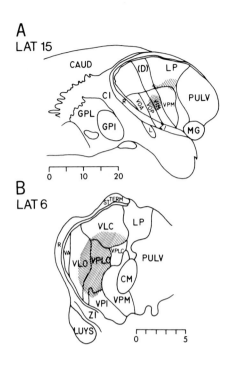

FIG. 3. A: Parasagittal section of human thalamus. (Redrawn from Albe-Fessard et al., ref. 2.) **B:** Parasagittal section of monkey thalamus. (Reconstructed from Olszewski ref. 22.) The shaded zones indicate where rhythmic bursting has been recorded in parkinsonian patients **(A)** and in monkeys with experimental rest tremor **(B)**.

thalamus (5 to 6 mm lateral to the midline). Often, these cells were encountered throughout a distance 5 to 6 mm long in the same vertical penetration. Figure 3B shows the region where these rhythmic units were encountered. The thalamic nuclei have been redrawn from Olszewski's atlas in a saggital plane, 6 mm from the midline where most of the units were found. This region is homologous to the thalamic area where neurons discharging in close association with tremor are found in parkinsonian patients (Fig. 3A) (1,2,9). It also corresponds exactly to the location of the neurons projecting to the arm area of the motor cortex (26).

Figure 4 illustrates this kind of abnormal rhythmic activity recorded in the VLo nucleus. In the lower trace, two units show sustained rhythmic firing at the same frequency. The autocorrelogram of the unit discharge (smaller spike, solid line) shows this frequency to be 3.7/sec. This is exactly the same frequency as that of the contralateral tremor shown by autocorrelation analysis of the EMG recording (dotted line) made in the same animal before paralysis. Sixty-two thalamic cells were submitted to this kind of analysis. About half of these cells showed bursting activity at the tremor frequency while the other half tended to fire at a frequency about 0.5 to 1 cycle/sec slower than the EMG tremor.

The effect of harmaline (5 mg/kg i.v.) on thalamic activity was assessed when conditions allowed prolonged recording of the same cell. The main effect of the drug on cells of the type shown in Figs. 1 and 2 (which are also found in

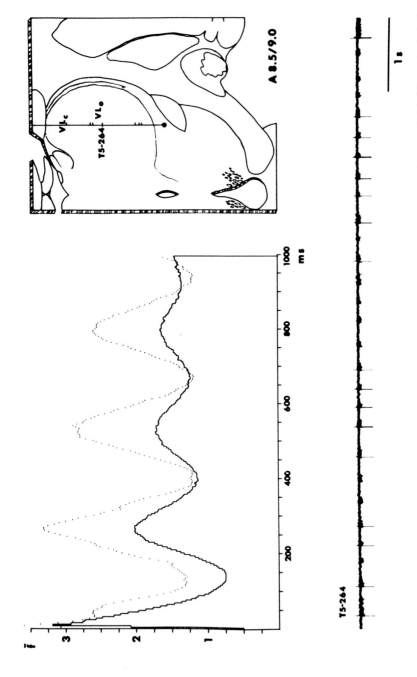

FIG. 4. Activity of thalamic neurons in paralyzed monkey. The lower trace shows the rhythmic activity recorded in VL_o as indicated in the right inset. Autocorrelation of the unit activity *(solid line)* shows a rhythmicity at 3.7/sec, which is exactly the same frequency as that of the tremor *(dotted line)* recorded in the contralateral arm before paralysis.

the normal animal) was an increase of the mean frequency of discharge and a disappearance of the bursting. However, the abnormal rhythmic activity recorded in lesioned monkeys did not disappear under harmaline and was often enhanced. This effect of the drug was particularly evident, as shown in Fig. 5, when the bursting was not initially sustained and regular.

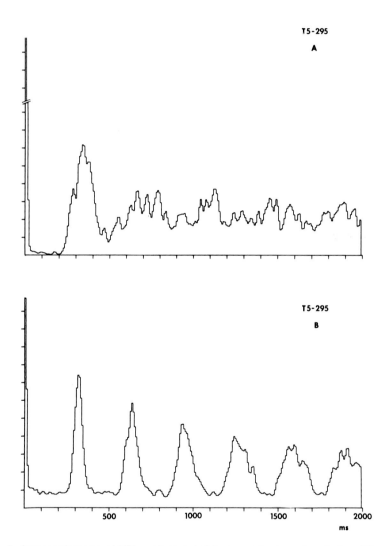

FIG. 5. Autocorrelograms of VPL_o unit recorded in a curarized monkey, before **(A)** and 15 min after **(B)** the administration of harmaline (5 mg/kg i.v.). This unit was recorded on the same side as a midbrain tegmentum lesion which had provoked a contralateral tremor of the arm. Harmaline enhanced the rhythmic bursting that occurred at 3.5/sec, the tremor frequency.

Motor Cortex Recordings

About 150 units were recorded in the arm area of the precentral cortex contralateral to the tremor. The cell shown in Fig. 6 was recorded in a paralyzed, undeafferented animal which had a contralateral tremor of the arm at 5/sec. In A, the spontaneous firing frequency is low at about 3.5/sec and there is no obvious rhythmicity. The other three recordings (B, C, and D) show that this unit had a tendency to fire rhythmically at about 5/sec when the discharge rate increased to 20–30/sec.

Figure 7 shows four examples of unit firing recorded in the arm area of the precentral cortex, contralateral to the deafferented upper limb in an unparalyzed animal. The rhizotomy was complete from C2 to T3. In each recording, the upper trace is the output of a transducer attached to the forearm; the middle trace is the EMG from the biceps (except for D where these two traces are reversed), and the lower trace is the unit activity. All these cells show episodes of rhythmic firing at the tremor frequency, which are particularly evident in A in the presence of tremor, and in D even in the complete absence of tremor. For some units, the relationship with tremor was very striking, as shown in Fig. 8. The EMG is from the contralateral triceps. The neuron fires synchronously with the tremor although not necessarily with each EMG burst. In C, the cortical rhythmic activity leads the tremor by a few cycles. Enhancement of the peripheral tremor is not necessarily concomitant with a more sustained

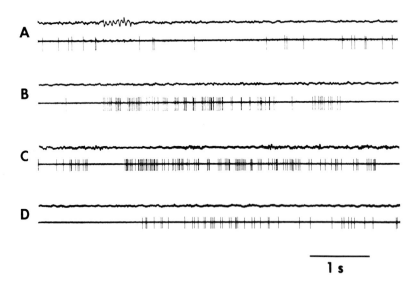

1 s

FIG. 6. A–D: Unit activity recorded in a paralyzed animal in the arm area of the precentral cortex, contralateral to the trembling limb. In each record, the upper trace is the motor cortex EEG and the lower trace is the unit activity. In **B, C,** and **D,** the cells show rhythmic activity at the tremor frequency (6/sec) despite motor paralysis.

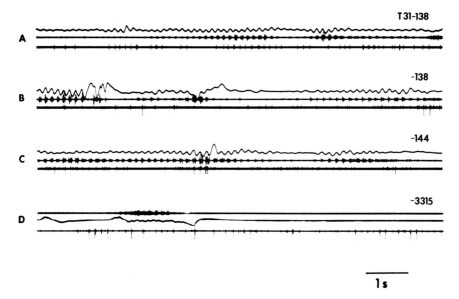

FIG. 7. A–D: Unit activity recorded in the arm area of the precentral cortex, contralateral to the deafferented trembling arm. In each record, the upper trace is the output of a transducer attached to the forearm, the middle trace is the EMG from the biceps (except in **D** where the traces are inverted), and the lower trace is the unit activity. All neurons show episodes of rhythmic firing at the tremor frequency.

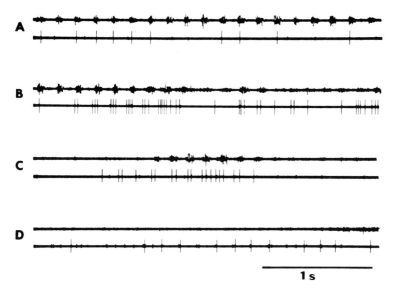

FIG. 8. A–D: Activity of a motor cortex neuron during tremor in the contralateral deafferented arm. The upper trace is the contralateral triceps EMG.

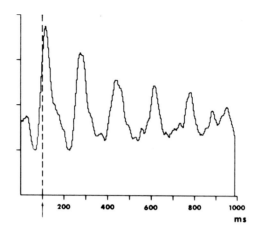

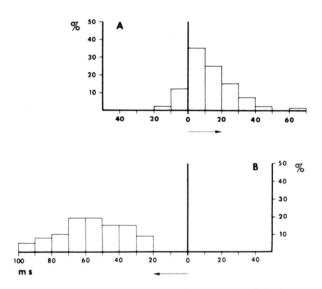

FIG. 9. Top: Cross-correlogram of the triceps EMG with neuronal discharges shown in Fig. 8. Time zero *(arrow)* indicates the onset of the EMG burst. **A** and **B:** The lower histograms (**A** and **B**) show the distribution of occurrences of the cortical spikes with respect to the onset (*vertical line at zero in* **A**) and to the end (*vertical line at zero in* **B**) of the EMG tremor bursts.

rhythmicity at the cortical level, and the cell can even be silent during pronounced tremor (A). This unit, as well as the other ones shown in Fig. 7, did not respond to passive movements of the limbs or to other natural stimulation such as stroking the skin or squeezing the muscles.

Autocorrelations of unit activity and EMG showed that both rhythmic events occurred at the same frequency: 5.9/sec. These two rhythmic phenomena were also phase locked as shown by the cross-correlogram (Fig. 9, top). The relationship between unit firing and the beginning or end of EMG burst activity is shown in Fig. 9 A and B. Histogram A shows the distribution of the cortical spikes with respect to the beginning of the burst of tremor which is indicated by the vertical line at zero. The distribution of the spikes in periods of 10 msec shows that 75% of the time the cortical unit discharge occurs either before or within the first 20 msec of the EMG bursts. In the lower histogram (B), the same measurements were made with respect to the end of the tremor bursts (vertical line at zero). The cortical cell never discharges any later than 20 msec before the end of the EMG bursts. From these observations, we conclude that peripheral feedback is not necessary for the appearance of cortical rhythmic bursting related to tremor, and that the cortical activity may itself result in the appearance of tremor.

DISCUSSION

The experimental results presented in this paper support the previously developed hypothesis of a thalamocortical mechanism involved in the generation of experimental Parkinson-like tremor in the monkey (4,12,14).

In paralyzed animals, we looked for rhythmic unit activity at the frequency of the tremor previously recorded in the same, unparalyzed animal. The assumption was made that a central mechanism responsible for the tremor would not be suppressed by a peripheral block of the movements or by the possible central action of the neuromuscular blocker (gallamine). In thalamic regions immediately in front of and above the lemniscal relay nuclei (VPL$_c$ and VP$_m$) we found a number of cells which displayed sustained rhythmic bursting at 3 to 6/sec. This pattern of discharge was independent of the level of vigilance, was little influenced by peripheral stimuli, and was often enhanced by the administration of harmaline (Fig. 5). The region where this rhythmic activity was recorded corresponds to the one where deep phasic responses were described in the monkey anesthetized with chloralose, and it is analogous to the thalamic regions where rhythmic activities were recorded in the parkinsonian patient (1,2,9). This type of sustained rhythmic activity was not observed in normal control monkeys (11). It is also of great significance that the thalamic region where abnormal rhythmicity was found corresponds exactly to the region identified by Strick (26) as containing the neurons which send axons to the arm area of the motor cortex in the monkey. All our animals showed tremor in the arms and, in rare instances where the legs were also involved, the tremor movements were always more marked in the upper limb.

In the motor cortex, rhythmic unit activity at the tremor frequency was also recorded in paralyzed animals. However, the paralyzed preparation is not entirely satisfactory and we were interested in recording tremor or other movements simultaneously with central unit activity but without peripheral feedback. This was achieved by surgical deafferentation. We confirmed the observation of Ohye et al. (21) that extensive dorsal rhizotomy does not abolish the experimental tremor in the monkey. In fact, an exaggeration of the tremor was sometimes evident. A number of cells discharging in relation to the tremor were found in the cortical representation area of the deafferented trembling limb. None of these units responded to passive movements of the limbs or to other natural stimuli, such as stroking the skin or squeezing the muscles.

These results as well as the relationship observed between the timing of the motor cortex and muscle activity (Fig. 9) strongly support the idea that rhythmical discharges of neurons in the motor cortex are causing the peripheral tremor rather than being the result of it.

It is currently impossible to make a definitive statement as to whether the motor cortex is merely driven by a thalamic "oscillator" or if both thalamus and cortex are actively involved, possibly by their interconnections (19). It has been observed that some thalamic cells, which were bursting regularly at the same frequency as the tremor, ceased to burst in a regular manner when the tremor was arrested by cooling the motor cortex (10), thus raising the possibility that the motor cortex may also play an active role in generating parkinsonian tremor (3).

Thalamic neurons can show rhythmic firing at the frequency of about 5/sec (11). This is a normal activity which is most prominent in the nuclei anterior to the ventrobasal complex and which is always concomitant with a state of relaxation (motor rest and decreased vigilance). This rhythmic activity, which can be quite sustained and regular, always occurs in the form of short-duration, high-frequency bursts. When the animal is aroused, the bursting disappears and is replaced by continuous firing of isolated spikes at a frequency of 10 to 30/sec (11).

In monkeys with brainstem lesions, the interruption of input to the thalamus, for instance by brain stem or lateral cerebellar lesions (7,16,18), could have profound effects on the complex organization of intrathalamic synaptic mechanisms. Hence, groups of thalamic cells could be shifted into a permanent state of rhythmic and synchronized bursting at 3 to 6/sec. Episodes of spontaneous tremor may then occur if a sufficiently large number of highly synchronized neurons is involved. Harmaline could enhance tremor by increasing the synchronization of thalamic bursting units, an effect that has been clearly demonstrated at the level of the inferior olive (6,13,20).

In summary, the results of the present study support the hypothesis that the experimental Parkinson-like tremor in the monkey is generated centrally by a thalamocortical mechanism. This does not require the integrity of peripheral feedback loops. A similar mechanism may be responsible for human parkinsonian tremor.

ACKNOWLEDGMENTS

This study was supported by grants to Yves Lamarre from the Medical Research Council of Canada. Y. Lamarre is the Director of the Medical Research Council of Canada Group in Neurological Sciences.

The authors acknowledge the competent technical help of Richard Bouchoux.

REFERENCES

1. Albe-Fessard, D. (1974): Thalamic activity and Parkinson's disease. In: *Central-Rhythmic and Regulation,* edited by W. Umbach and H. P. Koepchen, pp. 353–362. Hippokrates-Verlag, Stuttgart.
2. Albe-Fessard, D., Guiot, G., Lamarre, Y., and Arfel, G. (1966): Activation of thalamo-cortical projections related to tremorogenic processes. In: *The Thalamus,* edited by D. P. Purpura and M. D. Yahr, pp. 237–253. Columbia University Press, New York.
3. Alberts, W. W. (1972): A simple view of parkinsonian tremor. Electrical stimulation of cortex adjacent to the rolandic fissure in awake man. *Brain Res.,* 44:357–369.
4. Cordeau, J. P. (1961): Microelectrode studies in monkeys with a postural tremor. *Rev. Canad. Biol.,* 20:147–157.
5. Cordeau, J. P., Gybels, J., Jasper, H. H., and Poirier, L. J. (1960): Microelectrode studies of unit discharges in the sensorimotor cortex. Investigations in monkeys with experimental tremor. *Neurology,* 10:591–600.
6. de Montigny, C., and Lamarre, Y. (1973): Rhythmic activity induced by harmaline in the olivo-cerebello-bulbar system of the cat. *Brain Res.,* 53:81–95.
7. Goldberger, M. E., and Growden, J. H. (1971): Tremor at rest following cerebellar lesions in monkeys: effect of L-dopa administration. *Brain Res.,* 27:183–187.
8. Halpern, L. M., and Black, R. G. (1968): Gallamine triethiodide facilitation of local cortical excitability compared with other neuromuscular blocking agents. *J. Pharmacol. Exp. Ther.,* 162:166–173.
9. Jasper, H. H., and Bertrand, G. (1966): Thalamic units involved in somatic sensation and voluntary and involuntary movements in man. In: *The Thalamus,* edited by D. P. Purpura and M. D. Yahr, pp. 365–384. Columbia University Press, New York.
10. Jasper, H., Lamarre, Y., and Joffroy, A. (1972): The effect of local cooling of the motor cortex upon experimental Parkinson-like tremor, shivering, voluntary movements, and thalamic unit activity in the monkey. In: *Corticothalamic Projections and Sensorimotor Activities,* edited by T. Frigyesi, E. Rinvik, and M. D. Yahr, pp. 461–473. Raven Press, New York.
11. Joffroy, A. J., and Lamarre, Y. (1974): Single cell activity in the ventral lateral thalamus of the unanesthetized monkey. *Exp. Neurol.,* 42:1–16.
12. Lamarre, Y. (1975): Tremorgenic mechanisms in primates. In: *Advances in Neurology, Vol. 10,* edited by B. S. Meldrum and C. D. Marsden, pp. 23–34. Raven Press, New York.
13. Lamarre, Y., de Montigny, C., Dumont, M., and Weiss, M. (1971): Harmaline-induced rhythmic activity of cerebellar and lower brain stem neurons. *Brain Res.,* 32:246–250.
14. Lamarre, Y., and Joffroy, A. J. (1970): Thalamic unit activity in monkey with experimental tremor. In: *L-Dopa and Parkinsonism,* edited by A. Barbeau and F. H. McDowell, pp. 163–170. F. A. Davis Co., Philadelphia.
15. Lamarre, Y., and Joffroy, A. (1972): Rhythmic bursting of unit potentials in the ventrolateral thalamus of the monkey. In: *Corticothalamic Projections and Sensorimotor Activities,* edited by T. Frigyesi, E. Rinvik, and M. D. Yahr, pp. 273–278. Raven Press, New York.
16. Lamarre, Y., Joffroy, A. J., Dumont, M., de Montigny, C., Grou, F., and Lund, J. P. (1975): Central mechanisms of tremor in some feline and primate models. *Can. J. Neurol. Sci.,* 2:227–233.
17. Lamarre, Y. Joffroy, A. J., Filion, M., and Bouchoux, R. (1970): A stereotaxic method for repeated sessions of central unit recording in the paralyzed or moving animal. *Rev. Canad. Biol.* 29:371–376.

18. Larochelle, L., Bédard, P., Boucher, R., and Poirier, L. J. (1970): The rubro-olivo-cerebello-rubral loop and postural tremor in the monkey. *J. Neurol. Sci.,* 11:53–64.
19. Leblanc, F. E., and Cordeau, J. P. (1969): Modulation of pyramidal tract cell activity by ventrolateral thalamic regions. Its possible role in tremorogenic mechanisms. *Brain Res.,* 14:255–270.
20. Llinás, R., and Volkind, R. A. (1973): The olivo-cerebellar system: functional properties as revealed by harmaline-induced tremor. *Exp. Brain Res.,* 18:69–87.
21. Ohye, C., Bouchard, R., Larochelle, L., Bédard, P., Boucher, R., Raphy, B., and Poirier, L. J. (1970): Effect of dorsal rhizotomy on postural tremor in the monkey. *Exp. Brain Res.,* 10:140–150.
22. Olszewski, J. (1952): *The Thalamus of the Macaca Mulatta.* Karger, New York.
23. Poirier, L. J. (1960): Experimental and histological study of midbrain dyskinesias. *J. Neurophysiol.,* 23:534–551.
24. Poirier, L. J., Sourkes, T. L., Bouvier, G., Boucher, R., and Carabin, S. (1966): Striatal amines, experimental tremor and the effect of harmaline in the monkey. *Brain,* 89:37–52.
25. Pollock, L. J., and Davis, L. (1930): Muscle tone in parkinsonian states. *Arch. Neurol. Psychiatry (Chic.),* 23:303–319.
26. Strick, P. L. (1976): Anatomical analysis of ventrolateral thalamic input to primate motor cortex. *J. Neurophysiol.,* 39:1020–1031.

Advances in Neurology, Vol. 24, edited by
L. J. Poirier, T. L. Sourkes, and P. J. Bédard.
Raven Press, New York © 1979.

Functional Significance of Long Loop Reflex Responses to Limb Perturbation

J. T. Murphy, H. C. Kwan, and M. W. Repeck

Department of Physiology, University of Toronto, Toronto, Canada

The existence of long loop homonymous EMG responses to passive rotation of a limb part is now well established (8,9). External disturbances that activate cutaneous and joint mechanoreceptors as well as intramuscular stretch receptors when applied to the upper limb, typically produce reflex EMG responses at latencies above 40 msec. These are considered "long loop," in that they are clearly distinct from those responses at about 30 msec, which are considered segmental and primarily monosynaptic in origin. With ramp torque injections about the joint, the short latency reflex responses may be very weak or nonexistent. Because the long loop reflexes may have multiple independent components (8), we have termed these medium latency (ML) responses. These are to be distinguished from the short latency (SL), monosynaptic reflex responses, and the longer latency (LL) purely voluntary responses which may occur. The ML responses correspond directly to the M2, M3 forelimb responses described by Tatton and Lee (9), and are probably also analogous to the "functional stretch reflex" hindlimb responses of Melvill Jones and Watt (5).

There is a variety of evidence that the ML response has a transcortical component (Tatton et al., *this volume*). Most importantly, Tatton and Lee (9) have demonstrated that the ML response to imposed joint displacement may be significantly increased in patients with Parkinson's disease, a finding that has subsequently been confirmed (6). The increased ML response may in some instances be associated with and related to an increased background EMG activity (Evarts et al., *this volume*).

Whatever its cause in Parkinson's disease, the functional significance of the increased ML response remains obscure, precisely because the function of this response in normal subjects is unknown. In our laboratories, we have attempted to define this normal function, hoping thereby to clarify the pathophysiology of Parkinson's disease. Based on the notions that a critical parameter in the control of limb movement is stiffness (1–4,7) and that initial conditions of the limb must be known by the CNS for the organism to execute a successful movement, we hypothesized that the CNS functions to *pre-set* limb stiffness to a constant initial level, and that ML is causally related to this pre-setting.

It would follow that the later, voluntary EMG activity would then exert its effect on the basis of this known, pre-set stiffness.

METHODS

We examined predictions of the above hypothesis in 5 normal human subjects. Subjects were comfortably seated with the upper arm supported by a cast at a 90° angle to the longitudinal axis of the body. A torque motor was arranged to deliver torques in the flexion and extension directions about the elbow. Four parameters were monitored with 1-msec time resolution: (a) input voltage to the torque motor, V_i; (b) angular displacement, θ about the elbow; (c) torque, τ, generated by the forearm as measured with a strain gauge; and (d) surface triceps and biceps EMGs measured at a band width of 0.1 to 1.0 KHz. Initial joint position was set at 90° from full extension. Ramps of three different slopes were used as torque inputs. Subjects were instructed either to oppose the disturbance ("oppose" mode), or not to oppose it ("nonoppose" mode).

Limb stiffness, $\Delta\tau/\Delta\theta$, was directly computed as a function of time, using 5 msec time epochs. Because all events of interest occurred over a small ($< 10°$) angular displacement, high amplification of the latter was required, with corresponding amplification of noise levels. This necessitated a trade-off between a very short time epoch (high noise level) and a very long one (diminished time resolution). With the time epoch of 5 msec, computation of stiffness was practical beginning at 70 msec after displacement. This was satisfactory, since we were able to demonstrate by simulation studies that the inertial component of $\Delta\tau/\Delta\theta$ dominates in the period 0–70 msec. Beyond 70 msec, stiffness dominates.

RESULTS

Latency of ML

The latency of the reflex response will be dependent on the inputs used. With the present ramp inputs the mean onset latency for the 5 subjects was 77 ± 10 msec. SL EMG responses were extremely rare with these ramp inputs. Figure 1 shows examples of the EMG responses in the nonoppose and oppose modes.

The Stiffness Plateau

The hypothesis predicts that in the oppose mode, a reflex control signal, ML, will be generated, and constant level of stiffness will result. In the nonoppose mode, no reflex control signal would be observed, and no constant level of stiffness would be generated. This prediction was affirmed for all 5 subjects, as shown in Fig. 1 (pp. 126–127) and Fig. 2 (p. 128). Stiffness remained approximately constant until the LL, voluntary EMG activity began, at which period stiffness rose dramatically.

Casual Relationship of ML and Stiffness Plateau

If these two phenomena are causally related, as the hypothesis predicts, then two conditions must be met. The first is that ML must precede the onset of the stiffness plateau, and the second is that the onsets of ML and stiffness should covary. Predictions were sustained in all 5 subjects. Figure 2 shows examples of individual and averaged stiffness traces in relation to the ML and LL responses in a single subject. The delay between the electrical (ML) event and its mechanical (stiffness) effect was about 20 msec.

Simulation Study

To ensure that limb stiffness was indeed monitored in our experiments, simulation studies were carried out. To show the inertial component of the stiffness function, a rod with similar moment of inertia to the forearm was subjected to the identical perturbation and its stiffness function, $\Delta\tau/\Delta\theta$, was computed. The result was virtually identical to that for the human subjects in the nonoppose mode: early prominent inertial component (Figs. 1A and 2) (0–100 msec) followed by a rapid decay. This result emphasizes that the contribution of SL, which was rarely seen in these experiments, could not be assessed because SL occurs at a time when the inertial component of $\Delta\tau/\Delta\theta$ predominates. Adding a suitably chosen spring to the mechanical model resulted in a stiffness function similar to that of the human in the "oppose" mode. The results of these simulation studies validate the use of $\Delta\tau/\Delta\theta$ as an indicator of limb stiffness in our studies.

DISCUSSION

The potential importance of stiffness control in normal movement has been discussed previously (1–4,7). The present results provide a direct demonstration that stiffness is maintained at a constant level over a significant time period, prior to the release of a control program for voluntary movement. Moreover the data provide strong evidence that the ML reflex response is the causative agent in the generation of this stiffness plateau. Thus in our studies the *presence* of ML and the stiffness plateau were in all cases codependent, ML preceded the stiffness plateau, and the timing of each covaried. Hence the organism's response to a limb perturbation is to produce a long loop reflex EMG response, ML, which presets and stabilizes stiffness at a constant level upon which the subsequent voluntary movement can be superimposed.

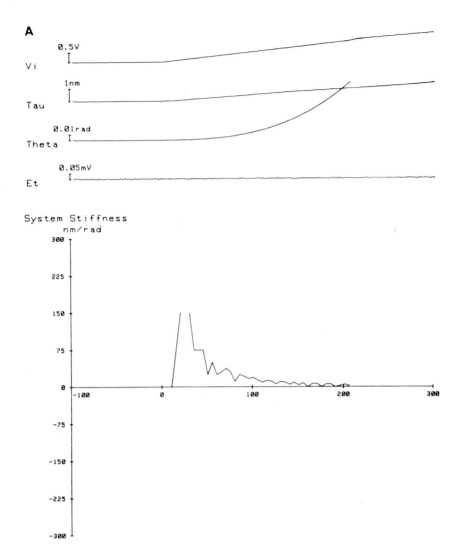

FIG. 1A. *(See legend facing page.).*

These observations on normal human subjects lend themselves immediately to predictions concerning the pathophysiology of parkinsonian symptoms, including rigidity. Alternations in the ML response to limb perturbation in Parkinson's disease, as shown by Tatton and Lee (9), would necessarily produce alteration in the stiffness plateau. An increase in stiffness would occur, which together with other abnormalities which can exist, might contribute to the genesis of clinical rigidity. These predictions await experimental tests.

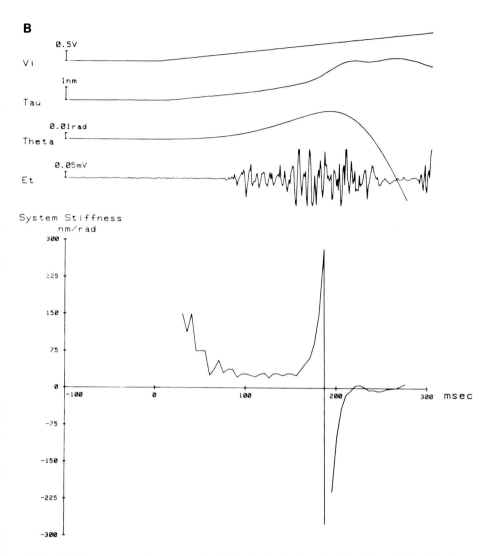

FIG. 1. Limb responses to ramp perturbation in the flexion direction. Records include the input control voltage (V_i), which starts at time 0; the torque applied to the limb system (tau); the angular displacement (theta); the surface triceps EMG (E_t); and the computed stiffness of the limb system stiffness in newton-meter/radian (nm/rad). **A:** In the nonoppose mode, there is an absence of triceps EMG, and a rapid decay of the stiffness of the limb system. **B:** In the oppose mode, prominent initial ML is seen in the EMG record, followed by a higher amplitude LL component. In the stiffness plot, the stiffness decay is arrested, and a constant stiffness plateau is observed. The later, rapid rise of the stiffness function from the plateau constitutes the effective opposition to the perturbation.

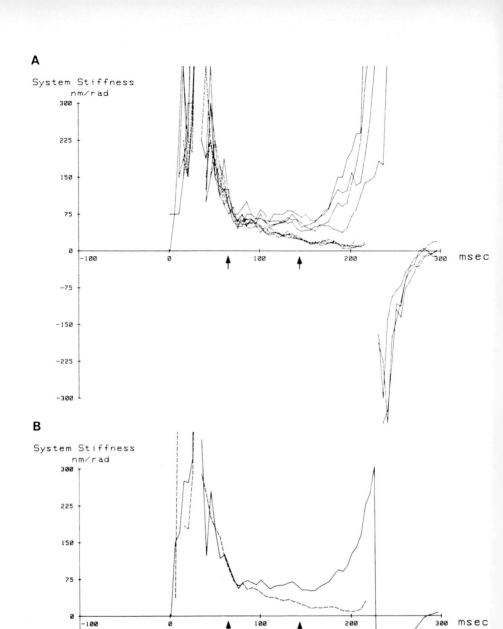

A

System Stiffness
nm/rad

B

System Stiffness
nm/rad

REFERENCES

1. Bizzi, E., Dev, P., Morasso, P., and Polit, A. (1978): Effect of load disturbances during centrally initiated movements. *J. Neurophysiol.,* 41:543–556.
2. Crago, P. E., Houk, J. C., and Hasan, Z. (1976): Regulatory actions of human stretch reflex. *J. Neurophysiol.,* 39:925–935.
3. Feldman, A. G. (1974): Changes in the length of the muscle as a consequence of a shift in equilibrium in the muscle-load system. *Biofizika,* 19:534–538.
4. Grillner, S. (1972): The role of muscle stiffness in meeting the changing postural and locomotor requirements for force development by the angle extensors. *Acta Physiol. Scand.,* 86:92–108.
5. Melvill Jones, G., and Watt, D. G. D. (1971): Observations on the control of stepping and hopping movements in man. *J. Physiol. (Lond.),* 219:709–727.
6. Mortimer, J. A., and Webster, D. D. (1978): Relationships between quantitative measures of rigidity and tremor and the electromyographic responses to load perturbations in unselected normal subjects and Parkinson patients. In: *Progress in Clinical Neurology, Vol. 4: Cerebral Motor Control in Man: Long Loop Mechanisms,* edited by J. E. Desmedt. Karger, Basel.
7. Nichols, T. R., and Houk, J. C. (1976): Improvement in linearity and regulation of stiffness that results from actions of stretch reflex. *J. Neurophysiol.,* 39:119–142.
8. O'Riain, M. D., Blair, R. D. G., and Murphy, J. T. (1978): The EMG responses to sudden stretches of limb muscles in normal human subjects. *Can. J. Physiol. Pharmacol.,* 56:771–776.
9. Tatton, W. G., and Lee, R. G. (1975): Evidence for abnormal long loop reflexes in rigid parkinsonian patients. *Brain Res.,* 100:671–676.

FIG. 2. A: Superimposed stiffness functions of the limb from four consecutive trials. *Left arrow* marks the mean ML onset time, and the *right arrow* the mean LL onset time for the trials. Solid traces were obtained when the subject was in the oppose mode, and dashed traces in the nonoppose mode. **B:** Averaged stiffness traces from both modes. After the initial inertial component, note definite departure between the two traces about 20 ms after the mean ML onset time *(left arrow).*

Advances in Neurology, Vol. 24, edited by
L. J. Poirier, T. L. Sourkes, and P. J. Bédard.
Raven Press, New York © 1979.

Motor Functions of the Basal Ganglia as Revealed by Studies of Single Cell Activity in the Behaving Primate

Mahlon R. DeLong and Apostolos P. Georgopoulos

Departments of Physiology and Neurology, The Johns Hopkins University School of Medicine, Baltimore, Maryland 21205

The role of basal ganglia in motor behavior has been the subject of continued study and speculation since the turn of the century. Several methods have been used to investigate the motor functions of the basal ganglia, including those of electrical stimulation and of ablation. The recently developed method of extracellular microelectrode recording of neuronal activity of electrical signs of the action potentials in behaving primates (11) has given new impetus to the research in this area. Studies of the activity of single neurons during movement confirmed the classical view that these nuclei participate in motor control, and led to the formulation of questions concerning specific aspects of their functional organization and of their relation to movement; namely, their somatotropic organization and the quantitative relations between neuronal activity and parameters of movement. We shall briefly review previous studies and present preliminary results of our current investigations of the motor functions of the globus pallidus, subthalamic nucleus, and substantia nigra obtained by single cell recording in behaving monkeys.

We have chosen the above structures for study because (a) the major outflow from the basal ganglia arises from the inner pallidum and the pars reticulata of the substantia nigra (28), (b) the subthalamic nucleus is intimately interconnected with the output nuclei (5,27) and appears to exert an important controlling influence (4,36) on these nuclei, and (c) the pars compacta of the substantia nigra appears to play a major role in motor behavior through the nigrostriatal dopaminergic system. The salient anatomic relations of the basal ganglia are summarized in Fig. 1.

SPONTANEOUS ACTIVITY

Most neurons in the globus pallidus discharge tonically at high rates during quiet wakefulness (7), in contrast to the low discharge rates observed in the striatum (9). Furthermore, the patterns of neuronal discharge differ between

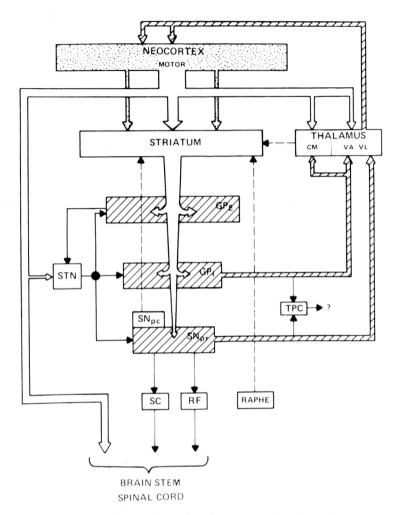

FIG. 1. Anatomic relations of the basal ganglia and their major afferent and efferent connections. GPe, external pallidal segment; GPi, internal pallidal segment; SNpr, substantia nigra pars reticulata; SNpc, substantia nigra pars compacta; STN, subthalamic nucleus; CM, centre median; VA, ventralis anterior; VL, ventralis lateralis; TPC, tegmenti pedunculopontinus pars compacta; SC, superior colliculus; RF, reticular formation.

the two pallidal segments. These patterns of discharge of cells of the external pallidal segment (GPe) are of two types: (a) with recurrent periods of high frequency discharge separated by periods of silence; and (b) with low mean frequency of discharge but with intermittent brief high frequency bursts of spikes. Approximately, 85% of GPe neurons are of the first type and 15% of the second type (7). In contrast, cells of the internal pallidal segment (GPi) show a sustained, high frequency bursting discharge without long interruptions. The clear difference in discharge patterns of GPe and GPi neurons provides additional evidence for the functional separation of the two pallidal segments which is suggested by their different anatomical connections (27).

Neurons located just below the pallidum, in the substantia innominata, and specifically in the nucleus basalis of Meynert and along the internal and external laminae of the pallidum ["border cells" (7)], exhibit a different pattern of discharge. It consists of sustained activity at frequencies lower than those of pallidal neurons proper with a gradual waxing and waning of the discharge over periods of time. The similarity of discharge rates and patterns between the "border," i.e., intralaminar, neurons and the n. basalis neurons, suggests that those border cells most probably correspond to the aberrant neurons of the n. basalis, which are found within the laminae of the pallidum, as originally described by Foix and Nicolesco (13) and subsequently by others (15,29,32). The studies of Poirier et al. (32) and Parent *(this volume)* provide additional information for several species on the relationship of n. basalis to the pallidum. The close proximity of the two nuclei and the extensive intermingling of pallidal and basalis neurons in the rat and cat, and to a lesser degree in the monkey, complicate greatly the interpretation not only of lesioning and stimulation studies of the globus pallidus, but also of single cell studies. It is obviously important to separate these two different populations in studies of the globus pallidus.

RELATION OF CELL DISCHARGE TO MOVEMENT

Self-Paced Limb Movements

In this study of neuronal activity in the basal ganglia during trained limb movements, monkeys performed self-paced alternating limb movements (push–pull or side-to-side) in order to obtain a liquid reward (7). The primary goals of that study were to determine (a) to what extent pallidal cells exhibited phasic modulations of discharge in relation to movement, and (b) whether their discharge was related to ipsilateral or contralateral limb movements. The results were unambiguous: many cells in each segment (GPe and GPi) exhibited clear modulation of discharge in relation to limb movements. Most (85%) of limb-related neurons discharged in association with contralateral limb movements. A degree of specificity for different directions of arm movements was indicated by the observation that the relation of neural activity to movement was usually stronger for either side-to-side or push–pull movement. Moreover, the activity of cells was related to either arm or leg movements but not to both. In addition to neurons related to movements of the limbs, many pallidal cells discharged in association with the delivery of juice, and as the animal licked spontaneously, chewed, or made mouth and tongue movements. These observations thus indicated a clear role of the pallidum in motor function of a rather specific nature.

In contrast to pallidal neurons, n. basalis and "border" cells did not discharge in association with limb movements, but many showed either an increase or a decrease in activity during the delivery of reward. However, unlike pallidal neurons, these cells did not discharge during spontaneous licking or chewing movements. The similarities in the functional properties of "border" and "basalis" neurons, and the differences of both groups from the pallidal neurons validated further the original proposal (7) based on the patterns of spontaneous activity, namely that (a) basalis and "border" neurons belong to the same entity, and that (b) these neurons form a population distinct from that of the pallidum proper.

Reaction Time Movements

An important question in understanding the role of the basal ganglia in motor control is whether these nuclei become active before the onset of movement, as shown for the motor cortex by Evarts (10) and for the cerebellum by Thach (34). An answer to that question was sought by studying the activity of single pallidal neurons during a reaction-time task in which monkeys reversed a steady force (greater than 200 *g*) with the arm in response to a visual stimulus (8). The activity of many cells in each pallidal segment, as well as in the putamen, was modulated before the earliest change in EMG activity of limb muscles and was better correlated with the onset of the movement than the visual stimulus. While it was not possible to determine from these studies whether the basal ganglia became active before the motor cortex, it was nevertheless clear that they participate in some aspects of the initiation of movement.

Slow Versus Fast Movements

In a later study (9), the hypothesis of Kornhuber (18) that the basal ganglia are primarily concerned with the generation of slow ("ramp") movements, and the cerebellum with the programming of fast ("ballistic") movements, was tested in monkeys trained to perform both fast and slow arm movements. The animals moved a lever in a push–pull direction between two zones, which were 1 cm wide and were separated by a distance of 5 cm. The animal had to move slowly (movement time greater than 600 msec) in response to a green light, or rapidly (movement time less than 140 msec) in response to a red light. The lever was allowed to pass through the target zone and hit against a mechanical stop. It was observed that of 187 neurons that were related to the task in the putamen, 45% showed a clear preferential activation during the slow movements, while less than 10% were activated preferentially during the fast movements; the remainder were related to both fast and slow movements. Similar but less remarkable results were obtained in the globus pallidus, where of 85 neurons that were related to the task, 17% were related preferentially to slow movements. In one animal, the neuronal activity in the deep cerebellar nuclei and the arm and shoulder area of the motor cortex was studied in the same task: none of 130 neurons in the motor cortex and only 3% of 107 cerebellar neurons discharged preferentially during slow movements. Extensive EMG studies were then performed in order to determine whether particular muscles might be selectively activated during slow movements in that task. While no such relation was observed in the arm musculature, the thoracic and lumbar paraspinal muscles were preferentially activated during the slow movements. It is possible, then, that the neurons of the basal ganglia, which were related preferentially to slow movements, might have in fact been concerned with the control of the axial musculature, rather than with the generation of slow arm movements per se. It should also be pointed out that an exclusive role of the basal ganglia in the generation of slow movements was ruled out by the results of this (9) and the preceding studies (7,8), in which it was shown that many of the neurons in these structures are related to fast arm movements as well.

CURRENT STUDIES

We recently began a study of the globus pallidus, subthalamic nucleus, and substantia nigra of the monkey. We characterized the functional properties of their neurons by observing the changes in neuronal activity during movements of specific parts of the body, and during "passive" manipulations of superficial (hair, skin) and deep (muscles, tendons, joints) structures. We also sought to define more precisely the relationship between neuronal discharge and specific parameters of movement (amplitude, velocity, acceleration) by studying the changes in the activity of neurons related to movements of the arm during the performance of a visuomotor arm tracking task.

RESULTS

Spontaneous Activity

The present studies confirmed the earlier observations concerning the distinctly different patterns of discharge in the two pallidal segments. The majority of neurons in the pars reticulata of the substantia nigra exhibited a sustained high frequency discharge similar to that of neurons in the internal pallidal segment, as described by Anderson (3) in the monkey, while those located in the pars compacta discharged at low rates (less than 10/sec). Some intermingling of high- and low-discharge rate neurons in the reticulata and compacta portions was observed. However, in the most rostral and lateral parts of the substantia nigra, where the pars reticulata is well developed and the pars compacta virtually absent, most of the neurons discharged at high rates, whereas in the caudal and medial parts where the pars compacta predominates, largely neurons with low discharge rates were observed.

In the rat it has been observed that neurons of the SNpc which discharge at low rates are dopaminergic (16). This probably holds as well for the primate on the basis of the present studies. Neurons located in the subthalamic nucleus exhibited a characteristic bursting pattern of discharge at moderate rates (average at 24/sec).

Functional Properties

Relation to Active Movements

The functional properties of 441 neurons isolated in 89 histologically identified penetrations in two monkeys were studied. Of these, 135 were located in GPe, 80 in GPi, 107 in subthalamic nucleus (STN), 93 in s. nigra, pars reticulata (SNpr), and 26 in s. nigra, pars compacta (SNpc). Many cells discharged during active movements of specific contralateral parts of the body, as follows: 36% in GPe, 29% in GPi, and 29% in STN were related to arm movements; 16% in GPe, 18% in GPi, and 22% in STN were related to leg movements; 10% in GPe, 18% in GPi, and 16% in STN were related to chewing or licking movements; 12% of the cells in GPe, 25% in GPi, and 19% in STN did not change their activity during movements or passive manipulations. The relation of neuronal discharge to movements of different parts of the body was rather specific for movements of one part of the body only (arm, leg, mouth). However, 16% of GPe cells discharged during both reaching and/or chewing. Such neurons are possibly related to cervical musculature since we observed in EMG studies that some cervical muscles were often activated during both of the above movements.

In the pars reticulata of the s. nigra only a small proportion (3%) of the neurons were related to limb movements, but 20% of the cells discharged during orofacial and/or lingual movements, as described by Mora et al. (26) in the monkey. Fifty-nine percent of the cells were not modulated during movements or passive manipulations and 3% were related to saccadic eye movements. In the pars compacta of the s. nigra, neurons with low discharge rates did not exhibit any phasic change of discharge during movements of the limbs or the mouth, nor during passive manipulations.

Responses to Passive Manipulations

In all structures, except the SNpc, weak responses to passive manipulations were observed in some neurons. They were much less strong than those observed during active movements and were frequently associated with manipulations of deep structures (muscles, tendons, joints) in and around the region of driving with active movements. Responses from superficial structures (skin, hair) were only rarely observed. No obvious responses to gross visual or auditory stimulation per se were observed in neurons in any of the above structures.

Somatotopic Organization

In the pallidum and the subthalamic nucleus, neurons related to specific parts of the body (e.g., arm) tended to cluster together. Moreover, a somatotopic organization was found within each nucleus. In each pallidal segment, neurons related to arm were generally located ventral to those related to leg [see also (7)] but dorsal to cells related to chewing or licking movements. This pattern of somatotopic organization reflects that of the somatotopic projection of the motor cortex to the putamen (20), where again arm is found ventral to leg but dorsal to face. Pallidal neurons related to limb or orofacial movements were distributed over a considerable rostrocaudal extent, although leg-related neurons were located mainly in the central portion of the nucleus. Neurons of the more rostral and dorsomedial parts of the pallidum, which receive projections from the caudate (33), were generally not modulated during movements or passive manipulations. A similar somatotopic organization was observed in the lateral part of the subthalamic nucleus: leg-related cells were located in the central part of the nucleus (in the rostrocaudal dimension) and at that level were dorsomedial to arm-related cells, which in turn were located dorsomedial to cells related to orofacial movements. In general, neurons of the medial part of STN were not related to the movements studied. In the pars reticulata of the s. nigra, the neurons related to orofacial and/or lingual movements were located primarily in its lateral part near the internal capsule.

Neuronal Activity During Visuomotor Arm Tracking

The activity of arm-related neurons in each pallidal segment ($n = 49$ for GPe, 23 for GPi) and the subthalamic nucleus (n = 31) was studied during the performance in a visuomotor arm-tracking task in which the monkey was required to follow a moving visual target with side-to-side movements of the arm. The manipulandum was a light-weight handle which the animal could grasp and move along a horizontal path with minimal friction. The display consisted of 2 rows of light emitting diodes (LEDs). Each row contained 128 LEDs (10/in.). The upper row indicated the position of the target and the lower the position of the handle. After holding in a starting position for at least 1 sec, step movements were elicited by suddenly jumping the target lamp to a new position, while pursuit movements were obtained by activating sequentially adjacent lamps. Data for spike and behavioral events and parameters of movement (position, velocity, and acceleration of the manipulandum) were collected and stored in a digital form for each trial. A trial-by-trial analysis of the data showed that most of the neurons in GPe, GPi, and STN were modulated in both the step and pursuit tasks. No preferential activation with either one of the tasks was observed. The percentage of neurons which showed significant changes in these tasks was highest in the subthalamic nucleus. Most cells were activated during either direction of movement but more strongly during the one or the other. A small proportion of neurons were significantly correlated with parameters of movement (amplitude, peak velocity, peak acceleration). In current studies, we are investigating this question more thoroughly with a more versatile apparatus which allows movement of the limb through greater amplitude, in different directions and under loads opposing or assisting the movement. EMG studies revealed no activation of axial musculature in either of the above tasks.

SUMMARY AND DISCUSSION

One of the results of the studies reviewed above is that a large proportion of neurons in the globus pallidus, subthalamic nucleus, and pars reticulata of the substantia nigra are related to active movements of specific parts of the body. While there is clear driving of some neurons by passive manipulations of joints, muscles, and tendons, this driving is weak compared to the neuronal changes observed during active movements. Responses to cutaneous, visual, or auditory stimuli are observed only rarely. These observations, combined with the fact that many neurons alter their activity prior to the onset of movement, emphasize the "motor" functions of a large part of the output nuclei of the basal ganglia and of the associated parts of the striatum (mainly the putamen in the monkey). It is interesting, on the other hand, that considerable emphasis has been placed on the "sensory" and/or "integrative" functions of the caudate nucleus (1,2,19), which in the monkey, receives projections primarily from the association cortex. In contrast to the abundance of cells related to movement in the output nuclei and the subthalamic nucleus, the absence of such phasic relation to movement in cells of the pars compacta of the s. nigra suggests that the nigrostriatal dopamine system may play a more general role in behavior. It is possible, nevertheless, that SNpc neurons may show subtle changes in discharge pattern during movement not yet detected in our studies. Since the projection of this system is topographically organized (12,25), it may also be possible that we have not sampled yet the relevant areas of the pars compacta.

The question of somatotopic organization within the basal ganglia has long been debated (4,6,22). The present study provides direct evidence that such an organization exists in the pallidum and the subthalamic nucleus in accordance with the orderly anatomical connections throughout the basal ganglia. A somatotopic organization of the putamen in the monkey has been suggested from anatomical studies (20), and recently confirmed in behaving monkeys (21). The observation that neurons related to orofacial lingual movements are located in the ventromedial part of the internal pallidal segment and in the lateral part of the pars reticulata of the substantia nigra, together with the striking similarities in the patterns of discharge, histologic appearance (14,24,29,30) and anatomic connections (23) of these two structures, leads us to propose that the internal pallidum may in fact be a lateral extension of the pars reticulata of the substantia nigra, the two structures being arbitrarily divided by the internal capsule. A similar view has been expressed previously on anatomical grounds alone (14, 24,29,30).

The importance of the subthalamic nucleus in motor activity was clearly revealed in the present studies: neurons of this nucleus were found to be the "most movement related" compared to those of the other structures studied.

The recent report of a sizeable projection from the motor cortex to the lateral part of the subthalamic nucleus in the monkey (17), together with earlier evidence (31), provides an anatomical basis for our observations. The size of this pathway might represent a development unique to primates and could be compared with the parallel increased projection of the motor cortex to the spinal cord: each of these two pathways may enable the motor cortex to gain direct control of the output of the basal ganglia and the spinal cord, respectively, a control needed perhaps for the performance of independent, skilled limb movements. This might explain the prevalence of dyskinesias of the limbs following lesions of the subthalamic nucleus in primates (35), in contrast to the difficulty of producing such dyskinesias in carnivores (36), where the subthalamic nucleus is small and receives only sparse projections from the motor cortex (Rinvik, this volume).

ACKNOWLEDGMENT

A part of the work presented here was supported by the National Institutes of Health Grant #5P01 NS06828–12.

REFERENCES

1. Albe-Fessard, D., Oswaldo-Cruz, E., and Rocha-Miranda, C. (1960): Activités évoquées dans le noyau caudé du chat en réponse à des types divers d'afférences. I. Etude macrophysiologique. *EEG Clin. Neurophysiol.,* 12:405–420.
2. Albe-Fessard, D., Rocha-Miranda, E., and Oswaldo-Cruz, E. (1960): Activités évoquées dans le noyau caudé du chat en réponse à des types divers d'afférences. II. Etude microphysiologique. *EEG Clin. Neurophysiol.,* 12:649–661.
3. Anderson, M. E. (1976): Tonic firing patterns of substantia nigra neurons in awake monkeys. *Neurosci. (Abstr.),* 2:59.
4. Carpenter, M. B., and Carpenter, S. C. (1951): Analysis of somatotopic relations of corpus luysi in man and monkey: relation between site of dyskinesia and distribution of lesions within subthalamic nucleus. *J. Comp. Neurol.,* 95:349–370.
5. Carpenter, M. B., and Strominger, N. L. (1967): Efferent fibers of the subthalamic nucleus in the monkey. A comparison of the efferent projections of the subthalamic nucleus, substantia nigra and globus pallidus. *Am. J. Anat.,* 121:471–472.
6. Davison, C., and Goodheart, S. P. (1940): Monochorea and somatotopic localization. *Arch. Neurol. Psychiatry,* 43:792–803.
7. DeLong, M. R. (1971): Activity of pallidal neurons during movement . *J. Neurophysiol.,* 34:414–427.
8. DeLong, M. R. (1972): Activity of basal ganglia neurons during movement. *Brain Res.,* 40:127–135.
9. DeLong, M. R., and Strick, P. L. (1974): Relation of basal ganglia, cerebellum and motor cortex units to ramp and ballistic limb movements. *Brain Res.,* 71:327–335.
10. Evarts, E. V. (1966): Pyramidal tract activity associated with a conditioned hand movement in the monkey. *J. Neurophysiol.,* 29:1011–1027.
11. Evarts, E. V. (1968): A technique for recording activity of subcortical neurons in moving animals. *EEG Clin. Neurophysiol.,* 24:83–86.
12. Fallon, J. H., and Moore, R. Y. (1978): Catecholamime innervation of the basal forebrain. *J. Comp. Neurol.,* 180:545–580.
13. Foix, C. E., and Nicolesco, J. (1925): *Anatomie Cérébrale, Les Noyaux Gris Centraux et la Région Mésencéphalo Sous Optique.* Masson, Paris.

14. Fox, C. A., Andrade, A. N., Lu Qui, I. J., and Rafols, J. A. (1974): The primate globus pallidus: a Golgi and electron microscopic study. *J. Hirnforsch.,* 15:75–93.
15. Gorry, J. D. (1963): Studies on the comparative anatomy of the ganglion basale of Meynert. *Acta Anat. (Basel),* 55:51–104.
16. Guyenet, P. G., and Aghajanian, G. K. (1978): Antidromic identification of dopaminergic and other output neurons of the rat substantia nigra. *Brain Res.,* 150:69–84.
17. Hartmann von Monakow, K., Akert, K., and Künzle, H. (1978): Projections of the precentral motor cortex and other cortical areas of the frontal lobe to the subthalamic nucleus in the monkey. *Exp. Brain Res.,* 33:395–403.
18. Kornhuber, H. H. (1971): Motor functions of cerebellum and basal ganglia: the cerebellocortical saccadic (ballistic) clock, the cerebellonuclear hold regulator, and the basal ganglia ramp (voluntary speed smooth movement) generator. *Kybernetik,* 8:157–162.
19. Krauthamer, G. M.: Sensory functions of the neostriatum. In: *The Neostriatum,* edited by I. Divac. Pergamon Press, New York *(in press).*
20. Künzle, H. (1975): Bilateral projections from precentral motor cortex to the putamen and other parts of the basal ganglia. An autoradiographic study in macaca fascicularis. *Brain Res.,* 88:195–209.
21. Liles, S. L. (1978): Unit activity in the putamen associated with conditioned arm movements: topographic organization. *Fed. Proc. Abstr.* 37:396.
22. Martin, J. P. (1967): *The Basal Ganglia and Posture.* Pitman Medical, London.
23. Mehler, W. R. (1971): Idea of a new anatomy of the thalamus. *J. Psychiatr. Res.,* 8:203–217.
24. Mirto, D. (1896): Contribute alla fina anatomia della substantia nigra di Sömmering e del pedunculo cerebralle dell'uomo. *Riv. Sper. Freniat.,* 22:197–210.
25. Moore, R. Y., Bhatnagar, R. K., and Heller, A. (1971): Anatomical and chemical studies of a nigro-neostriatal projection in the cat. *Brain Res.,* 30:119–135.
26. Mora, F., Mogenson, G. F., and Rolls, E. T. (1977): Activity of neurons in the region of the substantia nigra during feeding in the monkey. *Brain Res.,* 133:267–276.
27. Nauta, H. J. W., and Cole, M. (1978): Efferent projections of the subthalamic nucleus—an autoradiographic study in monkey and cat. *J. Comp. Neurol.,* 180:1–16.
28. Nauta, W. J. H., and Mehler, W. R. (1966): Projections of the lentiform nucleus in the monkey. *Brain Res.,* 1:3–42.
29. Olszewski, J., and Baxter, D. (1954): *Cytoarchitecture of the Human Brain Stem.* J. B. Lippincott, Philadelphia.
30. Parent, A., Poirier, L. J., Boucher, R., and Butcher, L. L. (1977): Morphological characteristics of acetylcholinesterase containing neurons in the CNS of DFP-treated monkeys. Part 2—diencephalic and medial telencephalic structures. *J. Neurol. Sci.,* 32:9–28.
31. Petras, J. M. (1972): Corticostriate and corticothalamic connections in the chimpanzee. In: *Corticothalamic Projections and Sensorimotor Activities,* edited by T. Frigyesi, E. Rinvik, and M. D. Yahr. Raven Press, New York.
32. Poirier, L. J., Parent, A., Marchand, R., and Butcher, L. L. (1977): Morphological characteristics of the acetylcholinesterase containing neurons in the CNS of DFP-treated monkeys. Part 1—extrapyramidal and related structures. *J. Neurol. Sci.,* 31:181–198.
33. Szabo, J. (1962): Topical distribution of the striatal efferents in the monkey. *Exp. Neurol.,* 5:21–36.
34. Thach, W. T. (1970): Discharge of cerebellar neurons related to two maintained postures and two prompt movements. I. Nuclear cell output. *J. Neurophysiol.,* 33:527–536.
35. Whittier, J. R. (1947): Ballism and subthalamic nucleus. *Arch. Neurol. Psychiatr.,* 58:672–692.
36. Whittier, J. R., and Mettler, F. A. (1949): Studies on the subthalamus of the rhesus monkey. II. Hyperkinesia and other physiologic effects of subthalamic lesions with special reference to the subthalamic nucleus of Luys. *J. Comp. Neurol.,* 90:319–372.

Advances in Neurology, Vol. 24, edited by
L. J. Poirier, T. L. Sourkes, and P. J. Bédard.
Raven Press, New York © 1979.

Altered Motor Cortical Activity in Extrapyramidal Rigidity

W. G. Tatton, P. Bawa, and I. C. Bruce

Playfair Neuroscience Unit, University of Toronto, Toronto, Ontario

In the seven decades since Gower (59) recognized muscular rigidity as a major deficit in Parkinson's disease, there has been a marked shift in our concepts of the neuronal mechanisms underlying movement control. Early investigators focused largely on reflex control (60) while in recent years increasing emphasis has been placed on the central programming of movements. Investigations of the numerically simpler motor systems in invertebrates have established that centrally encoded motor programs are activated by specific "command interneurons" and "played out" to the motoneurons through driver neurons and/or premotor networks without the necessity of reafferent information [see (30) for a detailed description of an invertebrate system]. The exact role that specific supraspinal and spinal neuronal populations play in central programming hierarchies is just beginning to be elucidated for mammalian motor control (53).

The shift in our concepts is perhaps best exemplified by the present view of the function of motor cortex, once considered to be the site of initiation of all voluntary movement. Studies of single nerve cell activity in trained monkeys have not supported a "command" role for the motor cortex (15) and indicate that at least some populations of motor cortical neurons function as driver neurons to integrate centrally programmed and reflex outputs at a level proximal to the motoneurons (16). Accordingly, basal ganglia neurons cannot necessarily be considered as functionally "downstream" to motor cortical neurons in a motor programming hierarchy. Even though progress has been made in elucidating the intrinsic and output connections of the basal ganglia (26,29,31,32,54), the functional role of basal ganglia neurons that output indirectly or directly to putative driver neurons in the motor cortex or the reticular formation is not understood (9). Despite the well-established evidence for nerve cell degeneration in the basal ganglia in Parkinson's disease, the uncertainty as to the functional relationship between so-called pyramidal and extrapyramidal neuronal populations in movement control has contributed to the comparatively slow evolution of our concepts regarding the pathophysiological basis of parkinsonian rigidity.

ABNORMAL STRETCH REFLEXES IN RIGIDITY

Similar to the early studies of pathological tone carried out in Gower's era (52), more recent investigations of parkinsonian rigidity have been largely directed toward uncovering abnormalities of stretch reflex function. Speculation that the rigidity of parkinsonism could be due to hyperactive stretch reflexes dates to the studies of Walshe (73). He showed that intramuscular procaine injection abolished the rigidity without affecting voluntary power in the muscle. Although Walshe's finding established that intact muscle afferent function was essential for the generation of rigidity, it did not provide an understanding of the abnormal central mechanisms underlying the pathological tone. Recognizing that rigidity must be related to increased alpha motoneuron output to the muscles perturbed by the mechanical displacement used to test tone, three general mechanisms could be consistent with Walshe's finding:

1. Increased responsiveness of muscle spindle endings to the mechanical disturbance to test tone. This would require a net increase in excitatory synaptic input to the gamma motoneurons innervating the intrafusal musculature.
2. Increased alpha motoneuron excitability due to increased net convergent excitatory synaptic input to the motoneurons from neuronal elements other than those in the reflex pathways activated by the mechanical disturbance used to test tone. Effectively, the proximal elements of the reflex pathways would be normally excitable and the rigidity would result from an increase in the general responsiveness of the "final common" elements, the alpha motoneurons, to excitatory input from any source.
3. Altered convergent synaptic input to interneurons linking the first order afferents to the alpha motoneurons. This could result in an increase in alpha motoneuron output that would be limited to the activation of selected reflex pathways whose interneurons were hyperexcitable without a generalized increase in alpha motoneuron responsiveness (47).

Investigations subsequent to Walshe's have been interpreted to support or deny all of the above mechanisms. Gamma motoneuron activity has been reported as increased in parkinsonian rigidity (12,58,69,71,72) supporting mechanism 1. In contrast, other workers have considered gamma motoneuron activity to be decreased (26) or within the normal range (2,36,76).

Other studies appear to support mechanism 2 (22,35,61,76,77) and suggest a sustained increase in supraspinal drive to the alpha motoneurons in rigidity. This would be in keeping with the finding of higher levels of baseline EMG activity in the majority of rigid parkinsonians as compared to age matched normals (E. V. Evarts et al., *this volume*).

Accepting the evidence for generalized increases in gamma and/or alpha motoneuron excitability as contributors to the generation of parkinsonian rigidity, hyperexcitability of those neurons alone does not provide a sufficient explanation for the selective alteration in some reflex functions considered to be dependent on muscle afferent input without the alterations of others. In keeping with the clinical observation that tendon jerks are usually normal in Parkinson's disease, the phasic stretch reflex has been found to be normal in parkinsonian rigidity (12,48). The rigidity is most evident in response to slower stretches (13) and is accompanied by increased electromyographic (EMG) activity during maintained muscle extension that evokes the static stretch reflex (2,11,13,59). These selective characteristics point to the possibility that mechanism 3 may play a significant role in the generation of the rigidity, and that polysynaptic reflexes activated by muscle stretch or joint displacement are responsible, rather than the monosynaptic reflex.

Recently it has been reported that the long latency components (LLC) of the stretch reflex are selectively increased as compared to the short latency components (SLC) in parkinsonian rigidity (6,37,51,68). Other workers have considered that the LLC are not increased out of proportion of levels of background alpha motoneuron excitability in accord with mechanism 2 (44). The LLC were initially observed in EMG recordings from human muscles stretched by imposed angular joint displacements (23,42,49). Computer averages of the EMG responses to the imposed displacements (45,51,67) and to punctate electrical stimulation of peripheral nerves (50,70) have revealed three major peaks of reflex activity. The three peaks appear to be homologous in man and monkeys for imposed displacements stretching the wrist muscles (65), and have been termed the M1, M2, and M3 peaks for convenience of description. Various lines of evidence have been interpreted as supporting the hypothesis that the LLC (the M2 and M3 peaks) are at least partially generated by polysynaptic reflexes (see 65 for details as to alternate mechanisms). Specifically, it has been suggested that the SLC represents the output of spinal reflexes (23) and LLC (most particularly the M2) is generated by transcortical pathway involving the motor cortex (1,41–43, 49,67).

A further abnormality in stretch reflex output in parkinsonian rigidity was initially recognized by Westphal (74) who reported a "paradoxical" contraction in the muscles shortened by an imposed displacement. Subsequent workers have shown a well-defined increase in EMG activity in the shortened muscle that consists of a dynamic component followed by a static component continuing as long as the shortening is maintained (2,11,58). Studies utilizing reversible ischemia or intramuscular procaine injections indicate that muscle afferent input from the stretched muscles is essential to the "paradoxical" reflex (2,57).

EMG RESPONSES TO IMPOSED DISPLACEMENTS IN PARKINSONIAN RIGIDITY

Figure 1 illustrates several of the essential differences in the reflex and voluntary responses to step load imposed displacement for a normal subject (traces a1, a2, and a3) and a rigid parkinsonian with bradykinesia, but with little or no 5-Hz rest tremor (traces b1, b2, and b3). In all of the studies reported in

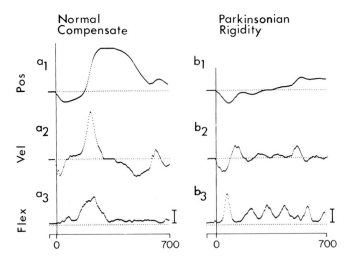

FIG. 1. Reflex and voluntary responses to imposed wrist displacements in a normal subject and a rigid parkinsonian subject. The traces are computer averages for 40 presentations of a 500-msec step load stretching the wrist flexors. The subjects were instructed to compensate for the imposed displacements. **a1 and b1:** Average wrist position traces with downward stretching the wrist flexors (maximum downward angular displacement in both traces is 20°). **a2 and b2:** Average velocity recording. **a3 and b3:** Averages of the rectified EMG recorded over flexor carpi ulnaris. Calibration bars equal 200 μV and time scales are in msec. Further details are included in the text.

this manuscript, human subjects or trained monkeys positioned a grasped handle attached to a computer-controlled torque motor in a narrow central zone. The axis of rotation of the torque motor was coaxial with the wrist joint, and the apparatus limited imposed displacements to that joint. Step loads of up to nine different magnitudes were presented in random sequence, at random intervals, and in random directions (flexion or extension). The subjects were instructed to compensate for the imposed displacement as quickly as possible (as in the compensate task of Fig. 1), or to passively allow the wrist to be fully displaced (passive task). The step loads were of random durations of 200 to 500 msec so as to avoid superimposition of EMG responses to step-on and step-off. The step loads could be superimposed on any constant baseline torque (preload).

In Fig. 1, the step load onset occurred at time 0. The initial downward displacement in the average wrist position traces, a1, and b1, stretched the wrist flexors. The maximum imposed angular displacement in both traces is about 20°. The velocity traces (a2 and b2) were obtained by computer differentiation of the position traces. The EMG activity was differentially recorded from small silver discs taped over the wrist flexor muscles. The EMG activity was rectified and computer averaged for 40 presentations of a single step load magnitude (identical loads were presented to both subjects). The greater stiffness of the parkinsonian muscles is evidenced by the lower velocity and increased time to maximum of the imposed displacement, as compared to that shown for the normal subject.

Even on the 700 msec timescale presented, three reflex peaks are evident in the initial 90 msec of the average EMG trace (a3) for the normal subject. The reflex output begins at 27 msec following the step load onset. These are immediately followed by an interval of strong "voluntary" EMG activity continuing to about 320 msec after the step load onset (see 65 for details regarding the identification and separation of reflex and voluntary components). The onset of the voluntary activity at a latency of 100 msec initiates a marked increase in the velocity of the return of the handle.

The parkinsonian subject shows a large and prolonged LLC beginning at the normal latency of the M2 peak (58 msec) continuing to 120 msec following the step load onset. Both the background EMG activity to the left of time 0 and the initial M1 component (the interval from 30 to 58 msecs) are within the range of normals. The size of all three reflex peaks in normals can be related to the level of background EMG activity and the initial velocity of the imposed displacements (64). Neither of these variables would appear to account for the increased responses over the interval of the LLC in the example presented. Further, they would be expected to increase the SLC in a proportional manner to the LLC (68).

The large reflex component appears to contribute to an initially increased velocity of return compared to the normal. The subsequent voluntary activity is slowly recruited, of comparatively low amplitude, and is characterized by an 8.0-Hz oscillation. The slow recruitment and relatively low amplitude of the voluntary activity is reflected in the low maximal velocities achieved in the voluntary return of the handle, and appears to correlate with degree of bradykinesia evident in a given patient.

Oscillations of the voluntary activity that are time-locked to the onset of the randomly presented imposed displacements, are frequently observed in rigid parkinsonian subjects, but are usually not as prominent as those in trace b3 (34,37). The oscillations together with deficits in the initiation and organization of fast or ballistic movements are considered in detail in other chapters of this volume (E. V. Evarts et al., *this volume*).

PHENOTHIAZINE INTOXICATION MODEL OF PARKINSONIAN RIGIDITY

Phenothiazines are known to induce so-called extrapyramidal or parkinsonian-like motor deficits in approximately 25% of human patients treated chronically with these agents (7). Accordingly we developed a model of parkinsonian rigidity in monkeys (*Macacca speciosa,* 3.0–5.0 kg) based upon chronic intoxication with acetylpromazine maleate. The dosage was gradually increased to a maximum of 12 to 18 mg/kg/day over a period of 12 days. By the fourth day of treatment, the monkeys developed bradykinesia, a flexor habitus, and detectable cogwheel rigidity. With continued treatment the deficits became increasingly apparent and an intermittent, low amplitude 5-Hz tremor became evident in the musculature of the extremities, particularly the more proximal muscle groups. Of importance to the present study the cogwheel rigidity was markedly evident in the wrist musculature.

The animals continued to be motivated by food rewards and maintained a good appetite, hence their metabolic state did not deteriorate over the 23 to 42 days of exposure to the drug. The motor deficits disappeared completely within 48 to 72 hr of discontinuing the phenothiazine.

We studied the EMG responses to imposed wrist displacements in the intoxicated monkeys. Figure 2 presents typical records for a monkey prior to (traces a1, a2, and a3), and on the 23rd day of phenothiazine intoxication (traces b1, b2, and b3). Traces a1 and b1 are average wrist position records, while a2 and b2 present average EMG traces for the stretched muscle, flexor carpi radialis (FCR) and a3 and b3, the shortened muscle extensor digitorum communis (EDC). The EMG activity was differentially recorded with pairs of fine intramuscular wires to eliminate the possibility of including activity from adjacent muscle groups. The normal compensating monkey shows well-defined reflex components over the initial 60 msec of the record for FCR (a2), which are immediately followed by well-organized voluntary output. The average EMG for EDC shows two intervals of reciprocal inhibition that correspond to the interval of reflex

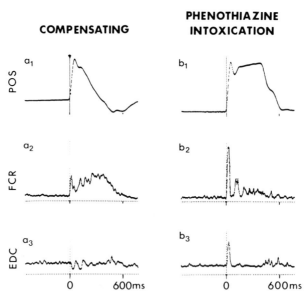

FIG. 2. Reflex and voluntary responses to imposed wrist displacement in a trained monkey prior to and during phenothiazine intoxication. The monkey was trained to compensate for the imposed displacements. **a1 and b1:** Average wrist position traces. **a2 and b2:** Averaged rectified EMG for flexor carpi radialis (FCR). **a3 and b3:** Averaged rectified EMG records for extensor digitorum communis (EDC). Upward deflections in the position traces stretch the wrist flexors. Maximum upwards displacement in both records is 40°. EMG records are matched in gain. Further details in text.

output (12 to 60 msec) and the onset of the voluntary output (60–150 msec).

In contrast, the records taken during the phenothiazine intoxication show: (a) markedly increased reflex components in FCR during the initial 60 msec following the step load onset (the inset EMG records in Fig. 5 illustrate that the increase predominantly involves the interval of the long-latency components); (b) poorly recruited "voluntary" output in FCR (beginning at an 80 msec latency) that is characterized by a damped 10 Hz oscillation; and (c) "paradoxical" reflex output in the shortened muscle during the initial 60 msec following the step load onset. Hence the intoxicated monkeys showed identical abnormalities to those in rigid parkinsonians on testing with step load imposed displacements together with reversal of the normal reciprocal inhibition of the shortened muscle (the Westphal phenomenon).

INPUT–OUTPUT RELATIONS FOR EMG RESPONSES TO IMPOSED DISPLACEMENTS

The EMG responses to the imposed displacements can only be unambiguously assessed by the construction of input–output plots for the peak components. The firing probabilities of the alpha motoneurons generating the EMG peaks have been shown to be graded monotonically with the magnitude of the step load imposing the displacement or the initial velocity of the imposed displacements (4). Furthermore, studies of the responses of single motor units to the imposed displacements in monkeys (65) have shown that the peaks in the averaged EMG response are largely generated by four separately responding "subpopulations" of alpha motoneurons. The four reflex intervals are illustrated in Fig. 3 which presents typical reflex responses for a monkey performing the passive task. In the passive task, the reflex output is not followed by the voluntary output after 60 msec. Each "subpopulation" only contributes to the generation

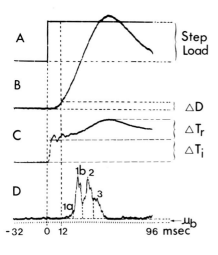

FIG. 3. Reflex responses to imposed wrist displacements in a trained monkey. The monkey was trained not to voluntarily resist the imposed displacements (passive task). A: All traces are averages for 25 presentations of the step load shown in trace A. B: Average position record with upward stretching the wrist flexors, $\Delta D = 4.2°$. C: Average net tension record. D: Average rectified EMG recorded from flexor carpi ulnaris. Further details presented in text.

of one of the three major peaks in average EMG response shown in trace D. Two subpopulations contribute to the M1 peak (over the intervals labeled 1a and 1b) while two other subpopulations generate the M2 (labeled 2) and M3 (labeled 3) peaks.

In Fig. 3, trace A shows the step load (onset at 0) imposing the average wrist displacement in trace B. The maximum imposed displacement in this example is 44.5°. Trace C presents the average net tension recording while trace D shows the averaged EMG responses. The tension recording can be separated into two portions labeled ΔT_i and ΔT_r. ΔT_i represents the tension imposed by the torque motor (the delay of about 3.5 msec required for ΔT_i to maximize is due to the inertia of the torque motor). ΔT_r represents the sum of the "tension" generated by the mechanical characteristics of the muscle–joint system being displaced, and the tension generated by the muscle contractions in response to the reflex alpha motoneuron output. Since the displacement continues during the EMG response, the two components of ΔT_r cannot be separated.

Figure 4 presents an input–output plot for the wrist flexor and extensor muscles in a normal compensating monkey. The average baseline EMG value (μ_b in Fig. 3) was computed in μVts/msec for the interval prior to the step load onset and used as a measure of baseline alpha motoneuron excitability.

Output was then determined by integrating the EMG response over each of the intervals shown in Fig. 3D, dividing the integrated value by the duration of the interval and subtracting μ_b to obtain M_i (for i = 1a, 1b, 2, and 3) in μVts/msec. Both M_i and μ_b were then normalized against the largest value for M_i (termed M_{max}) and plotted as M_i/M_{max} and μ_b/M_{max}.

The reciprocal inhibition in the antagonist muscles shortened by the imposed displacement was quantitated by measuring the integral of the decreased activity below μ_b over an interval encompassing the long latency components in the agonist muscle (as shown by the broken lines in the inset traces of Figs. 4 and 5). The integral was divided by the duration of the interval and normalized against the largest value obtained for the series of step loads.

The imposed input was determined by measuring the displacement over the initial 12 msec following the step load onset (ΔD in Fig. 3B). This measure was used to avoid including reafferent input generated by the reflex response as an input variable. The mechanical characteristics of the muscle–joint–cutaneous system displaced by the step load would be expected to remain constant as long as the EMG remains at baseline levels (until 13 msec in Fig. 3D). Following the onset of the reflex response, afferent activity due to the contraction of the stretched muscle and the relaxation of the shortened muscle would be superimposed on the input generated by the continuing imposed displacement. ΔD was then normalized against the largest value obtained for the series of step loads and plotted on the abscissa as $\Delta D/\Delta D_{max}$.

Three features are important to note in the input–output plot in Fig. 4 for the normal monkey: (a) the baseline EMG activity (μ_b/M_{max}) remains constant

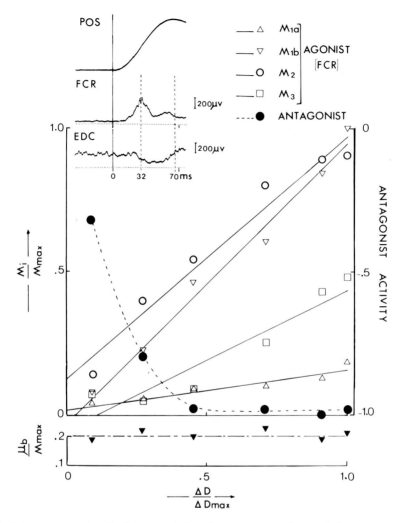

FIG. 4. Input–output plots for intervals of the reflex response to imposed displacements in a normal monkey. The monkey was trained in the compensate task. *Inset* shows average traces for wrist position (upward deflection stretches wrist flexors) and average rectified traces for flexor carpi radialis (FCR) and extensor digitorum communis (EDC). *Solid lines* are linear regression fits for the symbols plotted for each interval of the agonist activity (FCR). *Dotted line* is an arbitrary fit to the symbols for the antagonist activity (EDC). Further details in text.

with increasing $\Delta D/\Delta D_{max}$ ruling out changes in the net excitability of the alpha motoneurons as a factor in determining the input–output relationships; (b) the output of the stretched muscle increases monotonically with increasing initial displacement for all four intervals of the reflex response; and (c) the reciprocal inhibition of the shortened muscle is graded monotonically with increasing initial displacement until the muscle is completely silenced.

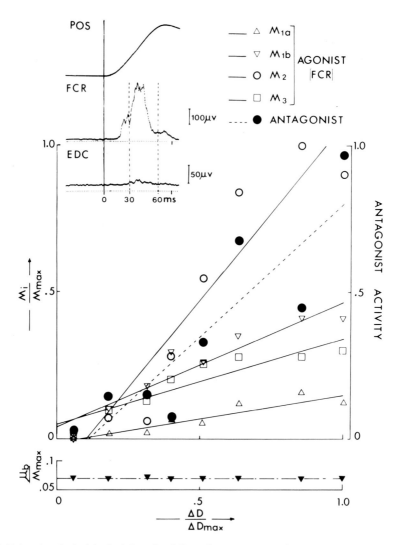

FIG. 5. Input–output plots for intervals of the reflex response to imposed displacements in a 23-day phenothiazine-intoxicated monkey. All features are identical to those in Fig. 4 except that the dotted line was fitted by linear regression to the symbols for the antagonist muscle. Further details in text.

Figure 5 presents the corresponding plot for the same monkey during the phenothiazine intoxication. The inset traces illustrate the marked increase in the amplitude and duration of EMG response over the interval of the LLC in the stretched muscle and the reversal of the reciprocal inhibition over a corresponding interval even for the smallest step loads presented.

Several features of the input–output plot differentiates it from that for the normal monkey: (a) the level of the baseline activity (normalized against M_{max})

is one-third that of the normal monkeys demonstrating that increased reflex response cannot be accounted for by increased alpha motoneuron excitability; and (b) the graded reflex inhibition of the shortened muscle has reversed to graded excitation over the interval of the long latency components.

ALTERED RESPONSES OF MOTOR CORTICAL NEURONS DURING PHENOTHIAZINE INTOXICATION

Microelectrode studies of motor cortical neurons (MCNs) in nonhuman primates under anesthesia have demonstrated potent inputs to those neurons from upper limb muscle afferents (27,40,56,75). Other investigations have examined the responses of MCNs in trained, awake monkeys to imposed angular displacements of different upper limb joints and with a variety of movement paradigms (8,17,38,39).

We studied the temporal relations between the responses of motor cortical neurons and the simultaneously recorded EMG responses to imposed displacements of the monkey wrist (66,67). A localized area or focus on the posterior bank and the crown of the precentral gyrus containing MCNs responding to imposed displacements of the wrist was mapped by systematic microelectrode penetrations in 3 monkeys. Approximately one-third of the MCNs within the focus showed identically timed excitatory peaks of firing on average response histogram (ARH) analysis. The excitatory ARH peaks had onset latencies of 22 to 25 msec following the step load onset and will be termed the reflex component (RC) [see Fig. 10 in (65)].

Intracortical stimulation maps (3) were superimposed over the maps for locations of MCNs showing RCs in the same animals. The superimposition established that the response focus corresponded to the microstimulation loci from which the EMG activity of the wrist flexors and extensor muscles could be driven at minimum latencies (8 msec) and minimum currents (8–12 μA). Microstimulation with higher currents (up to 25 μA) within the focus would drive other proximal or distal upper limb muscles, but at longer latencies (up to 200 msec). Microstimulation in the adjacent areas surrounding the focus drove either proximal or distal muscles at short latencies, as will be reported in detail elsewhere.

The onset and maximum of the RCs preceded onset and maximum of the simultaneously recorded M2 peak in the wrist muscles with a constant lead of 7 to 10 msec [see Fig. 9 (65)]. The intracortical microstimulation studies, electrical stimulation of the corticospinal tract, and the spike triggered averaging of MCN activity against EMG activity (18) all indicate the fastest conduction times from motor cortex to upper limb muscles range from 6 to 11 msec. Hence a major population of MCNs in a cortical area shown to project to wrist motoneurons at minimum latencies show spike activity that is exactly temporally appropriate to contribute to EMG activity over the interval of the M2 peak.

The RCs found for MCNs in normal monkeys can be reciprocal or uniform

(8) for imposed displacements in different directions (that is imposing wrist flexion or extension). The RCs of the MCN responses are followed by voluntarily generated activity (termed the voluntary component, VC) beginning at about 60 msec after the step load onset. This activity leads the voluntary activity of the EMG response (see Fig. $2a_2$) by about 10 msec. The RC and the VC can be separated by training monkeys in the compensate or the passive task. The separation together with examples of reciprocal and uniform RCs are illustrated in Fig. 6 (I and II).

Each group of histograms in Figure 6 was constructed for a single MCN and includes: (a) an autocorrelation histogram (ACH) constructed to display rhythmicities in the spontaneous or evoked firing of the MCNs; and (b) two pairs of ARH histograms, one pair constructed for a step load imposing wrist flexion (A and B in each group) and a second pair for a step load imposing wrist extension (C and D in each group). Each pair includes a histogram constructed with a bin width of 2.0 msec so as to allow the examination of the initial RC (A and C), and a second constructed with a bin width of 20 msec to facilitate examination of the VC. The time course of the step loads are shown below each histogram. The double terminations of the step loads indicates the minimum and maximum durations for step loads presented with a random duration.

Group I illustrates histograms constructed for a MCN with a reciprocally organized RC in a monkey performing the compensate task (as for Fig. 2, traces a1, a2, and a3). The autocorrelation histogram is flat and shows the MCNs' firing is random without any defineable rhythmicity. Histograms A and C show that the RCs in the first 60 msec have a 22 to 25 msec latency and are excitatory for a step load imposing wrist flexion and inhibitory for a step load imposing wrist extension. The corresponding histograms B and D show that the initial RCs are followed by excitatory activity or a period of inhibition that is appropriately timed to mediate the corresponding voluntary EMG activity in the wrist muscles (see Fig. 2). For example, the activity of this MCN would be appropriate to serve as a driver input, which would excite the flexor motoneurons in response to imposed displacements stretching the flexor muscles, and reciprocally reduce its tonic drive to the flexor motoneurons in response to displacements stretching the extensor muscles.

The histograms in group II are for an MCN in the response focus of a monkey performing the passive task. The ACH shows the MCN has no detectable rhythmicity in its firing. Histograms B and D demonstrate clear RCs in the initial 60 msec which are not followed by VCs similar to those found for MCNs in monkeys performing the compensate task. These MCN responses correspond to the EMG responses for the passive task in not showing voluntary activity (see Fig. 3). Histograms A and C show that the MCN responded with uniform RCs at a latency of 22–25 msec to either a displacement that stretched the flexors or the extensors. About one-half of responding MCNs in the focus were reflexly reciprocal and the other half were uniform in their RCs.

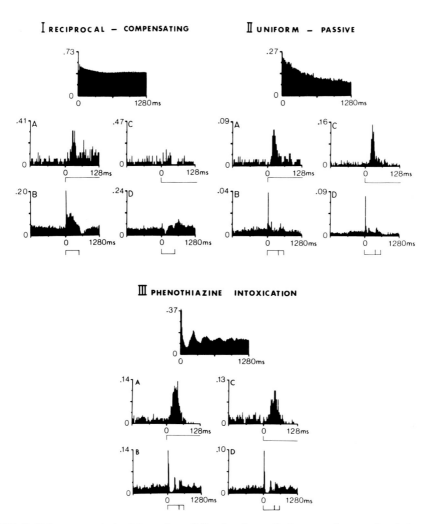

FIG. 6. Histogram analysis of the spike activity of motor cortical neurons in normal and pheno-thiazine intoxicated monkeys. Ordinates on all histograms present spikes/msec/step load presentation. The upper histogram in each group of five is an autocorrelation histogram, while the lower four are average response histograms for step load imposed displacements of the wrist. Time course and direction of the step load are denoted beneath the histograms (upward deflections stretched the wrist flexors). Each group was constructed for a single motor cortical neuron. Further details in text.

The histograms in group III were constructed for a MCN in a phenothiazine-intoxicated monkey. The ACH shows a prominent 4.3-Hz oscillation in the MCNs' activity which corresponds in frequency to the rest tremor found most prominently in the proximal limb musculature in the intoxicated monkey (see Lamarre and Joffroy, *this volume* for considerations regarding the role of the motor cortex in the generation of rest tremor). Histograms A and C show uniform excitatory reflex components with latencies of 22–25 msec. The 22–25 excitatory components show prolonged time courses as compared to those in normal monkeys (as compared to the responses in Fig. 6, I and II). For 117 MCNs analyzed from 2 intoxicated monkeys, we have not encountered a reciprocally responding MCN. All of the MCNs in the response focus show uniform excitatory RCs that were of prolonged duration similar to that in Fig. 6, III.

Furthermore, the MCNs in the intoxicated monkeys all showed low amplitude, poorly organized VCs. The majority also demonstrated a damped 10-Hz oscillation over the interval of the VC (as is illustrated in histograms III B and D), which corresponded in frequency to the oscillations in the voluntary portion of the simultaneously recorded EMG of the wrist muscles (see Fig. 2, trace b2).

In short, the MCN responses to imposed displacements are altered appropriately for the MCNs to serve as drivers of the abnormal reflex and voluntary EMG responses found in the phenothiazine monkeys. Further, the similarity of the abnormal EMG responses in the intoxicated monkeys and rigid parkinsonian's, together with the homology of the normal responses in the wrist muscles of humans and monkeys, supports a proposal that motor cortical output comprises one driver of the motoneuron activity generating parkinsonian rigidity. The proposal is in accord with Martin's suggestion, based largely upon clinical–pathological correlations, that motor cortical output forms the efferent limb of altered postural reflexes responsible for a number of parkinsonian deficits, including rigidity (46).

TENTATIVE MODEL FOR PYRAMIDAL–EXTRAPYRAMIDAL FUNCTION IN RIGIDITY

Studies of invertebrate motor systems suggest that proprioceptive reflexes serve to automatically adjust motoneuron output to "unexpected" conditions encountered during the execution of a centrally programmed movement (30). Yet if reflex gain (output/input) to a given muscle were limited to a single value, the automatic adjustments would not necessarily be appropriate to a number of motor programs with widely differing characteristics. For example, the wrist musculature in man is involved in motor acts as different as writing, lifting heavy objects, and hitting a badminton bird. Invertebrate systems have been shown to include specific "gain modulating" neurons that are controlled appropriately to the command interneuron enabling a given motor program (see ref. 69 for details of one system). The gain modulating neuron(s) adjust the excitability of proximal elements in the reflex pathway and thereby do not limit the output repertoire of the motoneurons. Hence, reflex gain is modulated without altering the general excitability of the motoneurons themselves.

Studies in humans and monkeys indicate that gain modulating mechanisms operate for upper limb reflexes. Hammond (24) reported that the LLC could be modulated according to prior instruction to resist or not to resist the imposed displacements. More recently it has been shown that the gain of input–output plots for the M2 portion of the LLC can be altered by prior instruction independently of the level of baseline alpha motoneuron excitability and the M1 portion of the response (64). The gain of the M2 portion appears to be adjustable to widely ranging values for a given muscle according to the characteristics of the motor act in progress (51; P. Bawa and W. G. Tatton, *unpublished observations*). The gain modulation of the M2 portion is shown schematically by the family of input-output relations labelled "normal" in Fig. 7.

Initially, rigid parkinsonians were reported to be unable to modulate the long latency components according to prior instruction (37,68). Subsequent investigations using more specific instruction sets (50) have shown the increased LLC in parkinsonians can be modulated. In accord with these findings, preliminary results in phenothiazine monkeys (see Fig. 5) and rigid humans (R. G. Lee and W. G. Tatton, *unpublished observations*) indicate that their input–output relations are steeper than most normals, as illustrated schematically in Fig. 7.

Previously it was proposed that basal ganglia output might function to modulate the gain of proprioceptive feedback through the motor cortex (20,37,68). The degeneration of specific neuronal populations in the basal ganglia in parkinsonism could then reduce the range of activity patterns available in the globus pallidus (GP) output to the motor cortex by way of the VL thalamic complex, and thereby limit the range of gain modulation of proprioceptive feedback through the motor cortex.

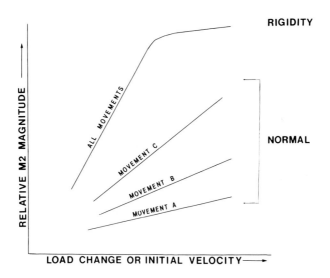

FIG. 7. Schematic for the modulation of the M2 portion of the stretch reflex according to the motor program being executed. Normal subjects are able to adjust input–output gain over a wide range for different movement conditions. Rigid parkinsonian subjects are limited to a narrow range of high gains irrespective of the movement being executed.

Prior instruction has been shown to modulate the responses of motor cortical neurons to proprioceptive inputs (63) and the activity patterns of GP neurons are known to be abnormal in a monkey model of parkinsonism (19). Motor cortical output has been shown to be altered by GP stimulation (55). Finally, the present studies indicate that motor cortical activity is appropriate to drive the abnormal responses to imposed displacements shown for extrapyramidal rigidity. The abnormal motor cortical drive could be expressed by modulating the excitability of spinal reflex pathways (10,21,28) or through direct motoneuron terminations (33).

All of the above are in accord with the tentative model but a number of questions essential to testing the model remain:

1. Are activity changes of GP neurons in normal monkeys appropriately-timed to modulate reflex gain?
2. Do the GP neurons showing the appropriately timed activity changes make output connections that can modulate the responses of MCNs to proprioceptive inputs?
3. Are the activity patterns of the GP neurons appropriately altered by the phenothiazine intoxication to fix the gain of MCN output to proprioceptive inputs at a high value?
4. Does the phenothiazine intoxication modify the reflexes by acting on basal ganglia neurons implicated in striatal dopamine depletion [most particularly on the nigrostriatal connections, see (31,32)], and is the effect of specific pharmacologic agents such as apomorphine and haloperidol in keeping with their known actions on basal ganglia neurons (7,62)?
5. Are motor cortical neurons the only neurons with activity that is appropriate to drive the abnormal EMG activity [see (38) for details as to the driver systems responsible for rest tremor]?

The model has to be extended beyond gain modulation in order to satisfy the paradoxical motoneuron output to the shortened muscle evidenced by the Westphal phenomenon in parkinsonians and the intoxicated monkeys. In some upper limb movements in normal humans, paradoxical reflex output in response to imposed displacements has been observed [(2); J. A. Mortimer, *personal communication*]. We have also been able to train monkeys in tasks that result in paradoxical reflex output (P. Bawa and W. G. Tatton, *unpublished observations*). Hence, paradoxical output may be a requirement of specific motor programs in normal animals. Accordingly, basal ganglia output could be postulated to control the switching of negative or positive proprioceptive feedback to any combination of agonist, synergist, and antagonist muscles appropriate to a given motor program. The switching might be achieved by altering the excitability of linking interneurons in the motor cortex or at a spinal level through motor cortical output convergence on interneurons in polysynaptic reflex pathways (21,28). Reflex output would then be adjusted both according to gain and distribution of muscles receiving excitation or inhibition according to the requirements of the motor program in progress. Failure of the adjustment could result in the fixed pattern of paradoxical output observed in extrapyramidal rigidity. Hence the degeneration of a basal ganglia system analogous to those in invertebrates (69) for adjusting reflex output to the motor program in operation would constitute one fundamental defect in parkinsonism.

ACKNOWLEDGMENTS

The research was supported by a Medical Research Council of Canada Grant (5218) to W.G.T. P.B. was supported by a Muscular Dystrophy Association Fellowship and I.C.B. was a Dystonia Foundation Fellow.

REFERENCES

1. Adam, J.; Marsden, D. C.; Merton, P. A., and Morton, H. B. (1976): The effect of lesions in the internal capsule and the sensorimotor cortex on servo action in the human thumb. *J. Physiol. (Lond.),* 254:27–28.
2. Andrews, C. J., Burke, D., and Lance, J. W. (1972): The response to muscle stretch and shortening in Parkinsonian rigidity. *Brain,* 95:795–812.
3. Asanuma, H., and Rosen, I. (1972): Topographical organization of cortical efferent zones projecting to distal forelimb muscles in the monkey. *Exp. Brain. Res.,* 14:243–256.
4. Bawa, P., and Tatton, W. G. (1977): Motor unit responses to angular wrist displacements in monkey and man. *Canada Physiol.,* 8:27.
5. Burke, D., Hagbarth, K. E., and Wallin, B. C. (1977): Reflex mechanisms in Parkinsonian rigidity. *Scand. J. Rehab. Med.,* 9:15.
6. Chan, C. W. Y., Kearney, R. E., and Melvill Jones, G. (1978): Electromyographic responses to sudden ankle displacement. *Soc. Neurosci. (Abstr.),* 4:292.
7. Chase, T. N. (1975): Extrapyramidal disorders induced by drugs. In: *The Nervous System, Volume 2: The Clinical Neurosciences,* edited by D. B. Towers, pp. 331–335. Raven Press, New York.
8. Conrad, B., Meyer-Lohmann, J., Matsunami, K., and Brooks, V. B. (1975): Precentral unit activity following torque pulse injections into elbow movements. *Brain Res.,* 94:219–236.
9. Delong, M. R. (1973): Putamen: activity of single units during slow and rapid arm movements. *Science,* 179:1240–1242.
10. Delwaide, P. J., Schab, R. S., and Young, R. R. (1974): Polysynaptic spinal reflexes in Parkinson's disease. *Neurology,* 24:820–827.
11. Denny-Brown, D. (1960): Diseases of the basal ganglia. Their relationship to disorders of movement. *Lancet,* 2:1099–1105, 1155–1162.
12. Dietrichson, P. (1971): Phasic ankle reflex in spasticity and Parkinson rigidity. The role of the fusimotor system. *Acta Neurol. Scand.,* 47:22–51.
13. Dietrichson, P. (1971): Tonic ankle reflex in parkinsonian rigidity and in spasticity. The role of the fusimotor system. *Acta Neurol. Scand.,* 47:163–182.
14. Dietrichson, P. (1973): The role of the fusimotor system in spasticity and parkinsonian rigidity. In: *New Developments in Electromyography and Clinical Neurophysiology, Vol. 3,* edited by J. E. Desmedt, pp. 496–507. Karger, Basel.
15. Evarts, E. V. (1975): The Third Stevenson Lecture. Changing concepts of central control of movement. *Can. J. Physiol. Pharmacol.,* 53:191–201.
16. Evarts, E. V., and From, C. (1978): The pyramidal tract neuron a summing point in a closed-loop control system in the monkey. In: *Progress in Clinical Neurophysiology, Vol. 4: Cerebral Motor Control in Man: Long Loop Mechanisms.* Edited by J. E. Desmedt, pp. 56–59. Karger, Basel.
17. Evarts, E. V., and Tanji, J. (1976): Reflex and intended responses in motor cortex pyramidal tract neurons of monkey. *J. Neurophysiol.,* 39:1069–1080.
18. Fetz, E. E., Cheney, P. D., and German, D. C. (1976): Corticomotoneuronal connections of

precentral cells detected by post-spike averages of EMG activity of behaving monkeys. *Brain Res.,* 114:505–510.

19. Filion, M. (1979): Globus pallidus unit activity during alterations of striatal dopaminergic mechanisms in monkeys. *Can. J. Neurol. Sci. (in press).*
20. Flowers, K. (1975): Ballistic and corrective movements on an aiming task. Intention tremor and parkinsonian movement disorders compared. *Neurology,* 25:413–421.
21. Fu, T. C., Hultborn, H., Larsson, R., and Lundberg, A. (1978): Reciprocal inhibition during the tonic stretch reflex in the decerebrate cat. *J. Physiol.,* 284:345–369.
22. Gassel, M. M., and Diamantopoulos, E. (1964): The Jendrassik maneuver. 1. The pattern of reinforcement of monosynaptic reflexes in normal subjects and patients with spasticity or rigidity. *Neurology (Minneap.),* 14:555–560.
23. Hammond, P. H. (1955): Involuntary activity in biceps following the sudden application of velocity to the abducted forearm. *J. Physiol. (Lond.),* 127:23–25.
24. Hammond, P. H. (1956): The influence of prior instruction to the subject on an apparently involuntary neuromuscular response. *J. Physiol. (Lond.),* 132:17–18.
25. Hassler, R. (1957): The pathological and pathophysiological basis of tremor and parkinsonism. In: *Proc. 2nd Int. Cong. Neuropathol. (Lond.),* 1:29–40. Exerpta Medica, Amsterdam.
26. Hassler, R. (1978): Striatal control of locomotion, intentional actions and of integrating and perceptive activity. *J. Neurol. Sci.* 36:187–224.
27. Hore, J., Preston, J. B., Durkovic, R. G., and Cheney, P. D. (1976): Responses of cortical neurons (areas 3a and 4) to ramp stretches of hindlimb muscles in the baboon. *J. Neurophysiol.,* 39:484–500.
28. Illert, M., Lundberg, A., and Tanaka, R. (1976): Integration in descending motor pathways controlling the forelimb in the cat. 2. Convergence on neurons mediating disynaptic corticomotoneuronal excitation. *Exp. Brain Res.,* 26:521–540.
29. Kemp, J. M., and Powell, T. P. S. (1971): The connexions of the striatum and globus pallidus: synthesis and speculation. *Philos. Trans. R. Soc. Lond. [Biol.],* 262:441–457.
30. Kennedy, D. (1969): The control of output by central neurons. In: *The Interneuron,* edited by M. A. B. Brazier, pp. 21–36. University of California Press, Berkeley.
31. Kitai, S. T., Kocsis, J. D., Preston, R. J., and Sugimori M. (1976): Monosynaptic inputs to caudate neurons identified by intracellular injection of horseradish peroxidase. *Brain Res.,* 109:601–606.
32. Kocsis, J. D., Sugimori, M., and Kitai, S. T. (1977): Convergence of excitatory synaptic inputs to caudate spiny neurons. *Brain Res.,* 124:403–413.
33. Kuypers, H. G. J. M. (1964): The descending pathways to the spinal cord, their anatomy and function. *Prog. Brain Res.,* 2:178–202.
34. Lance, J. W., Schwab, R. S., and Peterson, E. A. (1963): Action tremor and the cogwheel phenomenon in Parkinson's disease. *Brain,* 86:95–110.
35. Landau, W. M., Struppler, A., and Mehls, O. (1966): A comparative EMG study of the reactions to passive movement in parkinsonism and in normal subjects. *Neurology,* 16:34–48.
36. Landau, W. M., Weaver, R. A., and Hornbein, T. D. (1960): Fusimotor nerve function in man. *Arch. Neurol.,* 3:10–23.
37. Lee, R. G., and Tatton, W. G. (1975): Motor responses to sudden limb displacements in primates with specific CNS lesions and in human patients with motor system disorders. *Can. J. Neurol. Sci.,* 2:285–293.
38. Lemon, R. N., Hanby, J. A., and Porter, R. (1976): Relationship between the activity of precentral neurones during active and passive movements in conscious monkeys. *Proc. R. Soc. Lond. (Biol.),* 194:341–373.
39. Lemon, R. N., and Porter, R. (1976): Afferent input to movement-related precentral neurones in conscious monkeys. *Proc. R. Soc. Lond. (Biol.),* 194:313–339.
40. Lucier, G., Ruegg, D. G., and Wiesendanger, M. (1975): Responses of neurones in motor cortex and area 3a to controlled stretches of forelimb muscles in cebus monkeys. *J. Physiol. (Lond.),* 251:833–838.
41. Marsden, C. D., Merton, H. B., and Adam, J. (1977): The effect of lesions of the sensorimotor cortex and capsular pathways on servo responses from the human long thumb flexor. *Brain,* 100:503–526.
42. Marsden, C. D., Merton, P. A., and Morton, H. B. (1972): Servo action in human voluntary movement. *Nature (Lond.),* 238:140–143.

43. Marsden, C. D., Merton, P. A., and Morton, H. B. (1973): Is the human stretch reflex cortical rather than spinal? *Lancet,* 1:759–761.

44. Marsden, C. D., Merton, P. A.; Morton, H. B., and Adam, J. (1978): The effect of lesions of the central nervous system on long-latency stretch reflexes in the human thumb. In: *Prog. Clin. Neurophysiology,* Vol. 4: *Cerebral Motor Control in Man: Long Loop Mechanisms,* edited by J. E. Desmedt, pp. 334–341. Karger, Basel.

45. Marsden, C. D., Merton, P. A., Morton, H. B., Adam, J. E. R., and Hallet, M. (1978): Automatic and voluntary responses to muscle stretch in man. In: *Progress in Clinical Neurophysiology, Vol. 4: Cerebral Motor Control in Man: Long Loop Mechanisms,* edited by J. E. Desmedt, pp. 167–177. Karger, Basel.

46. Martin, J. P. (1967): *The Basal Ganglia and Posture.* Pitman, London.

47. Matthews, P. B. C. (1972): *Mammalian Muscle Receptors and Their Central Actions.* Williams and Wilkins, Baltimore.

48. McLellan, D. L. (1973): Dynamic spindle reflexes and the rigidity of Parkinsonism. *J. Neurol. Neurosurg. Psychiatry,* 36:342–349.

49. Melvill Jones, G., and Watt, D. G. D.: Observation on the control of stepping and hopping movements in man. *J. Physiol.,* 219:709–727.

50. Milner-Brown, H. S., Stein, R. B., and Lee, R. G. (1975b): Synchronization of human motor units. Possible role of exercise and supraspinal reflexes. *J. Neurol. Neurosurg. Psychiatry,* 38:245–254.

51. Mortimer, J. A., and Webster, D. D. (1978): Relationships between quantitative measures of rigidity and tremor and the electromyographic responses to load perturbations in unselected normal subjects and parkinson patients. In: *Progress in Clinical Neurophysiology, Vol. 4: Cerebral Motor Control in Man: Long Loop Mechanisms,* edited by J. E. Desmedt, pp. 342–360. Karger, Basel.

52. Mott, F. W., and Sherrington, C. S. (1895): Experiments upon the influence of sensory nerves upon movement and nutrition of the limbs. *Proc. R. Soc. Lond. (Biol.),* 57:481–488.

53. Mountcastle, V. B., Lynch, J. C., Georgopoulos, A., Sakata, H., and Acuna, C. (1975): Posterior parietal association cortex of the monkey: command functions for operations within extrapersonal space. *J. Neurophysiol.,* 38:871–908.

54. Nauta, W. J. H., and Mehler, W. R. (1969): Fiber connections of the basal ganglia. In: *Psychotropic Drugs and Dysfunction of the Basal Ganglia,* edited by G. Crane and R. Gardener, Jr., pp. 68–74. Public Health Services Pub. no. 1938, U.S. Government Printing Office, Washington, D.C.

55. Newton, R. A., and Price, D. D. (1975): Modulation of cortical and pyramidal tract induced motor responses by electrical stimulation of the basal ganglia. *Brain Res.,* 85:403–422.

56. Phillips, C. G. (1969): Motor apparatus of the baboon's hand. *Proc. R. Soc. Lond. (Biol.),* 173:141–174.

57. Rondot, P. (Sept.1971): Etude EMG de la reaction de raccourcissement. Presented at the Fourth International Congress of Electromyography, Brussels.

58. Rushworth, G. (1960): Spasticity and rigidity. An experimental study and review. *J. Neurol. Neurosurg. Psychiatry,* 23:99–118.

59. Rushworth, G. (1961): The gamma system in parkinsonisms. *Int. J. Neurol.,* 2:34–50.

60. Sherrington, C. S. (1906): *The Integrative Action of the Nervous System.* Scribners, New York.

61. Stephanis, C. N., and Matsouoka, S. (1965): Spinal motoneurone hyperexcitability in patients with Parkinson's disease as revealed by the recovery curve of the H-reflex. In: *Sixth International Congress of EEG and Clin. Neurophysiology,* pp. 625–626. Medizinische Akademie, Vienna.

62. Sourkes, T. L., and Poirier, L. J. (1966): Neurochemical bases of tremor and other disorders of movement. *Can. Med. Assoc. J.,* 94:53–60.

63. Tanji, J., and Evarts, E. V. (1976): Anticipatory activity of motor cortex neurons in relation to the direction of an intended movement. *J. Neurophysiol.,* 39:1062–1068.

64. Tatton, W. G., and Bawa, P. (1977): Input–output relations for "long-loop" reflexes. Alterations by pre-existing loads and volitional set. *Canada Physiol.,* 8:67.

65. Tatton, W. G., Bawa, P., Bruce I. C., and Lee, R. G. (1978): Long loop reflexes in monkeys: an interpretative base for human reflexes. In: *Progress in Clinical Neurophysiology, Vol. 4: Cerebral Motor Control in Man: Long Loop Mechanisms,* edited by J. E. Desmedt. pp 229–245. Karger, Basel.

66. Tatton, W. G., and Bruce, I. C. (1976): Temporal relations between motor cortical neuronal

responses and EMG responses to sudden load changes applied to the primate wrist. *Canada Physiol.,* 7:59.

67. Tatton, W. G., Forner, S. D., Gerstein, G. L., Chambers, W. W., and Liu, E. N. (1975): The effect of post-central cortical lesions on motor responses to sudden upper limb displacement in monkeys. *Brain Res.,* 96:108–113.
68. Tatton, W. G., and Lee, R. G. (1975): Evidence for abnormal long-loop reflexes in rigid Parkinsonian patients. *Brain Res.,* 100:671–676.
69. Tatton, W. G., and Sokolove, P. G. (1975): Analysis of postural motoneuron activity in crayfish abdomen. II. Coordination by excitatory and inhibitory connections between motoneurons. *J. Neurophysiol.,* 38(2).
70. Upton, A. R. M., McComas, A. J., and Sica, R. E. P. (1971): Potentiation of "late" responses evoked in muscles during effort. *J. Neurol. Neurosurg. Psychiatry,* 34:699–711.
71. Wallin, G. and Hagbarth, K. E. (1978): Muscle spindle activity in man during voluntary alternating movements. Parkinsonian tremor and clonus; In: *Progress in Clinical Neurophysiology,* Vol. 5: *Physiological Tremor, Pathological Tremors and Clonus,* edited by J. E. Desmedt, pp. 150–159. Karger, Basel.
72. Wallin, G., Hongell, A., and Hagbarth, K. E. (1973): Recordings from muscle afferents in parkinsonian rigidity. In *New Developments in Electromyography and Clinical Neurophysiology,* Vol. 3, edited by J. E. Desmedt, pp. 263–272. Karger, Basel.
73. Walshe, F. M. R. (1924): Observations on the nature of the muscular rigidity of paralysis agitans, and on it's relationship to tremor. *Brain,* 47:159–177.
74. Westphal, C. (1880): Uber eine art paradoxer muskelcontraction. *Arch. Psychiatr. NervKrankh.,* 10:243–248.
75. Wiesendanger, M. (1973): Input from muscle and cutaneous nerves of the hand and forearm to neurones of the precentral gyrus of baboons and monkeys. *J. Physiol. (Lond.),* 228:203–219.
76. Yap, C. B. (1967): Spinal segmental and long-loop reflexes on spinal motoneurone excitability in spasticity and rigidity. *Brain,* 90:887–896.
77. Zander, W., Olsen, P. and Diamantopoulos, E. (1967): Excitability of spinal neurons in normal subjects and patients with spasticity, parkinsonian rigidity, and cerebellar hypotonia. *J. Neurol. Neurosurg. Psychiatry,* 30:325–331.

Advances in Neurology, Vol. 24, edited by
L. J. Poirier, T. L. Sourkes, and P. J. Bédard.
Raven Press, New York © 1979.

Effects of Kinesthetic Inputs on Parkinsonian Tremor

H. Teräväinen, E. Evarts, and D. Calne

Laboratory of Neurophysiology, NIMH and Experimental Therapeutics Branch, NINCDS, Bethesda, Maryland 20014

Both the resting tremor in Parkinson's disease (PD) and clonus in patients with spasticity result from central disorders, but while clonus is associated with exaggerated segmental stretch reflexes and is commonly believed to involve oscillation within a reflex loop having excessively high gain, there is still considerable debate concerning the mechanisms underlying the resting tremor of PD. Certainly, the lack of abnormal segmental stretch reflexes in PD need not imply a lack of abnormality in *other* reflexes, and it follows that reflex factors in general cannot be assumed to be irrelevant to the resting tremor of PD. Indeed, recent observations on hyperactive long-loop reflexes in PD patients (12,21) have raised the possibility that PD resting tremor may be based on oscillations within an excessively high gain reflex loop containing both spinal and supraspinal components.

The present experiments sought to obtain data relevant to this hypothesis by determining the effects of displacing the tremulous limbs of PD patients at known phases of tremor. It was observed that such displacements could reset the phase of PD tremor, presumably by modifying the abnormal impulse patterns passing through the thalamic nucleus ventralis lateralis to motor cortex, and from motor cortex to spinal cord. Furthermore, it was found that displacements delivered to the limbs of patients without resting tremor could initiate tremor activity whose phase depended on the direction of the triggering displacement.

PATIENTS AND METHODS

Experiments on resting tremor were performed in 8 parkinsonian patients selected on the basis of having resting tremor on clinical examination; 7 were men (age range 30–70 years) and 1, a 64-year-old woman. Tremor amplitude varied in different patients and often in the same patient from slight and intermittent (grade 1) to constant and of large amplitude (grade 4). For comparative purposes, observations were obtained on "simulated tremor" in 8 normal volunteers 23 to 80 years of age. In addition, postural tremor was studied in 32 parkinson patients (7 women and 25 men with ages from 38 to 72 and mean age of 60.0 years). Additional data on postural tremor was obtained from 26 controls 38 to 80 years (mean 62.2 years) of age.

Resting Tremor

Subjects were seated with the forearm fixed in a closely fitting mold, which allowed flexion–extension movements of the wrist but prevented forearm movements. They grasped a handle which was designed so that their hand was sandwiched between two closely fitting vertical bars connected to the axle of a brushless DC torque motor (Aeroflex TQ 64). The position of the subject's hand was adjusted so that the axle of the torque motor was directly below the wrist joint: the rotation of the axle closely corresponded to the angle of the movement of the hand (Fig. 1). The axle of the torque motor was connected to a potentiometer for position recording, and fluctuations of axle position thus reflected tremor. EMG of the wrist extensors and flexors was recorded using bipolar surface EMG electrodes with amplifiers (Motion Control Corp.) positioned longitudinally on the extensor digitorum communis and palmaris longus muscles. The position and EMG data were recorded on paper for visual inspection and on magnetic tape together with code signals providing information on tremor detection and sites and directions of perturbations. Figure 2 illustrates the tremor and EMG recordings.

In order to deliver perturbations at specified phases of tremor, it was necessary

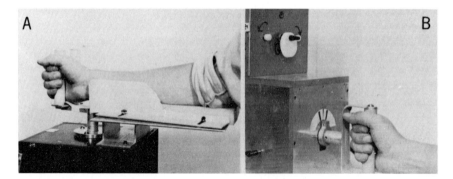

FIG. 1. Two postures adopted by subjects during tremor recording and delivery of limb displacements. **A:** Recording of resting wrist extension–flexion tremor. The elbow was flexed with the forearm resting in a support which immobilized it down to the wrist. The hand moved freely from the wrist joint and was sandwiched between two closely fitting vertical bars. These bars allowed the sudden displacements of the handle to cause hand movement without the patient needing to maintain a firm grip on the handle. The shaft of the torque motor was positioned directly below the wrist joint; thus, extension–flexion movements of the wrist caused a corresponding rotation of the shaft. Surface EMG electrodes (not shown) were positioned longitudinally over the extensor and flexor muscles. **B:** Posture used to study postural supination–pronation tremor. A steady state load required patients to activate or inhibit the biceps muscle to keep the handle vertical. Biceps EMG activity was recorded with surface electrodes overlying the muscle.

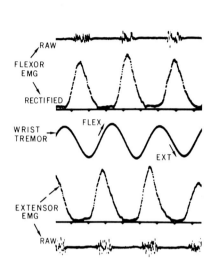

FIG. 2. Raw EMG data and corresponding summated, rectified and low-pass filtered EMG recordings are shown in relation to RC coupled wrist tremor in a patient with a large amplitude resting tremor. Extensor and flexor muscles operated in a reciprocal fashion to produce the tremor movement. Note that the extensor EMG activity peaked when the movement was in the direction of flexion, and that flexor EMG activity peaked when the movement was in the direction of extension. The peaks occurred at, or shortly after, the corresponding zero-crossings and were responsible for changing direction of the tremor movement. The phase relations between EMG and displacement during resting tremor are likely to be somewhat different from that shown in the figure, since, under the experimental conditions used, muscle activity had to counteract not only the inertia of the wrist itself but also the inertia of the moving parts (shaft and torque motor). In addition, RC coupling caused a slight phase shift in the measured tremor movement. This phase shift was measured from the above recordings by comparing to the RC position recordings with a direct-coupled position recording. The phase shift was about 15 msec for a 4-Hz tremor.

to detect tremor phase and set criteria for tremor amplitude. This was done by applying the tremor signal (RC coupled, time constant = 0.8 sec) to three analog comparators whose reference levels were adjusted to detect (a) a given amplitude of tremor in the flexion direction, (b) a given amplitude of tremor in the extensor direction, and (c) midpoints (i.e., zero-crossings) of the wrist position during tremor. Of course, as illustrated in Fig. 2, wrist position could cross zero in two directions depending on whether the crossing occurred as the wrist was being flexed or extended. When the amplitude of five successive cycles of tremor had exceeded the flexor and extensor comparator reference levels, a flip–flop was set to allow delivery of a perturbation either at the next positive-going zero-cross (when the wrist was being flexed) or at the next negative-going zero-cross (when the wrist was being extended). The displacement produced by these perturbations could be in either of two possible directions, retarding or accelerating the wrist movement occurring at the time perturbation occurred. The four possible combinations (two perturbation directions and two tremor directions) at which perturbation was delivered are illustrated in Fig. 3. For control data, the same tremor amplitude criteria necessary for delivery of perturbations were set, but no signal was delivered to the torque motor at the time when a perturbation would ordinarily have been given. Two control trials (one for positive-going zero-cross and one for negative-going zero-cross) were obtained for each set of four perturbations. In addition, strength (up to

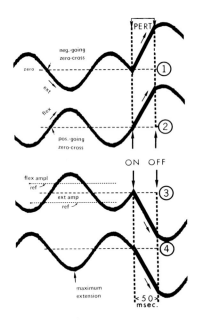

FIG. 3. The four possible combinations of the two perturbation directions and the two directions of resting tremor. An RC coupled tremor signal was fed to analog comparators to get midpoints ("zero-crossings") of the tremor in both extension (EXT) and flexion (FLEX) directions, as well as to detect a given tremor amplitude in extension and flexion directions ["amplitude reference" (AMPL REF)]. A ramp perturbation (PERT) of 50-msec duration was delivered after detection of five complete tremor cycles either to flex (1 and 2) or to extend (3 and 4) wrist at two different tremor phases: at the negative-going zero-crossing when the spontaneous tremor movement was in the extension (1 and 4), and at the positive-going zero-crossing when the movement was to flexion (2 and 3).

2 ft lb) and duration (between 20 and 300 msec) of the perturbations could be varied. Different perturbations occurred randomly at about 7-sec intervals provided that five full tremor cycles were detected by the comparators. Thus, perturbations did not occur unless tremor was present. Tremor was separately coded prior and after the perturbations, allowing later computer discrimination of immediate preperturbation tremor, immediate postperturbation tremor, and delayed (1 sec) postperturbation tremor.

After preliminary testing, both the force of the torque pulse (1.8 ft lb) and the duration of the perturbation (50 msec) were kept constant. This produced variable displacements relative to the tremor amplitude in different patients. Figure 4 illustrates this variability.

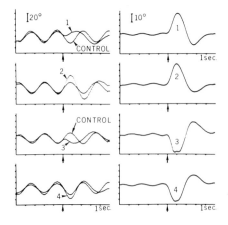

FIG. 4. Disturbances of the resting wrist tremor caused by perturbations schematically illustrated in Fig. 2. **Left:** A patient with a relatively large amplitude tremor (grade 3). **Right:** A patient with a small amplitude tremor (grade 2). In subjects with small amplitude tremor, the perturbations caused marked displacements relative to the tremor *(right)*. In contrast, the perturbations were considerably less effective when superimposed on high amplitude tremor *(left)*.

Postural Tremor

The condition commonly used for elicitation of postural tremor is maintenance of the outstretched arm against gravity. In our experiments, postural tremor was elicited by having the subject maintain active pronation or supination against a steady state torque either to pronate or supinate the forearm (Fig. 1B). Maintaining a stationary posture in the middle of the rotation of the torque motor shaft ($+45°$) required sustained one-sided muscular effort; for example, increased steady state activation of the supinators (e.g., biceps muscle) and inactivity of the muscles responsible for the pronation. This compares to the clinical examination, in which the patients are studied with their arms extended, a position requiring one-sided muscular effort to support the arm against a steady state force (gravity). By regulating the current through the motor, the experimenter could control the steady state activity of the muscles. During maintenance of the handle position against a steady state load, ramp perturbations were superimposed on the steady state torque either to pronate or supinate the forearm. Perturbations were randomly superimposed on the tremor and thus not triggered by known tremor phases, nor was tremor a necessary precondition for delivery of the stimuli, as was the case in the study on resting tremor. Biceps EMG activity was recorded using surface electrodes positioned longitudinally above the muscle.

RESULTS

Reflexes occurring after abrupt limb displacement during steady state muscular contraction against constant load are: (a) an increase of EMG activity due to monosynaptic stretch reflex in which muscle is stretched, and (b) a decrease of ongoing EMG activity due to the segmental unloading reflex in muscle which is shortened. The relations of perturbation-triggered reflex responses and ongoing muscle activity of the wrist extensor and flexor muscles during movement may be expected to be somewhat more complex than the relations at rest.

Resetting and Triggering Resting Tremor by Perturbation

All the results described below were obtained using perturbations of 50-msec duration, i.e., about one-fourth of the complete tremor cycle. This caused position changes of about 80-msec duration in normal subjects when the movement was not voluntarily resisted. In the patients, the tremor movement was either assisted or opposed by the perturbation, with the severity of the tremor modifying the effect of perturbation in assisting or opposing the ongoing movement. In the case of violent tremor (grade 4), the perturbation was relatively ineffective in changing the tremor movement. In somewhat less vigorous tremor, the perturbation could both stop the tremor when opposing the movement and also increase its amplitude when assisting the movement. When the tremor amplitude was small or moderate (grade 3 or less), the perturbation compared to the resistance supplied by the patient was strong enough to reverse the ongoing tremor movement (Fig. 4). Nevertheless, these short perturbations unquestionably caused tremor resetting in all but 2 patients. Both of these patients had large amplitude tremor, and though resetting was observed on some individual trials, the summated responses were inconclusive. In all patients with small to moderate tremor amplitude, resetting of the tremor was evident in both position recordings and recordings of the EMG activity. Changes in the EMG activity provide a clearer indication of perturbation-produced alterations in central nervous system activity, since changes in position are in part determined by the motor and limb inertia. For this reason, EMG data is used in preference to position data in presentation of the results.

Figure 5 shows extensor EMG activity and wrist tremor 1 sec before and after perturbations lasting 50 msec in a 64-year-old female with moderate resting tremor. Perturbations completely reversed or markedly assisted the tremor movement. The effects of the perturbations were either to shorten (Fig. 5A and

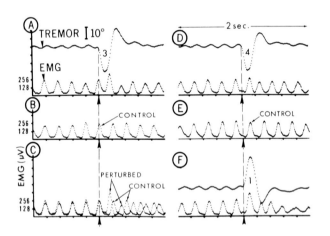

FIG. 5. Simultaneous recordings of the wrist tremor at rest (TREMOR) and extensor muscle EMG activity (EMG) in a patient with a grade 2 resting tremor. Tremor recording for 1 sec was followed by 50-msec perturbations *(arrows)* responsible for the displacements. **A** illustrates the effect of perturbations acting to extend the wrist and shorten the extensors at the time the extensors were active but the movement was flexion. The perturbation caused enhanced EMG activity beginning some 50 msec sooner than expected from the previous EMG cycles. **B** shows a control recording of tremor EMG without perturbation. Both the perturbed and control recordings are superimposed in C to illustrate that the resetting of the tremor phase was immediate and that the tremor continued after the disturbance in this new phase. **C** and **D** show effects of perturbations in opposite directions at the time the extensor muscles were inactive; when the wrist movement was extension, a perturbation either assisted **(D)** or reversed **(F)** the tremor movement. **E** is a control EMG for both the trials D and F. In **D**, the first EMG peak following a perturbation that shortened the extensors was not changed, but the second peak occurred some 55 msec sooner than in the control record **(E)**. When the extensors were stretched by the initial perturbation **(F)**, the first EMG peak occurred about 20 msec sooner than in the control record. Thus, the tremor phase was shifted *towards* the perturbations in all the above examples.

D), or stretch (Fig. 5F) the extensor muscles. In the first 2 cases, the initial effect of the perturbations was inhibition, and in the latter case an excitation. However, the EMG peaks came significantly sooner in all the cases than was to be expected from the control recordings (Fig. 5B and E) without perturbation. Furthermore, the subsequent peaks of EMG activity were shifted towards the perturbations compared to those of the control trials. This signified that the tremor phase was immediately changed and that the tremor continued thereafter in this new phase (e.g., Fig. 5C). That the tremor phase was shifted towards the perturbations, whether the muscles were stretched or shortened, is due to the fact that the initial perturbation triggers reciprocal changes in the activity of the agonist and antagonist muscles, with time delays quite different from those occurring during tremor. The details of these changes are rather complicated and will be dealt with in a subsequent report. Thus, the delays between peaks of muscle activity following perturbations in opposite directions may be considerably shorter (see Fig. 6) than those occurring between peaks of EMG activity in undisturbed resting tremor. Nevertheless, the direction of the perturbation did determine the sequence of the EMG responses as illustrated both in Fig. 6 (postural tremor) and in Figs. 5D and E (resting tremor) showing EMG responses to occur earlier if the muscle was initially stretched than if shortened.

There were differences in both timing and the extent of the tremor resetting

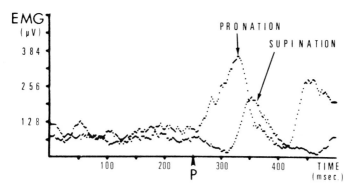

FIG. 6. Summated biceps EMG responses to perturbations either stretching (PRONATION) or shortening (SUPINATION) the biceps muscle when the patient was actively resisting a steady state load requiring biceps activation. The initial effect of pronating perturbations which stretched the biceps muscle was to elicit reflex activation with an onset latency of about 20 msec and a latency to peak of about 80 msec. Supinating perturbation which shortened the biceps muscle first caused inhibition (maximum at about 60 msec) followed by rebound excitation. This rebound peaked about 105 msec after the beginning of the perturbation. Thus, perturbations in opposite directions caused biceps activation whose temporal pattern depended on the direction of the perturbation. But it is important to note that the differences in the latencies to peak EMG responses to perturbations in opposite directions was only about 25 msec. Thus, the first peak in response to stretch occurred at a latency of 80 msec, while the rebound peak following the unloading reflex occurred at a latency of 105 msec. The short interval between those two peak EMG responses is similar to that observed in EMG responses occurring for perturbations delivered during resting tremor (Fig. 5).

in individual patients. The differences were in part related to variable latencies of the initial EMG responses (26 and 49 msec). In part, they were also due to the varying extent to which the perturbations disturbed the tremor activity (see Fig. 4). In some subjects devoid of any significant tremor, the perturbations could trigger large amplitude tremor for periods usually varying between 1 and 3 sec. In 1 subject with a relatively large amplitude tremor, the perturbations markedly suppressed tremor amplitude as well as disrupting its rhythm.

Triggering and Resetting Tremor During Maintained Posture

Figure 7 illustrates both triggering and resetting of the phase of tremor during maintained posture against a one-sided steady state load. The subject had a slight tremor prior to the displacement. The tremor EMG bursts were not related in time to the displacements, which were delivered at random with respect to the tremor. However, the EMG bursts after the displacement occurred with a consistent relation to the beginning of the perturbation and were also considerably increased in amplitude. The direction of the initial displacement determined the temporal sequence of the EMG responses (Fig. 6). Figure 7 also illustrates, as was most often but not always the case, that the perturbation to stretch of tonically active muscle (Fig. 7A) was more effective in tremor triggering than if the muscle had less steady state activity (Fig. 7B).

Of the 32 Parkinson patients studied, 11 had consistent postural tremor with

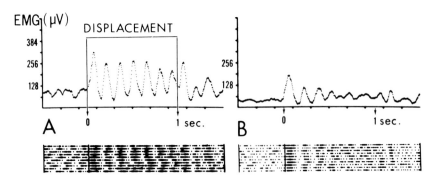

FIG. 7. Resetting and triggering of postural tremor. Biceps EMG activity was recorded during a maintained posture against a steady state load which required more **(A)** or less **(B)** biceps activation. A displacement in the handle position was produced by 1-sec perturbation which stretched the biceps muscle in both cases. It is evident from the figure that a perturbation which stretched the biceps when this muscle was actively resisting a steady state load **(A)** was more effective in triggering tremor than when the steady state load was acting in the opposite direction **(B)**. The cyclic activity of the biceps muscle during postural tremor prior to the perturbations is best seen in the raster display of tremor EMG activity in **A**. The initial stretch at time 0 synchronizes the poststimulus EMG activity with the stimulus, illustrating a resetting of the phase of postural tremor. The frequency of the postural tremor illustrated here is about 7 Hz, which is higher than that of 4.7-Hz resting tremor in the same patient (Fig. 5).

a frequency between 6 and 8 Hz. In 5 of the elderly normal volunteers (ages 61,71,71,75, and 80), the perturbation triggered oscillations during maintenance of the position with a frequency also of 6 to 8 Hz. These frequencies for the perturbation-triggered tremor were consistently higher than those of 3.8 to 5.1 Hz obtained for the resting parkinsonian tremor.

Bilateral Recordings of EMG Activity

Such reciprocity, as was usually the case between agonist and antagonist muscles, was not observed when the tremor of the right side was compared with the tremor of the left side. Bilateral EMG recordings from the extensor digitorum communis muscles were performed with 4 patients with bilateral resting tremor. In none of these patients was there synchronization of the EMG activity of the two sides during 12- to 15-min recording periods. In contrast to the resetting of the tremor of the perturbed hand, there was no effect on the EMG activity associated with the tremor of the contralateral limb.

DISCUSSION

The present results show that the *phase* of parkinsonian resting tremor can be reset by short external perturbations, provided that the perturbation is strong enough (in relation to the amplitude of the tremor) to cause a clear change in the limb position; for example, by reversing the direction of the tremor movement. The tremor resetting did not depend on the phase of the tremor at the time of the perturbation. Even if the perturbation was weak in relation to the force of the tremor, the displacement produced by the torque motor could still cause a change in the tremor *frequency* for a short period (usually less than 1 sec). Thus, inputs from peripheral receptors could markedly modify parkinsonian tremor, as has also been shown in the observations of Lee and Stein (11) reported at this same symposium.

Additional evidence in support of peripheral modulation of the large amplitude parkinsonian tremor has previously been presented. Stiles and Pozos (19) reported that by manually extending and flexing patients' hands with low frequency of oscillation of about 0.75 Hz, amplitude modulation of the tremor-related flexor and extensor EMG activity takes place. They also noted that the frequency of postural tremor in PD patients decreased by approximately one Hz for a 10-fold increase in displacement amplitude. Postural tremor may not operate on the same physiological basis as resting tremor, but the responses of PD tremor to large displacements was similar to responses of hand tremor in normal subjects in whom tremor had been induced by fatigue, thus suggesting the presence of both mechanical and reflex factors in the tremor (19). Several additional peripheral manipulations affect parkinsonian resting tremor amplitude and frequency, but have the disadvantage of being neurophysiologically complex and difficult to interpret. Thus, ischemia, tonic vibration, nerve block insufficent to decrease motor strength (18), and electrical stimulation of nerves (1,13,15, 17,18) or muscle (10) modulate resting tremor and, in the case of nerve stimulation, cause changes in the silent period and reset the tremor phase. In addition, Lee and Tatton (12) observed EMG oscillations after perturbation in a study involving active movement in a patient with resting tremor. Stimulations being randomly triggered, they concluded that "the peripheral mechanoceptor input may either reset an existing 5 Hz resting tremor, or initiate a 10 Hz oscillation."

The results that have now been summarized demonstrate resetting and triggering of tremor in PD patients and indicate that activity within the oscillatory tremorogenic loop is both modulated and triggered by peripheral proprioceptive input. Of course, this does not imply that the lesions responsible for the development of the parkinsonian tremor are not supraspinal. Instead, it is more likely that parkinsonian tremor results from a *failure* of normal CNS modulation of internal feedback signals within a supraspinal loop. The presence of "internal feedback" involving a supraspinal loop was suggested some time ago by Lundberg (14) and Oscarsson (16), and this concept is now supported by two new lines of neurophysiological evidence derived from studies on locomotion and scratching in the spinal animal. Arshavsky and co-workers (2–6) showed that in addition to modulation of spinal motoneurons by 1A afferent impulses, these same motoneurons are also modulated by central activity during "fictive locomotion." Modulation of both ventral spinocerebellar tract (VSCT) and dorsal spinocerebellar tract (DSCT) activity were observed in these experiments. DSCT modulation disappeared after peripheral deafferentation, whereas that of VSCT was preserved. It was concluded that VSCT is mainly concerned with centrally determined modulation, whereas DSCT is more concerned with peripherally determined modulation of motor activity. Similarly, by studying the scratch reflex in curarized spinal animal ("fictive scratching"), Arshavsky et al. (7,8) showed modulation of VSCT and cerebellar activity in the absence of peripheral afferent input. Taken broadly, the observations on VSCT modulation in deafferented preparations provide support for the concept of internal feedback. The existence of intrinsic oscillations within internal feedback loops in the absence of afferent input does not indicate that the afferent input is of no importance. On the contrary, when afferent input is present it can critically control the activity within the internal feedback circuits. The demonstration of this interaction of peripheral afferent input and internal rhythmic patterns has been made by Forssberg et al. (9) in the spinal cat showing that identical tactile stimuli applied to the dorsum of the foot in the middle of a step cycle could give rise to either a flexion or extension response, entirely depending on the phase of the step cycle in which the stimulus occurred. This demonstration of phase-dependent reflex reversal is another observation of centrally programmed movement subjected to peripheral afferent modifications, and is analogous to the resetting of tremor phase by external perturbations described in the present work.

From what is known of the anatomy and physiology of the CNS, the following hypothesis for mechanisms of parkinsonian tremor may be proposed: parkinsonian tremor is due to oscillations within a supraspinal loop involving proprioceptive impulses ascending via the VSCT to cerebellum, through nucleus ventralis lateralis (VL) of the thalamus to the motor cortex and returning back to spinal cord via the pyramidal tract. Figure 8 illustrates how ascending afferent inputs could impinge upon this circuit. The activity of VL nucleus is modulated by kinesthetic perturbations during limb movements (20), and it has a key position in this loop since it is a major point of convergence of both the cerebellar output and the output from the basal ganglia. Let us now assume that the "hyper-reflexia" leading to parkinsonian tremor is due to abnormal responses of the VL nucleus to the converging outputs of cerebellum and (diseased) basal ganglia; any output activating VL nucleus can generate, via motor cortex, a descending motor command which will, in turn, cause ascending internal feedback information in a loop which starts to oscillate. Oscillations in this loop can be set up both by internal feedback of impulses originating from the motor cortex, or by afferent inputs entering the same loop and triggering off the same type of oscillation. The present results on triggering and resetting the parkinsonian tremor can thus be considered as showing that stimuli injected into this hypothetical loop via peripheral pathways can trigger and/or modify its oscillatory activity.

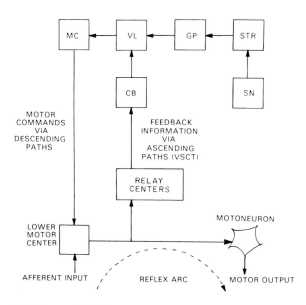

FIG. 8. A hypothetical supraspinal loop from the motor cortex (MC) to spinal cord and back to MC. Damage to the pathway from the substantia nigra (SN) to striatum (STR) leads to excessive output from the globus pallidus (GP) to the nucleus ventralis lateralis (VL) of the thalamus. Information arising both from MC and from afferent inputs converges in the spinal motor centers, and is then relayed upwards via ascending pathways through cerebellum (CB) to VL and MC. Either "internal feedback" arising from within the CNS, or external afferent input could trigger a hyperexcitable VL and set the loop into oscillation. Thus, while afferent input may not be necessary for the oscillations to occur within the loop, it can nevertheless modify or trigger activity within the inherently unstable loop.

SUMMARY

Single perturbations of 50-msec duration were delivered to flex or extend the wrist at known phases of resting parkinsonian tremor, either assisting or opposing ongoing tremor movements. The position of the wrist, and EMG of wrist extensor and flexor muscles, were recorded and subsequently analyzed by computer. Postural tremor was studied while patients resisted a steady state load and the tremor was disturbed by longer (1 sec) perturbations delivered at random in respect to the tremor. It was found for both resting and postural tremor that:

a) The phase of tremor can be reset by both sorts of perturbations.

b) Displacements delivered during absence of significant tremor can trigger tremor whose phases depended on the direction of the displacement.

c) Displacements usually increased tremor amplitude but could also stop tremor or disrupt its rhythm for short periods.

d) With a 50-msec perturbation, tremor frequency was not affected for more than 1 sec.

These results indicate the presence of a peripheral modulation of the parkinsonian tremor. Oscillation within a supraspinal internal feedback loop is suggested as a pathophysiological basis of the tremor, and it is proposed that afferent input can modify oscillatory activity within this loop.

REFERENCES

1. Alberts, W. W., Libet, B., Wright, Jr., E. W., and Feinstein, B. (1965): Physiological mechanisms of tremor and rigidity. *Confin. Neurol.,* 26:313–327.
2. Arshavsky, Yu. I., Berkinblit, M. B., Fukson, O. I., Gelfand, I. M., and Orlovsky, G. N. (1972): Activity of neurons of the DSCT during locomotion. *Biofizika,* 17:487–494.
3. Arshavsky, Yu. I., Berkinblit, M. B., Fukson, O. I., Gelfand, I. M., and Orlovsky, G. N. (1972): Activity of neurons of the VSCT during locomotion. *Biofizika,* 17:883–890.
4. Arshavsky, Yu. I., Berkinblit, M. B., Fukson, O. I., Gelfand, I. M., and Orlovsky, G. N. (1972): Activity of neurons of VSCT during locomotion of cats with deafferented hindlimbs. *Biofizika,* 17:1112–1118.
5. Arshavsky, Yu. I., Berkinblit, M. B., Fukson, O. I., Gelfand, I. M., and Orlovsky, G. N. (1972): Recording of neurons of the dorsal spinocerebellar tract during evoked locomotion. *Brain Res.,* 43:272–275.
6. Arshavsky, Yu. I., Berkinblit, M. B., Fukson, O. I., Gelfand, I. M., and Orlovsky, G. N. (1972): Origin of modulation in neurones of the ventral spinocerebellar tract during locomotion. *Brain Res.,* 43:276–279.
7. Arshavsky, Yu. I., Gelfand, I. M., Orlovsky, G. N., and Pavlova, G. A. (1975): Activity of neurones of the ventral spinocerebellar tract during "fictive scratching." *Biophysics,* 20:762–764.
8. Arshavsky, Yu. I., Gelfand, I. M., Orlovsky, G. N., and Pavlova, G. A. (1975): Origin of modulation in vestibulospinal neurons during scratching. *Biophysics,* 20:965–967.
9. Forssberg, H., Grillner, S., and Rossignol, S. (1976): Phase dependent reflex reversal during walking in chronic spinal cats. *Brain Res.,* 85:103–107.
10. Hufschmidt, H.-J. (1963): Proprioceptive origin of parkinsonian tremor. *Nature (Lond.),* 200:367–368.

11. Lee, R. G., and Stein, R. B. (1979): Reflex mechanisms in parkinsonian tremor and essential tremor. *Can. J. Neurol. Sci.,* 6.
12. Lee, R. G., and Tatton, W. G. (1975): Motor responses to sudden limb displacements in primates with specific CNS lesions and in human patients with motor system disorders. *Can. J. Neurol. Sci.,* 2:285–293.
13. Liberson, W. T. (1962): Monosynaptic reflexes and their clinical significance. *Electroenceph. Clin. Neurophys. (Suppl.),* 22:79–89.
14. Lundberg, A. (1966): Integration in the reflex pathway. In: *Muscular Afferents and Motor Control,* edited by R. Granit, pp. 275–305. Almqvist and Wiksell, Stockholm.
15. Mones, R. J., and Weiss, A. H. (1969): The response of the tremor of patients with parkinsonism to peripheral nerve stimulation. *J. Neurol. Neurosurg. Psychiatry,* 32:512–518.
16. Oscarsson, O. (1970): Functional organization of spinocerebellar paths. In: *Somatosensory System, Handbook of Sensory Physiology, Vol. 2,* edited by A. Iggo, pp. 121–127. Springer-Verlag, Berlin.
17. Renou, G., Rondot, P., and Bathien, N. (1973): Influence of peripheral stimulation on the silent period between bursts of parkinsonian tremor. In: *New Developments in Electromyography and Clinical Neurophysiology, Vol. 3,* edited by J. E. Desmedt, p. 635. Karger, Basel.
18. Rondot, P., and Bathien, N. (1976): Peripheral factors modulating parkinsonian tremor. In: *Advances in Parkinsonism,* edited by W. Birkmayer and O. Hornykiewicz, p. 269. Hoffman-La Roche and Co., Ltd., Basel.
19. Stiles, R. N., and Pozos, R. S. (1976): A mechanical-reflex oscillator hypothesis for parkinsonian hand tremor. *J. Appl. Physiol.,* 40:990–998.
20. Strick, P. L. (1976): Activity of ventrolateral thalamic neurons during arm movements. *J. Neurophysiol.,* 39:1032–1044.
21. Tatton, W. G., and Lee, R. G. (1975): Evidence for abnormal long-loop reflexes in rigid parkinsonian patients. *Brain Res.,* 100:671–676.

Advances in Neurology, Vol. 24, edited by
L. J. Poirier, T. L. Sourkes, and P. J. Bédard.
Raven Press, New York © 1979.

Single Unit Behavior in Human Muscle Afferent and Efferent Systems

Robert R. Young and Bhagwan T. Shahani

The Laboratory of Clinical Neurophysiology, Department of Neurology, Harvard Medical School, Massachusetts General Hospital, Boston, Massachusetts 02114

Physiologists study patients with various disorders of movement to understand in detail the abnormal behavior of the motor system. As a prerequisite, they should begin with even more detailed knowledge of normal physiology of the motor system but this is a state which is still far from being reached. Although important insights into the functional organization or "game plan" of the motor system may be obtained by studies of abnormal phenomena (indeed, practically all physiological experiments are carried out in animal preparations abnormally simplified by the artificial isolation of parts of the peripheral or central nervous system), neurophysiologists are obviously limited in their ability to explain or understand abnormal motor functions because sufficient understanding of the normal situation has not yet been achieved.

The contemporary clinical neurophysiologist may be differentiated from other neurophysiologists primarily in terms of the questions he asks; for example, the clinical neurophysiologist may concern himself with mechanisms underlying tremor, rigidity, and various normal and abnormal aspects of high level voluntary movement. Formerly, an important differentiating factor was the degree of precision of the experimental techniques available to, or employable by, one type of neurophysiologist or the other. Whereas even extracellular microelectrode recording from the human central nervous system is only very exceptionally undertaken and activity in dorsal root filaments is never recorded in man, techniques *have* been developed in the past decade by Hagbarth and Vallbo for the study of single unit behavior in the several human peripheral afferent systems (12,34). On the efferent side, reliable recordings of single motor unit activity during any other than weak tonic or "ramp" contractions remain impractical. However, computerized techniques have been developed during the 1970's by Freund, Andreassen, and others (2,8), which permit a quantitative description and statistical analysis of the discharge patterns of those single motor units which can be isolated during slow, nonphasic contractions.

We will now review certain aspects of the information gathered by the use of these single unit afferent recording techniques, and, in particular, recent contributions to our understanding of the function of the human motor system as it bears directly or indirectly upon the problems faced by patients with Parkinson's disease.

MUSCLE SPINDLE AFFERENT BEHAVIOR

There are several different types of tremor that are of clinical significance in patients with Parkinson's disease (11,19,28,29,31). Among these, the typical tremor-at-rest is still the primary symptom of Parkinson's disease which is most difficult to treat medically. When unaccompanied by an action tremor, it constitutes a primarily cosmetic disability or embarrassment to the patient though, at times, because of its dramatic appearance, it is deemed by patients to be responsible for their functional deficits which are, in fact, more accurately ascribed to akinesia. Nevertheless, tremor-at-rest remains one of the most troublesome aspects of Parkinson's disease even following the advent of dopaminergic therapies.

Although tremor-at-rest involves many regions of the peripheral and central nervous systems, the role played by muscle spindles and their afferent input in the genesis or modulation of this tremor has long been of interest. Earlier studies of the silent period produced by electrical stimulation (21) or sudden release of voluntarily contracting muscles (3,32) and experiments using local anesthetization of intramuscular nerves (27,35), yielded conflicting and necessarily indirect evidence as to the role of the muscle spindle in patients with Parkinson's disease. Following Merton's hypothesis concerning the production of movement around the so-called gamma loop (25), it became fashionable to consider that tremor and/or rigidity in Parkinson's disease reflected excessive activation of gamma efferent fibers to the muscle spindle, producing abnormal sensitivity of the static or phasic sensory endings on the intrafusal muscle fibers (see 9 for review). Evidence from ablative studies such as those of Foerster (7) or those with temporary block of conduction in peripheral nerves produced by local anesthetics (27,35) was taken to support the notion that an abnormality of muscle spindle afferent behavior was primarily involved in the production of symptoms and signs in patients with Parkinson's disease.

This assumption has not been supported by data emanating primarily from Hagbarth's laboratory (14) where the technique of *microneurography* was developed by Hagbarth and Vallbo (12). This involves recording single or multiunit afferent activity in human peripheral nerves by the introduction of a tungsten semimicroelectrode into the nerve under highly controlled conditions (see 34 for review). The activity recorded in this way is very similar to that which has been recorded in various animal laboratories for more than 40 years, principally from dorsal root filaments. As demonstrated in Fig. 1, muscle afferent activity is defined as coming from a muscle spindle when this activity (a) ceases during the initial phase of rising torque produced by an electrically induced twitch contraction of the extrafusal muscle fibers, and (b) begins again with a burst of discharges on the falling or relaxation phase of this twitch contraction.

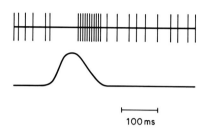

Fig. 1. Schematic drawing of impulses in a Ia primary spindle afferent ending *(upper line)* during an electrically induced twitch contraction of extrafusal fibers in the same muscle (movement produced by the muscle on *bottom line*). Calibration for this and subsequent figures is in milliseconds (ms). Note the pause in spindle afferent activity while the extrafusal fibers are actively contracting and one burst of afferent discharge as spindles are being passively stretched during the falling (relaxation) phase of the twitch.

The cessation of activity reflects the decrease in tension in intrafusal fibers produced by contraction of their extrafusal counterparts. As the extrafusal fibers relax and the muscle lengthens, intrafusal fibers are then stretched passively so that endings on their equatorial regions are stretched and impulses arise in the appropriate Ia fibers. There is *one* burst of Ia activity per twitch.

A different pattern of spindle afferent activity is recorded when the subject produces a brief voluntary twitch contraction of extrafusal fibers (Fig. 2). For each voluntary twitch, *two* bursts of activity are recorded in spindle afferent fibers. The second again reflects the passive stretch of the muscle spindle associated with relaxation of extrafusal fibers. However, the first burst of Ia activity occurs at roughly the same time as the EMG activity recorded from extrafusal fibers. This burst, associated with extrafusal muscle contraction, is due to so-called alpha–gamma linkage or coactivation (4,10,24). This first burst of Ia activity results from the fact that voluntary activation of alpha motoneurones in the anterior horn of the spinal cord is also accompanied by activation of gamma motoneurones in the same region. Therefore, gamma fusimotor outflow occurs at the same time and involves the same muscles as efferent activity in the alpha extrafusal system; this insures that the intrafusal endings will remain sensitive despite shortening of extrafusal fibers in parallel with them. There is evidence for the presence of beta motor outflow in cats where branches of one

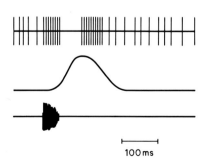

Fig. 2. Drawing of a recording similar to Fig. 1 but during a voluntary twitch contraction. *Upper line,* here as in Figs. 1–4, represents microneurographic recording of action potentials in Ia spindle afferent fibers. *Middle line,* as in Figs. 1–4, represents goniometric recording of movement produced by muscular activity. *Bottom line,* as in Figs. 2–4, represents EMG activity recorded from the muscle involved. Note two bursts of spindle afferent discharge: the one at about the same time as the voluntary EMG burst represents the results of alpha–gamma coactivation; and the second, at the same time as the one in Fig. 1, represents activity produced by passive stretch of the spindle.

alpha motor axone innervate both extra- and intrafusal fibers (6). Though this may occur in man, evidence to be reported elsewhere (D. Burke and K. -E. Hagbarth, *personal communication*) suggests that it may not be particularly significant. Careful analysis of the timing of the bursts of muscle spindle afferent activity reflecting alpha–gamma coactivation demonstrates that natural movements rarely, if ever, occur "around the gamma loop" by means of a follow-up servo-mechanism in the way first suggested by Merton (25), though servo-assistance via the segmental stretch reflex is an important element of motor control (15).

When normal subjects make voluntary sinusoidal tremorlike contractions of antagonist muscles at rates of 4 to 5 Hz, each cycle of this repetitive movement is also accompanied (as in Fig. 3) by two bursts of activity in the spindle primary afferents coming from one of these muscles (13). These are similar in origin to those depicted in Fig. 2. Hagbarth and colleagues have also shown clearly (14) that two similarly timed bursts of spindle afferent activity are seen per cycle of the typical tremor-at-rest of patients with Parkinson's disease whose tremulous movements are "involuntary" (similar to Fig. 3). It appears, therefore, that muscle spindle afferents *are* involved in the tremor-at-rest of Parkinson's disease, but that their behavior in terms of alpha–gamma coactivation is identical with what is recorded during normal voluntary tremorlike movements. It is as though (a) the tremor-at-rest of Parkinson's disease is being produced by descending volleys in motor system pathways ordinarily concerned with voluntary movements (1), and (b) the spinal segmental organization is utilized normally, at least in terms of fusimotor behavior (14). There is, then, no demonstrable abnormality in the behavior of muscle spindles in patients with the tremor-at-rest of Parkinson's disease [or in those with rigidity (see ref. 5 for review)]. Therefore, no contradiction exists between observations that the phase of tremor cycles in patients with Parkinson's disease can be reset by perturbations of the peripheral motor apparatus [produced by either an electrical twitch (18,21) or a mechanically induced change in length of extrafusal fibers (Teräväinen et al., *this volume*)], though the tremor-at-rest is not abolished by dorsal rhizotomy (7,20,26)—two observations which were surprisingly difficult to reconcile.

The following question then arises: Are all tremulous movements in humans

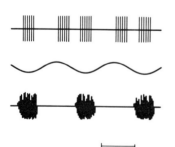

Fig. 3. Drawing of typical spindle afferent discharge, joint movement and EMG activity associated either with voluntary alternating 5-Hz rhythmic contraction or involuntary 5-Hz tremor-at-rest of Parkinson's disease. Note two bursts of spindle discharge per cycle of movement. The origin of each burst is similar to those in Fig. 2 and reflects alpha–gamma coactivation.

200 ms

associated with alpha–gamma coactivation? At least two types of tremulous movements have recently been demonstrated *not* to be associated with alpha–gamma coactivation. The first of these is clonus, in which Struppler and colleagues (33) as well as Hagbarth and his group (14) have demonstrated that muscle spindle afferent activity occurs in only one burst during each cycle of clonus (Fig. 4). This is the burst produced by passive lengthening of the muscle spindle as the extrafusal fibers relax; there is no evidence of contraction of intrafusal fibers. This is also true, of course, of electrically induced twitches, as demonstrated in Fig. 1, and of tendon jerks as well as the repeated stretch reflexes of clonus (Fig. 4). Apparently the spindle afferent activity, which enters the cord and is responsible for activation of alpha motoneurones in the segmental stretch reflex, does not coactivate gamma motoneurones.

Enhanced physiological tremor such as that produced by fatigue in normal subjects or in patients with Parkinson's disease, is the second example—and perhaps the first example of a true tremor—in which alpha–gamma coactivation is not present (15). Spindle afferent bursts, produced by passive stretch of intrafusal fibers during relaxation phases of the tremor in extrafusal fibers in that muscle, are able to affect the timing of discharges in a voluntarily activated motoneuron pool (Fig. 4)—voluntary background activation being necessary for demonstration of physiological tremor. Physiological tremor has been demonstrated by Schwab and colleagues (19,28) to occur in patients with Parkinson's disease as well as in subjects with normal motor systems. Therefore, it appears that patients with Parkinson's disease have at least two different mechanisms underlying two of their several different types of tremor—one with alpha–gamma coactivation and one without. Pharmacological or other manipulations can alter certain of the peripherally induced tremors such as those associated with anxiety (23) or the infusion of beta-adrenergic stimulating agents (22,36) in patients with Parkinson's disease, even though these same manipulations will not affect the centrally programmed and "normally mediated" tremor-at-rest, a symptom or sign of Parkinson's disease which *is* particularly well controlled by discrete stereotactic lesions of several targets deep in the cerebral hemisphere. In our experience, these CNS lesions do not, on the other hand, reduce the amplitude of peripherally induced tremors.

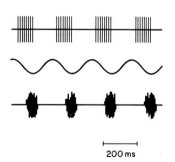

200 ms

Fig. 4. Drawing as in Fig. 3 but representing either the alternating contraction associated with clonus in a spastic patient or enhanced physiological tremor in a normal subject who is fatigued or who has received beta–adrenergic agonists. Note one burst of spindle discharge per cycle of movement. Each burst has an origin similar to that seen in Fig. 1; no evidence for gamma—fusimotor activation is seen. There *are* differences in the mechanisms underlying clonus (where the motoneurones are primarily activated by the Ia input) and enhanced physiological tremor (where discharges in voluntary activated motoneurones are timed by Ia input) (15).

SINGLE MOTOR UNIT BEHAVIOR

In comparison with microneurography, it is technically much easier to record activity of single or multiple motor units in human muscles, particularly those smaller motor units which are tonically recruited during voluntary or other contractions that produce little force. It still remains difficult, if not impossible, to obtain reproducible recordings of single motor unit activity from muscles during moderate or strong tonic contractions, or phasic contractions of any strength. Henneman's size principle (17) states that smaller diameter motoneurones with smaller diameter axons and fewer muscle fibers in their motor units are activated before larger motoneurones in voluntary or reflexly mediated contractions of extrafusal muscle. This is certainly true in normal subjects who produce either slow ramp contractions (16) or 4 to 5/sec repeated voluntary contractions mimicking tremor. Furthermore, as with the afferent activity described above, one finds elements of normal recruitment behavior of motoneurones in each of the bursts of EMG activity in the tremor-at-rest of Parkinson's disease (30,31,37). That is to say, smaller motor units are activated before larger ones in each burst (Fig. 5)—it appears as though "normal" descending motor system mechanisms are involved in the production of tremor-at-rest. This appears also to be true of enhanced physiological tremors; the lower amplitude physiological tremors are not associated with grouping of EMG discharges (15). However, in essential–familial types of tremor that are also common in patients with Parkinson's disease (11,28,29), a different pattern is seen during single motor unit analyses. During any given burst of EMG activity from extrafusal fibers in patients with essential tremor, larger motor units may be activated before smaller ones. As opposed to the tremor bursts in the tremor-at-rest of patients with Parkinson's disease in which each burst appears to arise *de novo,* it is as though the bursts of activity in patients with essential tremor reflect periodic interruptions in an ongoing background discharge—Fig. 6 illustrates this principle.

However, it must also be emphasized that at least two abnormal elements of recruitment behavior of single motor units are also recorded in patients with tremor-at-rest of Parkinson's disease or essential–familial tremor. The first concerns the instantaneous firing frequency (IFF) of single motor units. Normally, in ramp contractions with slowly increasing force or during maintenance of a

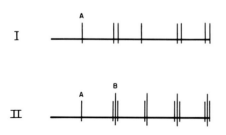

Fig. 5. Schematic drawing of the behavior of single motor unit (SMU) potentials in tremor-at-rest of Parkinson's disease. **I:** Recruitment of a low threshold SMU *(A).* Note high IFF in the second, fourth, and fifth tremor bursts. **II:** Additional recruitment of a higher threshold SMU *(B)* which follows a normal rank order of recruitment in each tremor burst. Calibration is 1 sec per total sweep.

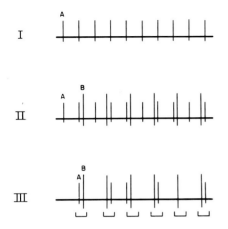

Fig. 6. A possible mechanism producing essential tremor (schematically depicted). I: Normal recruitment of a low threshold SMU *(A)*. II. Normal recruitment of an additional, larger amplitude, higher threshold SMU *(B)*. III. "Inhibition" of SMU discharge at regular intervals (between the brackets) produces appearance of the recruitment pattern seen in essential tremor. Note apparent failure of SMU to obey the "size principle" in each tremor burst *(bracketed)* with either unit A or B appearing to be recruited first. Calibration is 1 sec per total sweep.

steady output of force, motor units fire 8 to 12 times/sec and rarely can be recorded at firing rates in excess of 15 Hz. In patients with Parkinson's disease, the motor units activated at low tension levels can be seen to fire 2 or 3 times (IFF up to 50 Hz) during each tremor burst. During the tremor bursts in patients with essential–familial tremor, single motor units also may develop an abnormally high IFF (20–50 Hz). In normal subjects, such repetitive discharges at IFF's of 20–50 Hz are only seen during ballistic or quick phasic movements which are, at first glance at least, quite different from the settings in which tremor is seen in the 2 patient populations noted above.

The second abnormality concerns synchronization or temporal grouping of discharges of two or more separate motor units. Obviously *short-term* synchronization of independent motor units firing at about the same frequency will occur not infrequently "by chance," but these fortuitous groupings appear to be of no clinical consequence normally and are not even responsible for the production of physiological tremor (9,15). *Long-term* synchronization, on the other hand, is clearly abnormal. It is observed in the tremor-at-rest of Parkinson's disease and in the essential–familial tremors. It also can be produced in an active motoneurone pool in normal subjects by infusion of isoproterenol to stimulate intramuscular beta-adrenergic tremorogenic receptors or by vibration of the muscle. The detailed anatomy of these beta-adrenergic receptors and their normal functional significance remains to be demonstrated.

SUMMARY

In summary, therefore, both muscle spindle afferent activity and at least certain aspects of single motor unit behavior in the tremor-at-rest of Parkinson's disease appear to arise from the activity of perfectly normal mechanisms routinely employed in ordinary voluntary movement. This is not true for other types of human tremor; enhanced physiological tremor does not involve alpha–gamma coactivation and essential tremor does not appear to result from repeated renewed recruitment of motor units in each tremor burst. Though the implications for understanding the pathophysiology of Parkinson's disease or for its more effective treatment are not yet clear, there is little reason to doubt that increased understanding of the afferent and efferent unitary mechanisms involved will eventually be as useful as it is interesting at the present time.

ACKNOWLEDGMENTS

Supported by the Parkinson's Disease Project of the Massachusetts General Hospital.

REFERENCES

1. Alberts, W. W. (1972): A simple view of parkinsonian tremor. Electrical stimulation of cortex adjacent to the Rolandic fissure in awake man. *Brain Res.,* 44:357–369.
2. Andreassen, S. (1977): *Interval Pattern of Single Motor Units.* Technical University of Denmark, Copenhagen.
3. Angel, R. W. (1973): Spasticity and tremor. In: *New Developments in Electromyography and Clinical Neurophysiology,* edited by J. E. Desmedt, pp. 618–624. Karger, Basel.
4. Burke, D., Hagbarth, K.-E., and Löfstedt, L. (1978): Muscle spindle activity in man during shortening and lengthening contractions. *J. Physiol.,* 277:131–142.
5. Burke, D., Hagbarth, K.-E., and Wallin, B. G. (1977): Reflex mechanisms in parkinsonian rigidity. *Scand. J. Rehab. Med.,* 9:15–23.
6. Edmonet-Dénand, F., Jami, L., and Laporte, Y. (1975): Skeleto-fusimotor axons in hind-limb muscles of the cat. *J. Physiol.,* 249:153–166.
7. Foerster, O. (1936): Symptomatologie der Erkrankungen des Rückenmarks und seiner Wurzeln. In *Handbuch der Neurologie, Vol. 5,* edited by Bumke and Foerster, pp. 1–403. Springer-Verlag, Berlin.
8. Freund, H.-J., Budingen, H. J., and Dietz, V. (1975): Activity of single motor units from human forearm muscles during voluntary isometric contractions. *J. Neurophysiol.,* 38:933–946.
9. Freund, H.-J., and Dietz, V. (1978): The relationship between physiological and pathological tremor. In: *Physiological Tremor, Pathological Tremors and Clonus,* edited by J. E. Desmedt, pp. 66–89. Karger, Basel.
10. Granit, R. (1973): Linkage of alpha and gamma motoneurones in voluntary movement. *Nature (New Biol.),* 243:52–53.
11. Growden, J. H., Young, R. R., and Shahani, B. T. (1976): The differential diagnosis of tremor in Parkinson's disease. *Trans. Am. Neurol. Assoc.,* 150:197–199.
12. Hagbarth, K.-E., and Vallbo, Å. B. (1969): Single unit recordings from muscle nerves in human subjects. *Acta Physiol. Scand.,* 76:321–334.
13. Hagbarth, K.-E., Wallin, G., and Löfstedt, L. (1975): Muscle spindle activity in man during voluntary fast alternating movements. *J. Neurol. Neurosurg. Psychiatry,* 38:625–635.
14. Hagbarth, K.-E., Wallin, G., Löfstedt, L., and Aquilonius, S. M. (1975): Muscle spindle activity in alternating tremor of parkinsonism and in clonus. *J. Neurol. Neurosurg. Psychiatry,* 38:636–641.
15. Hagbarth, K.-E., and Young, R. R. (1979): Participation of the stretch reflex in human physiological tremor. *Brain (in press).*
16. Henneman, E., Shahani, B. T., and Young, R. R. (1976): The extent of voluntary control of human motor units. In: *The Motor System: Neurophysiology and Muscle Mechanisms,* edited by M. Shahani, pp. 73–78. Elsevier, Amsterdam.
17. Henneman, E., Somjen, G., and Carpenter, D. O. (1965): Functional significance of cell size in spinal motoneurons. *J. Neurophysiol.,* 28:560–580.
18. Hufschmidt, H. J. (1959): Über die reflektorische Grundlage des Parkinson-Tremors. *Dtsch. Z. Nervenheilk.,* 179:298–308.
19. Lance, J. W., Schwab, R. S. and Peterson, E. A. (1963): Action tremor and the cogwheel phenomenon in Parkinson's disease. *Brain,* 86:95–110.

20. Leriche, R. (1914): Radicotomie cervicale pour un tremblement parkinsonism. *Lyon Méd.,* 122:1075–1076.
21. Liberson, W. T. (1962): Monosynaptic reflexes and their clinical significance. *Electroenceph. Clin. Neurophysiol. (Suppl.),* 22:79–88.
22. Marsden, C. D., Foley, T. H., Owen, D. A. L., and McAllister, R. G. (1967): Peripheral beta-adrenergic receptors concerned with tremor. *Clin. Sci.,* 33:53–65.
23. Marsden, C. D., Gimlette, T. M. D., McAllister, R. G., Owen, D. A. L., and Miller, T. N. (1968): Effect of beta-adrenergic blockade on finger tremor and Achilles reflex time in anxious and thyrotoxic patients. *Acta Endocrinol.,* 57:353–362.
24. Matthews, P. B. C. (1972): *Mammalian Muscle Receptors and their Central Actions.* Arnold, London.
25. Merton, P. A. (1953): Speculations on the servo-control of movement. In: *The Spinal Cord,* edited by G. E. W. Wolstenholme, pp. 247–255. Churchill, London.
26. Pollock, L. J., and Davis, L. (1930): Muscle tone in parkinsonian states. *Arch. Neurol. Psychiatry,* 23:303–319.
27. Rondot, P. (1968): Physiopathologie du tremblement. *Gaz. méd. Fr.,* 20:75.
28. Schwab, R. S., and Young, R. R. (1971): Non-resting tremor in Parkinson's disease. *Trans. Am. Neurol. Assoc.,* 96:305–307.
29. Shahani, B. T., and Young, R. R. (1976): Physiological and pharmacological aids in the differential diagnosis of tremor. *J. Neurol. Neurosurg. Psychiatry,* 39:772–783.
30. Shahani, B. T., and Young, R. R. (1977): Specific abnormalities of single motor unit discharge patterns in tremor. *Neurology,* 27:354.
31. Shahani, B. T., and Young, R. R. (1978): Action tremors: a clinical neurophysiological review. In: *Physiological Tremor, Pathological Tremors and Clonus. Vol. 5: Progress in Clinical Neurophysiology,* edited by J. E. Desmedt, pp. 603–617. Karger, Basel.
32. Struppler, A., Burg, D., and Erbel, F. (1973): The unloading reflex under normal and pathological conditions in man. In: *New Developments in Electromyography and Clinical Neurophysiology,* edited by J. E. Desmedt, pp. 603–617. Karger, Basel.
33. Szumski, A. J., Burg, D., Struppler, A., and Velho, F. (1974): Activity of muscle spindles during muscle twitch and clonus in normal and spastic human subjects. *Electroencephalogr. Clin. Neurophysiol.,* 37:589–597.
34. Vallbo, Å. B., Hagbarth, K-E., Torebjörk, H. E., and Wallin, B. G. (1979): Proprioceptive somatosensory and sympathetic activity in peripheral human nerves. *Physiol. Rev.,* 59 (*in press*).
35. Walshe, F. M. R. (1924): Observations on the nature of the muscular rigidity of paralysis agitans, and on its relationship to tremor. *Brain,* 47:159–177.
36. Young, R. R., Growden, J. H., and Shahani, B. T. (1975): Beta-adrenergic mechanisms in action tremor. *New Engl. J. Med.,* 293:950–953.
37. Young, R. R., and Shahani, B. T. (1978): Analysis of single motor unit discharge patterns in different types of tremor. In: *Contemporary Clinical Neurophysiology (EEG Suppl. No. 34),* edited by W. A. Cobb and H. Van Duijn, pp. 527–528. Elsevier, Amsterdam.

Advances in Neurology, Vol. 24, edited by
L. J. Poirier, T. L. Sourkes, and P. J. Bédard.
Raven Press, New York © 1979.

Increased Dependence on Visual Information for Arm Movement in Patients with Parkinson's Disease

J. D. Cooke and J. D. Brown

Departments of Physiology and Clinical Neurological Sciences, University of Western Ontario, London, Canada

In patients with idiopathic or postencephalitic parkinsonism, it is well recognized that there may be day to day or even moment to moment changes in motor facility. As well, the presentation of tactile and visual cues or sudden other stimuli may allow or produce motor activity that otherwise would be impossible for the patient. Martin (9) documented this visual dependence in postencephalitic parkinsonian patients who seemed unable to walk or, at best, could make only short steps or shuffling movements. When presented with bold transverse lines in front of them, these same patients could then step out quite reasonably. Similarly, a small obstacle of any kind placed in front of these patients would enable them to start out and, at times, carry on without cues. Further, parkinsonian patients may climb stairs more easily than they can walk on the level.

In these patients, postural fixation of limbs has been shown to depend heavily on visual information. If Martin (9) asked his patients to reach out with their arms at shoulder height and touch, alternatively, the tips of the two forefingers held 9 to 15 inches apart, they were able to do so quite well for several minutes if their eyes were open. However, with eyes closed, the hand would almost immediately drop and the movement stop or gradually decrease. The subjective awareness of movement and relative limb position appeared intact in these same patients.

Hore et al. (7,8) have observed such an apparent reliance on visual cues for successful performance of motor activity in monkeys with reversible lesions in the globus pallidus. During cooling through a sheath implanted in the globus pallidus, the performance of simple step movements was impaired if the animal had no visual feedback of his arm position. Even with visual guidance, some impairment of motor performance remained during cooling. For example, movements were of a smaller amplitude and there was a tendency toward a flexion posture. Visual information, importantly, allowed the animals to improve their overall performance.

We describe here studies of patients with idiopathic parkinsonism, that indicate a similar increased dependence on visual information in the performance of simple arm movements. These studies have recently been published (1,2). The data to be presented are representative of the data obtained from 3 patients with idiopathic parkinsonism and 3 age-matched normal control subjects. Each of the patients' disability was assessed at the stage III level of Hoehn and Yahr (4). That is, there were some signs of impaired righting-reflexes, but each had some work potential and were physically capable of leading independent lives; their disability was mild to moderate. The particular patient discussed here was a 65-year-old man who was diagnosed as having Parkinson's disease in 1977. He showed normal mentation, reduction in facial expression, eye blink and associated movements and cogwheel rigidity of the neck and arms. The left side was more affected than the right and a resting tremor of the left hand was present. He was not on medication at the time of diagnosis or experimentation.

During the experiment, the subject was seated comfortably grasping a manipulandum handle (11) with his arm held horizontally and supported at the elbow. The subject's vision of his operant arm was blocked by a sheet. A continual record of handle (and thus forearm) position was obtained from a potentiometer at the handle pivot point. An oscilloscope placed at eye level approximately 1 m in front of the subject was used to present a visual display of handle position and/or target position. The target was displayed as a vertical bar; the width of the bar indicated the target width. The handle position was displayed as a vertical line. The targets were not mechanically detectable and were not bounded by mechanical stops. Target settings, visual display, etc., were controlled by a programmable analog-digital system (10). Data were recorded on an analog tape recorder (Honeywell 7600) and were digitized either on- or off-line with a PDP-11/40 system using a 200-Hz effective sampling rate.

The subject was required to perform two types of tracking movements by superimposing the handle bar on the target bar: (a) *step tracking,* where the target abruptly switched between two fixed positions every two seconds, and (b) *continuous tracking,* where the target to be tracked moved at constant velocity (ramp movement) between two fixed positions. For the step-tracking trials no restrictions were placed on movement times, reaction times, etc. The subjects were free to choose their own strategy of movement. The amplitude of target movement for all tests was 32° of arc. A movement was considered "in target" if the handle was within 6° of the target center.

In Fig. 1 are shown examples of the different types of tracking movements made by the patient with Parkinson's disease and by a normal subject. Both subjects were first required to track the target under visual guidance (VISION, left hand columns). After approximately 40 movements, the subject rested briefly. The handle cursor was then removed from the visual display (NO VISION, right hand columns) and a further 40 movements were recorded without any external cues of forearm position. Both the patient with Parkinson's disease

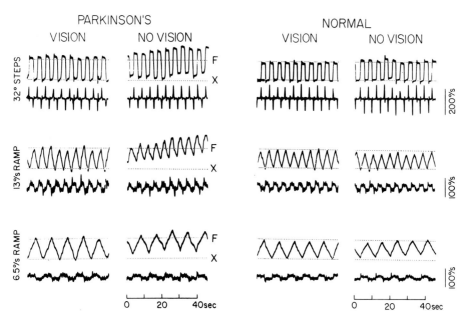

Fig. 1. Each pair of traces indicates handle position *(upper trace)* and velocity *(lower trace)* during performance of a tracking task. During the VISION trials, both handle and target cursors were visible to the subject; during the NO VISION trials, only the target cursor was visible. The traces on the left were obtained from the patient with Parkinson's disease and those on the right from the age-matched control. As indicated, an upward deflection of the position trace indicates a flexion movement. The *horizontal dotted lines* indicate the target centers for the step tracking trials and the maximum target movement for the ramp tracking trials. The distance between the dotted lines was 32° in each case (AG200477L, WS181077R). (From the *Canadian Journal of Neurological Sciences,* with permission.)

and the normal subject performed well under the "VISION" conditions. During step tracking the patient with Parkinson's disease showed a tendency for the arm to drift towards flexion while holding in the extension position between movements, this drift being interrupted periodically by a flexion movement. No overall change in limb position resulted during the course of the trial.

This tendency for flexion drift became more apparent if the handle cursor was not visible, i.e., the subject had to rely on proprioceptive information for limb positioning (Fig. 1; NO VISION). The patient with Parkinson's disease showed a progressive drift of arm position towards flexion during both step and continuous tracking.

Figure 2A shows mean end positions under the various conditions. For the step tracking movements the end position was taken as the mean arm position during holding between movements; for the continuous (ramp) tracking movements it was taken as the arm position when movement direction was reversed. As was indicated in Fig. 1, the patient with Parkinson's disease showed an

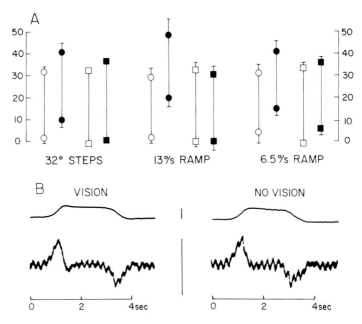

Fig. 2. A: Mean end positions of movements made with *(open symbols)* and without *(closed symbols)* the handle position being displayed. *Circles* show data obtained from the Parkinson patient and *squares,* from the normal control. Standard deviation bars are shown where greater than the plotted points. The vertical scale represents degrees with the target centers (steps) or maximum target movement (ramps) being at 0 and 32°. **B:** Step-tracking movements by the Parkinson patient during VISION and NO VISION trials. The *upper trace* is handle position and the *lower trace* velocity. Oscillations at approximately 5 Hz in the velocity record represent the Parkinson tremor. (From the *Canadian Journal of Neurological Sciences,* with permission.)

overall flexion drift when visual information about arm position was not given (NO VISION). The variability of arm positioning is indicated by the standard deviation bars. In contrast, the normal subject showed variably a flexion, an extension or no drift.

The increased variability in arm positioning during the NO VISION trials with the patient with Parkinson's disease was not associated with any overall change in movement amplitude (Fig. 2A), nor, as may be seen from the velocity records in Fig. 1 and in more detail in Fig. 2B, was there any marked change in the magnitude of the Parkinson's tremor during the "NO VISION" trials.

The present experiments thus reflect, in humans, the increased dependence on visual information observed in monkeys making accurate arm movements during basal ganglia dysfunction (6). In the present study, the subject with Parkinson's disease was unable to accurately maintain proper arm positioning in the absence of visual information about arm position. Since the forearm was fully supported, this cannot be attributed to loss of control of postural reflexes as was suggested by Martin (9) in explanation of some of his observations.

It has been suggested that the rigidity in idiopathic and other forms of parkinsonism may be related to selective increase in drive to the "static" fusimotor neurons (3), perhaps with an upper limb flexor bias. The flexion drift seen in the patients studied is, presumably, a reflection of this well-known clinical phenomenon. It must be emphasized, however, that in the absence of visual information about arm position, the Parkinson's patients did not correct for this flex or drift. Whether this was due to a lack of proprioceptive "awareness" of limb position is, as yet, uncertain.

In the examples shown in Fig. 1, the overall arm position was 10 to 20° in error by the end of the "NO VISION" trial. The rate of drift was about 0.3 to 0.5°/sec. At comparable angular velocities, normal subjects have been shown to detect passive angular displacements of less than 1° about the elbow (8) and of 3 to 4° about the knee (5) at the much slower velocity of 1°/min (5). In the absence of visual information, the patient with Parkinson's disease thus appeared unable to detect displacements, which were well in excess of the threshold for detection of passive displacements in normal humans. Care, however, must be taken in interpreting this as arising from some deficit in proprioceptive mechanisms; whether the flexion drift seen in the patient with Parkinson's disease may be equated with a passive displacement is uncertain. The former must arise from activity within the central nervous system and, as such, may not necessarily engage proprioceptive mechanisms in the same way or to the same extent as do externally applied displacements.

REFERENCES

1. Cooke, J. D., Brooks, V. B., Brown, J., and Lucier, G. (1977): Impaired awareness of arm position in Parkinson patients in the absence of visual feedback. *Soc. Neurosci. Abstr.,* 3:270.
2. Cooke, J. D., Brown, J. D., and Brooks, V. (1978): Increased dependence on visual information for movement control in patients with Parkinson's disease. *Can. J. Neurol. Sci.,* 5:413–415.
3. Dietrichson, P. (1971): *The Role of the Fusimotor System in Spasticity and Parkinsonian Rigidity,* p. 101. Universitetsforlaget, Oslo.
4. Hoehn, M. M., and Yahr, M. D. (1976): Parkinsonism: onset, progression, and mortality. *Neurology,* 17:427–442.
5. Horch, W., Clark, F. J., and Burgess, P. R. (1975): Awareness of knee joint angle under static conditions. *J. Neurophysiol.,* 38:1436–1447.
6. Hore, J., Meyer-Lohmann, J., and Brooks, V. B. (1977): Basal ganglia cooling disables learned arm movements of monkeys in the absence of visual guidance. *Science,* 195:584–685.
7. Hore, J., and Vilis, T. (1979): Monkey arm movement performance during basal ganglia dysfunction. *Can. J. Neurol. Sci.,* 6:48.
8. Laidlaw, R. W., and Hamilton, M. A. (1937): The quantitative measurement of apperception of passive movement. *Bull. Neurol. Inst. N.Y.,* 6:145–153.
9. Martin, J. P. (1967): *The Basal Ganglia and Posture.* Pitman Medical, London.
10. Thomas, J. S., and Cooke, J. D. (1976): A programmable analog-digital system for physiological and behavioural experiments. *J. Electrophysiol. Tech.,* 5:44–48.
11. Thomas, J. S., Croft, D., and Brooks, V. B. (1976): A manipulandum for human motor studies. *IEEE Trans. Biomed. Eng.,* 23:83–84.

Advances in Neurology, Vol. 24, edited by
L. J. Poirier, T. L. Sourkes, and P. J. Bédard.
Raven Press, New York © 1979.

Role of Dopamine in Substantia Nigra in the Regulation of Nigrostriatal Dopaminergic Neuron Activity

*A. Nieoullon, **A. Cheramy, and **J. Glowinski

*Institut de Neurophysiologie et Psychophysiologie du C.N.R.S., Département de
Neurophysiologie Générale, 13274 Marseille Cedex 2, France; and **Groupe NB, INSERM
U 114, Collège de France, 75231 Paris Cedex 5, France*

The concept of an autoregulation of dopaminergic neuron activity by dopamine (DA) itself at the level of the substantia nigra (SN) was first put forward by Aghajanian and Bunney (1). They suggested that DA in the SN has a physiological role since the iontophoretic application of DA reduces the firing of the dopaminergic cells and this effect is blocked by pretreatment with neuroleptics. A similar self-inhibitory mechanism was observed by Groves et al. (6) who reported that neurons in the SN pars compacta were inhibited by the local infusion of amphetamine. Therefore, it was proposed that DA in the SN could act on dopaminergic receptors located on the dopaminergic cells themselves.

BIOCHEMICAL EFFECT OF DOPAMINE IN THE SUBSTANTIA NIGRA ON THE ACTIVITY OF THE NIGRO-STRIATAL DOPAMINERGIC NEURONS

The effect of introducing exogenous DA in the SN on the activity of the nigrostriatal dopaminergic neurons was measured in our experimental model. We simultaneously used two push–pull cannulae in the same cat, either anesthetized with halothane, or "encéphale isolé" preparation. One cannula, placed in the caudate nucleus, is used to measure the release of ^{3}H-DA newly formed in the dopaminergic nerve terminals from L-^{3}H-tyrosine. The other cannula is placed at the level of the ipsilateral SN to pharmacologically modulate the activity of the dopaminergic neurons. The introduction of DA at low concentration (10^{-7}M) in the SN is followed by a significant decrease of ^{3}H-DA release from the corresponding caudate nucleus (Fig. 1). Thus, this result confirms that DA introduced into the SN inhibits the activity of the dopaminergic neurons, as suggested by the reduction of the amount of transmitter released from the axonal nerve endings. Moreover, this result is duplicated when the extraneuronal level of DA in SN is pharmacologically increased by nigral application of am-

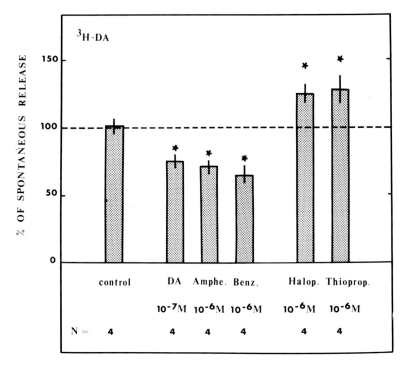

Fig. 1. Effect of superfusion of substantia nigra with DA and DA-related compounds on the release of ^{3}H-DA in the ipsilateral caudate nucleus. Two push–pull cannulae were simultaneously implanted into the left caudate nucleus and the left SN in cats. The cannula introduced into the caudate nucleus was continuously superfused with an artificial CSF containing L-3,5-^{3}H-tyrosine (25 μCi/500 μl/15 min). Three hours after the onset of the superfusion, DA (10^{-7}M) was added to the superfusing fluid of the SN. Hatched bars represent the quantity of ^{3}H-DA found in the superfusate fraction of the caudate nucleus during application of the drug in the SN. Data are the mean ± SEM of results obtained from groups of N animals. *p<0.05 compared with the corresponding control values. Similar experiments were performed with amphetamine (Amphe., 10^{-6}M), benztropine (Benz., 10^{-6}M), haloperidol (Halop., 10^{-6}M), and thioproperazine (Thioprop., 10^{-6}M).

phetamine (10^{-6}M) or benztropine (10^{-6}M), that act by facilitating the release mechanism and blocking the reuptake mechanism of the transmitter, respectively (Fig. 1).

In contrast, the application of antagonists of the dopaminergic receptors in SN causes activation of the dopaminergic neurons. This was shown by introducing haloperidol (10^{-6}M) into the superfusing fluid of the SN. This results in a significant increase of released ^{3}H-DA from the ipsilateral caudate nucleus. Similar results were obtained with another neuroleptic, thioproperazine (10^{-6}M) (Fig. 1).

These results are in agreement with the concept of autoregulation, as suggested by the finding in electrophysiological experiments. Therefore, DA in the SN seems to contribute to the regulation of the activity of the dopaminergic neurons by acting on dopaminergic receptors.

RELEASE OF DOPAMINE IN VIVO FROM THE CAT SUBSTANTIA NIGRA

The results obtained with amphetamine also extend to the findings of Björklund and Lindvall (2), who previously assumed that DA in the SN could be released from the dopaminergic neurons. From histochemical studies it was shown that numerous dendrites of the dopaminergic neurons in the rat brain course through the pars reticulata of the SN, and that DA could possibly be released from these dendrites. These results are supported by direct in vitro measurement of the release of DA from rat SN slices (5). Exogenous ^{3}H-DA previously taken up in the tissue was effectively released by potassium in a calcium-dependent mechanism.

In our cat model, the release of DA from SN was measured in vivo using the push–pull cannula technique and the continuous labeling of the dopaminergic

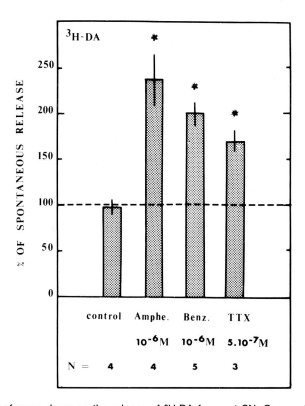

Fig. 2. Effect of some drugs on the release of ^{3}H-DA from cat SN. One push–pull cannula was introduced in SN and superfused with an artificial CSF containing L-3,5-^{3}H-tyrosine. Three hr after the beginning of the superfusion, amphetamine (Amphe., 10^{-6}M), benztropine (Benz., 10^{-6}M), or tetrodotoxine (TTX; 5.10^{-7}M) were added to the superfusing fluid. Hatched bars represent the quantity of ^{3}H-DA found in the superfusate of the SN during application of the drug in the structure. Results are expressed as in Fig. 1. * $p < 0.05$ when compared to corresponding control values.

cell bodies and dendrites with L-^{3}H-tyrosine. Under such conditions, it is possible to detect spontaneously released ^{3}H-DA in successive fractions of SN super-fusates. It reaches a steady state level after a short labeling period and is just slightly lower than that measured at the level of the nerve terminals in the caudate nucleus (10). In fact, the release of DA in the SN has certain characteristics in common with that observed in the striatum. It is activated by potassium (30 mM) added to the superfusing fluid, and also by amphetamine (10^{-6}M) or benztropine (10^{-6}M) delivered for a short period under the same conditions (Fig. 2).

Thus, these results strongly support the hypothesis in favor of a functional role of DA in the SN. DA released in the vicinity of the dopaminergic neurons may reduce the activity of these neurons by acting on dopaminergic receptors. However, two main problems raised by these results must be considered before discussing the physiological role of DA in the SN. First, where is the source of DA in the SN? Second, what is the mechanism by which DA reduces the activity of the nigrostriatal dopaminergic neurons?

ORIGIN OF DOPAMINE IN THE SUBSTANTIA NIGRA: A DENDRITIC RELEASE?

There are at least three possible sources of DA in the SN. First, DA could be released from dopaminergic axon terminals originating outside the SN and ending in this structure, or, DA release could involve a pool of intrinsic intra-nigral dopaminergic interneurons. Second, DA could be released from axonal recurrent collaterals originating from the axons of the nigrostriatal dopaminergic pathway and terminating in the SN. Finally, DA in the SN could be released from the dendrites of the dopaminergic neurons, as recently suggested by the histochemical studies of Björklund and Lindvall (2).

So far, it is impossible to identify the exact site of the release of DA in the SN. However, from one of our pharmacological experiments it seems that DA, in the mesencephalon, is not released from axonal nerve endings. In fact, tetrodo-toxin (TTX), which is known to reduce the release of ^{3}H-DA from nerve termi-nals in the caudate nucleus by blocking sodium channels and thus nerve activity in axons, has an opposite effect on the release of ^{3}H-DA in SN. The introduction of TTX for 1 hr into the superfusing fluid of the SN is followed by a marked increase of the ^{3}H-DA release (Fig. 2). This suggests that DA in the SN is not released by a mechanism involving sodium channels, as in axonal nerve endings. Therefore, with Björklund and Lindvall (2), we postulate that DA in the SN could be released from the dendrites of the dopaminergic neurons.

Two pieces of evidence support this hypothesis. Dendrodendritic synapses in the SN have been morphologically established (3,7,15) and such contacts between dopaminergic neurons could, therefore, support the lateral inhibition of these neurons, as suggested by the electrophysiological findings of Groves et al. (6). Llinas's results (9) are also in agreement with the concept of a dendritic release, and therefore, reinforce our results obtained with TTX. They showed that, contrary to the axons, spikes recorded intracellularly from dendrites of Purkinje cells in the avian cerebellum are absolutely not sensitive to the blocking of the sodium channels. This underlines the properties of some cells to conduct action potentials in dendrites, and therefore, the basic ionic mechanisms of this conduction are different in the dendritic and axonal parts of the neurons. Consequently, this could also be the case for the mechanisms responsible for the release of the transmitter from axonal nerve endings, on the one hand, and from dendrites on the other hand. Such mechanisms could explain our results with TTX on the nigral release of DA.

SOME ELEMENTS ON THE MECHANISMS OF AUTOREGULATION

The mechanism by which DA reduces the activity of the dopaminergic neurons is not fully understood. Two hypotheses are most often proposed. The effect of DA could be first mediated by the dopaminergic autoreceptors, as disclosed from the electrophysiological studies of Aghajanian and Bunney (1). In this case, the level of extraneuronal DA in the SN would determine the strength of an auto- or interinhibition of the dopaminergic neurons. A direct negative feedback mechanism would be involved in this regulation.

Nevertheless, certain facts suggest an alternative. DA released in the SN seems to control indirectly the activity of the dopaminergic neurons by presynaptically modulating the transmission at the level of their afferent inputs. More specifically, DA has been shown to modify the release of GABA from nigrostriatal fibers ending in the SN. In fact, the addition of exogenous DA in the superfusing fluid of rat nigral slices in vitro is followed by an increase release of ^{3}H-GABA. Similar results were obtained when the extraneuronal level of DA in the tissue slices was increased by amphetamine (14). On the other hand, we also obtained an increased release of ^{14}C-GABA continuously synthesized from ^{14}C-pyruvate in our *in vivo* experimental model when DA (10^{-7}M) was added for 1 hr to the superfusing fluid of the SN in the cat (C. Gauchy and A. Nieoullon, *unpublished data*). Therefore, the effect of DA may be mediated by the dopaminergic receptors located on nigral afferent fibers since a DA-sensitive adenylate cyclase is present in the SN and its activity is reduced after lesions are produced between the striatum and the SN, a procedure that reduces the level of GABA in the later structure (4); the DA-sensitive adenylate cyclase does not seem to be associated with the dopaminergic neurons since it is still present after the destruction of these neurons achieved by intranigral injection of 6-hydroxydopamine (13).

Moreover, it has also been demonstrated in experiments in vitro that GABA decreases the potassium-evoked release of substance P from rat nigral slices (8). Thus, DA possibly released from the dendrites of the dopaminergic neurons, may first presynaptically increase the release of GABA from strionigral afferent fibers by acting on dopaminergic receptors. Consequently, this increased release of GABA may induce a decreased release of substance P which acts as a facilitatory transmitter on the dopaminergic cells. Therefore, the increased release of DA leads to an indirect reduction of the facilitatory effect of substance P neurons on the dopaminergic cells. DA in the SN would decrease the activity of the dopaminergic neurons by reducing the excitatory effect on transmission or, in other words, by a dysfacilitating action (Fig. 3). However, this presynaptic control of the release of transmitters from nigral afferent fibers by DA is certainly not only restricted to the modulation of the release of the transmitters contained in the strionigral fibers, but DA may also regulate other messages delivered to the dopaminergic neurons, particularly those transmitters through the serotoninergic raphe–nigral projection. But very little evidence about the interactions of DA and serotonin in SN is available.

Moreover, in addition to this possible presynaptic control of the afferent information to the SN, DA could also interfere postsynaptically with the nondopaminergic nigrofugal neurons. Indeed, DA-sensitive cells are also found in the SN pars reticulata (1), from which originate at least the nigrothalamic and nigrotectal pathways. DA released from the dopaminergic neurons may thus control the activity of these pathways.

PHYSIOLOGICAL ROLE OF DOPAMINE IN THE SUBSTANTIA NIGRA

The results obtained in our experiments favor a physiological role of DA in the regulation of nigrostriatal dopaminergic neuron activity, since modifications of the DA level in SN induce corresponding changes in the activity of these cells, and since a spontaneous release of DA can be detected in the mesencephalon. This led to the assumption that the activity of the nigrostriatal dopaminergic neurons in physiological states is inversely correlated with the amount

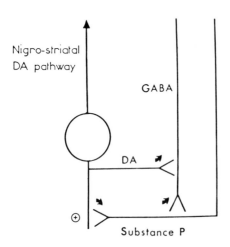

Nigro-striatal DA pathway

GABA

DA

Substance P

Fig. 3. Hypothetical model illustrating a possible mechanism of the action of DA in the SN. The activation (↑) of the dendritic release of DA in the SN may presynaptically increase the release of GABA from the nigrostriatal afferent fibers (↑). This in turn could result in a decreased release of substance P (↓), again by a presynaptic control of the nigrostriatal-substance P fibers. Thus, this leads to a suppression of an excitatory input to the dopaminergic neurons, in other words, to reduce activity by "dysfacilitation" and vice versa. However, this mechanism does not exclude the direct negative feedback process mediated through the dopaminergic autoreceptors located on dopaminergic neurons.

of DA released in the SN. When the level of extraneuronal DA in SN increases, this induces a decrease in the release of the transmitter at the level of the nerve terminals, and vice versa, when the level of DA in the SN decreases.

We have actually obtained results in agreement with this postulated mechanism. Changes in DA release in the SN are in the opposite direction of those found in the ipsilateral caudate nucleus following stimulation of cerebellar or sensory afferents. The electrical stimulation of the lateral cerebellar nucleus (the dentate nucleus) is followed by a decreased release of ^{3}H-DA in the contralateral SN, and this is associated with an increase of the transmitter release at the level of the corresponding caudate nucleus (11). Similar results were obtained after electrical stimulation of the ipsilateral forelimb paw (12). On the contrary, stimulation of the ipsilateral dentate nucleus or the contralateral forelimb is followed by an increased release of DA in the SN, and correspondingly, a decreased release of the transmitter in the caudate nucleus. Thus, this supports the hypothesis of the existence of a mechanism by which DA autoregulates the nigrostriatal dopaminergic neurons at the level of SN during physiological conditions.

ACKNOWLEDGMENTS

The authors wish to express their gratitude to C. Gauchy and V. Leviel for their collaboration during some experiments.

REFERENCES

1. Aghajanian, G. K., and Bunney B. S. (1973): Central dopaminergic neurons: neurophysiological identification and responses to drugs. In: *Frontiers in Catecholamine Research,* edited by E. Usdin and S. Snyder, pp. 643–648. Pergamon Press, London.
2. Björklund, A., and Lindvall, O. (1975): Dopamine in dendrites of substantia nigra neurons: suggestions for a role in dendritic terminals. *Brain Res.,* 83:531–537.
3. Cuello, A. C., and Iversen, L. L. (1978): Interactions of dopamine with other neurotransmitters in the rat substantia nigra: a possible functional role of dendritic dopamine. In: *Interactions Between Putative Neurotransmitters in the Brain,* edited by S. Garattini, J. F. Pujol, and R. Samanin, pp. 127–149. Raven Press, New York.
4. Gale, K. A., Guidotti, A., and Costa, E. (1977): Dopamine sensitive adenylate cyclase: location in the substantia nigra. *Science,* 195:503–505.
5. Geffen, L. B., Jessell, T. M., Cuello, A. C., and Iversen, L. L. (1976): Release of dopamine from dendrites in rat substantia nigra. *Nature,* 260:258–260.
6. Groves, P. M., Wilson, C. J., Young, S. J., and Rebec, G. V. (1975): Self-inhibition by dopaminergic neurons: an alternative to the "neuronal feed-back loop" hypothesis for the mode of action of certain psychotropic drugs. *Science,* 190:522–528.
7. Hajdu, F., Hassler, R., and Bak, I. J. (1973): Electron microscopic study of the substantia nigra and the strio-nigral projection in the cat. *Z. Zellforsch.,* 146:207–221.
8. Jessell, T. M. (1978): Substance P release from the rat substantia nigra. *Brain Res.,* 151:469–478.
9. Llinas, R., and Hess, R. (1976): Tetrodotoxin-resistant dendritic spikes in avian Purkinje cells. *Proc. Natl. Acad. Sci. USA,* 7:2520:2523.
10. Nieoullon, A., Cheramy, A., and Glowinski, J. (1977): Release of dopamine in vivo from cat substantia nigra. *Nature,* 266:375–377.
11. Nieoullon, A., Cheramy, A., and Glowinski, J. (1978): Release of dopamine in both caudate

nuclei and both substantia nigrae in response to unilateral stimulation of cerebellar nuclei in the cat: *Brain Res.,* 148:143–152.

12. Nieoullon, A., Cheramy, A., and Glowinski, J. (1978): Release of dopamine evoked by electrical stimulation of the motor and visual areas of the cerebral cortex in both caudate nuclei and in the substantia nigra in the cat. *Brain Res.,* 145:69–83.

13. Premont, J., Thierry, A. M., Tassin, J. P., Glowinski, J., Blanc, G., and Bockaert, J. (1976): Is the dopamine-sensitive adenylate cyclase in the rat substantia nigra coupled with "autoreceptors"? *FEBS Lett.,* 68:99–104.

14. Reubi, J. C., Iversen, L. L., and Jessell, T. M. (1977): Dopamine selectively increases ^{3}H-GABA release from slices of rat substantia nigra in vitro. *Nature,* 268:652–654.

15. Wilson, C. J., Groves, P. M., and Fifkova, E. (1977): Monoaminergic synapses, including dendro-dendritic synapses in the rat substantia nigra. *Exp. Brain Res.,* 30:161–174.

Advances in Neurology, Vol. 24, edited by
L. J. Poirier, T. L. Sourkes, and P. J. Bédard.
Raven Press, New York © 1979.

Studies on Different Types of Dopamine Nerve Terminals in the Forebrain and Their Possible Interactions with Hormones and with Neurons Containing GABA, Glutamate, and Opioid Peptides

*K. Fuxe, *K. Andersson, *R. Schwarcz, *L. F. Agnati, *M. Pérez de la Mora, *T. Hökfelt, **M. Goldstein, *L. Ferland, †L. Possani, and †R. Tapia

*Department of Histology, Karolinska Institute, Stockholm, Sweden; **Department of Psychiatry, New York University Medical Center, New York, New York 10016; and †Department of Experimental Biology, UNAM, Mexico

By means of the routine Falck–Hillarp procedure involving freeze-drying of brain tissue and paraffin sectioning, it has been possible to map out two types of dopamine (DA) nerve terminals within the tuberculum olfactorium, nucleus accumbens, and the neostriatum (33). In these areas it is possible to observe diffuse and dotted types of DA nerve terminals by fluorescence microscopy. The dotted type of DA nerve terminals form characteristic islands in the dorsal and anterior half of the neostriatum and marginal zones in the medial, dorsal, and lateral borders of this structure (17,21,33,41). In the neostriatum, these types of DA terminals are best demonstrated in the postnatal period, since they develop earlier than the diffuse type of neostriatal DA terminals. This is illustrated in Fig. 1 in which the islandic and marginal zone DA innervation is well illustrated using antibodies against tyrosine hydroxylase. The distribution of dotted and diffuse types of DA terminals in the nucleus accumbens and tuberculum olfactorium is illustrated in Fig. 2 and 3. As in the neostriatum, the diffuse type of DA terminals is in the vast majority, and the dotted type of DA terminals is confined mainly to the dorsal and caudal part of nucleus accumbens, and to the posterior and medial part of the tuberculum olfactorium. The fact that diffuse and dotted types of DA terminals can be distinguished could be related to the fact that there is less diffusion of DA out from the DA terminals of the dotted type. This probably explains why they appear dotted in the microscope. The reduced diffusion of DA from the dotted type of DA terminals during the routine Falck–Hillarp procedure may be due to the fact that DA has a higher affinity for the DA granules in these DA terminals than in the diffuse type of DA terminal. It is also possible that the dotted type of

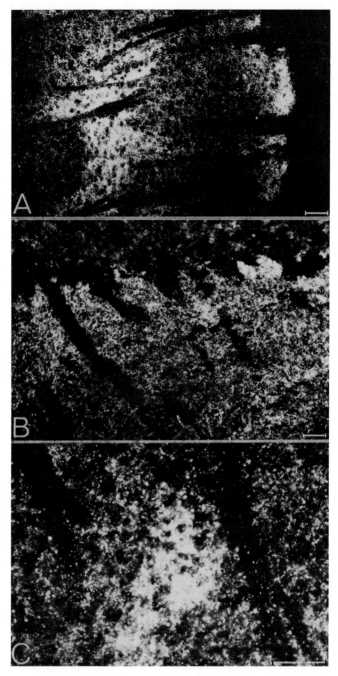

FIG. 1. Tyrosine hydroxylase immunofluorescence in neostriatum of a 7-day-old male rat. Tyrosine hydroxylase immunoreactivity is mainly found within DA nerve terminals forming islands in the nucleus caudatus and marginal zones in the borderline areas. Calibration bars in A, B, and C represent 50 μm.

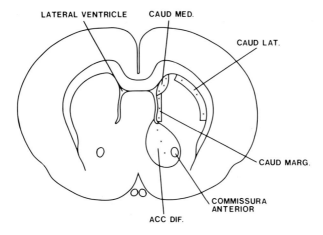

FIG. 2. DA nerve terminals studied at the rostral level of nucleus caudatus.

DA terminals contains a higher concentration of DA per varicosity, which may allow these terminals to be demonstrated as dots in spite of a diffusion of DA out of them during the preparation procedure.

An important observation obtained in our laboratory is that the dotted type of DA terminals appears to have a lower DA turnover than that of the diffuse type. Figure 4 shows that the dotted type of nerve terminals in the nucleus accumbens has a half-life of 98 min, which is significantly different from the half-life of DA found in the diffuse type of accumbens DA terminals (68 min). Furthermore, the results shown in Fig. 5 demonstrate that following treatment with the tyrosine hydroxylase inhibitor α-methyl-tyrosine methylester (H 44/68), there is also a reduced depletion of DA stores in the dotted type of DA

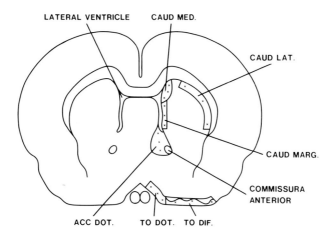

FIG. 3. DA nerve terminals studied at the caudal level of nucleus caudatus.

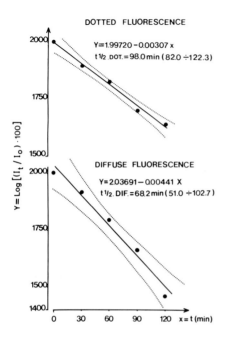

FIG. 4. DA fluorescence disappearance in the diffuse and dotted types of DA nerve terminals in the nucleus accumbens of normal male rats after tyrosine hydroxylase inhibition; $t\frac{1}{2}$ dot $\neq \frac{1}{2}$. Dif: $p < 0.05$. The rats were killed at various time intervals following the injection of α-methyl-tyrosine methylester (H 44/68, 250 mg/kg, i.p.). On the *y*-axis the log fluorescence values are shown in percent of the mean value for the untreated group. Every point represents the mean DA fluorescence of four to five rats. The line of best fit for these points is calculated by the least-squares method, and the 99% confidence interval around the line is also shown. The 95% confidence interval around the half-life obtained is shown. The half-lives found for the dotted and diffuse types of DA terminals are significantly different ($p < 0.05$) as demonstrated by Hollander test for the parallelism of two regression lines.

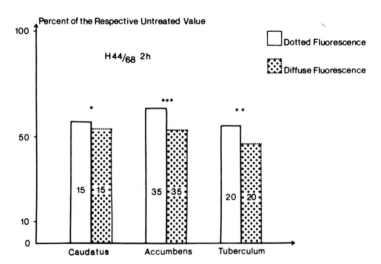

FIG. 5. DA fluorescence disappearance of diffuse and dotted types of DA nerve terminals following tyrosine hydroxylase inhibition in nuclei caudatus and accumbens, and tuberculum olfactorium. DA fluorescence was measured in untreated rats and in rats treated with α-methyl-tyrosine methylester (H 44/68, 250 mg/kg, i.p.) 2 hr before killing. The DA fluorescence values obtained are expressed in percent of the respective untreated group mean value. Number of animals studied are shown in each column. In the statistical analysis a nonparametric paired test was used. $^*p < 0.05$; $^{**}p < 0.01$; $^{***}p < 0.001$.

terminal within the nucleus caudatus, and within the tuberculum olfactorium. Thus, in these two regions the dotted type of DA terminal also seems to have a lower turnover than the diffuse type of DA terminal found in these areas. These results support the idea that the diffuse and dotted types of DA terminal may belong to different DA pathways ascending from the midbrain.

In this chapter, the possible origin of the DA nerve terminal systems in the forebrain and their possible regulation by glutamate, GABA, and endorphin-containing pathways and by hormones will be discussed.

ON THE ORIGIN OF DA NERVE TERMINALS IN THE FOREBRAIN

The Mesostriatal DA System

This DA system mainly originates from the substantia nigra [(2,34), A9 group according to Dahlström and Fuxe (9)]. Recently, however, evidence has been obtained that the DA cell bodies in the lateral part of the ventral tegmental area [A10 group according to Dahlström and Fuxe (9)] contribute to the DA innervation of the medial parts of the neostriatum (12,32). Furthermore, Nauta and Domesick (32) have reported that the DA cell bodies in the adjacent ventro-lateral reticular formation [group A8 according to Dahlström and Fuxe (9)] contribute to the DA innervation of the lateral parts of the neostriatum. Also, the dotted type of DA nerve terminal in the neostriatum originates from the ventral midbrain, since lesions in this area lead to disappearance of these DA nerve terminals. However, it is presently unclear whether the islandic and marginal zone DA innervation of the neostriatum mainly originates from the A9, A8, or A10 groups.

The Mesoaccumbens DA System

Most of the DA nerve terminals in the nucleus accumbens originate in the A10 cell group (3,32,44). Recent findings indicate that group A8 may participate in the innervation of this region (32). The exact origin of the diffuse and dotted types of DA terminals within these DA cell body regions is unknown.

The Mesotuberculum Olfactorium System

Most of the DA terminals within the tuberculum olfactorium originate in the A10 DA cell group in the ventral midbrain (3,32,44); also, in this case, the DA cell bodies in group A8 seem to contribute to the DA innervation of this area (32). The exact origin of the dotted and diffuse types of DA terminals within these DA cell groups is unknown. It must be underlined that the nigral DA cell bodies contribute very little to the innervation of the nucleus accumbens and the tuberculum olfactorium.

The Mesocortical DA System

The DA terminals in the limbic cortex, the prefrontal cortex, and in the septal area mainly originate within the ventral tegmental DA cell group (A10 group) (10,19,27,29,42). Recent studies, however, indicate that the DA innervation of the amygdaloid cortex, the prepyriform cortex, the suprarhinal cortex, and pyriform cortex also originates in a certain type of DA nerve cell of the substantia nigra (11). It is interesting to note that islands of DA terminals are formed within the ventral part of the entorhinal cortex. Neuroanatomically, this area is better defined as a transitional zone between the entorhinal cortex and the pyriform cortex. These islandic DA terminals seem to originate within the ventral tegmental DA cell group.

DIFFERENT TYPES OF NEOSTRIATAL DA RECEPTORS AND THEIR RELATION TO THE DIFFUSE AND ISLANDIC NEOSTRIATAL DA TERMINAL SYSTEMS

It has recently been demonstrated that an ergoline derivative, which selectively reduces DA turnover in the islandic and marginal DA terminal system, produces a similar peak activation of adenylate cyclase activity in striatal homogenates as does apomorphine (17). Thus, it seems possible that the DA receptors belonging to the islandic DA terminal system in the neostriatum are linked to the adenylate cyclase system. In contrast, DA receptors linked to the large diffuse type of DA terminal system in the neostriatum are probably, to a large extent, not linked to the adenylate cyclase but to another biological effector mechanism. These DA receptors are probably present on both axon terminals belonging to glutamate-containing cortical afferents as well as on some neostriatal interneurons (18,22,37,38). Thus, it seems as if most of the DA terminals release DA onto DA receptors that are not linked to the adenylate cyclase. Therefore, when looking for antiparkinsonian agents, it seems reasonable to look for DA receptor agonists which have DA agonistic activity especially at DA receptors not linked to the adenylate cyclase. The functional importance of the large diffuse DA terminal system versus the islandic DA terminal system also innervating the marginal zones remains to be established.

In support of the above suggestions is the fact that the DA receptor agonist bromocriptine, whose dopaminergic activity has been discovered in this laboratory in collaboration with Dr. Corrodi (7,26), exerts antiparkinsonian activity despite the fact that it probably acts mainly at DA receptors not linked to the adenylate cyclase. However, in vivo bromocriptine can increase cAMP levels in neostriatum (43).

It should be remembered that bromocriptine is not as powerful an antiparkinsonian agent as L-DOPA, which may be related to the fact that it does not stimulate all types of DA receptors. Again, it could be argued that it may not always be beneficial to activate all DA receptors over a prolonged period of time, since at some DA receptors this may produce a supersensitivity resulting in dyskinetic phenomena (28), while at others, a desensitization can occur resulting in a loss of the antiparkinsonian effects of the dopaminergic drugs (22,24).

POSSIBLE INTERACTION BETWEEN GLUTAMATE AND DA-CONTAINING NERVE TERMINALS IN THE NEOSTRIATUM

The available evidence indicates that a large number of the DA receptors in the neostriatum are located on cortical—possibly glutamate-containing—afferents innervating the neostriatum (37). Furthermore, glutamate seems capable of releasing DA via a glutamate receptor located on the DA bouton (23). However, glutamate receptors are probably also located on interneurons in the neostriatum: following a kainic acid-induced lesion in the striatum, Scatchard analysis reveals a 35% reduction in the number of binding sites for ^{3}H-kainic acid (see Fig. 6). In view of the fact that the kainic acid binding site is probably closely associated with the glutamate binding site, these results most likely support the existence of glutamate receptors on neostriatal interneurons. It therefore seems possible that one important action of DA is to influence glutamate release from axon terminals via presynaptic inhibition, in this way preventing excitation of certain types of neostriatal interneurons.

Studies using kainic acid have led to the hypothesis that Huntington's disease can be produced by overactivity in glutamate-containing pathways in the brain, the neuronal degeneration being produced by the continuous excitation of neostri-

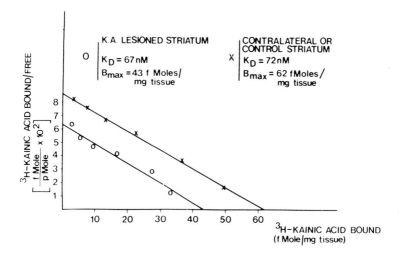

FIG. 6. Effects of intrastriatal injections of kainic acid on the binding characteristics of ^{3}H-kainic acid. A buffered solution of kainic acid (1 μg/0.5 μl) was injected unilaterally into the striatum. The animals were killed 2 weeks later, and the binding of ^{3}H-kainic acid in lesioned striata was compared to that in contralateral as well as intact control striata. Scatchard analysis reveals a reduction in the number of binding sites but no change in the dissociation constant (Schwarcz and Fuxe, *unpublished data*.)

atal neurons by means of enhanced glutamate receptor activity (8,30). It is presently unclear whether the change may be primarily in the glutamate receptor or in the presynaptic control of glutamate release. Of considerable interest is the fact that, 1 to 2 days following kainic acid injection, a dramatic increase of neostriatal DA turnover, probably as a response to the degeneration of interneurons in the neostriatum, can be observed. This increase of DA turnover may be partly due to the elicitation of an intrastriatal feedback mechanism. It is speculated that this marked release of DA could be at least in part responsible for the choreatic movements found in Huntington's disease (39).

POSSIBLE INTERACTIONS BETWEEN FOREBRAIN DA NERVE TERMINALS AND ENDORPHIN-CONTAINING NEURONS

Morphine increases DA turnover in the tuberculum olfactorium, nucleus accumbens, and neostriatum (13,25). These results indicate that opiate receptors can influence the activity of the forebrain DA nerve terminal systems. In view of the discovery of β-endorphin and enkephalin-containing neurons in the central nervous system, it seemed of interest to evaluate the effects of opiate peptides on DA turnover in discrete DA terminal systems of the neostriatum and the limbic forebrain. Available evidence suggests that met-enkephalin, enkephalin analogs, and β-endorphin can increase DA turnover in neostriatum and the limbic forebrain (1,5,6,17). As seen in Fig. 7, intraventricular infusion of met-

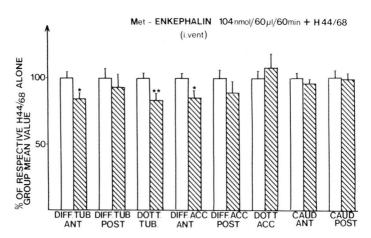

FIG. 7. Effects of met-enkephalin on the H 44/68 induced DA fluorescence disappearance in various DA nerve terminal systems of the forebrain of the male rat. Met-enkephalin or saline was infused in the lateral ventricle over a period of 1 hr and in a total volume of 60 μl. At the onset of the infusion, H 44/68 (250 mg/kg, i.p.) was given and the rats were killed 1 hr later. Means $\pm$ SEM (4–5 rats) are shown and given 1% of the saline (H 44/68-treated group mean value). Mann–Whitney U-test was used. $^*p < 0.05$; $^{**}p < 0.01$. For explanation of abbreviations used see legend to Fig. 9 (ant, anterior part; post, posterior part). (Fuxe et al., *unpublished data*.)

enkephalin (104 nmoles/rat) into Fluothane®–air anesthetized male rats produced a significant increase in DA turnover in the diffuse and dotted type of DA nerve terminal of the tuberculum olfactorium and in the diffuse type of DA nerve terminal of the nucleus accumbens. It is of particular interest to note that in a similar experiment with intraventricular infusion of 2 nmoles of β-endorphin, increases of DA turnover were also observed, but these were in other types of DA nerve terminal systems of the forebrain. Thus, as seen in Fig. 8, β-endorphin increased DA turnover exclusively in the diffuse type of DA terminal systems in the tuberculum olfactorium; the dotted type of DA terminals in this area was unaffected.

β-Endorphin also produced an increase of DA turnover in the posterior part of the nucleus caudatus. Thus, it seems as if β-endorphin and met-enkephalin produce differential effects on DA turnover in the DA terminal systems of the forebrain. This could be in part related to a difference of activation of various types of opiate receptor in the brain. Intraventricular injections of β-endorphin into awake male rats also produced a pattern of changes in DA turnover similar to those observed in the anesthetized rats (16). Thus, as seen

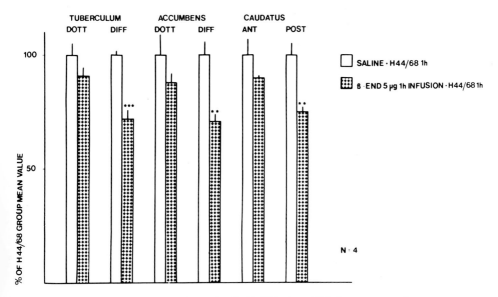

FIG. 8. The effect of β-endorphin on the H 44/68-induced DA fluorescence disappearance in various regions of the forebrain. β-Endorphin was infused during a period of 1 hr into the lateral ventricle, the total dose being 5 μg. At the onset of infusion the H 44/68 injection was made (250 mg/kg, i.p., 1 hr before killing). During the infusion period the saline- or β-endorphin-injected animals were in Fluothane®–air anesthesia. The fluorescence values are given in percent of H 44/68 alone-treated group. Within the tuberculum olfactorium and nucleus accumbens, the effects of β-endorphin were evaluated on both the diffuse and dotted types of DA nerve terminals. In the caudate nucleus, effects were evaluated in the anterior and posterior dorsal part of the nucleus. Means ± SEM are shown. Sample size is 4. Statistical analysis was made according to Mann–Whitney U-test. $**p < 0.01$; $***p < 0.001$.

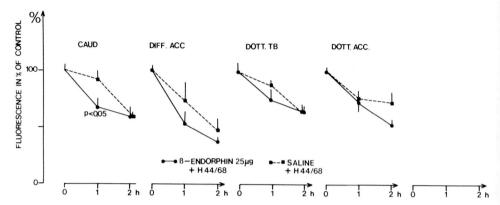

FIG. 9. The effects of β-endorphin on the H 44/68-induced fluorescence disappearance in DA nerve terminals of the forebrain. β-Endorphin (25 μg, 8 pmoles) or saline was given in a volume of 30 μl intraventricularly into the lateral ventricle of chronically implanted male rats. At the same time H 44/68 (250 mg/kg, i.p., 1 and 2 hr before killing) was given. Means ± SEM are shown (4–5 rats) and given in percent of untreated group mean value. Statistical analysis used was Mann–Whitney U-test. Diff. acc, diffuse type of DA fluorescence in anterior nucleus accumbens; caud, medial and anterior part of nucleus caudatus, diff TB, diffuse type of DA fluorescence in tuberculum olfactorium; dott. acc., dotted type of DA fluorescence in the posterior and dorsal part of nucleus accumbens; dott. TB, dotted type of DA fluorescence in the posterior and medial part of the tuberculum olfactorium (Fuxe et al., *unpublished data*).

in Fig. 9, the dotted type of DA terminal system in nucleus accumbens and tuberculum olfactorium is not significantly affected by β-endorphin, while the diffuse type of DA system in these regions is increased; this is true also for the DA terminals in nucleus caudatus. All the above findings, however, must be completed by studies involving the effect of met-enkephalin analogs, which are resistant to breakdown by peptidases and opiate receptor blocking agents such as naloxone. Although all areas studied are close to the ventricles or the subarachnoidal space, we must take into account that met-enkephalin may not reach the same regions as β-endorphin due to breakdown by peptidases. β-Endorphin, of course, is a much larger molecule. Naloxone treatment alone in doses of 5 to 10 mg/kg does not change DA turnover in the various DA nerve terminal systems of the forebrain, indicating that, in the normal male rat, the naloxone-sensitive opiate receptors do not play a major role in the control of DA activity. It should be mentioned that the β-endorphin-induced reduction of DA turnover in the median eminence is not blocked by pretreatment with 5 or 10 mg/kg of naloxone, indicating that opiate receptors resistant to naloxone can also participate in the control of the DA systems in the brain *(unpublished data)*. It seems likely that at least met-enkephalin-induced increases of DA turnover in the limbic forebrain observed in the present experiments could be related to stimulation of opiate receptors located on the limbic DA nerve terminals (6,35).

In collaboration with Professor Mutt, we have also analyzed the effects of vasoactive intestinal polypeptide (VIP) on DA turnover. This peptide is mainly present within intracortical neurons of the cerebral cortex (20). It was of considerable interest to see whether such a peptide also could influence the various DA terminal systems. Preliminary findings suggest that this peptide, too, when given intraventricularly in a dose of 16 nmoles/rat, can increase DA turnover in discrete DA terminal systems of the forebrain. The pattern of changes, however, as different from those found with met-enkephalin or with β-endorphin in the dose so far tested. Thus, an increase of DA turnover was found within the islandic and marginal zone DA nerve terminals and within the diffuse type of DA terminal in the tuberculum olfactorium. It will also be important to evaluate the specificity of the effects of this peptide. This will be performed *inter alia* by injections of glucagon, a peptide related to VIP.

INTERACTIONS BETWEEN DA NERVE TERMINALS AND GABA NEURONS IN THE FOREBRAIN

By means of immunohistochemistry using antibodies against glutamic acid decarboxylase (GAD), Roberts and collaborators (36) have mapped out a large number of terminal systems in the brain. In this laboratory in collaboration with Pérez de la Mora, Possani, and Tapia, immunohistochemical studies on GAD localization have also been performed. These studies have confirmed the work of Roberts et al. (36) and have also led to the mapping out of new types of GAD-containing nerve terminals. In Fig. 10 and 11 GAD-immunoreactive nerve terminals are demonstrated within the A10 DA cell group and the tuberculum olfactorium region. Thus, GABA-ergic mechanisms exist within both the DA cell body areas and the DA nerve terminal systems. Within the tuberculum olfactorium two types of GAD-positive nerve terminals exist. First, fine nerve terminal plexus can be shown in the molecular layer and within the cell body layer. Second, another type can be demonstrated in the medial forebrain bundle area and within the dorsal part of the island of Calleja. The latter terminals are strongly immunoreactive and fairly large. These latter terminals are the only ones that can be seen in Fig. 11 in view of the low magnification used. It should be underlined that these strongly immunoreactive GAD-positive terminals have a distribution different from that of the DA terminals. The latter are found mainly within the tuberculum olfactorium proper and only in low densities within the Calleja's islands. Thus, it does not seem likely that axo-axonic interactions occur between these types of GAD-positive terminals and the DA terminals in the tuberculum olfactorium.

Studies on the influence of GABA-ergic drugs on DA turnover in the forebrain indicate that GABA-ergic mechanisms can have both inhibitory and excitatory influences on the various DA terminal systems (15). Thus, muscimol in the low dose range can increase DA turnover in the nucleus caudatus. This could be explained on the basis of a preferential activation of those GABA receptors that have an excitatory influence on the DA systems. The specificity of these

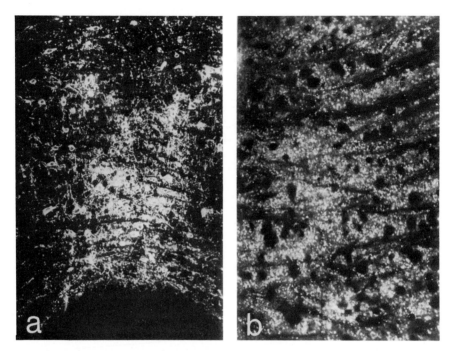

FIG. 10. A: Tyrosine hydroxylase immunofluorescence in the A10 DA cell group region. Strong specific immunofluorescence is observed within the DA cell bodies and their processes. ×90. **B:** Glutamic acid decarboxylase immunofluorescence within the A10 DA cell group area. A fairly dense plexus of GAD-positive nerve terminals are found in the neuropil, appearing as fine fluorescent dots. ×90.

results must be further tested by the use of other types of GABA receptor agonists as well as in studies with blockers of GABA receptors.

HORMONAL CONTROL OF THE TELENCEPHALIC DA TERMINAL SYSTEMS

Several findings in this laboratory suggest that prolactin can influence the turnover in certain types of mesostriatal and mesoaccumbens DA systems. Thus, in the hypophysectomized male rat, rat prolactin in a dose of 100 μg/kg given intravenously will acutely produce an increase of DA turnover in the dotted type of DA nerve terminals in the nucleus accumbens (see ref. 14). Furthermore, in the immature female rat, ovine prolactin given twice daily for 7 days in a dose of 0.5 μg/kg produces a reduction of DA turnover in the dotted and diffuse type of DA terminal in the nucleus accumbens, and within the diffuse type of DA terminal in the medial and anterior part of the nucleus caudatus. The islandic neostriatal DA terminals and the dotted type of DA terminals in the tuberculum olfactorium are not affected by treatment with these low doses

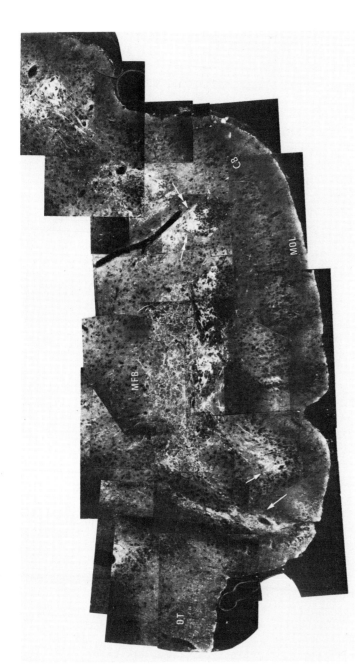

FIG. 11. Fontal section of the anterior telencephalon at the level of the tuberculum olfactorium. Two different patterns of GABA innervation can be visualized in this area: A fine plexus of GAD-containing nerve terminals innervating both the molecular layer and the cell body layer of the tuberculum olfactorium, and a very rich network of relatively coarse and strongly immunofluorescent GAD positive terminals innervating the region of the medial forebrain bundle (MFB). These terminals seem to establish synaptic contacts with nerve cells and dendrites, which also extend into the inner pool of the islands of Calleja *(double arrow)* and towards the cell body layer of the tuberculum olfactorium *(single arrow)*. CB, cell body layer; MFB, medial forebrain bundle; MOL, molecular layer; OT, tractus olfactorius. ×40.

of ovine prolactin. Following 2 weeks of treatment with the same dose of ovine prolactin, however, the effects of ovine prolactin had disappeared, and instead, an increase of DA turnover was observed in the dotted and diffuse types of DA terminals in the nucleus accumbens. DA terminals in the tuberculum olfactorium and the nucleus caudatus were not affected by the treatment. Finally, in castrated female rats having pituitary transplants under the renal capsule, a reduced DA turnover was observed in the diffuse type of DA terminal of the nucleus accumbens and of the anterior and medial part of the nucleus caudatus. The dotted type of DA terminal in the nucleus accumbens and the DA terminals of the neostriatal islands and of the marginal zones of the neostriatum were not influenced (see ref. 14). Thus, depending on the endocrine state of the animal and the treatment schedule used, prolactin will produce a reduction or an increase of DA turnover within the mesoaccumbens DA system and certain types of mesostriatal DA neurons. The islandic and marginal zone DA terminals of the neostriatum are unaffected. Thus, it is possible that there exist two types of prolactin receptor mechanisms within the brain, and that they induce excitatory or inhibitory influences on the ascending mesoaccumbens and mesostriatal DA systems. Under certain conditions such as in animals having pituitary transplants, prolactin may also induce oscillations in activity in some of the neostriatal DA terminal systems.

The mechanism for the prolactin-induced changes in DA turnover in discrete DA nerve terminal systems of the forebrain is unknown. It may be speculated, however, that the prolactin receptors are located within the preoptic and hypothalamic areas, and that the influence on the mesostriatal and mesoaccumbens DA systems is mediated through changes in activity of preoptic-nigral projections (40) and hypothalamic projections to the A10 and A8 groups (31). It seems clear that prolactin-induced changes in behaviors, especially maternal behaviors, can in part involve changes in activity in certain types of mesostriatal and mesoaccumbens DA systems. Other changes in the hormonal state, such as removal of the thyroid gland, will produce marked changes in discrete DA terminal systems in the forebrain (4).

At the present meeting it was reported that estrogens may have therapeutic effects in patients with L-DOPA-induced dyskinesias or tardive dyskinesias produced by neuroleptic drug treatment (see Bédard et al., *this volume*). These results suggest that estrogens may have antidopaminergic actions within the neostriatum. So far in this laboratory, estrogens given to castrated female rats have not been found to produce a change in DA turnover in the nucleus caudatus. Furthermore, the DA receptors did not appear to be clearly affected by repeated doses of estrogen in 4-week ovariectomized rats (25 μg/rat; daily s.c. for 3 days). Thus, in the vehicle-treated group the dissociation constant for ^{3}H-spiroperidol binding sites was 0.22 with a 95% confidence interval ranging from 0.15 to 0.40, while the dissociation constant in the estrogen-treated group was 0.23, the 95% confidence interval ranging from 0.16 to 0.84. There was a slight increase in the number of binding sites for ^{3}H-spiroperidol, however, since the

B_{max} value in the vehicle-treated group was 4.28, and in the estrogen-treated group, 5.79. It is important to underline, however, that the B_{max} values for ^{3}H-spiroperidol binding in the striatum in the ovariectomized female rat are far below those found in intact male rats ($B_{max} = 18$ pmoles/g), indicating an important role of hormones in the regulation of a number of DA receptors in the neostriatum.

SUMMARY

The regulation of the *diffuse* and *dotted* types of DA nerve terminals in the nucleus caudatus, tuberculum olfactorium, and nucleus accumbens has been analyzed. The dotted type of DA terminals has a lower amine turnover than the diffuse type. The DA receptors belonging to the islandic and marginal zone DA terminals of the neostriatum (dotted type) seem to be linked to an adenylate cyclase mechanism. Studies with kainic acid indicate that some glutamate receptors are located on neostriatal interneurons, and that prolonged activation of glutamate receptors, probably via a degeneration of neostriatal interneurons, can produce a dramatic increase of DA turnover in the nucleus caudatus. A feedback mechanism may be involved. Met-enkephalin and β-endorphin produce different patterns of increased DA turnover in the forebrain DA nerve terminal systems. GABA-ergic mechanisms exist in both DA cell body and DA nerve terminal-rich areas of the brain, as revealed by immunohistochemical studies on the localization of glutamic acid decarboxylase. GABA-ergic mechanisms seem capable of having both excitatory and inhibitory influences on DA turnover in the forebrain. Finally, the mesoaccumbens DA systems and certain types of mesostriatal DA systems are influenced by hormones such as prolactin. Thus, neuroendocrine-induced changes in behaviors may in part involve changes in activity of various types of ascending DA systems to the forebrain. These changes may in part be induced via descending hypothalamus and preoptic mesencephalic systems to the various DA cell bodies of the midbrain. The number of DA receptors may be controlled by the endocrine state.

ACKNOWLEDGMENTS

This work was supported by Grant 04X–715 from the Swedish Medical Research Council, Grant MH 25504–05 from the NIH, and a grant from Magn. Bergvalls Stiftelse.

REFERENCES

1. Algeri, S., Calderini, G., Consolazione, A., and Garattini, S. (1977): The effect of methionine-enkephalin and D-alanine methionine-enkephalinamide on the concentration of dopamine metabolites in rat striatum. *Eur. J. Pharmacol.,* 45:207–209.
2. Andén, N. -E., Carlsson, A., Dahlström, Ä., Fuxe, K., Hillarp, N. -Å., and Larsson, K., (1964): Demonstration and mapping out of nigro-neostriatal dopamine neurons. *Life Sci.,* 3:523–530.

3. Andén, N. -E., Dahlström, A., Fuxe, K., Larsson, K., Olson, L., and Ungerstedt, U. (1966): Ascending monoamine neurons to the telencephalon and diencephalon. *Acta Physiol. Scand.,* 67:313–326.
4. Andersson, K., Fuxe, K., Eneroth, P., Gustafsson, J. -Å., and Skett, P. (1978): On the catecholamine control of TSH secretion. Effects of thyroidectomy. *Neurosci. Lett. (Suppl.),* 1:S197.
5. Berney, S., and Hornykiewicz, O. (1977): The effect of β-endorphin and met-enkephalin on striatal dopamine metabolism and catalepsy: comparison with morphine. *Commun. Pharmacol.,* 1:597–604.
6. Biggio, G., Casu, M., Corda, M. G., Di Bello, C., Gessa, and Gessa, G. I. (1978): Stimulation of dopamine synthesis in caudate nucleus by intrastriatal enkephalins and antagonism by naloxone. *Science,* 200:552–554.
7. Corrodi, H., Fuxe, K., Hökfelt, T., Lidbrink, P., and Ungerstedt, U. (1973): Effect of ergot drugs on central catecholamine neurons: evidence for a stimulation of central dopamine neurons. *J. Pharm. Pharmacol.,* 25:409–412.
8. Coyle, J. T., and Schwarcz, R. (1976): Lesion of striatal neurons with kainic acid provides a model for Huntington's chorea. *Nature,* 263:244–246.
9. Dahlström, A., and Fuxe, K. (1964): Evidence for the existence of monoamine-containing neurons in the central nervous system. I. Demonstration of monoamines in the cell bodies of brain stem neurons. *Acta Physiol. Scand. (Suppl. 232),* 62:1–55.
10. Fallon, J. H., Koziell, D. A., and Moore, R. Y. (1978): Catecholamine innervation of the basal forebrain. II. Amygdala, suprarhinal cortex and entorhinal cortex. *J. Comp. Neurol.,* 180:509–532.
11. Fallon, J. H., and Moore, R. Y. (1978): Catecholamine innervation of the basal forebrain. III. Olfactory bulb, anterior olfactory nuclei, olfactory tubercle and piriform cortex. *J. Comp. Neurol.,* 180:533–544.
12. Fallon, J. H., and Moore, R. Y. (1978): Catecholamine innervation of the basal forebrain. IV. Topography of the dopamine projection to the basal forebrain and neostriatum. *J. Comp. Neurol.,* 180:545–580.
13. Fuxe, K., Agnati, L., Bolme, P., Everitt, B. J., Hökfelt, T., Jonsson, G., Ljungdahl, Å., and Löfström, A. (1975): The use of amine fluorescence histochemistry in the study of drugs, especially morphine, on the CNS. *Neuropharmacology,* 14:903–912.
14. Fuxe, K., Andersson, K., Hökfelt, T., Agnati, L. F., Ögren, S. -O., Eneroth, P., Gustafsson, J. -Å., and Skett, P. (1978): Prolactin–monoamine interactions in rat brain and their importance in regulation of LH and prolactin secretion. In: *Progress in Prolactin Physiology and Pathology,* edited by C. Robyn and M. Harter, pp. 95–109. Elsevier/North-Holland Biomedical Press, Amsterdam.
15. Fuxe, K., Andersson, K., Ögren, S. -O., Pérez de la Mora, M., Schwarcz, R., Hökfelt, T., Eneroth, P., Gustafsson, J. -Å., and Skett, P. (1978): GABA neurons and their interaction with monoamine neurons. An anatomical, pharmacological and functional analysis. In: *GABA-Neurotransmitters. Alfred Benzon Symposium XII.* Munksgaard, Copenhagen *(in press).*
16. Fuxe, K., Ferland, L., Agnati, L. F., Eneroth, P., Gustafsson, J. -Å., Labrie, F., and Skett, P. (1977): Effects of intraventricular injections of β-endorphin on dopamine levels and turnover in the unanesthetized male rat. Evidence for an increase of dopamine turnover in the caudatus and in the limbic forebrain and for a decrease of dopamine turnover in the median eminence. *Acta Pharmacol. Toxicol.,* 41 (Suppl. IV): 48.
17. Fuxe, K., Fredholm, B. B., Agnati, L. F., and Corrodi, H. (1978): Dopamine receptors and ergot drugs. Evidence that an ergoline derivative is a differential agonist at subcortical limbic dopamine receptors. *Brain Res.,* 146:295–311.
18. Fuxe, K., Fredholm, B. B., Agnati, L. F., Ögren, S. -O., Everitt, B. J., Jonsson, G., and Gustafsson, J. -Å. (1978): Interaction of ergot drugs with central monoamine systems. Evidence for a high potential in the treatment of mental and neurological disorders. *Pharmacology,* 16 (Suppl. 1): 99–134.
19. Fuxe, K., Hökfelt, T., Johansson, O., Jonsson, G., Lidbrink, P., and Ljungdahl, Å. (1974): The origin of the dopamine nerve terminals in limbic and frontal cortex. Evidence for mesocortico dopamine neurons. *Brain Res.,* 82:349–355.
20. Fuxe, K., Hökfelt, T., Said, S. I., and Mutt, V. (1977): Vasoactive intestinal polypeptide and the nervous system: immunohistochemical evidence for localization in central and peripheral neurons, particularly intracortical neurons of the cerebral cortex. *Neurosci. Lett.,* 5:241–246.
21. Fuxe, K., Hökfelt, T., and Ungerstedt, U. (1971): Localization of monoamines in the central

nervous system. In: *Monoamines, Noyaux Gris Centraux et Syndrome de Parkinson,* edited by J. de Ajuriaguerra and G. Gauthier, pp. 23–60. Georg & Cie., Genève.

22. Fuxe, K., Schwarcz, R., Agnati, L., Fredholm, B., Ögren, S. -O., Köhler, C., and Gustafsson, J. -Å. (1979): Actions of ergot derivatives at dopamine synapses. In: *Dopaminergic Ergot Derivatives and Motor Function,* edited by K. Fuxe and D. B. Calne. Pergamon Press, Oxford *(in press).*

23. Giorguieff, M. F., Kemel, M. L., and Glowinski, J. (1977): Presynaptic effect of L-glutamic acid on the release of dopamine in rat striatal slices. *Neurosci. Lett.,* 6:73–77.

24. Goldstein, M., Lew, J. Y., Engel, J., Nakamura, S., and Battista, A. (1979): The dopaminophilic properties of ergoline derivatives. In: *Dopaminergic Ergot Derivatives and Motor Function,* edited by K. Fuxe and D. B. Calne. Pergamon Press, Oxford *(in press).*

25. Gunne, L. -M., Jonsson, J., and Fuxe, K. (1969): Effects of morphine intoxication on brain catecholamine neurons. *Eur. J. Pharmacol.,* 5:338–342.

26. Hökfelt, T., and Fuxe, K. (1972): On the morphology and the neuroendocrine role of the hypothalamic catecholamine neurons. In: *Brain–Endocrine Interaction. Median Eminence: Structure and Function,* pp. 181–223. Karger, Basel.

27. Hökfelt, T., Fuxe, K., and Johansson, O. (1974): Pharmaco-histochemical evidence of the existence of dopamine nerve terminals in the limbic cortex. *Eur. J. Pharmacol.,* 25:108–112.

28. Klawans, H. L., and Rubovits, R. (1972): An experimental model of tardive dyskinesia. *J. Neurol. Trans.,* 33:235–246.

29. Lindvall, O., and Björklund, A. (1974): The organization of the ascending catecholamine neuron systems in the rat brain. *Acta Physiol. Scand. (Suppl.),* 412:1–48.

30. McGeer, E. G., and McGeer, P. L. (1976): Duplication of biochemical changes of Huntington's chorea by intrastriatal injection of glutamic and kainic acids. *Nature,* 263:517–519.

31. Nauta, W. J. H., and Domesick, V. B. (1978): Crossroads of limbic and striatal circuitry: hypothalamo-nigral connections. In: *Limbic Mechanisms,* edited by K. E. Livingston and O. Hornykiewicz. Plenum Press, London.

32. Nauta, W. J. H., and Domesick, V. B. (1979): The anatomy of the extrapyramidal system. In: *Dopaminergic Ergot Derivatives and Motor Function,* edited by K. Fuxe and D. B. Calne. Pergamon Press, Oxford *(in press).*

33. Olson, L., Seiger, Å., and Fuxe, K. (1972): Heterogeneity of striatal and limbic dopamine innervation. Highly fluorescent islands in developing and adult rats. *Brain Res.,* 44:283–288.

34. Poirier, L. J., and Sourkes, T. L. (1965): Contribution neuroanatomique et neurochimique à l'étude du tremblement de type Parkinsonien. *Actualité Neurophysiol.,* 6:167–181.

35. Pollard, H., Llorens, C., Bonnet, J. J., Constentin, J., and Schwartz, J. C. (1977): Opiate receptors on mesolimbic dopaminergic neurons. *Neurosci. Lett.,* 7:295–299.

36. Roberts, E. (1978): Immunocytochemical visualization of GABA neurons. In: *Psychopharmacology: A Generation of Progress,* edited by M. A. Lipton, A. DiMascio, and K. F. Killam, pp. 95–102. Raven Press, New York.

37. Schwarcz, R., Creese, I., Coyle, J. T., and Snyder, S. H. (1978): Dopamine receptors localized on cerebral cortical afferents to rat corpus striatum. *Nature,* 271:766–768.

38. Schwarcz, R., Fuxe, K., Agnati, L. F., and Gustafsson, J. -Å. (1978): Effects of bromocriptine on ^{3}H-spiroperidol binding sites in rat striatum. Evidence for actions of dopamine receptors not linked to adenylate cyclase. *Life Sci.,* 23:465–470.

39. Schwarcz, R., Fuxe, K., Hökfelt, T., Andersson, K., and Coyle, J. T. (1979): Dopamine and Huntington's disease: assessment using the kainic acid model. In: *Dopaminergic Ergot Derivatives and Motor Function,* edited by K. Fuxe and D. B. Calne. Pergamon Press, Oxford *(in press).*

40. Swanson, L. W. (1976): An autoradiographic study of the efferent connections of the preoptic region in the rat. *J. Comp. Neurol.,* 167:227–256.

41. Tennyson, V. M., Barrett, R. E., Cohen, G., Coté, L., Heikkila, R., and Mytilineou, C. (1972): The developing neostriatum of the rabbit: correlation of fluorescence histochemistry, electron microscopy, endogenous dopamine levels, and (^{3}H)dopamine uptake. *Brain Res.,* 46:251–285.

42. Thierry, A. M., Stinus, L., Blanc, G., and Glowinski, J. (1973): Some evidence for the existence of dopaminergic neurons in the rat cortex. *Brain Res.,* 50:230–234.

43. Trabucchi, M., Hofmann, M., Montefusco, O., and Spano, P. F. (1978): Ergot alkaloids and cyclic nucleotides in the CNS. *Pharmacology,* 16 (Suppl. 1): 150–155.

44. Ungerstedt, U. (1971): Stereotaxic mapping of the monoamine pathways in the rat brain. *Acta Physiol. Scand. (Suppl.),* 367:1–48.

Advances in Neurology, Vol. 24, edited by
L. J. Poirier, T. L. Sourkes, and P. J. Bédard.
Raven Press, New York © 1979.

Effect of Chronic Dopaminergic Agonism on Striatal Membrane Dopamine Binding

Harold L. Klawans, Ana Hitri, Paul M. Carvey, Paul A. Nausieda, and William J. Weiner

Department of Neurological Sciences, Rush University, Chicago, Illinois 60612

Two clinical situations are associated with chronic high-dose dopaminergic agonism. These are the long-term treatment of parkinsonism with levodopa, and the chronic abuse of amphetamine and related agents. Prolonged exposure of both levodopa and amphetamine is known to be associated with the onset of abnormal involuntary movements (drug-induced dyskinesias) and psychiatric disorders (1,3,4,11). The observation that these neurologic side-effects are usually related to chronic rather than acute administration of the offending agents suggests that the long-term exposure to dopaminergic agonists itself plays a role in the pathogenesis of these side-effects (6,7,14). It has been hypothesized that chronic dopaminergic agonism results in striatal dopamine receptor hypersensitivity, and that this may play a role in the neurologic and psychiatric effects of chronic dopaminergic agonism (6,7,10).

We have been using stereotyped behavior (SB) in rodents as a model of drug-induced dyskinesia. This model was chosen because SB is mediated by the activity of dopamine at striatal dopamine receptors. We have previously reported that both chronic levodopa and chronic *d*-amphetamine administration to guinea pigs produces increased behavioral response to the subsequent administration of apomorphine (10,15). The increased response to this drug supports the hypothesis that chronic exposure to dopaminergic agonists results in striatal dopaminergic receptor hypersensitivity. In order to investigate this possibility further, we have studied ^{3}H-dopamine binding to guinea pig striatal membranes after altered chronic levodopa or chronic *d*-amphetamine administration.

METHODS

Thirty-six pharmacologically virgin out-bred young male guinea pigs were housed six to a cage in environmentally controlled quarters lighted between 6 A.M. and 6 P.M. Animals were allowed free access to food and water. Prior to the chronic drug treatment, the animals were matched according to their initial behavioral response to apomorphine given at a low dose in order to ensure that each group of animals was started with chronic drug treatment at the same level of behavorial response (8).

The guinea pigs were divided into four groups. The first group was forced to swallow Sinemet tablets six times a week for 3 weeks, so that each animal received 200 mg levodopa/kg and 20 mg carbidopa/kg daily. The second group, the control animals, was force-fed a 10-mg/kg sugar tablet daily for 3 weeks. The third group was injected daily with 5 mg/kg of *d*-amphetamine sulfate for 4 weeks, and the fourth group received parallel saline injections.

During the 180 min following the administration of levodopa on days 1, 7, and 21, each animal was scored for stereotyped behavior at 10-min intervals using a six-point scale modified from Ernst (5); a score of zero signified normal behavior, while 5.0 represented continous noninterruptable chewing. By algebraically summing the recorded interval scores, a quantitative measure of drug response was produced. This was termed the "animal score" (AS). The amphetamine-treated animals were observed on the seventh day each week for amphetamine-induced stereotyped behavior using the above-mentioned rating scale.

Seven days after the final test injection, the animals were decapitated and the brains quickly removed and frozen on Dry Ice. The striata were dissected in a cold room (4°C) from serially sectioned brains, pooled by treatment group, and passed for binding studies to an investigator blind to the protocol. For binding studies the striatal tissues were homogenized in 40 volumes of ice-cold 50 mM TRIS HCl buffer, pH 7.4, containing 120 mM NaCl; 5 mM KCl, 2 mM $CaCl_2$, and 1 mM $MgCl_2$ according to the method of Creese et al. (3). The homogenate was centrifuged at $50,000 \times g$ for 10 min. The supernatant fluid was discarded and the pellet was rehomogenized in 100 volumes of the same buffer. One-milliliter aliquots corresponding to 10 mg (wet weight) of original tissue were incubated with various concentrations of ^{3}H-dopamine (0.1–20 nM), and with the same buffer as previously described for the tissue preparation with the addition of 0.1% ascorbic acid. The incubation was carried out at 4°C. After equilibration, the samples were rapidly filtered under vacuum through Whatman GF/B filters. Each filter was rinsed once with 5 ml of ice-cold buffer. The filters were counted by liquid scintillation spectrometry. Specific binding of ^{3}H-dopamine was measured as the excess radioactivity over blank tubes containing 200 nM apomorphine, whereas the stereospecific binding was determined as the excess over blank tubes containing 1 μM (+)-butaclamol as previously described by Creese et al. (3). ^{3}H-haloperidol binding was carried out under the same experimental conditions. The stereospecific ^{3}H-haloperidol binding was defined as excess over blank tubes containing 0.1 μM (+)-butaclamol.

RESULTS

Figure 1 shows the average interval scores of the levodopa-treated guinea pigs on days 1, 7, and 21. With day 1 serving as the base-line response, it can be seen that the chronic administration of levodopa causes an increase in SB

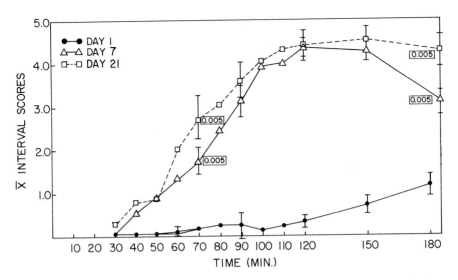

FIG. 1. Effect of chronic levodopa/carbidopa administration on stereotyped behavior of guinea pigs. Statistical analysis was performed using a one-tailed Mann-Whitney student test.

when observed on days 7 and 21. Figure 1 also demonstrates a significant difference in the latency [as defined by the 60-min interval score (U' 60 = 47 and 4.5.5 < 55; $N'/N-$ 16/15, $p < 0.005$)] and duration of the response for the 7 and 21 day observations.

Statistical analysis of animal scores for each week demonstrated that the response rates are significantly different from the base line [U' A.S. = 5, 10, and 5, respectively, < 55; N'/N = 16/15, $p < 0.005$] indicating that chronic administration of 200 mg levodopa/kg combined with 20 mg carbidopa/kg increases the magnitude of SB in young male guinea pigs when compared to base-line response.

Figure 2 contrasts the mean interval scores of the chronic *d*-amphetamine-treated animals and the control animals. The maximum degree of hypersensitivity appears to develop after 3 weeks of chronic *d*-amphetamine administration. As can be seen, the scores of animals treated for the second, third, and fourth weeks with amphetamine are significantly different from the first week's scores, whereas comparison of the weekly animal scores for control animals (data not presented) shows no statistical difference among the four testings.

Evidence of stereospecific ^{3}H-dopamine binding to mature guinea pig striatal membranes is shown in Fig. 3. The Scatchard and Lineweaver-Burk plots (insert) revealed two distinct binding sites for ^{3}H-dopamine in the striatal membranes. The first has a high affinity for ^{3}H-dopamine with an association constant (K_a) of 1×10^9 M and binding site concentration of 26 pmoles/g. The second or low-affinity binding site for ^{3}H-dopamine is characterized by a K_a of 1×10^8 M and with a binding site concentration of 51 pmoles/g.

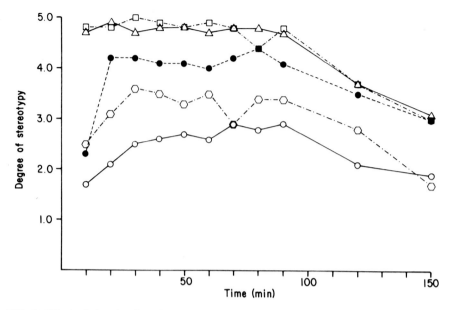

FIG. 2. Effect of chronic *d*-amphetamine administration on stereotyped behavior of guinea pigs. For statistical evaluation the one-tailed Mann-Whitney student test was used. Control: *open circles,* week one: *open hexagons,* week two: *closed circles,* week three: *open triangles,* week four: *open squares.* 1 wk: $N/N' = 6/12$, $U' = 16$, ns; 2 wks: $N/N' = 6/12$, $U' = 14.5$, ns; 3 wks: $N/N' = 6/12$, $U' = 0.5$, $p < 0.005$; 4 wks: $N/N' = 6/12$, $U' = 0.0$, $p < 0.005$.

Figure 4 demonstrates the effect of chronic *d*-amphetamine and levodopa/carbidopa pretreatment on ^{3}H-dopamine stereospecific binding at the high affinity binding site. As can be seen, chronic *d*-amphetamine resulted in a threefold increase in the affinity without changing the number of binding sites. Similarly, levodopa/carbidopa increased the affinity fourfold without affecting the binding site concentration.

The effect of *d*-amphetamine and levodopa/carbidopa on ^{3}H-dopamine stereospecific binding at the low affinity binding site is illustrated in Fig. 5. As can be seen, *d*-amphetamine produced a 33% increase and levodopa/carbidopa a fourfold increase in the number of binding sites without changing the affinity.

Figure 6 demonstrates the effect of levodopa pretreatment on ^{3}H-haloperidol stereospecific binding characteristics in the guinea pig striatal membranes. In contrast to ^{3}H-dopamine binding, ^{3}H-haloperidol binding displayed only one binding site with K_a 1×10^7 M and binding site concentration of 61 pmoles/g. This was not affected by chronic levodopa/carbidopa treatment.

DISCUSSION

The results presented here clearly demonstrate that chronic levodopa/carbidopa treatment and chronic *d*-amphetamine treatment both result in behavioral

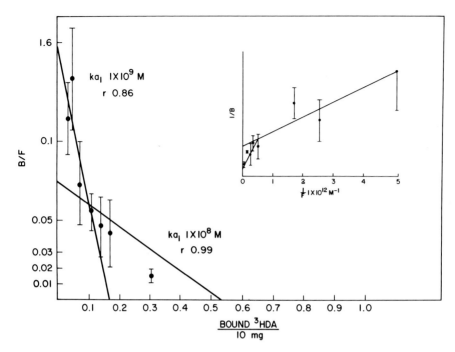

FIG. 3. Scatchard plot of ³H-dopamine stereospecific binding to guinea pig striatal membranes. Insert shows the data presented in Lineweaver Burk plot. The curved binding line on each plot was broken down into two straight lines by a stepwise linear regression analysis. Each point is the mean of four separate experiments and standard deviations of the means are represented by the bars.

supersensitivity to each agent, and that this supersensitivity is associated with alterations in ³H-dopamine binding to isolated striatal membranes. Our studies also indicate the existence of two distinct binding sites for ³H-dopamine in guinea pig striatal membranes, and that these two types of dopamine receptors are not affected identically by chronic *d*-amphetamine or levodopa treatment. Several clinical observations support the concept that different striatal neurons may have different types of dopamine receptors (9,13). The first is the observation that levodopa-induced dyskinesias and levodopa-induced improvement of parkinsonism symptoms can occur independently. A patient can manifest such dyskinesia, thought to reflect increased dopaminergic activity within the striatum, without any improvement in his parkinsonian state, as a result of decreased dopaminergic activity. A second clinical observation is that choreatic movement can be improved in patients with Huntington's chorea without the production of drug-induced parkinsonism. These observations are also consistent with the findings of York that there are two separate striatal nerve cell populations: a dopamine-facilitated nerve cell population that possesses predominantly facilitatory dopamine receptors, and a nerve cell population with inhibitory dopamine

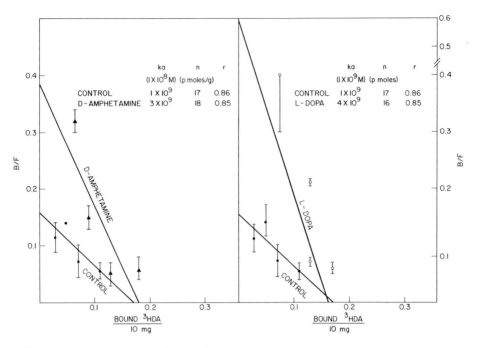

FIG. 4. Scatchard analysis of the effect of chronic *d*-amphetamine and levodopa/carbidopa pretreatment on ³H-dopamine stereospecific binding at the high-affinity binding site.

receptors (12,16). Along this line, Cools and colleagues presented evidence that hyperstimulation of both types of receptor in the caudate nucleus of the cat results in the appearance of athetoid choreiform movements of the forelimbs, whereas hyperstimulation of only the dopamine inhibitory bilateral system within the anterodorsal part of the caudate nucleus of the cat results in oro–facial–lingual dyskinesias (2).

In the work presented here the chronic administration of both *d*-amphetamine and levodopa produced a proliferation of the dopamine binding sites only at the low affinity binding site. It is possible that this low affinity binding site represents the dopamine inhibitory receptors, the proliferation of which may be responsible for the increased stereotyped chewing behavior of the guinea pigs. This SB may of course be considered to be a model of human oral–facial–lingual dyskinesias. Chronic *d*-amphetamine and levodopa treatment produced changes at both receptor sites, with increased numbers of receptors being produced at the low-affinity site, and increased affinity at the high-affinity site. It is uncertain which of these changes is related to the drug-induced behavioral sensitivity.

Our results also suggest that dopamine receptor site assays employing the naturally occurring agonist ³H-dopamine differ from assays employing ³H-haloperidol. The same tissue preparation showed two separate ³H-dopamine sites

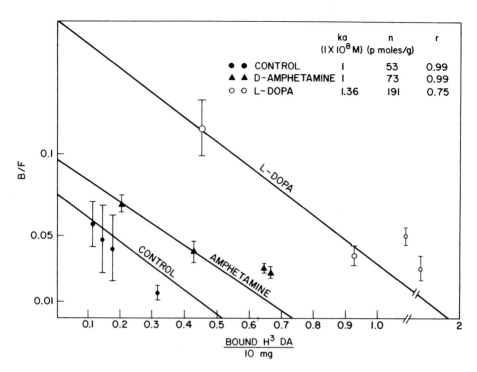

FIG. 5. Scatchard analysis of the effect of *d*-amphetamine and levodopa/carbidopa on ³H-dopamine stereospecific binding at the low-affinity binding site.

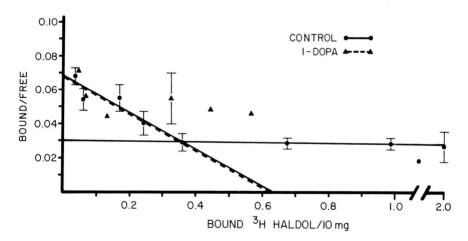

FIG. 6. Scatchard analysis of the effect of levodopa/carbidopa pretreatment on ³H-haloperidol stereospecific binding in guinea pig striatal membranes.

but only one binding site for ³H-haloperidol, and this binding, unlike the ³H-dopamine binding, was not affected by chronic levodopa treatment. The fact that there is a direct correlation between the behavorial supersensitivity induced by chronic agonist administration and increased ³H-dopamine binding characteristics supports our view that assays employing the naturally occurring agonist may be more specific for dopamine receptors than synthetic dopamine receptor agonists or antagonists.

ACKNOWLEDGMENTS

This work was supported by grants from the United Parkinson's Foundation, Chicago, and the Boothroyd Foundation, Chicago.

REFERENCES

1. Barbeau, A. (1971): A long term side effect of L-dopa. *Lancet,* 1:395.
2. Cools, A. R. (1975): Basic considerations of the role of concertedly working dopaminergic, GABA-ergic, cholinergic and serotonergic mechanisms within the neostriatum motor activity, stereotyped gnawing, turning and dyskinesia activity in cocaine and other stimulants. In: *Advances in Behavioral Biology, Vol. 21,* edited by E. H. Ellinwood and M. M. Kilby, pp. 97–141. Pergamon Press, New York.
3. Creese, I., Burt, D. R., and Snyder, S. H. (1975): Dopamine receptor binding: differentiation of agonist and antagonist states with ³H-dopamine and ³H-haloperidol. *Life Sci.,* 17:993–1002.
4. Ellinwood, E. H. (1967): Amphetamine psychosis, I. Description of the individuals and process. *J. Nerv. Ment. Dis.,* 144:273–283.
5. Ernst, A. M.: Mode of action of apomorphine and dexamphetamine on gnawing compulsion in rats. *Psychopharmacologia,* 10:316–323, 1967.
6. Klawans, H. L. (1975): Amine precursors in neurologic disorders and the psychosis. In: *Biology of the Major Psychoses,* edited by O. X. Freedman, H. L. Klawans, C. Goetz, P. A. Nausiela, and W. F. Weiner, pp. 259–276. New York, Raven Press.
7. Klawans, H. L., et al. (1977): Levodopa-induced dopamine receptor hypersensitivity. *Ann. Neurol.,* 2:125–129.
8. Klawans, H. L., Hitri, A., Carvey, P., Nausieda, P. A., and Weiner, W. J.: The effect of chronic *d*-amphetamine exposure on striatal dopamine receptors *(submitted for publication).*
9. Klawans, H. L., Ilahi, M. M., and Ringel, S. P. (1971): Toward an understanding of the pathophysiology of Huntington's Chorea. *Confin. Neurol.,* 33(5):297–303.
10. Klawans, H. L., and Margolin, D. I. (1975): Amphetamine-induced dopaminergic hypersensitivity in guinea pigs. *Arch. Gen. Psychiatry,* 32:725–732.
11. Kramer, J., Fishman, V. S., and Littlefield, D. S. (1967): Amphetamine abuse pattern and effects of high dose taken intravenously. *J.A.M.A.,* 201:305–309.
12. McLennan, H., and York, D. H. (1967): The action of dopamine on neurons of the caudate nucleus. *J. Physiol. (Lond.),* 189:393–402.
13. Moskovitz, C., Moses, H., and Klawans, H. L. (1978): Levodopa-induced psychosis: a kindling phenomenon. *Ann. Psychiatry,* 135:6.
14. Randrup, A., and Munkvad, I. (1966): Dopa and other naturally occurring substances as causes of stereotypy and rage in rats. *Acta Psychiatr. Scand. (Suppl.),* 42:191–193.
15. Rubovits, R., and Klawans, H. L. (1972): Implications of amphetamine induced stereotyped behavior as a model of tardive dyskinesia. *Arch. Gen. Psychiatry,* 27:502–507.
16. York, D. H. (1970): Possible dopaminergic pathway from substantia nigra to putamen. *Brain Res.,* 20:233–249.

Advances in Neurology, Vol. 24, edited by
L. J. Poirier, T. L. Sourkes, and P. J. Bédard.
Raven Press, New York © 1979.

Dendroaxonic Transmission and its Implications for the Therapy of Parkinson's Disease

P. L. McGeer, E. G. McGeer, and V. T. Innanen

Kinsmen Laboratory of Neurological Research, Department of Psychiatry, University of British Columbia, Vancouver, British Columbia, Canada, V6T 1W5

The focus of attention in Parkinson's disease is dopaminergic cells of the substantia nigra. Prevention of the disease probably depends on eliminating their loss while treatment is aimed at compensating for their deficit. The main pharmacological approaches include supplementing dopamine, stimulating its receptor sites, or blocking cholinergic receptor sites. The latter approach, arrived at empirically in the 19th century, was the only widely used treatment until a few years ago. It was the basis of the original hypothesis of a cholinergic–dopaminergic balance in the neostriatum (23), advanced shortly after it was realized dopamine might be a transmitter or neuronal modulator. Paradoxically, there had existed in the literature a report that nicotine improved the clinical status in post-encephalitic parkinsonism (26). This treatment method has not been pursued, no doubt because of the toxicity of nicotine. Nevertheless, its unexpected efficacy poses an important theoretical problem, the solution of which could open new avenues for treatment. Moreover, it might lead to an explanation of why smokers have less tendency to develop the disease. This negative correlation between smoking and Parkinson's disease has been demonstrated in at least three large-scale studies (12,17,18).

We report in this chapter the unexpected finding of apparent nicotinic binding sites on dopaminergic afferents to the neostriatum. This is in contrast to muscarinic binding sites, which appear to be mainly on neostriatal neurons. We hypothesize that the nicotinic binding sites may be for dendro-axonic, or reverse, neurotransmission across the dopaminergic-cholinergic synapse in the neostriatum, and may account for the extrapyramidal actions of nicotine. Similarly, we report spiroperidol binding sites on descending striato-nigral afferents which contact dopaminergic dendrites. Again, their presence is hypothesized to be for dendro-axonic transmission, which may be a general phenomenon in the CNS and not just restricted to nigro-striatal dopaminergic neurons.

The concept that dendrites can release as well as receive neurotransmitters is not entirely new (32). Some neurons lack axons altogether, and in such circumstances dendrites would have to initiate activity or else the neuron would be a communication's sink. In other circumstances dendrites can be seen to be presynaptic to other dendrites. But such morphological features are exceptional. Even in areas where only the usual axodendritic and axosomatic synapses can be seen, however, histochemical methods for neurotransmitters, or their synthetic enzymes, have generally shown them to occur prominently in dendrites. This is true, for example, for serotonin and the catecholamines (1,4,33), tyrosine hydroxylase (TH) (28,29), dopa decarboxylase (11), tryptophan hydroxylase (29), and choline acetyltransferase (CAT), the synthetic enzyme for acetylcholine (14). Glutamic acid decarboxylase (GAD) is more readily localized to nerve endings than to cell soma or dendrites by immunohistochemical procedures, but it also has been found in dendrites under special circumstances where axonal transport has been inhibited (31).

While several theories could be advanced as to the reason why neurotransmitters and their synthetic enzymes should exist in dendrites, one possibility is that the neurotransmitters are released to act on axonal endings, thus providing reverse neurotransmission across the synapse. If this is the case, there should be binding sites for the transmitters on the afferent neurons.

The nigro-striatal dopaminergic system can be used as a model to test this hypothesis. There are descending GABA (6,13) and probably substance P (16) tracts which make contact with dopaminergic dendrites in the substantia nigra (SN). In the neostriatum, dopaminergic nerve endings make contact with cholinergic dendrites (14). If dopamine is released from dendrites in the SN to affect axonal connections, there should be a reduction in dopaminergic receptor sites following lesions which destroy the descending pathways but spare dopaminergic cells. On the other hand, there should be no reduction in such receptor sites when the descending pathways are spared but dopaminergic cell bodies are destroyed. Intrastriatal injections of kainic acid will produce a destruction of GABA and substance P cell bodies which send axons to the SN, while leaving dopaminergic cell bodies in the SN intact (2,16). On the other hand, intraventricular injections of 6-hydroxydopamine (6-OHDA) will destroy the nigrostriatal dopaminergic tract while preserving the descending pathways (22). A combination of the two toxins will produce varying amounts of pre- and postsynaptic destruction. Accordingly, we measured dopaminergic receptor binding in the SN using ^{3}H-spiroperidol after varying doses of kainic acid and/or 6-OHDA.

Similarly, intrastriatal kainic acid injections will destroy structures in the neostriatum postsynaptic to dopaminergic nerve endings, but will spare the endings themselves. Intraventricular 6-OHDA will destroy the dopaminergic nerve endings, but spare the cholinergic and other postsynaptic structures (22). If acetylcholine was being released from dendrites to act on dopaminergic nerve endings, there should be a drop in cholinergic receptor sites following 6-OHDA. A drop following kainic acid administration, on the other hand, would signify loss of receptors on striatal neurons postsynaptic to the cholinergic interneurons and/or autoreceptors. ^{3}H-QNB and ^{125}I-α-bungarotoxin (α–Btx) were used to measure the muscarinic and nicotinic receptors, respectively, in the neostriatum.

TH, CAT, and GAD activities in the neostriatum were used as indices of the injury to the various neuronal systems.

METHODS

Male Wistar rats weighing 300 g were given unilateral injections of 2 to 5 nmoles of kainic acid into the striatum, followed 1 week later, in some cases, by intraventricular injections of 200 to 250 μg of 6-OHDA 30 min after an intraventricular injection of 5 mg tranylcypromine sulfate/kg. All animals were sacrificed 10 to 15 days postoperatively, and the striata were individually assayed for TH, GAD, CAT, and protein by a previously reported method (21,24). In some instances, the individual striatal homogenates were used for the preparation of synaptic membrane preparations for binding assays through freezing, centrifugation, and polytroning, while in others (used to obtain the data for Scatchard plots), the striata were combined according to the measured enzyme activities and/or the operative procedures. Because of their small size, two or three SNs were combined according to treatment before being assayed for spiroperidol binding.

^{3}H-Spiroperidol (specific activity, 32 Ci/mm), ^{3}H-QNB (specific activity, 27 Ci/mm), and α-Btx (specific activity, 6–14 mCi/mg) were obtained from New England Nuclear. The incubation procedures used in the binding assays were, respectively, those of Creese and Snyder (3), Yamamura and Snyder (36), and De Belleroche and Bradford (5).

RESULTS

The kainic acid and 6-OHDA injections were purposely done with varying doses so that various degrees of neuronal destruction were produced. This is reflected in the range of enzyme activities evident in Fig. 1 to 3. The data were analyzed for significant correlations between the binding and enzyme activities in the homogenates.

Figure 1 shows QNB binding versus residual GAD and TH activities in the neostriata of rats. The figure demonstrates that there is no correlation between QNB binding and TH levels, indicating that an appreciable population of muscarinic receptor sites probably does not exist on dopaminergic afferents to this structure. The figure indicates, however, a strong correlation between QNB binding and GAD levels, suggesting, as previously reported (2), that most of the muscarinic binding sites are on neurons destroyed by the kainic acid injections. Following kainic acid, a number of neuronal systems in the striatum are destroyed (2). CAT levels, for example, dropped in parallel with GAD levels in these animals (correlation coefficient, 0.88). Thus, it is not possible to distinguish which neuronal population(s) contain the muscarinic receptors.

The results with α-Btx on individual striata were quite different. Figure 2

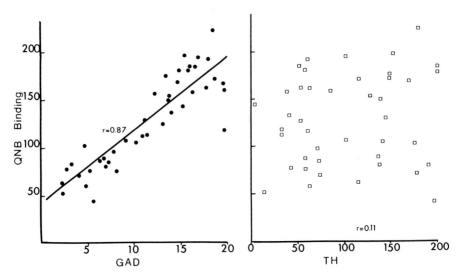

FIG. 1. Saturable ³H-QNB binding (cpm/20 μg protein) in rat neostriatum as a function of GAD (in μm/hr, 100 mg protein) and TH (in nm/hr, 100 mg protein) activities. All data are from the same neostriata of rats treated with kainic acid, 6-OHDA, or both agents.

shows that there was a strong correlation between residual TH activity and binding whether or not the rats received kainic acid; there was no significant correlation with residual GAD (or CAT) activities. Thus, it would appear as if nicotinic receptors exist on dopaminergic afferents to the striatum but not on neurons with their perikarya in that structure. Scatchard plots suggested that the reduction in α-Btx binding following 6-OHDA injections was not due to a reduction in affinity but in numbers of receptors.

Figure 3 indicates a significant correlation of ³H-spiroperidol binding in the SN with striatal GAD levels but not with striatal TH levels. This suggests that spiroperidol is not binding to dopaminergic dendrites in the SN but to afferents descending from the striatum. It cannot be certain that these are GABA neurons because substance P pathways are also known to descend from the striatum and to be affected by intrastriatal injections of kainic acid (7); the possibility remains that there are other descending systems as well.

DISCUSSION

It has been previously reported that dopamine-sensitive adenylate cyclase activity in the SN disappears when brain lesions are performed that eliminate the descending afferents from the neostriatum (7,35). Adenylate cyclase is believed to be the second messenger for dopamine and, although there is not always complete parallelism between dopamine-sensitive adenylate cyclase activity and spiroperidol binding, there appear to be qualitatively similar changes in these lesions.

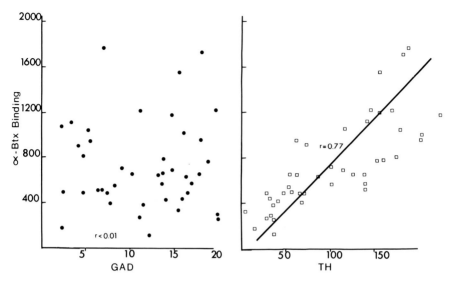

FIG. 2. Saturable ^{125}I-α-Btx binding (cpm/2 mg protein) in rat neostriatum as a function of GAD and CAT activities. Units of activity and rat treatments as in Fig. 1.

The possibility has been suggested that the dopamine-sensitive adenylate cyclase in the SN is postsynaptic to axo-axonic synapses from recurrent dopaminergic axons. This hypothesis seems unlikely, however, since axo-axonic synapses are rarely, if ever, seen in the SN in electron microscopic studies, and such electron microscopic studies in rats treated with 6-OHDA have never revealed degenerating nerve endings in the SN (14). Moreover, lesions of the nigro-striatal dopaminergic tract lead to retrograde, as well as anterograde degeneration (22). All of these indications militate against the existence of dopamine boutons within the SN and therefore against the hypothesis that the dopamine-sensitive adenylate cyclase (and the spiroperidol binding sites) are postsynaptic to such boutons.

Other types of evidence suggest that there is, in fact, dendritic storage and release of dopamine in the SN, and such storage and release are consistent with the hypothesis that there is a dialogue rather than a monologue across these synapses with the dopamine receptors being located on the presynaptic membrane. Hefti and Lichtensteiger (15) concluded from subcellular studies in the rat that at least 40 to 50% of nigral dopamine seems to be localized in dendrites and probably occurs largely in particles that they termed "dendrosomes," since they behave like synaptosomes on density gradient centrifugation. Antidromic activation of the medial forebrain bundle region *in vivo* results in accumulation of DOPAC in nigral tissues (19,20). Similarly, stimulation of the SN leads to the appearance of dopamine in nigral push–pull cannulae (27). Stimulation of SN slices *in vitro* by a high potassium concentration also causes the appearance of dopamine and its metabolites in extracellular fluid, and this

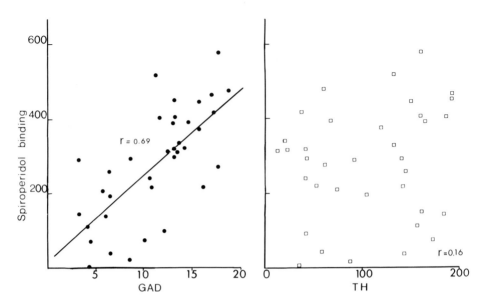

FIG. 3. Saturable ^{3}H-spiroperidol binding (cpm/mg protein) in substantia nigra plotted against the average GAD and TH activities in the corresponding striata. Units of activity and rat treatments as in Fig. 1.

evoked release is dependent on calcium and inhibited by magnesium, just as is the exocytotic release of vesicle-bound transmitter from presynaptic nerve endings (8). Furthermore, dopamine is recaptured by dendrites through an active uptake process (1,8,34) such as occurs in dopaminergic nerve endings. The possibility that dendritically released dopamine affects the release of GABA from nigral nerve endings is suggested by the study of Reubi et al. (30) who found that dopamine selectively increases the release of ^{3}H-GABA from slices of rat SN *in vitro.*

Evidence also exists suggesting a direct influence of acetylcholine on dopaminergic nerve endings in the neostriatum. In isolated striatal tissues, it has been shown that acetylcholine increases the release of ^{3}H-dopamine previously synthesized from ^{3}H-tyrosine (10). This has been attributed to a nicotinic effect in synaptosomes (5) and to both nicotinic and muscarinic effects in slices (9,10). Since the dopaminergic nerve endings are cut off from their cell bodies in such preparations, the data cannot be explained on the basis of interneuronal loops acting back on the SN. Nor can the data be explained on the basis of axo-axonic synapses, since these have never been observed in the striatum. They can be explained on the hypothesis that acetylcholine is released from dendrites and that the dendritically released acetylcholine is able to act directly on dopaminergic nerve endings. The apparent association of α-Btx binding sites in the striatum with dopaminergic systems is consistent with this explanation.

The quantities of α-Btx that are bound in the striatum, and of spiroperidol in the substantia nigra, would suggest that far fewer receptor sites exist on afferent neurons than on dendrites. For example, the maximal amount of α-Btx bound in the striatum, presumably to presynaptic binding sites, was 16 to 24 fmoles/mg of protein. This may be compared to 600 fmoles for QNB which presumably binds postsynaptically. Similarly, the maximal spiroperidol binding in the SN was approximately 20 fmoles/mg of protein, while in the striatum it was roughly 400 fmoles. Considered another way, the α-Btx binding to afferent dopaminergic neurons in the striatum is 16 to 24 fmoles/mg, while spiroperidol binding to receptors for those nerve endings is approximately 400 fmoles/mg. The difference implies a bias in synaptic "crosstalk" in favor of axodendritic as opposed to dendroaxonic movement of transmitters. Such a bias would account for the paucity of storage vesicles seen in dendrites as opposed to nerve endings.

The available chemical and morphological data are not conclusive but they suggest a direct action of dendritically released transmitter on axonal endings, possibly modulating the amount of presynaptic transmitter released following repeated axonal stimulation. The evidence concerns only acetylcholine and dopamine in the extrapyramidal system, but the possibility exists that such synaptic dialogues may be a more or less general phenomenon in the CNS.

Apart from this fundamental question, the hypothesized synaptic dialogue across synapses in the neostriatum might provide a rational explanation for the apparent beneficial effects of nicotine in Parkinson's disease (26) and argue for further trials of nicotinic agents. The literature and data presented here would suggest that nicotine could cause enhanced dopamine release from dopaminergic nerve endings in the striatum by action at the α-Btx binding sites. Much more needs to be learned about the nature of cholinergic receptors on dopaminergic neurons and the types of agents that will act on them to promote dopamine release. It is even conceivable that the efficacy of atropine-like agents is indirectly connected to these receptors. By blocking muscarinic receptors postsynaptic to neostriatal cholinergic cells, acetylcholine production might be increased, thus permitting more to be released from dendrites to act on nicotinic receptors on dopaminergic neurons.

The possibility that nicotine, or some other component of tobacco, might function as a stimulant to dopaminergic cells and thus ward off Parkinson's disease is even more intriguing. It is known that nigrostriatal dopaminergic cells are particularly vulnerable to aging. At birth there are roughly 400,000 cells in each human SN. This number drops to approximately 250,000 by age 65. Parkinsonians usually have less than 150,000 (25). The processes by which cell death occurs might be entirely different in the two circumstances, but extrapolation of nigrostriatal cell counts versus age suggest that parkinsonism could become almost universal with a sufficiently elderly population. Thus, the loss of dopaminergic cells in the SN is a concern for normal individuals as well as parkinsonians, and methods of prevention should be pursued. The negative correlation of smoking and Parkinson's disease, while only slight (12,17,18) is an indication that such a goal might be feasible.

ACKNOWLEDGMENT

This research was supported by grants from the Medical Research Council of Canada, the W. Garfield Weston Foundation, and the Province of British Columbia. Mrs. Edith Singh provided excellent technical assistance.

REFERENCES

1. Bjorklund, A., and Lindvall, O. (1975): Dopamine in dendrites of substantia nigra neurons: suggestions for a role in dendritic terminals. *Brain Res.,* 83:531–537.
2. Coyle, J. T., McGeer, E. G., McGeer, P. L., and Schwarcz, R. (1978): Neostriatal injections: a model for Huntington's chorea. In: *Kainic Acid as a Tool in Neurobiology,* edited by E. G. McGeer, J. W. Olney, and P. L. McGeer, pp. 139–160. Raven Press, New York.
3. Creese, J., and Snyder, S. H. (1977): A simple and sensitive radioassay for antischizophrenic drugs in blood. *Nature,* 270:180–183.
4. Dahlstrom, A., and Fuxe, K. (1964): A method for the demonstration of monoamine containing fibers in the central nervous system. *Acta. Physiol. Scand.,* 60:293–295.
5. De Belleroche, J., and Bradford, H. F. (1978): Biochemical evidence for the presence of presynaptic receptors on dopaminergic nerve terminals. *Brain Res.,* 142:53–68.
6. Fonnum, F., Grofova, I., Rinvik, E., Storm-Mathison, J., and Waldberg, F. (1974): Origin and distribution of glutamate decarboxylase in substantia nigra of the cat. *Brain Res.,* 71:77–92.
7. Gale, K., Guidotti, A., and Costa, E. (1977): Dopamine sensitive adenylate cyclase location in substantia nigra. *Science,* 195:503–505.
8. Geffen, L. B., Jessell, T. M., Cuello, A. C., and Iversen, L. L. (1976): Release of dopamine from dendrites in rat substantia nigra. *Nature,* 260:258–260.
9. Giorguieff, M. F., Le Floc'h, M. L., Glowinski, J., and Besson, M. J. (1977): Involvement of cholinergic presynaptic receptors of nicotinic and muscarinic types in the control of spontaneous release of dopamine from striatal dopaminergic terminals in the rat. *J. Pharmacol. Exp. Ther.,* 200:535–544.
10. Giorguieff, M. F., Le Floc'h, M. L., Westfall, T. C., Glowinski, J., and Besson, M. J. (1976): Nicotinic effect of acetylcholine on the release of newly synthesized [^{3}H]dopamine in rat striatal slices and cat caudate nucleus. *Brain Res.,* 106:117–131.
11. Goldstein, D., Fuxe, K., and Hokfelt, T. (1972): Characterization and tissue localization of catecholamine synthesizing enzymes. *Pharmacol. Rev.,* 24:293–309.
12. Hammond, E. C. (1966): Smoking in relation to the death rates of one million men and women. In: Epidemiological approaches to the study of cancer and other chronic diseases. *National Cancer Institute Monograph, No. 19,* Washington GPO, 127–204.
13. Hattori, T., Fibiger, H. C., and McGeer, P. L. (1975): Demonstration of a pallidonigral projection innervating dopaminergic neurons. *J. Comp. Neurol.,* 162:487–504.
14. Hattori, T., Singh, V. K., McGeer, E. G., and McGeer, P. L. (1976): Immunohistochemical localization of choline acetyltransferase containing neostriatal neurons and their relationship with dopaminergic synapses. *Brain Res.,* 102:164–173.
15. Hefti, F., and Lichtensteiger, W. (1978): Subcellular distribution of dopamine in substantia nigra of the rat brain: Effects of γ-butyrolactone and destruction of noradrenergic afferents suggest formation of particles from dendrites. *J. Neurochem.,* 30:1217–1230.
16. Hong, J., Yang, H. Y. T., Racagni, G., and Costa, E. (1977): Projections of substance P containing neurons from neostriatum to substantia nigra. *Brain Res.,* 122:541–544.
17. Kahn, H. A. (1966): The Dorn study of smoking and mortality among U.S. veterans. In: Epidemiological approaches to the study of cancer and other chronic diseases. *National Cancer Institute Monograph, No. 19,* Washington GPO, 1–25.
18. Kessler, I. I., and Diamond, E. L. (1971): Epidemiologic studies of Parkinson's disease. I. Smoking and Parkinson's disease: a survey and explanatory hypothesis. *Am. J. Epidemiol.,* 94:16–25.
19. Korf, J., and Zieleman, M. (1976): Dopamine release in substantia nigra? *Nature,* 260:257–258.

20. Korf, J., Zieleman, M., and Westerink, B. H. C. (1977): Metabolism of dopamine in the substantia nigra after antidromic activation. *Brain Res.,* 120:184–187.
21. Lowry, O. H., Rosebrough, H. J., Farr, A. L., and Randall, R. J. (1951): Protein measurement with the Folin phenol reagent. *J. Biol. Chem.,* 193:265–275.
22. McGeer, E. G., Fibiger, H. C., McGeer, P. L., and Brooke, S. (1973): Temporal changes in amine synthesizing enzymes of rat extrapyramidal system after hemitransections or 6-hydroxydopamine administration. *Brain Res.,* 52:289–300.
23. McGeer, P. L., Boulding, J. E., Gibson, W. C., and Foulkes, R. G. (1961): Drug-induced extrapyramidal reactions. Treatment with diphenhydramine hydrochloride and dihydroxyphenylalanine. *J.A.M.A.,* 177:665–670.
24. McGeer, P. L., and McGeer, E. G. (1976): Enzymes associated with the metabolism of catecholamines, acetylcholine and GABA in human controls and patients with parkinsonism and Huntington's chorea. *J. Neurochem.,* 26:65–76.
25. McGeer, P. L., McGeer, E. G., and Suzuki, J. S. (1977): Aging and extrapyramidal function. *Arch. Neurol.,* 34:33–35.
26. Moll, H. (1926): The treatment of post-encephalitic parkinsonism by nicotine, *Br. Med. J.,* 1079–1081.
27. Nieoullon, A., Cheramy, A., and Glowinski, J. (1977): Release of dopamine in vivo from cat substantia nigra. *Nature,* 266:375–377.
28. Pickel, V. M., Tong, H. J., and Reis, D. J. (1975): Ultrastructural localization of tyrosine hydroxylase in noradrenergic neurons of brain. *Proc. Natl. Acad. Sci. U.S.A.,* 72:659–663.
29. Pickel, V. M., Tong, H. J., and Reis, D. J. (1976): Monoamine synthesizing enzymes in central dopaminergic, noradrenergic and serotonergic neurons. *J. Histochem. Cytochem.,* 24:792–806.
30. Reubi, J. C., Iversen, L. L., and Jessell, T. M., (1977): Dopamine selectively increases ^{3}H-GABA release from slices of rat substantia nigra in vitro. *Nature,* 268:653–654.
31. Ribak, C. E., Vaughn, J. E., Sato, K., Barber, R., and Roberts, E. (1977): Glutamate decarboxylase localization in neurons of the olfactory bulb. *Brain Res.,* 126:1–18.
32. Roberts, E. (1966): The synapse as a biochemical self-organizing microcybernetic unit. *Brain Res.,* 2:117–166.
33. Sladek, J. R., Jr., and Parnavelas, J. G. (1975): Catecholamine-containing dendrites in primate brain. *Brain Res.,* 100:657–662.
34. Sotelo, C. (1971): The fine structural localization of norepinephrine ^{3}H in the substantia nigra and area postrema of the rat. An autoradiographic study. *J. Ultrastruct. Res.,* 36:824–841.
35. Spano, P. F., Trabucchi, M., and Di Chiara, G. (1977): Localization of nigral dopamine-sensitive adenylate cyclase on neurons originating from the corpus striatum. *Science,* 196:1343–1345.
36. Yamamura, H. I., and Snyder, S. H. (1974): Muscarinic cholinergic binding in rat brain. *Proc. Natl. Acad. Sci. U.S.A.,* 71:1725–1729.

Advances in Neurology, Vol. 24, edited by
L. J. Poirier, T. L. Sourkes, and P. J. Bédard.
Raven Press, New York © 1979.

Presynaptic and Postsynaptic Effects of Dopamine Receptor Blocking Agents

*Nils-Erik Andén and Maria Grabowska-Andén

Department of Pharmacology, University of Göteborg, S-400 33 Göteborg, Sweden

In recent years it has been demonstrated that dopamine (DA) receptors occur not only on postsynaptic neurons of the DA synapses but also on the nerve terminals and the cell bodies of the DA neurons (for reviews see refs. 6,7,20). The latter receptors have been called presynaptic receptors or autoreceptors. Neuroleptic drugs can block both types of DA receptors. It is not known, however, if the various neuroleptic drugs might differ in their relative ability to block post- and presynaptic DA receptors. In the present work we have investigated how haloperidol, clozapine, pimozide, and the pimozide analog R 28935 (erythro-1-{1-[2-(1,4-benzodioxan-2-yl)-2-hydroxyethyl] -4-piperidyl} -2-benzimidazolinone) (25) interfere with post- and presynaptic effects of the DA receptor agonist apomorphine in the rat corpus striatum. Similarly to neuroleptic drugs, morphine has been reported to cause catalepsy, rigidity, and increased turnover of dopamine in rats (for review see ref. 16). Therefore, the possible effects of morphine on pre- and postsynaptic DA receptors have been analyzed in ways similar to those of neuroleptics.

MATERIALS AND METHODS

Apomorphine-Induced Rotation

On the day before the experiment, guide cannulae were implanted bilaterally by means of a stereotaxic instrument when the rats (male Sprague–Dawley weighing about 200 g) were anesthetized with pentobarbital sodium. Just before the start of the recording of the rotation, 1 µl 25% KCl was injected during 45 sec into the corpus striatum on one side by means of a guide cannula. Simultaneously, an equimolar amount of NaCl (1 µl 20%) was given into the corpus striatum on the opposite side. Thirty seconds after the completion of the intrastriatal injections of 25% KCl and 20% NaCl, apomorphine was given intraperitoneally at a dose of 2 mg/kg, and the rats were placed in plastic cylinders with a diameter of 50 cm. The number of complete rotations around

---

* Present address: Department of Medical Pharmacology, Box 573, S-751-23 Uppsala, Sweden.

a vertical axis to the KCl- or to the NaCl-treated side was counted during 5-min periods for 45 min. All rats were treated with reserpine (10 mg/kg i.p.) 4 hr before·the start of the recording.

The rats injected with 1 μl 25% KCl into the corpus striatum on one side reacted by turning to the KCl-treated side following apomorphine, and from the KCl-treated side following neuroleptic drugs (22). These drug-induced asymmetries are similar to those seen after unilateral removal of the corpus striatum (2,5). Therefore, it is likely that the hypertonic KCl injection inactivates the corpus striatum on the treated side.

Since the rats were pretreated with reserpine, the effects of apomorphine were, in all probability, the result of stimulation of postsynaptic DA receptors. The apomorphine-induced rotation of rats with the corpus striatum inactivated on one side is due to asymmetry in muscle tone, combined with increase in motor activity evoked by stimulation of postsynaptic DA receptors in the corpus striatum and in the nucleus accumbens, respectively (1). In the experimental model used, the sensitivity of the postsynaptic DA receptors should not deviate very much from normal, particularly since the time of pretreatment with reserpine was short.

Accumulation of DOPA

The *in vivo* tyrosine hydroxylase activity of the corpus striatum was determined by the accumulation of DOPA following inhibition of the DOPA decarboxylase by 3-hydroxybenzylhydrazine (NSD 1015; 100 mg/kg i.p., 30 min) (8). DOPA was determined spectrofluorimetrically after homogenization, cation exchange chromatography, and oxidation (12).

The γ-hydroxybutyrate precursor γ-butyrolactone (GBL) blocks the nerve impulse flow of the nigroneostriatal DA neurons both normally and when it is accelerated by neuroleptic drugs (19,24). The accumulation of DOPA in the corpus striatum induced by a DOPA decarboxylase inhibitor is enhanced by GBL (19), as well as by axotomy (13). The effect of GBL or axotomy on the DA synthesis is completely antagonized by apomorphine (13,19,24). Since this effect of apomorphine occurs in the absence of nerve impulses in the DA neurons, and since axo-axonal synapses are very rare in the corpus striatum (14), the apomorphine-induced inhibition of the increased DOPA accumulation following GBL is probably caused by stimulation of DA receptors located on the DA nerve terminals (presynaptic DA receptors).

RESULTS

Apomorphine-Induced Rotation

The reserpine-pretreated rats injected with 1 μl 25% KCl into the corpus striatum on one side, turned their heads and tails to the NaCl-treated side,

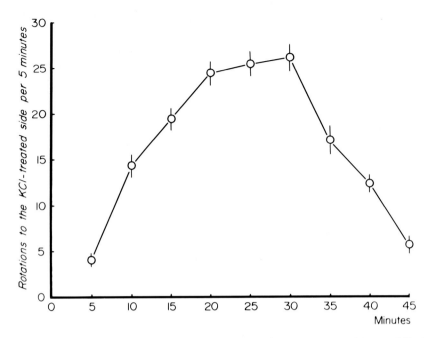

FIG. 1. Time-course for the rotation induced by apomorphine (2 mg/kg i.p.) in rats following unilateral injection of 1 μl 25% KCl into the corpus striatum. The rats were pretreated with reserpine (10 mg/kg i.p., 4hr). The values are means $\pm$ SEM of 23 experiments.

i.e., contralaterally to the KCl-treated side. Apomorphine at a dose of 2 mg/ kg i.p. turned the rats from the NaCl-treated to the KCl-treated side and they started to rotate. The rotation was maximal after 15 to 30 min and it ceased after about 45 min (Fig. 1). The effect was dose-dependent with a peak following 2 mg/kg i.p. (data not shown).

Apomorphine-Induced Inhibition of the Accumulation of DOPA

The synthesis of DA in the rat corpus striatum, measured as the accumulation of DOPA following inhibition of the DOPA decarboxylase by NSD 1015, was increased by GBL (750 mg/kg i.p., 35 min before sacrifice) to about 300% of the NSD 1015 control (Fig. 2). Apomorphine (2 mg/kg i.p., 40 min before sacrifice) given in combination with GBL reduced the DA synthesis to values even below those of the NSD 1015 control (Fig. 2). The peak effect was seen after about 2 mg/kg apomorphine i.p. (18).

Haloperidol

Haloperidol injected intraperitoneally 15 min before apomorphine inhibited the apomorphine-induced rotation of reserpine-pretreated rats in a dose-depen-

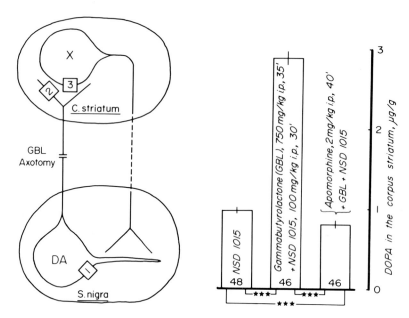

FIG. 2. Left: Three possible locations of dopamine receptors regulating the turnover of the dopamine in the corpus striatum. **Right:** Accumulation of DOPA induced by NSD 1015 following GBL and apomorphine plus GBL. The values are means ± SEM of 46–48 experiments. Statistical significances were calculated by Student's t-test (*** $p < 0.001$). The inhibitory effect of apomorphine is probably due to stimulation of dopamine receptor 2 on the dopamine nerve terminals in the corpus striatum.

dent manner (Fig. 3). The apomorphine-induced inhibition of the DA synthesis of the GBL-treated rats was also antagonized by haloperidol, although somewhat higher doses were needed than those in the rotation experiments. Haloperidol enhanced the accumulation of DOPA following only NSD 1015, and this effect had a dose-response relationship similar to that of the inhibition of the rotation.

Clozapine

Clozapine markedly antagonized the apomorphine-induced rotation but it only weakly interfered with the apomorphine-induced inhibition of the DA synthesis (Fig. 4).

Pimozide

Pimozide was much more potent in reducing the apomorphine-induced rotation than in inhibiting the apomorphine-induced effect on DA synthesis (Fig. 5). The accumulation of DOPA following only NSD 1015 was increased by intermediate doses of pimozide.

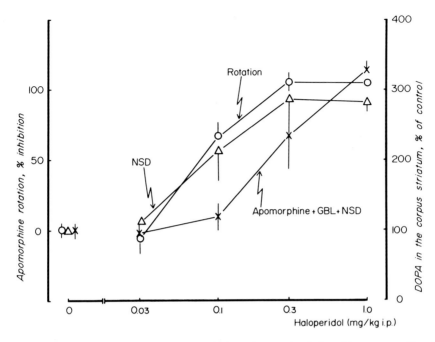

FIG. 3. Effects of different doses of haloperidol on the rotation induced by apomorphine (2 mg/kg i.p.) and on the accumulation of DOPA in the corpus striatum following NSD 1015 (100 mg/kg i.p., 30 min before sacrifice) or following apomorphine (2 mg/kg i.p., 40 min before sacrifice) plus GBL (750 mg/kg i.p., 35 min before sacrifice) plus NSD 1015 (100 mg/kg i.p., 30 min before sacrifice). Haloperidol was given 15 min prior to the injection of apomorphine (rotation) or of NSD 1015 (DOPA accumulation). The values are means ± SEM of 3 to 13 experiments.

R 28935

R 28935 was also much more potent in counteracting the apomorphine-induced rotation than the apomorphine-induced inhibition of DA synthesis (Fig. 6). It enhanced the synthesis of DA at somewhat lower doses than those necessary to inhibit the effect of apomorphine on the synthesis of DA.

Morphine

Morphine (30 mg/kg i.p., 30 min before apomorphine) completely prevented the apomorphine-induced rotation (0 ± 0.0 rotations per 45 min, $N = 6$). Inhibition of DA synthesis by apomorphine was not reversed by morphine (30 mg/kg i.p.); actually there was a tendency to a potentiation of the apomorphine effect (Fig. 7). Morphine by itself stimulated the synthesis of DA by means of a mechanism sensitive to the opiate receptor antagonist naloxone.

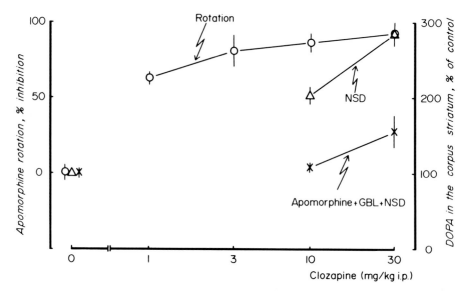

FIG. 4. Effects of different doses of clozapine on the rotation induced by apomorphine and on the accumulation of DOPA in the corpus striatum following NSD 1015 or following apomorphine plus GBL plus NSD 1015 (see Fig. 3). Clozapine was given 30 min prior to the injection of apomorphine (rotation) or of NSD 1015 (DOPA accumulation). The values are means ± SEM of 3 to 8 experiments.

DISCUSSION

The blockade of the postsynaptic and presynaptic DA receptors in the corpus striatum by the five drugs studied has been investigated by means of the effects of the DA receptor agonist apomorphine on the rotation and on the DA synthesis following GBL, respectively. In both models, the dose of apomorphine was just supramaximal, i.e., 2 mg/kg i.p. Haloperidol, clozapine, pimozide, and R 28935 inhibited both the presynaptic and the postsynaptic effects of apomorphine. The ED_{50}s calculated from Figs. 3 to 6 are presented in the first and third columns of Table 1. Haloperidol appeared to block the presynaptic receptors almost as effectively as the postsynaptic receptors, as seen in the fourth column of Table 1. The other three drugs were clearly much more active on the postsynaptic than on the presynaptic DA receptors. It is of interest that R 28935 previously has been found to be more effective on postsynaptic than on presynaptic α-adrenoreceptors in the central nervous system (3).

Haloperidol, clozapine, pimozide, and R 28935 by themselves also increased the synthesis of DA, and the calculated ED_{50}s are presented in the second column of Table 1. In all cases, somewhat higher doses were needed in order to antagonize the effect of apomorphine on the synthesis of DA than to stimulate the synthesis of DA, probably due to a more powerful DA receptor stimulation

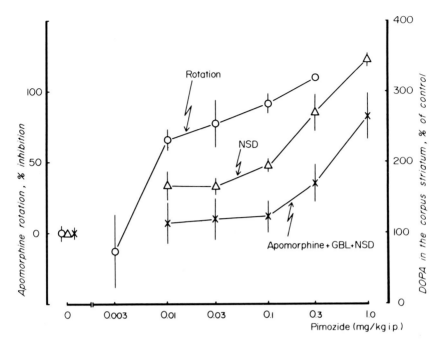

FIG. 5. Effects of different doses of pimozide on the rotation induced by apomorphine and on the accumulation of DOPA in the corpus striatum following NSD 1015 or following apomorphine plus GBL plus NSD 1015 (see Fig. 3). Pimozide was given 2 hr prior to the injection of apomorphine (rotation) or of NSD 1015 (DOPA accumulation). The values are means ± SEM of 3 to 15 experiments.

following administration of apomorphine (column 5 in Table 1). The similar ratios between doses increasing the synthesis of DA in the presence and absence of apomorphine might indicate that the presynaptic effect is more important than the postsynaptic for the normal increase in the DA synthesis by neuroleptic drugs, although a postsynaptic receptor blockade naturally might contribute.

A presynaptic blockade of DA receptors by a neuroleptic drug might cause disadvantages in therapy. It is generally assumed that neuroleptic-induced tardive dyskinesia is caused by an increased sensitivity of the DA receptors of the effector cells, perhaps as a compensation to long-term blockade of the DA receptors (9,11,15,17,21,23). The influence of DA on the effector cells should be even more pronounced following neuroleptics inhibiting post- as well as presynaptic DA receptors, since these drugs also facilitate the release of DA by nerve impulses. On the other hand, it has been reported that presynaptic DA receptors can also develop supersensitivity (18). This mechanism should counteract the postsynaptic supersensitivity. In clinical practice, the first factor might be more important since it has been reported that clozapine, acting preferentially post-synaptically, does not cause tardive dyskinesia during long-term treatment and

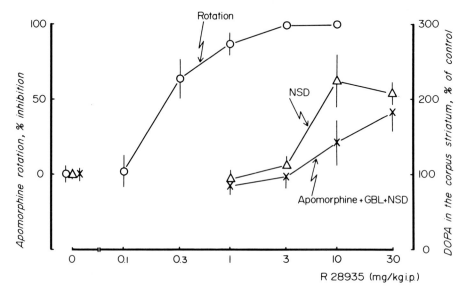

FIG. 6. Effects of different doses of R 28935 (erythro-1-[1-[2-(1,4-benzodioxan-2-yl)-2-hydroxy-ethyl]-4-piperidyl]-2-benzimidazolinone) on the rotation induced by apomorphine and on the accumulation of DOPA in the corpus striatum following NSD 1015 or following apomorphine plus GBL plus NSD 1015 (see Fig. 3). R 28935 was given 15 min prior to the injection of apomorphine (rotation) or of NSD 1015 (DOPA accumulation). The values are means ± SEM of 3 to 13 experiments.

readily antagonizes the dyskinesia seen after chronic treatment with haloperidol (10).

Morphine completely inhibited the apomorphine-induced rotation but it did not reverse the apomorphine-induced inhibition of DA synthesis. From these data it might be inferred that morphine selectively blocks postsynaptic DA receptors. However, morphine (30 mg/kg i.p.) does not cause asymmetry of rats with the corpus striatum inactivated on one side, whereas haloperidol produces a marked turning of the head and tail from the KCl-treated side under the same conditions. Furthermore, morphine completely inhibits the haloperidol-induced turning when given before or after haloperidol (4). Therefore, it appears that morphine causes muscular rigidity by an action outside the corpus striatum, and that a blockade of DA receptors is not involved in this action. Likewise, the morphine-induced stimulation of the DA turnover does not seem to be mediated via DA receptors. All the actions of morphine are probably due to activation of opiate receptors, since these actions are blocked by naloxone (4).

ACKNOWLEDGMENTS

This work was supported by the Swedish Medical Research Council (04X–502). For generous gifts of drugs, we thank Janssen Pharmaceutica, Beerse (haloperidol, pimozide, R 28935); Sandoz, Basle (clozapine); CIBA-Geigy, Möln-

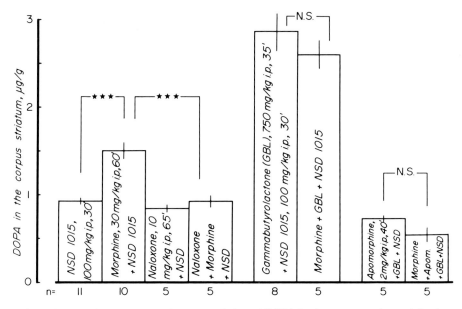

FIG. 7. Effects of morphine on the accumulation of DOPA in the corpus striatum following NSD 1015, naloxone plus NSD 1015, γ-butyrolactone (GBL) plus NSD 1015 and apomorphine plus γ-butyrolactone plus NSD 1015. The values are means $\pm$ SEM of 5 to 11 experiments. Statistical significances were calculated by Student's t-test (*** $p < 0.001$; N. S., not significant, $p > 0.05$).

TABLE 1. *Approximate potencies of four drugs in stimulating dopamine synthesis and in inhibiting apomorphine-induced rotation*

	ED50 (mg/kg i.p.)			Ratio between ED50	
Drug	Apo + GBL + NSD[a]	NSD 1015	Rotation	Apo + GBL + NSD / Rotation	Apo + GBL + NSD / NSD
Haloperidol	0.20	0.08	0.08	2.5	2.5
Clozapine	>30	10	<1	>30	>3
Pimozide	0.40	0.10	0.008	50	4
R 28935	12.5	4	0.25	50	3

[a] Apomorphine + gammabutyrolactone + NSD 1015.

dal (reserpine); and Endo, Garden City (naloxone). Skillful technical assistance was provided by Maria Lindbäck and Inger Oscarsson.

REFERENCES

1. Andén, N.-E. (1976): Animal models of brain dopamine function. In: *Advances in Parkinsonism*, edited by W. Birkmayer and O. Hornykiewicz, pp. 169–177. Editions "Roche," Basle.
2. Andén, N.-E., Dahlström, A., Fuxe, K., and Larsson, K. (1966): Functional role of the nigro-neostriatal dopamine neurons. *Acta Pharmacol. (Kbh.),* 24:263–274.

3. Andén, N.-E, Gomes, C., Persson, B., and Trolin, G. (1978): R 28935 and prazosin: effects on central and peripheral alpha-adrenoreceptor activity and on blood pressure. *Naunyn Schmiedebergs Arch. Pharmacol.,* 302:299–306.
4. Andén, N.-E., and Grabowska-Andén, M. (1978): Morphine-induced changes in striatal dopamine mechanisms not evoked from the dopamine nerve terminals. *J. Pharm. Pharmacol.,* 30:732–734.
5. Andén, N.-E., Rubenson, A., Fuxe, K., and Hökfelt, T. (1967): Evidence for dopamine receptor stimulation by apomorphine. *J. Pharm. Pharmacol.,* 19:627–629.
6. Bunney, B. S., and Aghajanian, G. K. (1975): Evidence for drug actions on both pre- and postsynaptic catecholamine receptors in the CNS. In: *Pre- and Postsynaptic Receptors,* edited by E. Usdin and W. E. Bunney, Jr., pp. 89–122. Marcel Dekker, New York.
7. Carlsson, A. (1975): Receptor-mediated control of dopamine metabolism. In: *Pre- and Postsynaptic Receptors,* edited by E. Usdin and W. E. Bunney, Jr., pp. 49–65. Marcel Dekker, New York.
8. Carlsson, A., Davis, J. N., Kehr, W., Lindqvist, M., and Atack, C. V. (1972): Simultaneous measurement of tyrosine and tryptophan hydroxylase activities in brain in vivo using an inhibitor of the aromatic amino acid decarboxylase. *Naunyn Schmiedebergs Arch. Pharmacol.,* 275:153–168.
9. Gianutsos, G., Drawbaugh, R. B., Hynes, M. D., and Lal, H. (1974): Behavioural evidence for dopaminergic supersensitivity after chronic haloperidol. *Life Sci.,* 14:887–899.
10. Hippius, H. (1976). On the relations between antipsychotic and extrapyramidal effects of psychoactive drugs. In: *Antipsychotic Drugs: Pharmacodynamics and Pharmacokinetics,* edited by G. Sedvall, B. Uvnäs and Y. Zotterman, pp. 437–445. Pergamon Press, Oxford.
11. Jackson, D. M., Andén, N.-E., Engel, J., and Liljeqvist, S. (1975): The effect of long-term penfluridol treatment on the sensitivity of the dopamine receptors in the nucleus accumbens and in the corpus striatum. *Psychopharmacologia,* 45:151–155.
12. Kehr, W., Carlsson, A., and Lindqvist, M. (1972): A method for the determination of 3,4-dihydroxyphenylalanine (DOPA) in brain. *Naunyn Schmiedebergs Arch. Pharmacol.,* 274:273–280.
13. Kehr, W., Carlsson, A., Lindqvist, M., Magnusson, T., and Atack, C. (1972): Evidence for a receptor-mediated feed-back control of striatal tyrosine hydroxylase activity. *J. Pharm. Pharmacol.,* 24:744–747.
14. Kemp, J. M., and Powell, T. P. S. (1971): The synaptic organization of the caudate nucleus. *Philos. Trans. R. Soc. Lond. Biol.,* 262:403–412.
15. Klawans, H. L., and Rubovits, R. (1972): An experimental model of tardive dyskinesia. *J. Neural Trans.,* 33:235–246.
16. Kuschinsky, K. (1976): Actions of narcotics on brain dopamine metabolism and their relevance for "psychomotor" effects. *Arzneimittel-Forsch.,* 26:563–567.
17. Möller-Nielsen, I., Fjalland, B., Pedersen, V., and Nymark, M. (1974): Pharmacology of neuroleptics upon repeated administration. *Psychopharmacologia,* 34:95–104.
18. Nowycky, M. C., and Roth, R. H. (1977): Presynaptic dopamine receptors. Development of supersensitivity following treatment with fluphenazine decanoate. *Naunyn Schmiedebergs Arch. Pharmacol.,* 300:247–254.
19. Roth, R. H., Walters, J. R., and Aghajanian, G. K. (1973): Effect of impulse flow on the release and synthesis of dopamine in the rat striatum. In: *Frontiers in Catecholamine Research,* edited by S. H. Snyder and E. Usdin, pp. 567–574. Pergamon Press, New York.
20. Roth, R. H., Walters, J. R., Murrin, L. C., and Morgenroth III, V. H. (1975): Dopamine neurons: role of impulse flow and pre-synaptic receptors in the regulation of tyrosine hydroxylase. In: *Pre- and Postsynaptic Receptors,* edited by E. Usdin and W. E. Bunney, Jr., pp. 5–48. Marcel Dekker, New York.
21. Sayers, A. C., Bürki, H. R., Ruch, W., and Asper, H. (1975): Neuroleptic-induced hypersensitivity of striatal dopamine receptors in the rat as a model of tardive dyskinesias. Effects of clozapine, haloperidol, loxapine and chlorpromazine. *Psychopharmacologia,* 41:97–104.
22. Stock, G., Magnusson, T., and Andén, N.-E. (1973): Increase in brain dopamine after axotomy or treatment with gammahydroxybutyric acid due to elimination of the nerve impulse flow. *Naunyn Schmiedebergs Arch. Pharmacol.,* 278:347–361.
23. Tarsy, D., and Baldessarini, R. J. (1974): Behavioural supersensitivity to apomorphine following chronic treatment with drugs which interfere with the synaptic function of catecholamines. *Neuropharmacology,* 13:927–940.

24. Walters, J. R., and Roth, R. H. (1976): Dopaminergic neurons: an *in vivo* system for measuring drug interactions with presynaptic receptors. *Naunyn Schmiedebergs Arch. Pharmacol.,* 296:5–14.
25. Wellens, D., DeWilde, A., van Bogaert, A., van Bogaert, P. P., Wouters, L., Reneman, R. S., and Janssen, P. A. J. (1975): Unusual mechanism of hypotensive activity exerted by erythro-1-[1-[2-(1,4-benzodioxan-2-yl)-2-OH-ET]-4-piperidyl]-2-benzimidazolinone (R 28935). *Arch. Int. Pharmacodyn.,* 215:91–103.

Advances in Neurology, Vol. 24, edited by
L. J. Poirier, T. L. Sourkes, and P. J. Bédard.
Raven Press, New York © 1979.

Dopamine Agonists: Antiparkinsonian Efficacy in Experimental Animal Models and Binding to Putative Dopamine Receptors

*M. Goldstein, *J. Y. Lew, **S. Nakamura, and **A. F. Battista

*Departments of *Psychiatry and **Neurosurgery, Neurochemistry Laboratories, New York University Medical Center, New York, New York 10016*

Monkeys with ventromedial tegmental (VMT) lesions that develop sustained postural tremor (12) were used as models for evaluation of antiparkinsonian efficacy of drugs (3). In monkeys with VMT lesion, L-DOPA relieves the surgically induced tremor and concomitantly evokes abnormal involuntary movements (AIMs) similar to those observed in man (4). Ergot alkaloids such as bromocriptine and lergotrile relieve the tremor in monkeys with VMT lesions (9,11) and clinical studies indicate that they are of therapeutic value in some parkinsonian patients (8,9).

More recently we have tested the antiparkinsonian efficacy of some newer ergoline derivatives in experimental animal models (14). The antiparkinsonian efficacy of ergoline derivatives was compared with their potencies of binding to putative dopamine receptors.

MATERIALS AND METHODS

Ergoline derivatives were gifts from the Eli Lilly Research Laboratories, Indianapolis, Indiana, and from Schering Ltd., Berlin. The turning behavior in rats with unilateral lesions of the nigrostriatal dopamine (DA) pathway was determined as previously described (14). The antitremor efficacy and occurrence of AIMs in monkeys with VMT lesions was evaluated by published procedures (4). The structures and the serial numbers of the tested ergoline derivatives are presented in Fig. 1. The availability of binding assays with specific radioligands for measuring the affinities of drugs to putative postsynaptic DA receptors, has made it possible to investigate the interactions of ergoline derivatives with DA receptors (1).

EFFECT OF ERGOLINE DERIVATIVES ON RELIEF OF TREMOR AND ON THE OCCURRENCE OF AIMs IN MONKEYS WITH VMT LESIONS

The results presented in Table 1 show the effects of putative DA agonists on surgically induced tremor and on the occurrence of AIMs in monkeys with

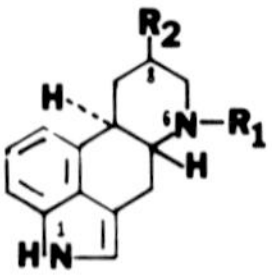

R_2 / R_1	$-CH_2OH$	$-CH_2OCH_3$	$-CH_2SCH_3$	$-CH_2CH_2SOCH_3$	$-NCON(C_2H_5)_2$
$-CH_3$	184-1	169B	062	196B	Lisuride
$-C_2H_5$			158A		
$-C_3H_7$	96A		141B	155B	

FIG. 1. Chemical structures and serial numbers of ergoline derivatives.

VMT lesions. Bromocriptine and lergotrile relieve tremor for a longer time period than L-DOPA. These ergot derivatives initially evoke sedation and less-pronounced AIMs than L-DOPA or piribedil. Lisuride, N-methylergoline 062, N-ethylergoline 158-A, and N-propylergoline 141-B have a long-lasting anti-tremor efficacy, but these ergots also evoke long-lasting AIMs of Types I and II (Table 1).

TABLE 1. *Effect of L-DOPA and of putative DA agonists on postural tremor and on the occurrence of AIMs in monkeys with VMT lesions*

	Pharmacological response		
		AIM[a]	
Drug (mg/kg)	Relief of tremor (hr)	Type	Duration (hr)
L-DOPA (100) + MK 486 (10)	0.5–2	I, II	1–2
Piribedil (3)	3–4	I, II	2–4
Bromocriptine (8)	2–6	I	1–2
Lergotrile (5)	2–5		
Lisuride (0.5)	3–8	I, II	8–12
Ergoline 062 (1.0)	8–24	I, II	8–24
Ergoline 158-A (0.4)	7–24	I, II	4–5
Ergoline 141-B (1.0)	<72	I, II	7–24

[a] AIM I: Restlessness and aggressiveness. AIM II: Chorea-like movements, various types of stereotyped movements.

DOPAMINE RECEPTOR BINDING AND PHARMACOLOGICAL POTENCIES OF ERGOTS

Ergots displace DA agonists and antagonists from striatal membrane sites, which indicates that these drugs are mixed agonists–antagonists at the DA receptors (7). The effects of ergoline derivatives on the binding of ^{3}H-spiroperidol (Spi) or of ^{3}H-DA are shown in Table 2. The ergoline derivatives displace ^{3}H-DA more effectively and ^{3}H-Spi less effectively from the striatal membrane sites than bromocriptine. The N-propylergoline derivative is a more potent displacer of ^{3}H-DA binding than the corresponding N-ethyl or N-methyl derivative (Table 2). The affinity of the ergoline derivatives for the DA receptors seems to correlate with their potencies to relieve tremor in monkeys with VMT lesions or to induce rotation in rats with lesions of the nigrostriatal DA pathway. Thus, N-propylergoline 96-A or N-propylergoline 141-B is a more potent displacer of ^{3}H-DA binding, and elicits at a lower dose, a rotation in rats with unilateral 6 OHDA lesions of the nigrostriatal pathway than the corresponding N-methylergoline 184-1 or N-methylergoline 062, respectively. The tremor in monkeys with VMT lesions is also relieved by N-propylergoline 141-B at lower dose than by N-methylergoline 062 (Table 2).

DA RECEPTOR SUBSENSITIVITY AFTER CHRONIC TREATMENT WITH ERGOLINE 141-B

The degeneration of DA neuronal systems or chronic treatment with neuroleptics results in supersensitivity of the DA receptors. Since most of the available DA agonists have a relatively short duration of action, it was difficult to assess the effects of their long-term exposure on the activity state of DA receptors. The availability of long-acting DA agonists such as ergolines has made it now possible to determine the effects of repeated administration of these drugs on the DA receptors.

Rats were treated for 2 weeks twice daily with ergoline 141-B (0.2 mg/kg;

TABLE 2. *Inhibition of dopaminergic receptor binding by ergoline derivatives and their potencies to elicit rotation in rats or to relieve tremor in monkeys*

Ergoline	Ki(nM)[a]		MED[b](mg/kg)	
	^{3}H-DA	^{3}H-Spi	Rotation[c]	Tremor[d]
062	89.2 ± 5.5	171.0 ± 11.0	0.5	0.5
158-A	20.4 ± 1.6	215.0 ± 14.5	0.1	0.2
141-B	12.8 ± 0.8	34.2 ± 2.4	0.05	0.1

[a] The values are the means from at least three experiments $\pm$ SEM.
[b] Minimum effective dose (MED).
[c] MED which elicited rotation in six out of nine tested rats with 6-OHDA lesions.
[d] MED which relieved tremor for at least 1 hr in two tested monkeys with VMT lesions.

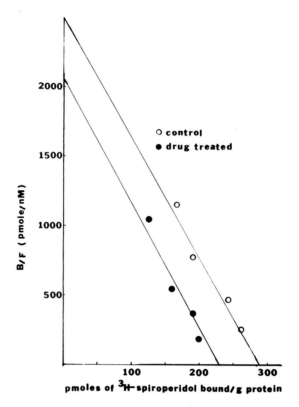

FIG. 2. Scatchard analysis of specific ³H-spiroperidol binding in rat striatal membrane of control and ergoline 141-B-treated animals. Binding was measured at four concentrations of ³H-spiro-peridol (0.125–0.1 nM) and the experiments were repeated three times.

i.p.). Five days after terminating the chronic treatment there was a significant decrease (15–25%) in the binding of ³H-Spi. Scatchard plot analysis revealed that chronic treatment with ergoline 141-B has no effect on the dissociation constant for ³H-Spi binding. However, there was a significant decrease in the total number of binding sites (control: binding = 292 ± 12 pmole per g protein; ergoline 141-B treatment: binding = 230 ± 11 pmole per gram protein) (Fig. 2). These results show that chronic treatment with a long-acting DA agonist produces subsensitivity at the DA receptors.

DISCUSSION

The central DA agonist activities of ergot alkaloids is based on the following pharmacological profile: (a) decrease in pituitary prolactin and ACTH secretion; (b) reduced DA turnover in the CNS; (c) binding interactions with putative dopamine receptors; (d) contralateral turning behavior in rats with unilateral 6-OH dopamine lesions of the nigrostriatal DA pathway; (e) relief of tremor in monkeys with VMT lesions; and (f) antiparkinsonian efficacy in man.

It is somewhat surprising that in the majority of parkinsonian patients it was not possible to totally replace levodopa or levodopa plus carbidopa with bromocriptine (8). The weak antiparkinsonian action of bromocriptine in man may be attributed to the relatively weak DA agonist activity of the drug (7), or it might be due to preferential stimulation by the ergot alkaloids of a DA receptor population that functionally differs from the other populations of DA receptors.

Recent studies have shown that ergots do not stimulate DA-sensitive adenylate cyclase (5). DA receptors localized on cerebral cortical afferents to the striatum are not linked to DA-sensitive adenylate cyclase (13) and, therefore, one is tempted to suggest that ergots interact preferentially with these receptors. To test this hypothesis we are now determining the effects of cortical ablation on the binding affinities of ergots to striatal DA receptors.

Of considerable interest are the findings that there is a good correlation between the affinities of ergoline derivatives for DA receptor binding sites and their potencies in behavioral tests for DA agonists activity. The aliphatic substitution of the nitrogen at the six position seems to be of importance in determining the DA agonist potency of ergoline derivatives. Thus, the potencies of ergolines for displacing ^{3}H-DA binding from striatal membrane sites and for their effectiveness in the behavioral tests for DA agonists can be ranked in the following order: N-propyl, > N-ethyl, > N-methyl.

The aliphatic substitution of the nitrogen seems to enhance not only the DA agonist potencies of ergolines but also of other DA agonists. It was reported that N-propylnorapomorphine has a longer lasting effect on rotational behavior in rats than apomorphine (10). In a previous study we have shown that the intraventricular administration of epinine (30–50 μg) to monkeys with VMT lesions results in the relief of the surgically induced tremor (2). More recently it was reported that the addition of N-dimethyl groups to geometric isomers of 2-amino-1(3,4-dihydroxyphenyl)cyclobutane increases their affinity for DA binding sites (6). It seems, therefore, possible to synthesize more potent DA agonists by N-substitution of DA analogs.

The question is now whether ergoline derivatives, which are potent DA agonists, will be better antiparkinsonian agents than L-DOPA or than bromocriptine. It is still not known whether a potent DA agonist is an ideal antiparkinsonian drug. Potent DA agonists may produce undesirable side-effects such as AIMs. Furthermore, it is evident from the results of this study that chronic treatment with ergolines produces subsensitivity at the DA receptors. Hopefully, clinical trials with ergoline derivatives will establish whether potent long-acting DA agonists are useful drugs in treatment of Parkinson's disease and/or other extrapyramidal dysfunctions.

ACKNOWLEDGMENTS

This work was supported by National Institute of Neurological and Communicative Disorders and Stroke Grant NS-06801 and National Institute of Mental Health Grant MH-02717.

REFERENCES

1. Burt, D. R., Creese, I., and Snyder, S. H. (1976): Properties of (^{3}H) haloperidol and (^{3}H) dopamine binding associated with dopamine receptors in calf membranes. *Mol. Pharmacol.,* 12:800.
2. Goldstein, M., Anagnoste, B., Battista, A. F., Nakatani, S., and Ogawa, M. (1973): Biochemical aspects of experimentally induced Parkinsonism. In: *Neurotransmitters, vol. 50,* edited by I. J. Kopin, pp. 434–447. Research Publications, Assoc. for Research in Nervous and Mental Disease. Williams & Wilkins, Baltimore.
3. Goldstein, M., Battista, A. F., Nakatani, S., and Anagnoste, B. (1970): Drug induced relief of experimental tremor in monkeys. *Neurology (Minneap.),* 20 (11), Part 2:89–95.
4. Goldstein, M., Battista, A. F., Ohmoto, T., Anagnoste, B., and Fuxe, K. (1973): Tremor and involuntary movements in monkeys: effect of L-DOPA and of a dopamine receptor stimulating agent, *Science,* 179:816.
5. Govoni, S., Iuliano, E., Spano, P. F., and Trabucchi, M. (1977): Effect of ergotamine and dihydroergotamine on dopamine-stimulated adenylate cyclase in rat caudate nucleus. *J. Pharm. Pharmacol.,* 29:45–47.
6. Komiskey, H. L., Bossart, J. F., Miller, D. D., and Patil, P. N. (1978): Conformation of dopamine at the dopamine receptor. *Proc. Natl. Acad. Sci. U.S.A.,* 75:2641–2643.
7. Lew, J. Y., Hata, F., Ohashi, T., and Goldstein, M. (1977): The Interactions of bromocriptine and lergotrile with dopamine and α-adrenergic receptors. *J. Neural Transm.,* 41:109–121.
8. Lieberman, A., Kupersmith, M., Estey, E., and M. Goldstein. (1976): Treatment of Parkinson's disease with bromocriptine. *N. Engl. J. Med.,* 295:1400–1404.
9. Lieberman, A., Miyamoto, T., Battista, A., and M. Goldstein. (1975): Studies on the antiparkinsonian efficacy of lergotrile. *Neurology (Minneap.),* 25:459–462.
10. Mendez, J. S., Cotzias, G. C., Finn, B. W., and Dahl, K. (1975): Rotatory behavior induced in nigra-lesioned rats by N-propylnorapomorphine, apomorphine, and levodopa. *Life Sci.,* 16:1737–1742.
11. Miyamoto, T., Battista, A., Goldstein, M., and K. Fuxe. (1974): Long-lasting antitremor activity induced by 2-Br-α-ergocryptine in monkeys. *J. Pharm. Pharmacol.,* 26:452–454.
12. Poirier, L. J., Sourkes, T. L., Bouvier, G., Boucher, R., and Carabin, S. (1966): Striatal amines, experimental tremor and the effect of harmaline in the monkey. *Brain,* 89:37–52.
13. Schwarcz, R., Creese, I., Coyle, J. T., and Snyder, S. H. (1978): Dopamine receptors localised on cerebral cortical afferents to rat corpus striatum. *Nature,* 271:766–768.
14. Ungerstedt, U. (1970): Mechanism of action of L-DOPA studied in an experimental Parkinson model. In: *Monoamines, Noyaux Gris Centraux et Syndrome de Parkinson (Bel-Air Symposium IV),* edited by J. de Ajuriaguerra and G. Gauthier, p. 165. Masson, Paris.

Advances in Neurology, Vol. 24, edited by
L. J. Poirier, T. L. Sourkes, and P. J. Bédard.
Raven Press, New York © 1979.

GABA and GABA-ergic Medication: Relation to Striatal Dopamine Function and Parkinsonism

*G. Bartholini, *K. G. Lloyd, *P. Worms, **J. Constantinidis, and **R. Tissot

*Research Department, Synthélabo-L.E.R.S., 75013 Paris, France; and **University Psychiatric Clinic, Geneva, Switzerland

Evidence from postmortem studies (5,9; Lloyd and Davidson, *this volume*) and experiments with animal models (4,7,11) suggests that neurons utilizing γ-aminobutyric acid (GABA) as their neurotransmitter are involved in neurological and psychiatric disorders such as epilepsy, Huntington's chorea, Parkinson's disease, and possibly schizophrenia. Also, iatrogenic disorders—neuroleptic-induced tardive dyskinesias and involuntary movements in parkinsonian patients treated with L-DOPA—may involve alterations in GABA function. However, no clear clinical data support this hypothesis, due mainly to the lack of safe and specific GABA-ergic drugs (3). This article describes the biochemical effects in animals and preliminary clinical results in parkinsonian patients of a new GABA receptor agonist, SL 76 002 [α-(chloro-4-phenyl) fluoro-5-hydroxy-2-benzylidene-amino-4-butyramide].[1] The lack of toxicity of this compound in animals predicts a large safety margin in humans; SL 76 002 may, therefore, help in assessing both the role of GABA in various human diseases and the therapeutic potential of GABA-ergic drugs.

METABOLISM OF SL 76 002 AND RELATION TO GABA NEURONS

SL 76 002 is a Schiff's base derived from GABAmide and an ortho-hydroxy-benzophenone. Upon administration to rats, SL 76 002 is rapidly transformed into SL 75 102[1], GABAmide, and GABA itself (Fig. 1). Shortly after oral administration of radiolabeled SL 76 002, all four products are found in both plasma and brain (1). As GABA and GABAmide virtually do not cross the blood–brain barrier, their formation must occur in the cerebral tissue. SL 75 102 is probably formed both centrally and peripherally (A. C. Durand and L. G. Dring, *in preparation*).

SL 76 002 is a broad-spectrum anticonvulsant, enhances catalepsy due to haloperidol (reversed by bicuculline) and diminishes the firing rate of the dorsal

---

[1] Synthesized by Dr. J. P. Kaplan, Chemistry Dept., Synthélabo-L.E.R.S., Paris.

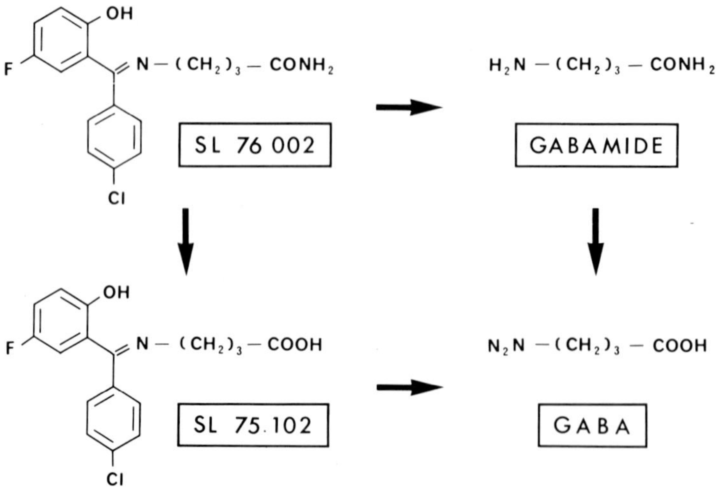

FIG. 1. Structural formula and possible metabolic pathways of SL 76 002.

Deiter's neurons (also bicuculline-sensitive) (6). In man, SL 76 002 is an effective antiepileptic agent and is of therapeutic benefit in an early phase of Huntington's chorea (1). The chemical structure, pharmacological spectrum, and metabolism of SL 76 002 suggest that this compound exerts its action via stimulation of GABA receptors. This hypothesis is supported by the observation that SL 76 002 and its metabolites displace ^{3}H-GABA from binding sites of membranes prepared from either human cerebellar cortex or whole rat brain (1). Neither SL 76 002 nor SL 75 102 inhibits GABA transaminase or GABA uptake (1).

These results indicate that SL 76 002 can be considered as a precursor of GABA receptor agonists (including GABA itself) as well as a GABA receptor stimulant in its own right.

EFFECT OF SL 76 002 ON THE ACTIVITY OF DOPAMINE NEURONS

Systemically administered SL 76 002 diminishes release and synthesis of dopamine (DA). Thus, SL 76 002 decreases the rate of DA disappearance due to α-methyl-p-tyrosine (αMT). This effect occurs in the striatum but not in limbic areas (nucleus accumbens + olfactory tubercle + nucleus striae terminalis + septum) (1). Furthermore, SL 76 002 decreases the amount of DA released into the perfusate of the cat striatum implanted with the push–pull cannula (1) (Fig. 2). SL 76 002 also reduces striatal DA synthesis as estimated by either DOPA accumulation *in vivo* (1) or by the formation of $^{14}CO_2$ from 1-^{14}C-tyrosine in slices, an effect which is picrotoxin-sensitive (Zivkovic and Scatton, *in preparation*).

When the activity of DA neurons is enhanced (e.g., by neuroleptics), the effects of SL 76 002 become more marked. Thus, SL 76 002 blocks, in a dose-dependent manner, the haloperidol-induced increase in the rate of disappearance of striatal DA after αMT pretreatment in the rat. A similar effect is now also seen in limbic areas, but only after high doses of SL 76 002 (1). The haloperidol-induced increase in tyrosine hydroxylase activity is reversed by SL 76 002 and this effect is more pronounced in the striatum than in the olfactory tubercle (1). In experiments using the push–pull cannula (Fig. 2), SL 76 002 completely prevents the chlorpromazine-induced increase in DA release from the cat caudate nucleus.

These results indicate that SL 76 002 diminishes (as probably GABA neurons do) DA synthesis and release via a reduction of DA neuron activity. This has direct relevance to the therapeutic potential of GABA mimetics in general, and of SL 76 002 in particular, in parkinsonian patients for L-DOPA-induced involuntary movements, which are probably connected to an excess of DA at the receptors. Thus, assuming that the bulk of DA formed from L-DOPA originates from the remaining DA nerve terminals, the DA release—susceptible to control by GABA-ergic means—should be reduced with consequent amelioration of dyskinesias. However, if the GABA-mediated control is entirely located presynaptically to the DA terminal, then GABA mimetic drugs would likely not

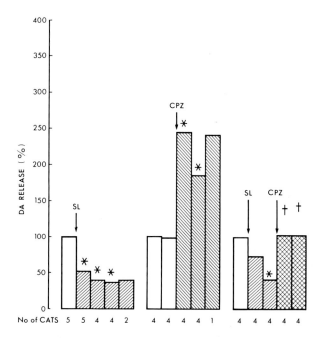

FIG. 2. Effect of SL 76 002 on the release of dopamine in the cat caudate nucleus. The caudate nucleus of the gallamine-immobilized cat was perfused by means of the push–pull cannula; DA was measured in the perfusate by a radioenzymatic assay (2). SL 76 002 (SL, 50 mg/kg) or chlorpromazine (CPZ, 10 mg/kg) were injected i.v. *(arrows).* Results are expressed as percent (mean with SEM) of preinjection (control) collection period (=100). Each collection period = 60 min. $*p < 0.05$ vs. control period; $\dagger p < 0.05$ vs. CPZ alone.

TABLE 1. *Effect of SL 76 002 on the stereotypies induced in rats by apomorphine*

	Dose of SL 76 002 (mg/kg i.p.)				
	0	50	100	200	400
Mean stereotypy score after apomorphine	13.0 ± 0.5	12.0 ± 0.5	10.0 ± 0.3	7.0 ± 0.5	6.0 ± 0.6
No. of rats	30	30	30	24	16
Significance vs. apomorphine alone	—	ns	<0.5	<0.01	<0.01

Animals were injected with SL 76 002 and apomorphine (0.25 mg/kg s.c.) at time 0. Stereotypy scores were assessed every 10 min during the following 60 min (10). Significance was determined by the two-tailed Student's *t*-test.

only reduce the L-DOPA-induced dyskinesias but also aggravate the parkinsonian symptoms.

However, the possibility exists that, in addition to its presynaptic control of DA neurons, GABA affects the function of the striatum distally to the DA receptor. Accordingly, SL 76 002 blocks the stereotypies induced in the rat by apomorphine (Table 1), which is thought to act via stimulation of postsynaptic striatal DA receptors (8). Therefore, the apomorphine-induced stereotypies may be used as an animal model for L-DOPA dyskinesias, and the inhibition by SL 76 002 suggests a useful role for GABA mimetics in this condition. Furthermore, assuming that the action of GABA postsynaptic to DA neurons prevails on the presynaptic action, the reduction of the L-DOPA-induced dyskinesias should not be accompanied by an aggravation of the parkinsonian syndrome.

CLINICAL RESULTS

Preliminary clinical results indicate that SL 76 002 affects striatal function. Thus, SL 76 002 has been administered to four parkinsonian patients affected by severe L-DOPA-induced involuntary movements. In one subject treated with 1,000 mg L-DOPA (+ 625 mg benserazide), 600 mg daily of SL 76 002 caused both the disappearance of involuntary movements and an aggravation of the parkinsonian syndrome. This patient refused to continue the treatment. In contrast, in two other patients, 300 mg of SL 76 002 led to a complete disappearance of dyskinesias without aggravation of parkinsonism; furthermore, in these two subjects and for the 3 months to date, it was possible to increase the daily dose of L-DOPA from 300 to 400 and 625 to 875 mg, respectively (and the associated benserazide dose from 75 to 100 and 625 to 750 mg/day, respectively): this caused a significant amelioration of parkinsonian symptoms without the reappearance of involuntary movements. Finally, in a fourth patient in whom L-DOPA had been completely discontinued due to the severity of dyskinesias, 300 mg daily of SL 76 002 allowed the reinstatement of the L-DOPA regimen

(300 mg + 75 mg benserazide) with amelioration of parkinsonism in the absence of involuntary movements (1 month treatment to date).

SUMMARY AND CONCLUSIONS

The activity of the nigrostriatal DA pathway appears to be controlled, *inter alia,* by inhibitory GABA inputs, as evidenced by reduction in the synthesis and release of striatal DA induced by SL 76 002, a putative GABA mimetic; the DA neurons appear to be more sensitive to this GABA input when they are in an activated state. In addition to this presynaptic control of DA neurons, GABA likely plays a role in modifying striatal mechanisms postsynaptic to the DA-receptor, as evidenced by the reduction of apomorphine stereotypies by SL 76 002. According to these two sites of action, SL 76 002 should decrease L-DOPA-induced dyskinesias in parkinsonian patients. Preliminary clinical trials confirm this view.

REFERENCES

1. Bartholini, G., Scatton, B., Zivkovic, B., and Loyd, K. G. (1979): On the mode of action of SL 76 002, a new GABA receptor agonist. In: *GABA-Neurotransmitters,* edited by H. Kofod, P. Krogsgaard-Larsen, and J. Scheel-Krüger, pp. 326–339. Munksgaard, Copenhagen.
2. Bartholini, G., and Stadler, H. (1977): Evidence for an intrastriatal GABA-ergic influence on dopamine neurons of the cat. *Neuropharmacology,* 16:343–347.
3. Chase, T. N., and Taminga, C. A. (1979): GABA system participation in human motor, cognitive and endocrine function. In: *GABA-Neurotransmitters,* edited by H. Kofod, P. Krogsgaard-Larsen, and J. Scheel-Krüger, pp. 283–294. Munksgaard, Copenhagen.
4. Coyle, J. T., Biziere, K., Campochiaro, P., Schwarcz, R., and Zaczek, R. (1979): Kainic acid-induced lesion of the striatum as an animal model for Huntington's disease. In: *GABA-Neurotransmitters,* edited by H. Kofod, P. Krogsgaard-Larsen, and J. Scheel-Krüger, pp. 419–431. Munksgaard, Copenhagen.
5. Iversen, L. L. (1978): Biochemical psychopharmacology of GABA. In: *Psychopharmacology: A Generation of Progress,* edited by M. A. Lipton, A. Di Mascio, and K. F. Killam, pp. 25–38. Raven Press, New York.
6. Lloyd, K. G., Worms, P., Depoortere, H., and Bartholini, G. (1979): Pharmacological profile of SL 76 002, a new GABA mimetic drug. In: *GABA-Neurotransmitters,* edited by H. Kofod, P. Krogsgaard-Larsen, and J. Scheel-Krüger, pp. 308–325. Munksgaard, Copenhagen.
7. Meldrum, B. S. (1975): Epilepsy and γ-aminobutyric acid-mediated inhibition. *Int. Rev. Neurobiol.,* 117:1–36.
8. Ungerstedt, U., Ljungberg, J., and Schultz, W. (1978): Dopamine receptor mechanisms: behavioural and electrophysiological studies. In: *Dopamine,* edited by P. J. Roberts, G. N. Woodruff, and L. L. Iversen, pp. 311–321. Raven Press, New York.
9. Van Gelder, N. M., Sherwin, A. M., and Rasmussen, T. (1972): Amino acid content of epileptogenic human brain: focal versus surrounding regions. *Brain Res.,* 40:385–393.
10. Worms, P., and Lloyd, K. G. (1979): Predictability and specificity of behavioural screening tests for neuroleptics. In: *Pharmacological Methods in Toxicology,* edited by G. Zbinden and F. Gross. Pergamon Press, London *(in press).*
11. Worms, P., Willigens, M. T., and Lloyd, K. G. (1978): GABA involvement in neuroleptic-induced catalepsy. *J. Pharm. Pharacol.,* 30:716–718.

Advances in Neurology, Vol. 24, edited by
L. J. Poirier, T. L. Sourkes, and P. J. Bédard.
Raven Press, New York © 1979.

Responses of Brain Neurochemistry to Levodopa Treatment in Parkinson's Disease

U. K. Rinne, V. Sonninen, and H. Laaksonen

Department of Neurology, University of Turku, Turku, Finland

It is now generally accepted that the loss of dopaminergic substantia nigra neurons and dopamine deficiency in the corpus striatum play an essential role in the pathophysiology of Parkinson's disease. This was well established in the pioneer study by Ehringer and Hornykiewicz (5) and has subsequently been confirmed by several studies showing a decrease of dopamine and its metabolite, homovanillic acid (HVA), in the brain (2,9,20,26,27,29) and that of HVA in the cerebrospinal fluid (1,7,24,25). However, nondopaminergic neuronal systems may also be involved in the pathophysiology of Parkinson's disease (12,13,16, 22,23,29).

The therapeutic action and clinical effects of levodopa as dopamine replacement therapy are well established. Furthermore, biochemical studies on postmortem brains by us (26,27,29) and others (6,10) have provided direct evidence of increased formation of dopamine in the parkinsonian striatum during levodopa treatment, suggesting that at least a part of the therapeutic effect of levodopa may be mediated through the correction of dopamine deficiency. The present paper is concerned with further studies of biochemical changes of dopamine and GABA neurons in the postmortem brain samples of parkinsonian patients who had undergone treatment with levodopa alone or combined with a decarboxylase inhibitor. Special attention has been paid to receptors and to analyzing the possible correlations between neurochemical changes and clinical responses to treatment.

RESULTS

Dopamine Neurons

DOPA and 3-O-Methyldopa

As can be seen from Table 1, we did not find DOPA or its metabolite, 3-O-methyldopa, in the brain samples of control or parkinsonian patients who had not been treated with levodopa. In the brains of patients treated with levodopa there were, however, detectable concentrations of DOPA and especially

TABLE 1. *Concentration (μg/g) of DOPA and 3-O-methyldopa in brain regions of parkinsonian patients and control subjects*

Brain region	Dopa			3-O-Methyldopa		
		Parkinsonism			Parkinsonism	
	Control	Without levodopa	With levodopa	Control	Without levodopa	With levodopa
Caudate nucleus	nd (4)	nd (3)	0.74 ± 0.38 (7)	nd (4)	nd (3)	5.97 ± 4.84 (7)
Putamen	nd (4)	nd (4)	0.51 ± 0.50 (4)	nd (4)	nd (4)	2.57 ± 1.1 (4)
Cerebral cortex	nd (4)	nd (3)	0.60 ± 0.20 (7)	nd (4)	nd (4)	3.74 ± 3.06 (7)

Values given as mean ± SEM. Number of patients in parentheses.
nd, not detectable.

of 3-O-methyldopa, not only in the striatum but also in the cerebral cortex. These concentrations were highly dependent on the dose and also on the interval between the last dose and the death of the patients.

Dopamine

Table 2 shows that there was a significant mean increase in the concentration of dopamine in the brain of parkinsonian patients treated with levodopa as compared with nontreated parkinsonian patients. Changes were more pronounced in the extrapyramidal brain regions, but there was a clearly increased concentration of dopamine also in the cerebral cortex. However, the mean concentrations of dopamine after combined treatment with levodopa and a decarboxylase inhibitor were lower than after levodopa alone, except in the hypothalamus.

On the other hand, the individual cases showed great variation in the responses of brain dopamine to levodopa treatment. The concentration of dopamine varied from rather high amounts to values as low as those found in untreated parkinsonian patients. This variation was clearly related to the size of the dose and also to the interval between death and administration of the last dose of the drug. However, statistical analyses showed that concentrations of dopamine in the extrapyramidal brain regions of parkinsonian patients treated with levodopa, alone or combined with a decarboxylase inhibitor, were not correlated with the clinical responses to treatment.

Homovanillic Acid

Table 3 shows that, as in the case of dopamine, the concentration of its main metabolite HVA also increased significantly in the brain regions of parkinsonian patients treated with levodopa alone. This increase was more marked

TABLE 2. Concentration (µg/g) of dopamine in brain regions of parkinsonian patients and control subjects

Group	Caudate nucleus	Putamen	Pallidum	Substantia nigra	Hypothalamus	Cerebral cortex
Controls	1.75 ± 0.29 (49)	2.40 ± 0.34 (48)	0.63 ± 0.07 (43)	0.61 ± 0.10 (29)	0.33 ± 0.10 (28)	0.20 ± 0.04 (48)
Parkinsonian patients						
Without levodopa	0.50 ± 0.20 (20)	0.57 ± 0.17 (21)	0.31 ± 0.12 (17)	0.14 ± 0.05 (11)	0.22 ± 0.09 (15)	0.12 ± 0.03 (20)
With levodopa	1.22 ± 0.30 (21)	1.16 ± 0.31 (21)	1.01 ± 0.35 (19)	1.09 ± 0.51 (11)	0.32 ± 0.11 (14)	0.46 ± 0.15 (20)
With levodopa + decarboxylase inhibitor	0.46 ± 0.11 (22)	0.55 ± 0.14 (24)	0.38 ± 0.08 (21)	0.51 ± 0.16 (12)	0.54 ± 0.19 (16)	0.18 ± 0.04 (24)

Values given as mean ± SEM. Number of patients in parentheses.

TABLE 3. *Concentration (μg/g) of HVA in brain regions of parkinsonian patients and control subjects*

Group	Caudate nucleus	Putamen	Pallidum	Substantia nigra	Hypothalamus	Cerebral cortex
Controls	3.41 ± 0.24 (61)	5.87 ± 0.38 (61)	2.97 ± 0.18 (59)	2.06 ± 0.20 (45)	0.60 ± 0.10 (35)	0.16 ± 0.04 (58)
Parkinsonian patients						
Without levodopa	1.55 ± 0.25 (23)	1.62 ± 0.31 (24)	1.15 ± 0.18 (23)	0.81 ± 0.13 (15)	0.48 ± 0.18 (21)	0.15 ± 0.05 (23)
With levodopa	5.25 ± 0.85 (22)	8.07 ± 1.46 (22)	5.37 ± 1.30 (22)	5.27 ± 1.35 (17)	2.00 ± 0.44 (21)	1.61 ± 0.44 (22)
With levodopa + decarboxylase inhibitor	3.97 ± 0.58 (32)	5.21 ± 0.85 (32)	2.91 ± 0.33 (32)	2.45 ± 0.34 (26)	0.96 ± 0.15 (28)	0.33 ± 0.06 (32)

Value given as mean ± SEM. Number of patients in parentheses.

than that of dopamine. Although in these patients the extrapyramidal brain regions had the highest concentrations, HVA increased significantly also in the other brain regions studied.

As in the case of dopamine, the concentration of HVA in the cerebral cortex after combined treatment with levodopa and a decarboxylase inhibitor was significantly lower than after levodopa alone. Corresponding differences were also found in other brain regions studied, although they were considerably less marked than that in the cerebral cortex. The individual data show that, as with dopamine, there was great variation in the concentration of HVA, depending on the dosage and the time of the last administration of the drug. However, HVA seemed to remain in the brain considerably longer than dopamine. As with the concentration of dopamine, there was no significant correlation between HVA levels and the clinical responses of the patients.

Enzymes

In agreement with recent studies (10,15), it was found that the activity of tyrosine hydroxylase (TH) was significantly reduced in all extrapyramidal nuclei analyzed in comparison with the controls (Table 4). Furthermore, in our studies it was found that the clinical picture of the disease had significant influences on the TH activity in some extrapyramidal brain regions analyzed. TH activity in the substantia nigra was negatively correlated with the duration of the disease. Moreover, striatal TH activity was correlated negatively with the disability of the patients and with the severity of hypokinesia and rigidity. There was no clear correlation between TH activity and the severity of tremor.

Levodopa treatment with or without a decarboxylase inhibitor did not have significant effect on TH activity, although there was a trend toward decreased activity. However, there was a negative correlation between the duration of levodopa treatment and striatal TH activity. Moreover, the improvement of total disability was negatively correlated with TH activity in the caudate nucleus and putamen.

Similarly to other reports (11,12), it was found that the activity of dopa decarboxylase (DDC) was decreased significantly in the extrapyramidal nuclei of the parkinsonian brain compared with the controls (Table 5). Levodopa treatment with or without a decarboxylase inhibitor did not have any significant effect on DDC activity.

Dopamine Receptors

As can be seen from Table 6, the highest number of binding sites for ^{3}H-spiroperidol in the basal ganglia of controls was found in the caudate nucleus and putamen as compared with that in the pallidum. There was no sex difference.

The specific binding of ^{3}H-spiroperidol was significantly reduced in the caudate nucleus ($p < 0.01$) and putamen ($p < 0.05$) of parkinsonian patients who had

TABLE 4. *Activity (nmoles/g protein per hr) of tyrosine hydroxylase in brain regions of parkinsonian patients and control subjects*

Group	No. of patients	Caudate nucleus	Putamen	Pallidum	Substantia nigra
Controls	26	7.4 ± 0.7	8.7 ± 0.7	4.3 ± 0.5	15.8 ± 2.3
Parkinsonian patients					
Without levodopa	13	5.6 ± 1.3	4.8 ± 1.2	2.1 ± 0.5	9.6 ± 0.3
With levodopa	27	4.0 ± 0.5	2.6 ± 0.6	1.8 ± 0.3	5.2 ± 1.0
All cases	40	4.6 ± 0.5	3.3 ± 0.6	1.9 ± 0.3	6.6 ± 1.2
Controls vs. all cases of Parkinson's disease		$p < 0.01$	$p < 0.001$	$p < 0.001$	$p < 0.001$
Controls vs. without levodopa			$p < 0.01$	$p < 0.01$	$p < 0.05$
Controls vs. with levodopa		$p < 0.001$	$p < 0.001$	$p < 0.001$	$p < 0.001$

Values given as mean ± SEM.

TABLE 5. *Activity (nmoles/g protein per hr) of dopa decarboxylase in brain regions of parkinsonian patients and control subjects*

Group	No. of patients	Caudate nucleus	Putamen	Pallidum	Substantia nigra
Controls	19	284.9 ± 50.3	213.7 ± 47.7	79.3 ± 25.8	229.3 ± 77.1
Parkinsonian patients					
Without levodopa	13	116.0 ± 34.5	90.6 ± 28.5	49.9 ± 20.9	80.9 ± 40.4
With levodopa	28	157.8 ± 28.6	73.8 ± 18.4	37.8 ± 8.6	67.6 ± 15.6
All cases	41	144.6 ± 22.4	78.9 ± 15.3	41.6 ± 8.8	71.9 ± 16.5
Controls vs. all cases of Parkinson's disease		$p < 0.05$	$p < 0.01$		
Controls vs. without levodopa		$p < 0.01$	$p < 0.05$		
Controls vs. with levodopa		$p < 0.05$	$p < 0.01$		$p < 0.05$

Values given as mean $\pm$ SEM.

not received any levodopa therapy (Table 6). However, in the pallidum there was no significant change in the ^{3}H-spiroperidol binding. To determine whether the decrease in ^{3}H-spiroperidol binding in the parkinsonian striatum was due to a change in dissociation constant or a change in number of receptors, a Scatchard analysis was carried out. The results showed that there was merely a decrease in receptor number, but no significant change in dissociation constant.

Parkinsonian patients suffering from psychotic episodes and treated with neuroleptic drugs before death had significantly higher binding of ^{3}H-spiroperidol in the caudate nucleus ($p < 0.05$) and putamen ($p < 0.05$) than in nonpsychotic parkinsonian patients without neuroleptic treatment. Scatchard analysis showed that there was an increase in receptor number. There were no significant differences between these two parkinsonian patient groups in regard to other clinical variables.

As shown in Table 6, levodopa treatment did not have any significant effect on the binding of ^{3}H-spiroperidol in the parkinsonian striatum. However, again in levodopa-treated psychotic patients who had received neuroleptic medication, there was significantly increased ^{3}H-spiroperidol binding in the caudate nucleus ($p < 0.001$) and putamen ($p < 0.01$). Moreover, there were more involuntary movements in these patients than in the former ones; but there were no other significant differences between these patient groups in regard to other clinical variables or responses to levodopa treatment.

GABA Neurons

Glutamic Acid Decarboxylase

There is evidence of possible alterations of GABA neurons in Parkinson's disease. For example, there is decreased activity of glutamic acid decarboxylase (GAD) in the extrapyramidal brain regions of parkinsonian patients (12,15,22). In our recent material the decrease of GAD activity as compared with the controls reached the level of statistical significance in the substantia nigra, pallidum, and caudate nucleus, as well as in the cerebral and cerebellar cortex (Table 7). Moreover, it was found that the duration of the disease and the disability of the patients showed a positive correlation with the activity of GAD in the extrapyramidal brain regions. Of the parkinsonian symptoms, only the severity of tremor correlated positively with GAD activity in the striatum, whereas rigidity and hypokinesia did not bear any relationship to GAD activity.

Levodopa treatment did not cause any significant effect on the activity of GAD. However, the improvement of total disability, rigidity and hypokinesia showed a negative correlation with GAD activity in the substantia nigra. A similar correlation was also found between GAD activity in the pallidum and the improvement of total disability and rigidity. In the case of the other brain

TABLE 6. *Specific ³H-spiroperidol binding (fmoles/mg protein) in parkinsonian and control brains*

Group	No. of patients	Caudate nucleus	Putamen	Pallidum
Controls	17	154 ± 19	159 ± 24	40 ± 7
Parkinsonian patients				
Nontreated	6	74 ± 15	88 ± 23	51 ± 7
With neuroleptics	5	262 ± 76	317 ± 87	127 ± 53
With levodopa	5	70 ± 14	110 ± 36	32 ± 4
With levodopa and neuroleptics	5	222 ± 19	276 ± 32	77 ± 20
Controls vs. nontreated		$p < 0.01$	$p < 0.05$	
Controls vs. with levodopa		$p < 0.01$		
Nontreated vs. with neuroleptics		$p < 0.05$	$p < 0.05$	
With levodopa vs. with levodopa and neuroleptics		$p < 0.001$	$p < 0.01$	

Values given as mean ± SEM.

areas analyzed, there was no statistically significant correlation between GAD activity and the improvement of the parkinsonian symptoms.

GABA

Both in the controls and parkinsonian patients, the highest level of GABA was in the pallidum and substantia nigra (Table 8). The concentration of GABA was significantly decreased in the cerebral and cerebellar cortex of parkinsonian patients compared with the controls, but there were no significant changes in the extrapyramidal nuclei. However, the level of GABA in the caudate nucleus and putamen showed positive correlation with the duration of the disease and the concentration of GABA in the substantia nigra with the disability of the patients. Moreover, there was a negative correlation between the severity of tremor and the level of GABA in the substantia nigra.

Levodopa treatment did not significantly change the level of GABA in the brain. However, the improvement of total disability during levodopa treatment correlated negatively with the level of GABA in the substantia nigra and that of hypokinesia with the level of GABA in the caudate nucleus.

GABA Receptors

The possible involvement of GABA neurons in Parkinson's disease has recently been supported by findings (14,21) of decreased GABA receptor binding in the substantia nigra of the parkinsonian brain. As shown in Table 9, GABA receptor binding was significantly ($p < 0.05$) less in the substantia nigra of the parkinsonian patients than in that of the controls. In the other brain regions,

TABLE 7. Activity (nmoles/100 mg protein per hr) of GAD in brain regions of parkinsonian patients and control subjects

Group	No. of patients	Caudate nucleus	Putamen	Pallidum	Substantia nigra	Cerebral cortex	Cerebellar cortex
Controls	38	621 ± 90	500 ± 71	806 ± 115	931 ± 143	365 ± 55	615 ± 65
Parkinsonian patients							
Without levodopa	22	337 ± 92	355 ± 93	466 ± 107	421 ± 119	177 ± 61	366 ± 79
With levodopa	33	581 ± 101	577 ± 104	723 ± 118	584 ± 111	333 ± 65	574 ± 74
All cases	55	483 ± 72	488 ± 74	620 ± 84	520 ± 82	269 ± 47	491 ± 56
Controls vs. all cases					$p < 0.05$		
Controls vs. without levodopa		$p < 0.05$		$p < 0.05$	$p < 0.01$	$p < 0.05$	$p < 0.05$

Values given as mean ± SEM.

TABLE 8. Concentration (nmoles/mg protein per hr) of GABA in brain regions of parkinsonian patients and control subjects

Group	No. of patients	Caudate nucleus	Putamen	Pallidum	Substantia nigra	Cerebral cortex	Cerebellar cortex
Controls	31	29.1 ± 1.8	35.8 ± 1.8	60.6 ± 3.3	43.2 ± 3.0	15.6 ± 1.1	14.2 ± 0.9
Parkinsonian patients							
Without levodopa	17	25.2 ± 2.5	35.0 ± 2.3	56.3 ± 4.6	43.0 ± 3.2	11.7 ± 0.9	10.4 ± 0.9
With levodopa	30	28.1 ± 1.5	36.9 ± 1.8	67.1 ± 3.5	47.3 ± 3.5	11.8 ± 0.7	11.0 ± 0.8
All cases	47	27.1 ± 1.3	36.2 ± 1.4	63.2 ± 2.9	45.8 ± 2.5	11.8 ± 0.6	10.8 ± 0.6
Controls vs. all cases						$p < 0.01$	$p < 0.01$
Controls vs. without levodopa						$p < 0.01$	$p < 0.01$
Controls vs. with levodopa						$p < 0.01$	$p < 0.05$

Values given as mean ± SEM.

TABLE 9. *Specific receptor binding of ³H-GABA (fmoles/mg protein) in parkinsonian and control brains*

Group	No. of patients	Caudate nucleus	Putamen	Pallidum	Substantia nigra	Cerebral cortex	Cerebellar cortex
Controls	11	283 ± 20	245 ± 16	112 ± 22	85 ± 11	787 ± 74	1838 ± 114
Parkinsonian patients							
Without levodopa	7	257 ± 31	226 ± 36	100 ± 17	52 ± 11	619 ± 68	1818 ± 232
With levodopa	5	281 ± 68	243 ± 39	74 ± 14	38 ± 15[a]	678 ± 130	1570 ± 366
All cases	12	267 ± 32	233 ± 25	89 ± 12	46 ± 9[a]	644 ± 64	1715 ± 197

[a] $p < 0.05$ as compared with controls.
Values given as mean ± SEM.

however, there were no significant changes, although a trend toward decreased binding did occur in the pallidum.

There was no clear relationship between GABA binding and the duration or severity of the disease, nor did the severity of individual parkinsonian symptoms correlate with GABA receptor binding either. Moreover, levodopa treatment did not have any significant effect on GABA binding in the parkinsonian brain.

DISCUSSION

There is no doubt that the progressive loss of dopaminergic substantia nigra neurons and deficiency of striatal dopamine play an essential role in the pathophysiology of Parkinson's disease. Moreover, decreased activities of TH and DDC in the extrapyramidal nuclei of parkinsonian patients correlate well with dopamine deficiency. However, activities of these enzymes are relatively high as compared to the great loss of dopaminergic substantia nigra neurons. These findings suggest that the remaining neurons of the substantia nigra may be hyperactive, which is also indicated by the fact that the HVA–dopamine ratio in the basal ganglia is greater in parkinsonian patients than in controls (9,26,27).

Correlations found in the present study between activities of TH and clinical parameters of Parkinson's disease give further support to the existence of a link between the striatal dopamine deficiency and the main clinical symptomatology of the disease (2). The present results clearly suggest that hypokinesia and rigidity are symptoms that originate primarily in the dopaminergic system. Also, levodopa treatment gives the best results with these parkinsonian symptoms, and in some patients tremor did not improve at all (30), indicating that there may also be neural mechanisms other than dopaminergic ones in the pathophysiology of tremor. Indeed, the present results gave some evidence that GABA neurons may be involved.

Results of the present study give further support to the possible involvement of GABA neurons in the neuronal interaction of the extrapyramidal system in Parkinson's disease either primarily or as a secondary consequence. Changes of GABA neurons in the cerebral and cerebellar cortex are further evidence that in Parkinson's disease there are pathophysiological manifestations outside the extrapyramidal system. Obviously, the etiological factor(s) may cause a general brain defect, although it seems to have a greater affinity to the dopaminergic neurons in the substantia nigra.

Findings on the binding of ^{3}H-spiroperidol showed that in Parkinson's disease there is not only a degeneration of dopaminergic substantia nigra neurons, but also a progressive loss of postsynaptic dopamine receptor sites in the striatum. It has been suggested that this alteration may contribute to the decreased response of parkinsonian patients to chronic levodopa therapy (19). In the present material, however, there was no clear relationship between therapeutic response and ^{3}H-spiroperidol binding.

Our patients were relatively severely disabled and showed deteriorating responses to levodopa. In contrast, neuroleptic medication with or without levodopa seems to increase dopamine-receptor binding in the striatum. This agrees with recent findings in animals (3,17) and in schizophrenic patients (18). These results, together with the increased ^{3}H-haloperidol binding demonstrable in the putamen of parkinsonian patients, support the theory of dopaminergic supersensitivity in Parkinson's disease (8). It has yet to be clarified, though, whether the psychosis, the use of neuroleptics, or the Parkinson's disease process itself forms the basis for increased dopamine-receptor binding. Of course, the increased occurrence of involuntary movements in the parkinsonian patient group treated with levodopa and neuroleptics argues in favor of increased dopaminergic neurotransmission.

Analysis of brain dopamine and HVA provided direct evidence of increased formation of dopamine in the brain of parkinsonian patients treated with levodopa alone (9,26,27) or combined with a decarboxylase inhibitor (26,29). Thus, although the dopaminergic substantia nigra–striatum system is severely damaged in parkinsonian patients, it still can produce dopamine. This seems to indicate that at least a part of the therapeutic effect of levodopa may be mediated through the correction of dopamine deficiency in the nigrostriatal neurons, but the possible effects of other metabolic processes cannot be ruled out.

Exogenous levodopa seems to be metabolized in all the brain regions but, according to the results of the present study, levodopa combined with a decarboxylase inhibitor increases dopamine turnover more selectively in the substantia nigra–striatum system than levodopa alone. Indeed, there is experimental evidence (4) that the decarboxylase in the capillary walls in various brain regions shows variation in sensitivity to a decarboxylase inhibitor, resulting in differences in the penetration of levodopa into the brain. Moreover, part of the dopamine and HVA found after treatment with levodopa alone may be derived from the dopamine metabolism in the brain capillary walls.

The increased concentration of dopamine or HVA in the brain showed no significant correlation with the therapeutic responses to levodopa therapy. This finding, together with observed changes in plasma levodopa concentrations (28,31), suggests that the brain mechanisms are more important for the therapeutic response than the amount of levodopa entering the brain. Probably in each individual parkinsonian patient under levodopa treatment there is an optimal level of levodopa in the brain which causes saturation of the functional extrapyramidal system. By giving more levodopa it would be possible to induce higher levels of levodopa in the brain, but instead of any further benefit, there would merely occur a greater frequency of side-effects. It therefore seems important to avoid overdosage of levodopa and it is better to treat patients with the lowest dosage that will restore adequate functional performance capacity.

SUMMARY

Levodopa treatment increases the concentration of dopamine and homovanillic acid in the parkinsonian brain. Levodopa combined with a decarboxylase inhibitor increases dopamine turnover more selectively in the nigrostriatal system than levodopa alone. These results seem to indicate that at least part of the therapeutic effect of levodopa may be mediated through the correction of the deficiency of striatal dopamine in the parkinsonian brain.

The activities of TH and DDC were decreased in the basal ganglia of the parkinsonian brain. Levodopa treatment did not have a significant effect on them. However, there was a trend towards decreased TH activity and a significant negative correlation between the duration of levodopa treatment and striatal TH activity.

The specific binding of ^{3}H-spiroperidol was significantly reduced in the caudate nucleus and putamen of the parkinsonian patients. Thus in Parkinson's disease, there is not only a degeneration of dopaminergic substantia nigra neurons but also a loss of postsynaptic dopamine-receptor sites in the striatum. Levodopa treatment did not affect dopamine receptor binding but neuroleptic medication increased it significantly.

The activity of glutamic acid decarboxylase was decreased in the parkinsonian extrapyramidal nuclei as well as in the cerebral and cerebellar cortex but the content of GABA decreased only in the cerebral and cerebellar cortex. GABA receptor binding was significantly decreased in the substantia nigra of the parkinsonian brain. These findings suggest the involvement of GABA neurons in the neuronal interaction of the extrapyramidal system in Parkinson's disease.

ACKNOWLEDGMENT

This study was supported by a grant from the Sigrid Jusélius Foundation.

REFERENCES

1. Bernheimer, H., Birkmayer, W., and Hornykiewicz, O. (1966): Homovanillinsäure im Liquor cerebrospinalis: Untersuchungen beim Parkinson-Syndrom und anderen Erkrankungen des ZNS. *Wien. klin. Wochenschr.,* 78:417–419.
2. Bernheimer, H., Birkmayer W., Hornykiewicz, O., Jellinger, K., and Seitelberger, F. (1973): Brain dopamine and the syndromes of Parkinson and Huntington. *J. Neurol. Sci.,* 20:415–455.
3. Burt, D. R., Creese, I., and Snyder, S. H. (1977): Antischizophrenic drugs: chronic treatment elevates dopamine receptor binding in brain. *Science,* 196:326–328.
4. Constantinidis, J., Bartholini, G., Geissbuhler, G., and Tissot, R. (1970): La barrière capillaire enzymatique pour DOPA au niveau de quelques noyaux du tronc cérébral du rat. *Experientia (Basel),* 26:381.
5. Ehringer, H., and Hornykiewicz, O. (1960): Verteilung von Noradrenalin und Dopamine (3-hydroxytyramin) im Gehirn des Menschen und ihr Verhalten bei Erkrankungen des extrapyramidalen Systems. *Klin. Wochenschr.,* 38:1236–1239.
6. Greer, M., Collins, G. H., and Anton, A. H. (1971): Cerebral catecholamines after levodopa therapy. *Arch. Neurol.,* 25:461–467.
7. Johansson, B., and Roos, B. E. (1965): Acid monoamine metabolites in the cerebrospinal fluid of patients with Parkinson's syndrome. *Proceedings of the Eighth International Congress of Neurology (Vienna),* p. 141.
8. Lee, T., Seeman, P., Rajput, A., Farley, I. J., and Hornykiewicz, O. (1978): Receptor basis for dopaminergic supersensitivity in Parkinson's disease. *Nature,* 273:59–61.
9. Lloyd, K. G., Davidson, L., and Hornykiewicz, O. (1973): Metabolism of levodopa in the human brain. In: *Advances in Neurology, Vol. 3,* edited by D. B. Calne, pp. 173–188. Raven Press, New York.

10. Lloyd, K. G., Davidson, L., and Hornykiewicz, O. (1975): The neurochemistry of Parkinson's disease: effect of L-DOPA therapy. *J. Pharmacol. Exp. Ther.,* 195:453–464.
11. Lloyd, K. G., and Hornykiewicz, O. (1972): Occurrence and distribution of aromatic L-amino acid (L-DOPA) decarboxylase in the human brain. *J. Neurochem.,* 19:1549–1559.
12. Lloyd, K. G., and Hornykiewicz, O. (1973): L-glutamic acid decarboxylase in Parkinson's disease: effect of L-DOPA therapy. *Nature,* 243:521–523.
13. Lloyd, K. G., Möhler, H., Heitz, P., and Bartholini, G. (1975): Distribution of choline acetyl-transferase and glutamate decarboxylase within the substantia nigra and in other brain regions from control and parkinsonian patients. *J. Neurochem.,* 25:789.
14. Lloyd, K. G., Shemen, L., and Hornykiewicz, O. (1977): Distribution of high affinity sodium-independent (^{3}H)gamma-aminobutyric acid (^{3}H-GABA) binding in the human brain: alterations in Parkinson's disease. *Brain Res.,* 127:269–278.
15. McGeer, P. L., and McGeer, E. G. (1976): Enzymes associated with the metabolism of catecholamines, acetylcholine and GABA in human controls and patients with Parkinson's disease and Huntington's chorea. *J. Neurochem.,* 26:65–76.
16. McGeer, P. L., McGeer, E. G., and Wada, J. A. (1971): Glutamic acid decarboxylase in Parkinson's disease and epilepsy. *Neurology (Minneap.),* 21:1000–1007.
17. Muller, P., and Seeman, P. (1978): Brain neurotransmitter receptors after long-term haloperidol: dopamine, acetylcholine, serotonin, alfa-noradrenergic and naloxone receptors. *Life Sci.,* 21:1751–1758.
18. Owen, F., Cross, A. J., Grow, T. J., Longden, A., Poulter, M., and Riley, G. J. (1978): Increased dopamine-receptor sensitivity in schizophrenia. *Lancet,* 8083:223–226.
19. Reisine, T. D., Fields, J. Z., and Yamamura, H. I. (1977): Neurotransmitter receptor alterations in Parkinson's disease. *Life Sci.,* 21:335–344.
20. Riederer, P., and Wuketich, St. (1976): Time course of nigrostriatal degeneration in Parkinson's disease. *J. Neural Transm.,* 38:277–301.
21. Rinne, U. K., Koskinen, V., Laaksonen, H., Lönnberg, P., and Sonninen, V. (1978): GABA receptor binding in the parkinsonian brain. *Life Sci.,* 22:2225–2228.
22. Rinne, U. K., Laaksonen, H., Riekkinen, P., and Sonninen, V. (1974): Brain glutamic acid decarboxylase activity in Parkinson's disease. *Eur. Neurol.,* 12:13–19.
23. Rinne, U. K., Riekkinen, P., Sonninen, V., and Laaksonen, H. (1973): Brain acetylcholinesterase in Parkinson's disease. *Acta Neurol. Scand.,* 49:215–226.
24. Rinne, U. K., and Sonninen, V. (1968): Dopamine and Parkinson's disease. *Ann. Med. Intern. Fenn.,* 57:105.
25. Rinne, U. K., and Sonninen, V. (1972): Acid monoamine metabolites in the cerebrospinal fluid of patients with Parkinson's disease. *Neurology (Minneap.),* 22:62–67.
26. Rinne, U. K., and Sonninen, V. (1973): Brain catecholamines and their metabolites in parkinsonian patients. Treatment with levodopa alone or combined with a decarboxylase inhibitor. *Arch. Neurol.,* 28:107–110.
27. Rinne, U. K., Sonninen, V., and Hyyppä, M. (1971): Effect of L-DOPA on brain monoamines and their metabolites in Parkinson's disease. *Life Sci.,* 10:549–557.
28. Rinne, U. K., Sonninen, V., and Marttila, R. (1977): Brain dopamine metabolism and the relief of parkinsonism. In: *Parkinson's Disease—Concepts and Prospects,* edited by J. P. W. F. Lakke, J. Korf, and H. Wesseling, pp. 73–83. Excerpta Medica, Amsterdam.
29. Rinne, U. K., Sonninen, V., Riekkinen, P., and Laaksonen, H. (1974): Postmortem findings in parkinsonian patients treated with L-DOPA: biochemical considerations. In: *Current Concepts in the Treatment of Parkinsonism,* edited by M. D. Yahr, pp. 211–233. Raven Press, New York.
30. Rinne, U. K., Sonninen, V., and Siirtola, T. (1970): L-DOPA treatment in Parkinson's disease. *Eur. Neurol.,* 4:348–369.
31. Rinne, U. K., Sonninen, V., and Siirtola, T. (1973): Plasma concentration of levodopa in patients with Parkinson's disease. *Eur. Neurol.,* 10:301–310.

Advances in Neurology, Vol. 24, edited by
L. J. Poirier, T. L. Sourkes, and P. J. Bédard.
Raven Press, New York © 1979.

Compensatory Biochemical Changes at the Striatal Dopamine Synapse in Parkinson's Disease— Limitations of L-DOPA Therapy

Oleh Hornykiewicz

Institute of Biochemical Pharmacology, University of Vienna, Vienna, Austria

In addition to the crucial role of the striatal dopamine (DA) deficiency for the pathophysiology and extrapyramidal symptomatology of the parkinsonian condition (4,7), the severe dysfunction of the nigrostriatal DA system has at least two functionally consequential results: first, it leads to pre- and postsynaptic alterations within the still-functioning DA neurons; and second, it most probably is one of the important causes for the altered activity in the basal ganglia, of some of the neuronal systems utilizing putative neurotransmitters other than DA, notably acetylcholine, gamma-aminobutyric acid, serotonin, and noradrenaline (cf. ref. 8). Thus, the loss of striatal DA function seems to elicit a "chain-reaction" in the parkinsonian brain, altering the state of activity of both the remaining DA system itself as well as other functionally interrelated neuronal systems. These events illustrate the fact that, in general, the brain always tends to function as a whole; and since several of the neurotransmitter-related changes probably represent measures of the parkinsonian brain directed at correcting the functional consequences of the dopaminergic dysfunction, they also throw light on the wide range of the brain's capacity for compensation of lost function.

In the following discussion, I intend to concentrate on (a) the changes that take place in Parkinson's disease within the presynaptic as well as the postsynaptic portions of the striatal DA synapse complex; and (b) the effect of L-DOPA treatment on these compensatory changes in relation to the (long-term) effectiveness of this drug therapy. The main points of the discussed material are summarized in Table 1.

STRIATAL DOPAMINE DEFICIENCY: COMPENSATORY CHANGES AT THE LEVEL OF THE DOPAMINE SYNAPSE

Presynaptic Changes

In Parkinson's disease, the remaining nigrostriatal DA neurons are in a state of functional overactivity. This can be concluded from the following observations.

(a) In the parkinsonian striatum the ratio DA to homovanillic acid (HVA) is definitely shifted in favor of the metabolite (4). This indicates an increase of turnover, i.e., synthesis and release, of striatal DA. In addition, it can be assumed that this increase in DA turnover, especially DA release, results in a corresponding decrease of the actual DA storage capacity within the functionally still-intact DA neurons. (b) In one of the two available studies on DA synthesizing enzymes, it was found that in Parkinson's disease, L-tyrosine hydroxylase was less severely reduced than L-DOPA decarboxylase (12). This can be interpreted as an induction of the rate-limiting enzyme activity in the still-functioning DA neurons. This interpretation is consistent with the above conclusion that these neurons are in a state of overactivity, forming and releasing increased amounts of DA per unit time.

Analogous conclusions have been drawn from animal experiments showing that after partial lesions of the nigrostriatal DA pathway in the rat, there was an increase in the rate of formation of DA from ^{3}H-tyrosine in the striatum homolateral to the lesion, as compared with the striatum of the unlesioned side (1).

From a physiological point of view, development of overactivity of the remaining neurons in partially denervated tissues is an easily acceptable concept, its apparent role being the maintenance of normal function by compensating for the loss of a larger number of a given neuronal population. Since the remaining DA neurons in the parkinsonian striatum are most probably the principal sites of DA formation from therapeutically administered L-DOPA, their overactivity can be assumed to play an important role in determining L-DOPA's therapeutic efficacy.

Postsynaptic Changes

It is known that in the mammalian nigrostriatal complex there exist two distinct types of postsynaptic DA receptor: the adenylate cyclase-coupled receptor, which is specifically stimulated by DA (9); and the DA receptor, which is characterized by its affinity to neuroleptics such as haloperidol (13). In this respect, it is probable that these two types of postsynaptic DA receptor are localized to different morphological elements within the nigrostriatal complex. In Parkinson's disease, both of these postsynaptic DA receptors seem to undergo typical alterations.

DA Receptors Characterized by ^{3}H-Haloperidol Binding

In analogy to the well-known phenomenon of "denervation supersensitivity," the dopaminergic denervation of the striatum in Parkinson's disease can be expected to result in a development of supersensitivity to DA of at least some of the postsynaptic DA receptor sites. Direct evidence for the existence of supersensitivity to DA in the parkinsonian striatum has recently been obtained by

TABLE 1. *Parkinson's disease—compensatory biochemical changes at the level of the striatal dopamine synapse*

	Presynaptic	Postsynaptic
Biochemical change(s)	Ratio DA:HVA shifted in favor of HVA (4)	Increased binding of ³H-haloperidol to striatal membrane preparations (11)
Functional correlate	Increased DA turnover = overactivity of remaining DA neurons (4)	"Supersensitivity" of haloperidol-binding DA receptors
Pathophysiological significance	(a) Maintainance of function despite major DA neuron loss; (b) more DA formed and released per unit time during L-DOPA therapy	Maximal effectiveness of endogenous DA as well as DA formed from therapeutically administered L-DOPA
Effect of L-DOPA therapy	Elimination by the accumulating DA	Elimination by the accumulating DA

Additional postsynaptic biochemical change: Decreased basal and DA-stimulated adenylate cyclase activity (14); Functional correlate: "Subsensitivity" of the adenylate cyclase-coupled DA receptors; Pathophysiological significance: ? (See text); Effect of L-DOPA therapy: ?

References to literature are given in parentheses.

measuring, in striatal membrane preparations, the specific binding of ^{3}H-haloperidol or other neuroleptics so as to tag those DA receptor sites that show a particularly high affinity for these compounds. By means of this DA receptor assay it was shown (11) that in the parkinsonian striatum (especially the putamen) the values for the specific ^{3}H-haloperidol binding were about 70% above the levels found in control subjects. From this finding the conclusion can be drawn that in the parkinsonian striatum there is an increased number (or affinity for DA) of this particular type of postsynaptic DA receptor. This typical finding can be taken as evidence for the existence of denervation supersensitivity to DA of the parkinsonian striatum. Interestingly, analogous assays using ^{3}H-apomorphine which, in contrast to haloperidol, tags (under certain experimental conditions) preferentially presynaptic DA sites, demonstrated a decreased binding of this ligand in the parkinsonian striatum; this is not surprising in view of the severe loss of presynaptic dopaminergic elements in this disorder.

The finding of a denervation type of supersensitivity to DA in the parkinsonian striatum explains two earlier clinicopharmacological observations. (a) Patients with severe akinesia were found to respond more sensitively to an i.v. test dose of L-DOPA than patients with mild akinesia (4). Since the degree of akinesia correlates positively with the degree of striatal DA loss (4), L-DOPA sensitivity of the patients was apparently determined by the degree of dopaminergic denervation of their striatal tissue. (b) Therapeutic doses of L-DOPA seem to induce dyskinesias more readily in parkinsonian patients than in nonparkinsonian subjects (cf. ref. 3). Since the L-DOPA-induced dyskinesias are, in all probability, striatal in origin and mediated by (excess of) DA, this observation again supports the notion of supersensitivity of the striatal DA receptors in Parkinson's disease.

It is obvious that together with the overactivity of the remaining presynaptic DA terminals, the development of supersensitive postsynaptic DA receptors provides for a maximal degree of utilization of the endogenous DA as well as the DA formed from exogenous L-DOPA.

Adenylate Cyclase-Coupled DA Receptors

In contradistinction to the behavior of the DA receptors with specific binding affinity to neuroleptics, the adenylate cyclase-coupled DA receptors seem to be reduced in the parkinsonian striatum. Thus, in a recent study it was found (14) that in the parkinsonian caudate nucleus the basal activity of adenylate cyclase was approximately 56% of control ($p < 0.001$), and in the putamen 58% of control ($p < 0.005$); even more markedly reduced was the activity of the DA-stimulated adenylate cyclase, being only 18% of control for the caudate nucleus ($p < 0.001$) and 25% of control for the putamen ($p < 0.01$).

At present no explanation can be offered for this functional disturbance of the adenylate cyclase-coupled DA receptor sites in the parkinsonian striatum. However, it is tempting to speculate that the opposite behavior of the ^{3}H-haloperidol binding sites and the DA-stimulated adenylate cyclase, as the two types of distinct postsynaptic DA receptor, may be related to the possibility of DA exerting opposite physiological effects in the striatum. Recently, the existence of excitatory and inhibitory DA receptors in the cat striatum has been postulated (6); also, neurophysiological observations point to inhibitory (5) as well as excitatory (10) functions of the nigrostriatal DA pathway on the firing rate of striatal units. In view of these possibilities, it could be that the adenylate cyclase-coupled DA receptors in the striatum normally subserve functions whose reduction may offer an advantage in counteracting some of the extrapyramidal symptoms in Parkinson's disease.

EFFECT OF L-DOPA ON THE COMPENSATORY CHANGES IN THE STRIATAL DOPAMINE SYSTEM—L-DOPA AS A SELF-LIMITING DRUG

L-DOPA's high efficacy as an antiparkinsonian drug seems to be determined by three factors: (a) preservation of a minimum number of striatal DA terminals permitting the transformation of L-DOPA to DA [in this respect, the high degree of divergence of the dopaminergic innervation of the striatum (2) is a crucial physiological factor, safeguarding the striatum, up to a critical point, against an early loss of function]; (b) the overactivity of the remaining nigrostriatal DA neurons, permitting higher than normal amounts of DA to be formed and released per unit time; and (c) development of supersensitivity to DA of the striatal postsynaptic DA receptors (as measured by specific ^{3}H-haloperidol binding), which potentiates the physiological effect of a given amount of DA.

The dependence of L-DOPA's efficacy in Parkinson's disease on the compensatory mechanisms at the level of the striatal DA synapse, clearly points out the limits set to successful long-term L-DOPA treatment. It seems obvious from a pharmacological point of view that all those compensatory changes, which are due to the partial dopaminergic denervation of the striatum, will be reversed when the striatal DA levels are increased during successful L-DOPA therapy (12). In this respect, a loss of postsynaptic sensitivity of the striatal DA receptor sites in L-DOPA-treated patients has been directly demonstrated by means of the ^{3}H-haloperidol binding assay. In contrast to the increased binding in homogenates of the striatum from untreated parkinsonian patients (see above) this index of postsynaptic receptor sensitivity to DA was found to be within normal limits in those patients who had been treated with L-DOPA until death (11).

It is evident that with the nigral neurons being progressively reduced in number during the natural course of the disease, the L-DOPA-induced elimination of the compensatory mechanisms will eventually result in a substantial loss of the drug's effectiveness. Obviously, as an antiparkinson agent, L-DOPA is a self-limiting drug. In addition, it is not known at present in what way the probable "shutting off" by L-DOPA of the activity of the remaining nigrostriatal DA neurons may affect the physiological properties, or even survival, of these neurons. It is possible that low dose or intermittent L-DOPA administration may better preserve the compensatory overactivity of the DA neurons as well as the supersensitivity of the DA receptors, thus assuring a better long-term effectiveness of L-DOPA as an antiparkinsonian drug.

SUMMARY

The DA deficiency in the striatum in Parkinson's disease has two functional consequences, at the level of the striatal DA synapse, that have to be considered as compensatory in nature. These compensatory mechanisms seem to subserve the purpose of maintaining, in a disease that basically is both degenerative and progressive, a critical minimum of function for as long periods of time as possible. These two functional changes are: (a) overactivity of the remaining striatal (presynaptic) DA neurons; and (b) supersensitivity of the striatal (post-synaptic) DA receptors. Effective L-DOPA therapy in Parkinson's disease has been shown to increase the levels of the striatal DA. This DA accumulation can be expected to reduce, via the known negative feedback loop, the activity of the remaining DA neurons, thus eliminating one important compensatory mechanism. Likewise, the striatal DA receptors may become desensitized by the synaptically accumulating DA. There is evidence to show that the latter event in fact takes place in the striatum of patients on long-term L-DOPA therapy. The desensitization of the striatal DA receptors may represent an important factor limiting the success of long-term L-DOPA therapy. This may help to explain the clinical observation that, with time, the patients' response to L-DOPA markedly declines. As an antiparkinsonian drug L-DOPA is a self-limiting drug. Perhaps low-dose or intermittent L-DOPA therapy would better preserve the responsivity of parkinsonian patients to dopaminergic drug therapy.

REFERENCES

1. Agid, Y., Javoy, F., and Glowinski, J. (1973): Hyperactivity of remaining dopaminergic neurons after partial destruction of the nigro-striatal dopaminergic system in the rat. *Nature (New Biol.)*, 245:150–151.
2. Andén, N.-E., Fuxe, K., Hamberger, B., and Hökfelt, T. (1966): A quantitative study of the nigro-neostriatal dopamine neuron system in the rat. *Acta Physiol. Scand.*, 67:306–312.
3. Barbeau, A. (1969): L-DOPA therapy in Parkinson's disease: a critical review of nine years experience. *Can. Med. Assoc. J.*, 101:791–800.
4. Bernheimer, H., Birkmayer, W., Hornykiewicz, O., Jellinger, K., and Seitelberger, F. (1973): Brain dopamine and the syndromes of Parkinson and Huntington. *J. Neurol. Sci.*, 20:415–455.
5. Connor, J. D. (1970): Caudate nucleus neurons: correlation of the effects of substantia nigra stimulation with iontophoretic dopamine. *J. Physiol., (Lond.)*, 208:691–703.
6. Cools, A. R., and Van Rossum, J. M. (1976): Excitation-mediating and inhibition-mediating dopamine receptors: a new concept towards a better understanding of electrophysiological, biochemical, pharmacological, functional and clinical data. *Psychopharmacologia*, 45:243–254.
7. Hornykiewicz, O. (1973): Parkinson's disease: from brain homogenate to treatment. *Fed. Proc.*, 32:183–190.
8. Hornykiewicz, O. (1976): Neurochemical interactions and basal ganglia function and dysfunction. In: *The Basal Ganglia*, edited by M. D. Yahr, pp. 269–278. Raven Press, New York.

9. Kebabian, J. W., Petzold, G. L., and Greengard, P. (1972): Dopamine-sensitive adenylate cyclase in caudate nucleus of rat brain and its similarity to the "dopamine receptor." *Proc. Natl. Acad. Sci. U.S.A.,* 69:2145–2149.
10. Kitai, S. T., Sugimori, M., and Kocsis, J. D. (1976): Excitatory nature of dopamine in the nigro-caudate pathway. *Exp. Brain Res.,* 24:351–363.
11. Lee, T., Seeman, P., Rajput, A., Farley, I. J., and Hornykiewicz, O. (1978): Receptor basis for dopaminergic supersensitivity in Parkinson's disease. *Nature,* 273:59–61.
12. Lloyd, K. G., Davidson, L., and Hornykiewicz, O. (1975): The neurochemistry of Parkinson's disease: effect of L-DOPA therapy. *J. Pharmacol.,* 195:453–464.
13. Seeman, P., Chau-Wong, M., Tedesco, J., and Wong, K. (1975): Brain receptors for antipsychotic drugs and dopamine: direct binding assays. *Proc. Natl. Acad. Sci. U.S.A.,* 72:4376–4380.
14. Shibuya, M. (1979): Dopamine-sensitive adenylate cyclase activity in the striatum in Parkinson's disease. *J. Neural Transm.,* 44:287–295.

Advances in Neurology, Vol. 24, edited by
L. J. Poirier, T. L. Sourkes, and P. J. Bédard.
Raven Press, New York © 1979.

Catecholamine-Related Enzymes in the Brain of Patients with Parkinsonism and Wilson's Disease

*Toshiharu Nagatsu, *Takeshi Kato, **Ikuko Nagatsu, **Yukari
Kondo, **Shinobu Inagaki, †Reiji Iizuka,
and ††Hirotaro Narabayashi

*Laboratory of Cell Physiology, Department of Life Chemistry, Tokyo Institute of
Technology, Yokohama, Japan; **Department of Anatomy, Fujita-Gakuen University
School of Medicine, Toyoake, Aichi, Japan; and Departments of †Psychiatry and
††Neurology, Juntendo University School of Medicine, Tokyo, Japan

In patients with parkinsonism the concentration of dopamine in the nigro-striato-pallidal complex of the brain is greatly reduced (1). This reduction of dopamine in the dopaminergic neurons appears to be due to reduction of the activity of dopamine-synthesizing enzymes, since the activities of DOPA decarboxylase (DDC) (4) and tyrosine hydroxylase (TH) (3,6,8,9) were found to be decreased.

We have previously examined most of the enzymes related to catecholamines such as TH, DDC, dopamine β-hydroxylase (DBH), phenylethanolamine-N-methyltransferase (PNMT), monoamine oxidase (MAO) (type A and type B) (8,9), and dopamine-stimulated adenylate cyclase (7) in parkinsonian brains. We have further examined these catecholamine-related enzymes in brains from more parkinsonian patients and from patients who had Wilson's disease and Huntington's chorea. The activity of cyclic AMP-dependent protein kinase, which may be associated with the molecular events underlying the process of synaptic transmission (2), has also been examined.

MATERIALS AND METHODS

Data on the patients examined are shown in Table 1. The control human brains and parkinsonian brains from cases 1 to 3 were reported in our previous papers (8,9). Five more parkinsonian cases and single cases of Wilson's disease and Huntington's chorea were examined. The ages and postmortem periods of controls were similar to those of parkinsonian patients. The parkinsonian patients had not taken L-DOPA during the last 6 months before death. The analytical methods used to assay the enzymes have been reported (5,6). DDC activity was measured both by the previously reported radiochemical method with DL-(1-^{14}C)-DOPA as substrate and by a new method, in which L-DOPA or D-

TABLE 1. *Case histories of parkinsonian patients*

Case	Sex/Age	Cause of death	Postmortem period (hr)
Parkinsonism			
1 S.M.	M/73	Pneumonitis	4
2 I.N.	F/63	Unknown	6
3 M.O.	F/58	Heart failure	2
4 O.T.	F/78	Heart failure	10
5 M.S.	M/63	Heart failure	2.5
6 S.H.	F/61	Heart failure	6
7 N.O.	M/72	Peritonitis	1.5
8 S.K.	F/82	Heart failure	1
Wilson's disease			
T.S.	M/22	Pulmonary embolism	3
Huntington's chorea			
A.K.	F/53	Subdural hygroma	2

DOPA serves as substrate for the experiment or control, respectively; dopamine formed was assayed by high-performance liquid chromatography with an electrochemical detector (Yanaco L-2000 with VMD-101 voltammetry detector, Kyoto, Japan).

RESULTS AND DISCUSSION

The activities of TH, DDC, and DBH in terms of pmoles (min) (mg protein) or nmoles (hr) (g tissue) are shown in the Tables 2 to 4. TH activity (Table 2) in all eight parkinsonian patients was markedly decreased (3–10% of the controls) especially in the caudate nucleus and putamen. It was also significantly reduced in the pallidum, substantia nigra, and locus ceruleus. This result supports our previous conclusion that TH activity in parkinsonian brain is greatly decreased (8,9).

DDC activity (Table 3), especially in parkinsonian cases 2 to 5, was decreased in the caudate nucleus, putamen, pallidum, and subtantia nigra, but the activity in cases 1, 7, and 8 was similar to or even higher than that in controls. Therefore, the mean values of all eight parkinsonian brains were not significantly different from those of controls. This supports our previous observation on the presence of parkinsonism with low TH and yet normal DDC activity. We had reported for the first time a case of parkinsonism (case 1) with low TH and normal DDC (8,9) and two more such cases have been found in this study. Histopathological study is now under way in order to determine the morphological differences in the brain of parkinsonian patients with low TH and low DDC, and with low TH and normal DDC, respectively.

The activity of human brain DDC is very low as compared with that in other animals. This is not due to the presence of endogenous inhibitors (8,9). When DDC activity was assayed by our new method (see above), values similar to those obtained by radiochemical assay with DL-(1-^{14}C)-DOPA as substrate were observed. Moreover, the individual variation of DDC activity was high, suggesting that postmortem stability of the enzyme may affect the activity.

DBH activity in different regions of the brains from parkinsonian patients has also been examined for the first time in our previous (8,9) and present studies. DBH activity was high in the locus ceruleus and hypothalamus, but it was lower in parkinsonian patients than in the controls. This suggests that moderate impairment may also exist in the noradrenergic neurons in parkinsonism.

We had reported that PNMT activity in the adrenergic neurons was also significantly reduced in the hypothalamus of parkinsonian patients (8,9). Therefore, it is conceivable that not only severe damage in the nigrostriatal dopaminergic neurons, but also moderate damage of central noradrenergic and adrenergic neurons may exist in parkinsonism.

Although only single cases of Wilson's disease and Huntington's chorea were examined, TH and DDC in the brains from these two patients appear to be within normal range in most structures studied (Tables 2 and 3). Normal TH activity in Huntington's chorea had been reported by McGeer and McGeer (6). It was our interest to see the change in DBH activity in a case of Wilson's disease, since DBH is a copper enzyme. As shown in Table 5, copper concentrations in the brain were found to be greatly increased in the patient with Wilson's disease, but DBH activity was rather low in the hypothalamus. The copper concentration in the thalamus was lower in parkinsonian patients than in controls; the significance of this finding remains for further investigation.

We had previously reported that the activity of dopamine-stimulated adenylate cyclase in the caudate nucleus was higher in parkinsonian patients, who had not taken L-DOPA, than in controls (7). Since cyclic AMP-dependent protein kinase appears to be associated with the molecular events underlying the process of synaptic transmission (2), we have measured cyclic AMP-dependent protein kinase activity in the caudate nucleus of parkinsonian patients. As shown in Table 6, basal and cyclic AMP-dependent protein kinase activities were not significantly different between age-matched controls and parkinsonian patients. This may suggest that only the dopamine receptor is supersensitive in the postdopaminergic neurons of the caudate nucleus of parkinsonian patients who did not receive L-DOPA treatment. Supersensitivity of dopamine receptors in the caudate nucleus and putamen of parkinsonian patients without L-DOPA treatment has also been confirmed by specific ^{3}H-haloperidol binding (5).

SUMMARY

Although it is evident that further work on more cases is needed to establish our conclusions, present results may be tentatively summarized as shown in Table 7. TH activity in the nigrostriatal dopaminergic neurons is greatly decreased in parkinsonism, and this may be enough to explain the decrease in

TABLE 2. *Tyrosine hydroxylase activity in brain regions*

Brain region	Activity (mean ± SE)			
	Controls	Parkinsonism	Wilson's disease	Huntington's chorea
	pmoles (min) (mg protein)			
Caudate nucleus	10.22 ± 2.82 (7)	0.89 ± 0.35 (8)[b] (1.32,0.29,0.20,0.00, 1.13,1.05,3.00,0.15)	4.22	3.96
Putamen	15.16 ± 6.37 (8)	0.36 ± 0.19 (8)[a] (0.38,0.00,1.39,0.00, 0.93,0.00,0.16,0.00)	4.24	4.11
Pallidum	8.92 ± 2.27 (6)	1.42 ± 0.90 (8)[b] (1.62,0.00,1.27,0.00, 0.92,0.06,7.49,0.00)	8.59	0.65
Substantia nigra	18.49 ± 5.37 (6)	2.70 ± 1.22 (8)[b] (6.40,1.34,2.68,0.00, 1.11,0.16,9.50,0.37)	51.9	3.06
Locus ceruleus	36.00 ± 6.32 (4)	6.54 ± 3.52 (7)[b] (21.2,3.10,15.7,—, 1.31,0.84,3.52,0.14)	—	—
Hypothalamus	2.82 ± 0.67 (7)	1.72 ± 0.72 (8) (5.38,0.00,2.23,0.00, 1.11,0.73,4.15,0.14)	3.37	0.49

nmoles (hr) (g tissue)

Caudate nucleus	52.3 ± 11.5 (7)	4.8 ± 1.8 (8)[b] (6.5,1.3,0.9,0.0, 8.5,5.2,14.9,0.8)	19.8	20.9
Putamen	76.0 ± 26.9 (8)	2.1 ± 1.1 (8)[a] (2.2,0.0,7.3,0.0, 6.5,0.0,0.8,0.0)	18.8	23.1
Pallidum	49.5 ± 11.7 (6)	7.1 ± 4.6 (8)[b] (5.9,0.0,6.3,0.0, 5.7,0.35,38.3,0.0)	40.3	4.3
Substantia nigra	99.7 ± 27.6 (6)	15.4 ± 7.5 (8)[b] (35.0,6.2,13.1,0.0, 6.1,1.1,60.0,2.0)	210	17.1
Locus ceruleus	153.6 ± 25.4 (4)	28.1 ± 13.6 (7)[b] (86.7,10.5,73.7,—, 6.8,4.0,14.3,0.7)	—	—
Hypothalamus	13.4 ± 3.4 (7)	9.5 ± 4.1 (8) (32.3,0.0,11.0,0.0, 7.5,3.8,20.6,0.7)	17.6	2.4

Numbers of samples and the individual activities for each patient are given in parentheses.
[a] $p < 0.05$ for difference between controls and parkinsonism.
[b] $p < 0.01$ for difference between controls and parkinsonism.

TABLE 3. *DOPA decarboxylase activity in brain regions*

Brain region	Activity (mean ± SE)			
	Controls	Parkinsonism	Wilson's disease	Huntington's chorea
	pmoles (min) (mg protein)			
Caudate nucleus	8.60 ± 5.06 (8)	7.55 ± 3.09 (8) (21.3,0.4,1.7,4.6, 0.25,2.7,20.8,8.6)	20.0	37.0
Putamen	11.87 ± 8.47 (6)	4.35 ± 1.56 (8) (10.3,0.3,1.3,9.1, 0.25,0.3,8.7,4.5)	19.4	22.5
Pallidum	4.82 ± 4.22 (6)	5.24 ± 2.51 (8) (12.9,0.3,3.6,2.1, 0.3,0.6,19.5,2.8)	32.5	2.0
Substantia nigra	2.54 ± 2.02 (6)	6.45 ± 3.66 (8) (13.0,0.3,2.1,3.5, 0.4,0.4,29.9,2.0)	189	18.9
Locus ceruleus	9.35 ± 6.28 (5)	22.73 ± 7.06 (6) (42.2,0.8,16.1,—, —,7.3,40.0,30.1)	—	—
Hypothalamus	6.72 ± 3.22 (7)	11.03 ± 4.81 (8) (21.1,0.3,6.4,7.5, 0.4,0.3,39.6,12.7)	31.1	2.5

nmoles (hr) (g tissue)

Caudate nucleus	42.0 ± 22.0 (8)	38.3 ± 15.4 (8) (107,2.1,7.9,24.7, 1.9,13.1,103,46.6)	96.3	193
Putamen	55.9 ± 36.1 (6)	23.8 ± 8.6 (8) (60.2,1.3,7.1,48.1, 1.7,1.7,45.0,25.5)	89.0	125
Pallidum	25.4 ± 21.9 (6)	24.8 ± 12.0 (8) (48.0,1.3,17.8,11.9, 1.7,3.2,100,14.5)	160	13.1
Substantia nigra	13.5 ± 10.7 (6)	38.2 ± 22.9 (8) (72.1,1.5,9.8,19.7, 2.3,2.2,187,10.7)	699	105
Locus ceruleus	38.6 ± 25.0 (5)	97.7 ± 28.4 (6) (168,2.7,79.4,—, —,34.8,163,139)	—	—

Numbers of samples and the individual activities for each patient are given in parentheses.

TABLE 4. Dopamine β-hydroxylase activity in brain regions

Brain region	Activity (mean ± SE)			
	Controls	Parkinsonism	Wilson's disease	Huntington's chorea
	pmoles (min) (mg protein)			
Hypothalamus	58.9 ± 17.9 (9)	15.1 ± 4.4 (8)[a] (33.3,16.9,12.3,5.8, 2.8,0.0,19.1,30.7)	9.6	37.7
Thalamus	6.00 ± 2.36 (7)	4.09 ± 0.80 (8) (4.93,4.92,1.44,2.2, 2.4,3.0,8.3,5.5)	3.5	34.5
Locus ceruleus	188 ± 76 (2)	23.3 ± 8.4 (4)[a] (—,—,—,—, 15.3,48,3.13.8,15.7)	—	36.2
	nmoles (hr) (g tissue)			
Hypothalamus	264.3 ± 79.9 (9)	83.5 ± 25.1 (8)[a] (177,89.6,58.8,34.3, 18.9,0.0,95.7,194)	51.4	248
Thalamus	41.4 ± 13.8 (7)	28.3 ± 4.4 (8) (32.2,32.0,10.4,15.8, 18.5,39.4,46.4,31.8)	19.0	223
Locus ceruleus	876 ± 348 (2)	109 ± 41 (4)[a] (—,—,—,—, 74.2,231,56.6,72.6)	—	204

Numbers of samples and the individual activities for each patient are given in parentheses.
[a] $p < 0.05$ for difference between controls and parkinsonism.

TABLE 5. *Copper concentrations in human brain*

Brain region	Copper concentration (μg/g tissue, mean $\pm$ SE)		
	Controls (5)	Parkinsonism (5)	Wilson's disease
Thalamus	3.98 $\pm$ 0.51	2.33 $\pm$ 0.48 [a]	70.3
Hippocampus	4.30 $\pm$ 0.73	3.21 $\pm$ 1.36	39.8

[a] $p < 0.05$ for difference between controls and parkinsonism.

TABLE 6. *Basal and cyclic AMP-dependent protein kinase activity in the caudate nucleus of normal controls and parkinsonian patients*

Samples	Protein kinase activity [pmoles (min) (mg protein) mean $\pm$ SE]		
	cAMP	+ 2 μM cAMP	Increase due to cAMP
Controls (5)	100 $\pm$ 18	196 $\pm$ 31	96 $\pm$ 16
Parkinsonism [a] (3)	110 $\pm$ 38	204 $\pm$ 58	94 $\pm$ 21

[a] Cases 1, 2, and 3.

TABLE 7. *Probable changes in catecholamine-related enzymes in parkinsonian brain*

Enzymes	Changes
Tyrosine hydroxylase	Greatly decreased
Dopa decarboxylase	Greatly decreased, decreased, or normal
Dopamine β-hydroxylase	Decreased
Phenylethanolamine-N-methyl-transferase	Decreased
Monoamine oxidase (A and B)	Normal (decreased in hypothalamus)
Dopamine-dependent adenylate cyclase	Increased
Cyclic AMP-dependent protein kinase	Normal

dopamine. DDC activity appears to be also decreased in many, but there may be some cases of parkinsonism with low TH and normal DDC. DBH and PNMT activities in parkinsonian brains may also be moderately decreased, indicating partial impairment of noradrenergic and adrenergic neurons in parkinsonian brain. These changes in catecholamine-synthesizing enzymes may not occur in Wilson's disease or Huntington's chorea. Dopamine-stimulated adenylate cyclase may be increased in the caudate nucleus of parkinsonian patients without

L-DOPA treatment, but the activity of cyclic AMP-dependent protein kinase may not change.

REFERENCES

1. Ehringer, H., and Hornykiewicz, O. (1960): Verteilung von Noradrenalin und Dopamin (3-Hydroxytyramin) im Gehirn des Menschen und ihr Verhalten bei Erkrankungen des Extrapyramidalen Systems. *Klin. Wochenschr.,* 38:1236–1239.
2. Greengard, P. (1978): Phosphorylated proteins as physiological effectors. *Science,* 199:146–152.
3. Lloyd, K. G., Davidson, L., and Hornykiewicz, O. (1975): The neurochemistry of Parkinson's disease: effect of L-DOPA therapy, *J. Pharm. Exp. Ther.,* 195:453–464.
4. Lloyd, K. G., and Hornykiewicz, O. (1970): Parkinson's disease: activity of L-DOPA decarboxylase in discrete brain regions. *Science,* 170:1212–1213.
5. Lee, T., Seeman, P., Rajput, A., Farley, I. J., and Hornykiewicz, O. (1978): Receptor basis for dopaminergic supersensitivity in Parkinson's disease. *Nature,* 273:59–61.
6. McGeer, P. L., and McGeer, E. G. (1976): Enzymes associated with the metabolism of catecholamines, acetylcholine and GABA in human controls and patients with Parkinson's disease and Huntington's chorea. *J. Neurochem.,* 26:65–76.
7. Nagatsu, T., Kanamori, T., Kato, T., Iizuka, R., and Narabayashi, H. (1978): Dopamine-stimulated adenylate cyclase activity in the human brain: changes in Parkinsonism. *Biochem. Med.,* 19:360–365.
8. Nagatsu, T., Kato, T., Numata (Sudo), Y., Ikuta, K., Sano, M., Nagatsu, I., Kondo, Y., Inagaki, S., Iizuka, R., Hori, A., and Narabayashi, H. (1977): Phenylethanolamine-N-methyltransferase and other enzymes of catecholamine metabolism in human brain. *Clin. Chim. Acta,* 75:221–232.
9. Nagatsu, T., Kato, T., Numata, Y., Sano, M., Nagatsu, I., Kondo, Y., Inagaki, S., Iizuka, R., Hori, A., and Narabayashi, H. (1976): Phenylethnanolamine-N-methyltransferase and other catecholamine enzymes in human brain. *Bull. Jpn. Neurochem. Soc.,* 15:68–71; Abstract in *Neurochem. Res.,* 2:335.

Advances in Neurology, Vol. 24, edited by
L. J. Poirier, T. L. Sourkes, and P. J. Bédard.
Raven Press, New York © 1979.

Involvement of GABA Neurons and Receptors in Parkinson's Disease and Huntington's Chorea: A Compensatory Mechanism?

*Kenneth G. Lloyd and Lynne Davidson

Department of Psychopharmacology, Clarke Institute of Psychiatry, Toronto, Canada M5T 1R8

The principle of homeostasis is well accepted for the maintenance of sympathetic and/or parasympathetic mediated events (e.g., regulation of cardiovascular function, temperature, or respiration). However, there is no reason a priori to suggest that similar principles are not applicable to higher nervous system function. A logical candidate for a CNS system that undergoes compensatory changes would appear to be the nigrostriato-nigral circuit. Within the striatum it appears very likely that the nigrostriatal dopamine (DA) neurons terminate *(inter alia)* on cholinergic interneurons, which themselves participate in the local control of striatal DA release (cf. 20). Other neurons controlling striatal DA release probably include those using GABA or glutamate (20,31). Additionally, there is a complex feedback loop from the caudate–putamen–pallidum to the substantia nigra with GABA, substance P, and probably other transmitters participating in the regulation of DA cell body activity (7,17,20).

Evidence from animal experiments suggests that the nigrostriato–nigral circuit can, in response to various insults, undergo compensatory changes that allow the system as a whole to function normally. For example, the tolerance to haloperidol catalepsy observed on chronic administration is highly correlated with a specific alteration in striatal acetylcholine synthesis. This suggests that compensatory changes in striatal cholinergic neuron activity participate in the reduction of catalepsy (28).

The present study has tried to determine if alterations in GABA neuron function in extrapyramidal diseases (e.g., Parkinson's disease, Huntington's chorea) are part of a homeostatic compensation mechanism or if they are a reflection of cell loss.

MATERIALS AND METHODS

Human brains were collected, frozen, and dissected as described previously (21). L-Glutamic acid decarboxylase (GAD) activity was estimated by the pro-

---

* Present address: Department of Biology, Neuropharmacology Unit, Synthélabo-L.E.R.S., 31, ave Paul Vaillant Couturier, 92220 Bagneux, France.

duction of $^{14}CO_2$ from glutamic acid-1-$^{14}COOH$ (24) and ^3H-GABA binding was measured by a modification (27) of the procedure of Enna and Snyder (11). For incubation of the membranes for ^3H-GABA binding with Triton-X-100 (0.02%) or phospholipase C (0.001 U, Serdary Research Laboratories), the frozen cerebellar tissue was homogenized (Polytron) in potassium phosphate buffer (0.02 M, pH 7.0) containing either Triton-X-100 or phospholipase C and then incubated for 30 min at 37°C. The material was then centrifuged (48.000 $\times$ g $\times$ 15 min) and the normal assay procedure continued.

RESULTS AND DISCUSSION

Parkinson's Disease

There is evidence that compensation can occur in response to nigrostriatal DA neuron loss [the underlying neurochemical deficit in Parkinson's disease, (14,21)]. Thus, clinically evident symptoms of Parkinson's disease are usually seen with a striatal DA loss of 60% or greater (cf. 19), implying that the brain can compensate for the loss of a large number of DA neurons before clinical pathology becomes evident. This compensation probably involves hyperactivity of the remaining DA neurons as suggested by the elevation in the ratios of homovanillic acid (HVA):DA and tyrosine hydroxylase:DOPA decarboxylase in striatum and substantia nigra from parkinsonian brains, as compared to controls (Table 1). This implies that DA is being synthesized, released, and metabolized more rapidly in the parkinsonian brain, a conclusion supported by the observation that after partial lesion by 6-OHDA of the nigrostriatal DA tract in the rat, the remaining DA neurons are hyperactive (1).

Although these observations indicate that compensation for DA neuron loss can take place, they do not provide evidence that GABA is involved. There are ample data showing that a GABA-mediated inhibitory path originates in the striatum-pallidum and terminates in the substantia nigra (cf. 26). Furthermore, these strionigral GABA neurons terminate *(inter alia)* on DA cell bodies as indicated by the loss of ^3H-GABA receptor binding in parkinsonian substantia nigra (27,36), where the major morphological alteration is the loss of DA cell bodies (14). This alteration in ^3H-GABA binding is not reversed by the administration of antiparkinsonian drugs (36) (Table 2). Such a loss of ^3H-GABA binding is not observed in the caudate nucleus or putamen from parkinsonian patients (27,35,36). Evidence from animal models supports the hypothesis that GABA-mediated events are involved in the regulation of extrapyramidal function: (a) the catalepsy induced by haloperidol is augmented by diverse GABA mimetics (which alone are devoid of cataleptogenic activity), and compounds that reduce GABA-ergic transmission reduce haloperidol-induced catalepsy (39); (b) when administered alone, muscimol (a GABA-mimetic) does not alter the firing rate of DA neurons in the substantia nigra, but is effective in reversing the enhanced firing rate induced by haloperidol (38); (c) compensation occurs

TABLE 1. Ratios of HVA:DA and tyrosine hydroxylase:DOPA decarboxylase (TH:DOPA D) in striatum and substantia nigra from control and parkinsonian patients[a]

	Caudate nucleus		Putamen		Substantia nigra	
	Control	Parkinson's disease (nonDOPA)	Control	Parkinson's disease (nonDOPA)	Control	Parkinson's disease (nonDOPA)
HVA:DA ratio	0.83 ± 11 (15)	16.9 ± 6.3[c] (3)	0.89 ± 0.10 (15)	8.76 ± 3.6[c] (3)	1.94 (1)	15.50 (1)
% control						799
TH:DOPA D ratio	0.062 ± 0.010 (10)	0.170 ± 0.026[c] (3)	0.052 ± 0.011 (10)	0.218 ± 0.069[b] (3)	—	—
% control		274		419		

[a]Results expressed as mean ± SEM. Number of brains examined is in parentheses. Data from ref. 19.
[b]$p < 0.05$ vs. controls.
[c]$p < 0.01$ vs. controls.

TABLE 2. *Analysis of ³H-GABA binding in the substantia nigra of parkinsonian patients[a]*

Patient group	³H-GABA binding (fmoles/mg protein)	% Control	Significance
Controls	30.8 ± 5.0 (11)	100	—
Parkinson's disease			
untreated	nd	0	
amantadine	3.7	12.0	
anticholinergics	8.3	26.9	
receiving L-DOPA	15.4 ± 1.8 (3)	50.0	<0.05
all Parkinson's disease	9.7 ± 2.9 (6)	31.5	<0.001

[a] Data expressed as mean $\pm$ SEM. Number of brains examined is in parentheses. nd, not detectable.

to the acute L-DOPA or haloperidol-induced alterations in nigral GABA levels, as shown by the tolerance observed on chronic daily administration of these drugs (25).

It has been reported by several independent investigators that GAD, the enzyme that synthesizes GABA from glutamate, is deficient in some extrapyramidal regions of brains from non-L-DOPA treated parkinsonian patients (4,26, 30,37). These alterations are most notable in the caudate nucleus, putamen, and substantia nigra, although they also occur in the globus pallidus. In patients treated chronically with L-DOPA, the activity of GAD in the striatum is greater than in nonDOPA-treated patients (23) and these changes in GAD activity are positively correlated with the duration of L-DOPA therapy ($p < 0.02$) (Fig. 1). Since there is no consistent neuropathology of the striatum in Parkinson's disease (31), it is possible that reintroduction of DA receptor stimulation leads to an activation of quiescent striatal GABA neurons (see below).

From these observations it is proposed that *(inter alia)* the nigral DA cell bodies are normally inhibited by a GABA-mediated synapse, likely of striatal and/or pallidal origin. In cases of hypofunction of the DA nigrostriatal system (as in parkinsonism), there is a compensatory decrease of the GABA-mediated inhibition allowing the DA neurons to fire more rapidly, releasing more DA in an attempt to overcome the deficit at the striatal DA synapse. Interference with this compensatory mechanism (e.g., by maintaining GABA-receptor stimulation by GABA agonists) enhances the extrapyramidal dysfunction.

Huntington's Chorea

Huntington's chorea is an inherited disorder for which the neuropathology (severe neuronal loss and gliosis in the striatum) and symptomatology (hyperkinetic movements and dementia) are in marked contrast to those observed in the parkinsonian patient. Furthermore, in Parkinson's disease, the nigrostriatal DA path has degenerated (14,21), whereas in Huntington's chorea the concentrations of DA, its metabolites, and related enzymes appear to be within the normal

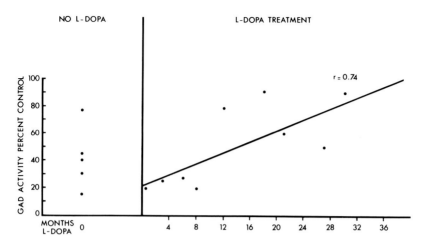

FIG. 1. GAD activity in the putamen of patients with Parkinson's disease. (Data from refs. 23 and 24.)

range or at most slightly decreased (5,6,30). However, in both Huntington's chorea (6,30) and Parkinson's disease (see above) similar alterations in GAD activity occur in the striatum and substantia nigra. As GABA cell bodies are said to be densely concentrated in the striatum (29), and as most striatal neurons (32) as well as GAD activity are lost in Huntington's chorea, it follows that a primary loss of striatal GABA neurons occurs in this disease. This is in contrast to the proposed compensatory decrease in GABA neuron activity (but not actual loss) occurring in Parkinson's disease (see above).

If the above reasoning is correct, then GABA-replacement therapy appears a logical proposal in Huntington's chorea. However, dipropylacetate (a GABA transaminase inhibitor), imidazoleacetic acid and muscimol (direct GABA agonists), and GABA itself have all failed to ameliorate Huntington's chorea (8,9). On the other hand, isoniazid (a GABA transaminase inhibitor) (34) and SL 76 002 (a GABA mimetic) (3) have been reported to be of benefit. It is noteworthy that in the latter study only patients with recently emerged disease benefited from treatment, whereas chronic patients were not aided.

The general lack of clinical effect of GABA-related drugs could be due to the loss of GABA receptors as part of the disease process. Although the initial report (10) on ^{3}H-GABA binding indicated a nonsignificant decrease, a second study (23) showed a large, highly significant loss of ^{3}H-GABA binding sites in the caudate nucleus and putamen. Recently, a third study has appeared indicating a variable but severe loss of ^{3}H-GABA binding sites in the striatum (16). A loss of striatal GABA receptors is consistent with the massive striatal degeneration occurring in Huntington's disease, and with the observation that after chronic degeneration of the striatum following kainic acid treatment (an animal model for Huntington's chorea), there is a large loss of ^{3}H-GABA binding sites (40). A progressive loss of striatal GABA receptors may explain the success of GABA mimetics in early therapy of Huntington's disease and their ineffectiveness in chronic patients.

In order to study the functional state of the remaining GABA receptors in the Huntington's brain the cerebellar cortex has been used. This is necessary as, owing to massive degeneration, there is insufficient striatal material to perform a kinetic analysis. This tissue has previously been utilized for the pharmacological characterization of ^{3}H-GABA binding in the human brain (15,22). In membranes prepared from cerebellar cortex from Huntington's patients, the affinity of ^{3}H-GABA binding (analyzed by IC_{50}, Lineweaver-Burk or Scatchard plots) is significantly enhanced (Table 3) as compared to that in normal brains. This suggests that in the Huntington's brain, the GABA receptor is functional at the lower concentrations of GABA that occur in this disease (33). This affinity change could be either a compensatory mechanism (i.e., supersensitivity) to the decreased GABA neuron function or it could be an integral part of the disease process.

This question may be partially answered by studying the effect of Triton-X-100 on ^{3}H-GABA binding in Huntington's disease. In the rat brain (12) and normal human brain (22) (Table 3), low concentrations (0.02–0.05%) of this nonionic detergent greatly increase the affinity of ^{3}H-GABA binding. The resultant K_d is very similar to that observed for Huntington's brains (Table 3). When membranes from Huntington's cerebellar cortex are treated with Triton-X-100 the affinity of ^{3}H-GABA binding is unaltered. This suggests that the membrane component extracted from the control membranes by Triton-X is missing or altered in the Huntington's material. As Triton-X-100 will remove lipids from the membranes, the effect of phospholipase C on ^{3}H-GABA binding was assessed. Preincubation with this enzyme markedly increased the affinity of ^{3}H-GABA

TABLE 3. *Dissociation constants for ^{3}H-GABA binding to cerebellar membranes prepared from control or Huntington's patients: effect of Triton-X-100 or phospholipase C pretreatment*

Pretreatment	Control patients			Huntington's chorea		
	IC_{50} (nM)	K_d (LWB) (nM)	K_d (Scatchard) (nM)	IC_{50} (nM)	K_d (LWB) (nM)	K_d (Scatchard) (nM)
Untreated tissue	171 ± 13 (29)	179 ± 30 (9)	200 ± 69 (9)	39 ± 7[b] (21)	36 ± 6[b] (8)	39 ± 7[a] (8)
Triton-X-100 (0.02%)	42 ± 5[d] (4)	29 ± 6[d] (4)	34 ± 4[c] (4)	43 ± 7 (5)	32 ± 4 (5)	32 ± 3 (5)
Phospholipase C (0.001 U)	39 ± 5[d] (4)	49 ± 4[d] (4)	43 ± 7[c] (4)	37 ± 2 (5)	26 ± 5[a] (5)	25 ± 4[a] (5)

Results are expressed as mean ± SEM with number of brains examined in parentheses. LWB, Lineweaver-Burk plot.
[a] $p < 0.05$ as compared to controls.
[b] $p < 0.01$ as compared to controls.
[c] $p < 0.05$ as compared to untreated patients.
[d] $p < 0.01$ as compared to untreated patients.

binding to control membranes but only slightly altered ^{3}H-GABA binding to Huntington's membranes (Table 3). Such an effect of phospholipase C on binding of ^{3}H-GABA to rat membranes (using a different preparation) has previously been noted (13).

These findings would indicate that the changes observed in ^{3}H-GABA binding in Huntington's chorea are associated with an alteration in a lipid component of the membrane, possibly a phospholipid. It is possible that the accessibility to the GABA site of highly lipophobic molecules (such as GABA) is controlled by these phospholipids, and their removal results in easier access to the GABA site, with an apparent change in binding affinity. Such a physiological regulation of receptor function does not seem limited to GABA, since other neurotransmitter receptors are also influenced by changes in their phospholipid milieu (e.g., 2,18).

CONCLUSIONS

In Parkinson's disease, the decreases in striatal and nigral GAD activity observed in non-L-DOPA-treated patients appear to be a compensatory change, an attempt to maintain nigrostriatal DA transmission. In contrast, the loss of GAD activity in Huntington's chorea is likely due to a primary loss of GABA neurons. The alterations of ^{3}H-GABA binding in the substantia nigra in Parkinson's disease likely reflects the loss of DA cell bodies with attached GABA receptors. In Huntington's chorea the affinity changes in ^{3}H-GABA binding may be caused by the alterations in the phospholipids of the membrane near the receptor. This could imply that phospholipids normally play a role in the functional activity of the GABA receptor.

REFERENCES

1. Agid, Y., Javoy, F., and Glowinski, J. (1973): Hyperactivity of remaining dopaminergic neurons after partial destruction of the nigrostriatal dopaminergic system in the rat. *Nature (New Biol.)*, 245:150–151.
2. Aronstam, R. S., Abood, L. G., and Baumgold, J. (1977): Role of phospholipids in muscarinic binding by neural membranes. *Biochem. Pharmacol.*, 26:1689–1695.
3. Bartholini, G., Scatton, B., Zivkovic, B., and Lloyd, K. G. (1979): On the mode of action of SL 76 002, a new GABA receptor agonist. In: *GABA-Neurotransmitters*, edited by H. Kofod, P. Krogsgaard-Larsen, and J. Scheel-Kruger, pp. 326–339. Munksgaard, Copenhagen.
4. Bernheimer, H., and Hornykiewicz, O. (1962): Das Verhalten einiger Enzyme im Gehirn normaler und Parkinsonkranken Menschen. *Arch. Exp. Pathol.*, 243:295.
5. Bernheimer, H., and Hornykiewicz, O. (1973): Brain amines in Huntington's chorea. In: *Advances in Neurology, Vol. 1: Huntington's Chorea, 1872–1972*, edited by A. Barbeau, T. N. Chase, and G. W. Paulson, pp. 525–531. Raven Press, New York.
6. Bird, E. D, and Iversen, L. L. (1974): Huntington's chorea. *Brain*, 97:457–472.
7. Brownstein, M. J., Mroz, E. A., Tappaz, M. L., and Leeman, S. E. (1977): On the origin of substance P and glutamic acid decarboxylase (GAD) in the substantia nigra. *Brain Res.*, 135:315–323.
8. Chase, T. N., and Tamminga, C. A. (1979): GABA system participation in human motor, cognitive and endocrine function. In: *GABA-Neurotransmitters*, edited by H. Kofod, P. Krogsgaard-Larsen, and J. Schell-Kruger, pp. 283–294. Munksgaard, Copenhagen.

9. Chase, T. N., and Walters, J. R. (1976): Pharmacologic approaches to the manipulation of GABA-mediated synaptic function in man. In: *GABA in Nervous System Function,* edited by E. Roberts, T. N. Chase, and D. B. Tower, pp. 497–513. Raven Press, New York.

10. Enna, S. J., Bennett, J. P., Bylund, D. B., Snyder, S. H., Bird, E. D., and Iversen, L. L. (1976): Alterations of brain neurotransmitter receptor binding in Huntington's chorea. *Brain Res.,* 116:531–537.

11. Enna, S. J., and Snyder, S. H. (1975): Properties of gamma-aminobutyric acid (GABA) receptor binding in rat brain synaptic membrane fractions. *Brain Res.,* 100:81–98.

12. Enna, S. J., and Snyder, S. H. (1977): Influences of ions, enzymes and detergents on gamma-aminobutyric acid-receptor binding in synaptic membranes of rat brain. *Molec. Pharmacol.,* 13:442–453.

13. Giambalvo, C. T., and Rosenberg, P. (1976): The effect of phospholipases and proteases on the binding of gama-aminobutyric acid to functional complexes of rat cerebellum. *Biochem. Biophys. Acta,* 436:741–756.

14. Hornykiewicz, O. (1966): Dopamine (3-hydroxytyramine) and brain function. *Pharmacol. Rev.,* 18:925–964.

15. Iversen, L. L. (1978): The biochemical psychopharmacology of GABA. In: *Psychopharmacology: A Generation of Progress,* edited by M. A. Lipton, A. DiMascio, and K. F. Killam, pp. 25–38. Raven Press, New York.

16. Iversen, L. L., Bird, E. D., and Spokes, E. G. (1978): GABA in Huntington's disease and schizophrenia. *Seventh International Congress of Pharmacology,* Abstract No. 2475.

17. Kanazawa, I., Emson, P. C., and Cuello, A. C. (1977): Evidence for the existence of substance P-containing fibres in striato-nigral and pallido-nigral pathways in rat brain. *Brain Res.* 119:447–453.

18. Limbird, L. E., and Lefkowitz, R. J. (1976): Adenylate cyclase-coupled beta adrenergic receptors: effect of membrane lipid-pertubing agents on receptor binding and enzyme stimulation by catecholamines. *Mol. Pharmacol.,* 12:559–567.

19. Lloyd, K. G. (1977): Neurochemical compensation in Parkinson's disease. In: *Parkinson's Disease: Concepts and Prospects,* edited by J. P. W. F. Lakke, J. Korf, and H. Wesseling, pp. 61–72. Excerpta Medica, Amsterdam.

20. Lloyd, K. G. (1978): Neurotransmitter interactions related to central dopamine neurons. In: *Essays in Neurochemistry and Neuropharmacology, Vol. 3,* edited by M. B. H. Youdim, W. Lovenberg, D. F. Sharman, and J. R. Lagnado, pp. 129–207. Wiley, New York.

21. Lloyd, K. G., Davidson, L., and Hornykiewicz, O. (1975): The Neurochemistry of Parkinson's disease: effect of L-DOPA therapy, *J. Pharmacol. Exp. Ther.,* 195:453–464.

22. Lloyd, K. G., and Dreksler, S. (1979): Analysis of ^{3}H-gamma-aminobutyric acid (GABA) binding in the human brain. *Brain Res.,* 163:77–87.

23. Lloyd, K. G., Dreksler, S., and Bird, E. D. (1977): Alterations in ^{3}H-GABA binding in Huntington's chorea. *Life Sci.,* 21:747–754.

24. Lloyd, K. G. and Hornykiewicz, O. (1973): L-Glutamic acid decarboxylase in Parkinson's disease: effect of L-DOPA therapy. *Nature,* 243:521–523.

25. Lloyd, K. G., and Hornykiewicz, O. (1977): Effect of chronic neuroleptic or L-DOPA administration on GABA levels in the rat substantia nigra. *Life Sci.,* 21:1489–1496.

26. Lloyd, K. G., Möhler, H., Bartholini, G., and Hornykiewicz, O. (1976): Pathological alterations in glutamic acid decarboxylase activity in Parkinson's disease. In: *Advances in Parkinsonism,* edited by W. Birkmayer and O. Hornykiewicz, pp. 186–192. Editions Roche, Basle.

27. Lloyd, K. G., Shemen, L., and Hornykiewicz, O. (1977): Distribution of high affinity sodium-independent [^{3}H] gamma-aminobutyric acid ([^{3}H]GABA) binding in the human brain: alterations in Parkinson's disease. *Brain Res.,* 127:269–278.

28. Lloyd, K. G., Shibuya, M., Davidson, L., and Hornykiewicz, O. (1977): Chronic neuroleptic therapy: tolerance and GABA systems. In: *Advances in Biochemical Psychopharmacology, Vol. 16,* edited by E. Costa and G. L. Gessa, pp. 409–415. Raven Press, New York.

29. McGeer, P. L., and McGeer, E. G. (1975): Evidence for glutamic acid decarboxylase-containing interneurons in the striatum. *Brain Res.,* 91:331–335.

30. McGeer, P. L., and McGeer, E. G. (1976): Enzymes associated with the metabolism of catecholamines, acetylcholine and GABA in human controls and patients with Parkinson's disease and Huntington's chorea. *J. Neurochem.,* 26:65–76.

31. McGeer, P. L., McGeer, E. G., Scherer, U., and Singh, K. (1977): A glutaminergic corticostriatal path? *Brain Res.,* 128:369–373.

32. Oppenheimer, D. R. (1976): Diseases of the basal ganglia, cerebellum and motor neurons. In: *Greenfield's Neuropathology,* edited by W. A. Blackwood and J. A. N. Corsellis, pp. 608–651. Arnold, London.
33. Perry, T. L., Hansen, S., Lesk, D., and Kloster, M. (1973): Amino acids in plasma, cerebrospinal fluid and brain of patients with Huntington's chorea. In: *Advances in Neurology, Vol. 1: Huntington's Chorea, 1872–1972,* edited by A. Barbeau, T. N. Chase, and G. W. Paulson, pp. 609–618. Raven Press, New York.
34. Perry, T. L., MacLeod, P. M., and Hansen, S. (1977): Treatment of Huntington's chorea with isoniazid, *N. Engl. J. Med.,* 297:840.
35. Reisine, T. D., Fields, J. Z., Yamamura, H. I., Bird, E. D., Spokes, E., Schreiner, P. S., and Enna, S. J. (1977): Neurotransmitter receptor alterations in Parkinson's disease, *Life Sci.,* 21:335–344.
36. Rinne, U. K., Roskinen, V., Laaksonen, H., Lönnberg, P., and Sonninen, V. (1978): GABA receptor binding in the parkinsonian brain, *Life Sci.,* 22:2225–2228.
37. Rinne, U. K., Sonninen, V., Riekkenen, P., and Laaksonen, H. (1974): Dopaminergic nervous transmission in Parkinson's disease. *Med. Biol.,* 52:208–217.
38. Walters, J. R., Lakoski, J. M., and Eng, N. (1978): Effect of muscimol, AOAA and Na valproate on the activity of dopamine neurons and dopamine synthesis. In: *GABA-Neurotransmitters, Vol. 30,* edited by H. Kofod, P. Krogsgaard-Larsen, and J. Scheel-Kruger, pp. 716–718. Munksgaard, Copenhagen.
39. Worms, P., Willigens, M. T., and Lloyd, K. G. (1978): GABA involvement in neuroleptic-induced catalepsy. *J. Pharm. Pharmacol.,* 30:716–718.
40. Zaczek, R., Schwarcz, R., and Coyle, J. T. (1978): Long-term sequelae of striatal kainic lesion. *Brain Res.,* 152:626–632.

Advances in Neurology, Vol. 24, edited by
L. J. Poirier, T. L. Sourkes, and P. J. Bédard.
Raven Press, New York © 1979.

Analysis of Hydroxylase Cofactor Activity in the Cerebrospinal Fluid of Patients with Parkinson's Disease

*,†R. A. Levine, **A. C. Williams, †D. S. Robinson, **D. B. Calne, and †W. Lovenburg

†*Section on Biochemical Pharmacology, National Heart, Lung, and Blood Institute;*
***Experimental Therapeutics Branch, IRP, National Institute of Neurological and Communicative Disorders and Stroke, NIH, Bethesda, Maryland 20014*

The neurological manifestations of Parkinson's disease are thought to be largely related to the loss of dopaminergic function in the central nervous system. It is now well known that the synthesis of dopamine is dependent upon the activity of tyrosine hydroxylase, and this in turn, is regulated by the concentration of hydroxylase cofactor in the cells (11). Tetrahydrobiopterin (BH_4) is thought to be the naturally occurring cofactor (1). In recent studies in our laboratory, we have established an assay procedure that is sufficiently sensitive to measure the hydroxylase cofactor activity in cerebrospinal fluid (CSF) (12). Since the cofactor content of the CSF may reflect numbers of aminergic neurons or the activity state of these neurons, it was of interest to examine CSF cofactor content in patients with Parkinson's disease and in age-matched normal subjects. In the current work we have observed that while there is an inverse correlation of hydroxylase cofactor activity in the CSF with age, there is also a significant reduction in CSF hydroxylase cofactor in patients with Parkinson's disease.

METHODS

Patients

The patient population consisted of patients with untreated Parkinson's disease. The control subjects had no neurological or psychiatric disease. Patients and controls were excluded if their CSF protein or cell count was abnormal.

Specimens

CSF was obtained by lumbar puncture, which was performed at 9 A.M. after overnight bedrest. All patients and controls had been on a standard diet with

---

* A predoctoral student in the Department of Pharmacology, The George Washington University Medical Center, Washington, D.C.

a low monoamine content for the previous 48 hr. A series of 2-ml aliquots of CSF were collected from each patient, immediately frozen on Dry Ice, and placed in liquid nitrogen storage until the time of assay. The 4th to the 6th ml of CSF removed were used for the homovanillic acid (HVA) and 5-hydroxyindoleacetic acid (5-HIAA) estimations, and the 13th to the 15th ml for the hydroxylase cofactor determinations. Five milligrams of ascorbic acid were placed in the tube containing the HVA and 5-HIAA aliquot. Clinical information was withheld from the analytical laboratory until assays were completed.

Assays

The assay for hydroxylase cofactor content in the CSF was a modification of the radioenzymatic method described by Guroff et al. (6). This assay, which utilizes a phenylalanine hydroxylation system, has been modified to obtain the necessary sensitivity for measuring cofactor content in the CSF. Details of this assay will be described elsewhere (12). HVA and 5-HIAA levels were measured by a gas chromatographic–mass spectroscopic method (4,14).

RESULTS

This modified hydroxylation system provided the necessary sensitivity to determine hydroxylase cofactor activity in all CSF samples assayed. As seen in Table 1, the cofactor content in the CSF of parkinsonian patients was significantly lower than in control patients ($p < 0.001$). These data represent only those parkinsonian patients for whom there were age-matched controls. The mean for the normal subjects was 17.7 pmoles/ml with a range of 10.3 to 25.2 pmoles/ml. The mean for the patients with Parkinson's disease was 8.9 pmoles/ml with a range of 7.2 to 14.4 pmoles/ml.

In an attempt to determine whether a relationship exists between hydroxylase cofactor in the CSF and central aminergic activity, we measured the CSF content of HVA and 5-HIAA. (These compounds are the major metabolites of dopamine and serotonin, respectively.) In this study we combined parkinsonian patients and normal subjects regardless of age. With 35 subjects there was a significant correlation of cofactor and HVA content ($r = 0.73$, $p < 0.001$) but not with cofactor and 5-HIAA.

In Fig. 1, CSF cofactor content has been analyzed as a function of age in the normal controls. There is a significant correlation with age ($r = -0.48$, $p < 0.01$) with a trend for levels to decline between the ages of 20 and 60.

DISCUSSION

The low hydroxylase cofactor levels seen in the CSF of patients with Parkinson's disease, a disease known to be associated with degeneration of dopaminergic neurons, supports the suggestion that this measurement could be used as a

TABLE 1. *Hydroxylase cofactor activity in the CSF of age-matched parkinsonian patients and control subjects*

	Mean age	BH$_4$ equivalents (pmoles/ml)
Normal ($n = 10$)	52 ± 2.6	17.72 ± 1.7
Parkinsonian ($n = 10$)	52 ± 4.0	8.93 ± 0.95

The hydroxylase cofactor activity of CSF was quantified by comparison to BH$_4$ standards. The samples were analyzed in triplicate and are given as the mean $\pm$ SEM for each group of age matched patients.

reflection of central aminergic activity. Corroborative evidence is derived from the good correlation between CSF cofactor content and levels of HVA, the major metabolite of dopamine. The lack of correlation with the predominant metabolite of serotonin, 5-HIAA, is at first glance surprising, since BH$_4$ is also the hydroxylase cofactor involved in the synthesis of serotonin. However, two possible explanations for this discrepancy arise. First, there is evidence that CSF 5-HIAA may be a poor reflection of the metabolic turnover of serotonin (5). Second, it has been suggested, based on a variety of experimental evidence, that BH$_4$ may be of less critical importance for serotonin synthesis than it is for dopamine synthesis (2).

The decreased CSF cofactor levels seen in Parkinson's disease are most likely

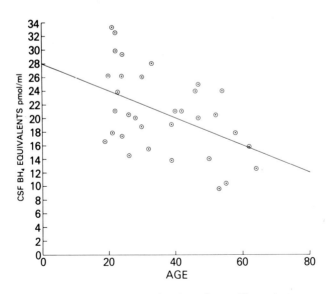

FIG. 1. Hydroxylase cofactor activity as a function of age. The cofactor was analyzed as described in the Methods section and expressed as tetrahydrobiopterin equivalents based on the use of authentic tetrahydropterin standards.

to reflect reduced dopamine metabolism resulting from a loss of dopaminergic neurons from an unknown cause. However, a more fundamental role for BH_4 should be considered. For instance, low BH_4 levels due to a failure of its synthesis could lead to reduced dopamine synthesis, and conceivably eventual death of dopaminergic neurons and clinical parkinsonism. It is of interest in this regard that two rare forms of phenylketonuria have been described (7,8). One is caused by a genetic deficiency of quinoid dihydropteridine reductase; this enzyme is required for the regeneration of active BH_4 from its inactive oxidized state. The children with this disease (8) have low HVA and 5-HIAA in both CSF and brain, although they do not exhibit parkinsonian features or any response to L-DOPA therapy. More recently, a patient with another variant form of phenylketonuria having reduced tissue content of hydroxylase cofactor has been described (7); this patient had severe neurological deficiencies without definite parkinsonism, although it is of interest that he developed dyskinesia upon treatment with L-DOPA. It is possible that in some patients with Parkinson's disease, similar but less severe mechanisms are involved.

The possibility of attempting to alter brain BH_4 levels for therapeutic purposes should be considered as increased dopamine synthesis after intraventricular injection of BH_4 has been demonstrated in animals (9). Increasing BH_4 levels in patients with Parkinson's disease might increase dopamine synthesis, and hopefully, the firing rates of the surviving dopaminergic neurons. BH_4 does not readily cross the blood–brain barrier; hence, systemic therapy is unlikely to be effective unless a more lipophilic active analog could be developed. Alternatively, one might be able to increase synthesis of BH_4 by increasing the brain concentration of its precursors or by increasing the activity of the synthetic enzymes involved. It is of interest that Leeming et al. (10) have recently shown that administration of phenylalanine elevates serum levels of biopterin, possibly by stimulating its biosynthesis. Lastly, it might be possible to increase the rate of reduction of the inactive pterin to active BH_4 by increasing the activity of the enzyme quinoid dihydropteridine reductase.

The reduction of CSF hydroxylase cofactor levels with age is of interest as it provides *in vivo* confirmation of the previously reported reduction of dopaminergic neurons, tyrosine hydroxylase activity, and dopamine concentration in brain with increasing age (3,13). Whether this natural loss of dopaminergic neurons is due to some intrinsic property of these cells or due to their increased or selective vulnerability to some external agent is unclear. It is also uncertain whether this normal loss of dopaminergic neurons with age is of any functional importance, since there may be compensatory mechanisms such as the loss of other neuronal systems with age. It would be of interest to determine if in Parkinson's disease this rate of loss of dopaminergic neurons was accelerated. If this were the case, it would imply that there was an active pathological process at work rather than a normal aging process superimposed upon a deficit of dopaminergic cells acquired at some time earlier in life.

ACKNOWLEDGMENT

We should like to thank our patients for their cooperation in this study and Nancy Salamandra who gave excellent secretarial assistance.

REFERENCES

1. Brenneman, A. R., and Kaufman, S. (1964): The role of tetrahydropteridines in the enzymatic conversion of tyrosine to dopa. *Biochem. Biophys. Res. Comm.,* 17:177–183.
2. Bullard, W. P., Guthrie, P. B., Russo, P. B., and Mandell, A. J. (1978): Regional and subcellular distribution and some factors in the regulation of reduced pterins in rat brain. *J. Pharmacol. Exp. Ther.,* 206:4–20.
3. Carlsson, A., and Winblad, B. (1976): Influence of age and time interval between death and autopsy on dopamine and 3-methoxytyramine levels in human basal ganglia. *J. Neural Transm.,* 38:271–276.
4. Gordon, E. K., Oliver, J., Black, K., and Kopin, I. J. (1974): Simultaneous assay by mass fragmentography of vanillyl mandelic acid, homovanillic acid, and 3-methoxy-4-hydroxy-phenyl-ethylene glycol in cerebrospinal fluid and urine. *Biochem. Med.,* 11:32–40.
5. Green, A. R., Grahame-Smith, D. G. (1975): 5-Hydroxytryptamine and other indoles in the central nervous system. In: *Handbook of Psychopharmacology,* edited by L. L. Iverson, S. D. Iverson, and S. H. Snyder, pp. 169–245. Plenum Press, New York.
6. Guroff, G., Rhoads, C. A., and Abramowitz, A. (1967): A simple radioisotope assay for phenyl-alanine hydroxylase cofactor. *Anal. Biochem.,* 21:273–278.
7. Kaufman, S., Berlow, S., Summer, G., Milstien, S., Schulman, J., Orloff, S., Spielberg, S., and Pueschel, S. (1978): Hyperphenylalinemia due to a deficiency of biopterin. *N. Engl. J. Med.,* 299; 673–679.
8. Kaufman, S., Holtzman, N. A., Milstien, S., Butler, I., and Krumholz, A. (1975): Phenylketon-uria due to a deficiency of dihydropteridine reductase. *N. Engl. J. Med.,* 293:785–790.
9. Kettler, R., Bartholini, G., and Pletscher, A. (1974): *In vivo* enhancement of tyrosine hydroxyl-ation in rat striatum by tetrahydrobiopterin. *Nature,* 249:476–478.
10. Leeming, R. J., Blair, J. A., Green, A., and Raine, D. N. (1976): Biopterin derivatives in normal and phenylketonuric patients after oral loads of L-phenylalanine, L-tyrosine, and L-tryptophan. *Arch. Dis. Child.* 51:771–777.
11. Lovenberg, W., Ames, M. M., and Lerner, P. (1978): Mechanisms of short-term regulation of tyrosine hydroxylase. In: *Psychopharmacology: A Generation of Progress,* edited by M. A. Lipton, A. DiMascio, and K. F. Killam, pp. 247–259. Raven Press, New York.
12. Lovenberg, W., Levine, R. A., Robinson, D. R., Ebert, M., Williams, A. C., and Calne, D. B. (1979): Hydroxylase cofactor activity in cerebrospinal fluid of normal subjects and patients with Parkinson's disease. *Science,* 204:624–626.
13. McGeer, P. L., McGeer, E. G., and Suzuki, J. S. (1977): Aging and extrapyramidal function. *Arch. Neurol.,* 34:33–35.
14. Watson, E., Wilk, S., and Roboz, J. (1974): Derivatization and gas chromatographic determina-tion of some biologically important acids in cerebrospinal fluid. *Anal. Biochem.,* 59:441–451.

Advances in Neurology, Vol. 24, edited by
L. J. Poirier, T. L. Sourkes, and P. J. Bédard.
Raven Press, New York © 1979.

Plasmatic Renin Activity in Parkinsonism

*H. Allain, *J. Van den Driessche, and **O. Sabouraud

*Laboratoire de Pharmacologie, Faculté de Médecine, and **Service de Neurologie, Hôpital
Pontchaillou, Rennes 35000, France

The role of the central nervous system in the regulation of the secretion of renin by the kidney is supported by both pharmacological (6) and electrophysiological evidence (18,21,25,30,31). This regulation brings into play the orthosympathetic nervous system, which stimulates the secretion of renin (20,31). In animals, the administration of L-DOPA in association with an inhibitor of DOPA decarboxylase (IDC) decreases the orthosympathetic tonicity (4,22,29) and the secretion of renin (5). The central effect of the catecholamines is different from the peripheral effect produced by L-DOPA alone (5), dopamine (17), and adrenaline or noradrenaline (27), which, on the contrary, stimulate the secretion of renin by a direct effect on the vessels of the kidney. The dual effect obtained from these experiments explains why inconclusive or contradictory results have been reported concerning the effect of L-DOPA without an inhibitor on plasmatic renin activity (PRA) (24). Therefore, the existence of the relationship between the central catecholaminergic mechanisms and the renal juxtaglomerular system (5) as demonstrated in animals, seemed to justify a new study of PRA in parkinsonism in order to attempt to answer the following questions: (a) Do the variations of PRA represent a reliable criterion for the assessment of the disturbances of the central catecholaminergic activity in untreated parkinsonians? (b) Does L-DOPA–IDC decrease the PRA in patients as it does in animals? (c) If so, does the comparison between the effect of the latter treatment and that of other dopamine agonists contribute to determine whether the central effect is dopaminergic? (d) Could the variations of PRA induce in turn functional side-effects?

METHODOLOGY

PRA was evaluated by radioimmunological assay of the angiotensin I (CIS pack). The results are expressed in nanograms per milliliter per hour of angiotensin I. Eighty-six individuals were involved in this study. The control group includes 17 persons selected from either the families of the patients or other patients receiving no drug and hospitalized for causes not known to affect PRA. In another group of 40 parkinsonians, the basic activity of PRA was measured (static study). This group was divided into three subgroups: 12 patients were untreated; 14 were parkinsonian patients chronically treated by L-DOPA–IDC (they were markedly improved without any side-effects); and 14 were parkinsonians who displayed L-DOPA-induced dyskinesia, although none presented the therapeutic criteria of the "onset and end of dose dyskinesia" (13). The intensity of the dyskinesia was recorded on an arbitrary scale of 0 to 4. No drug other than L-DOPA–IDC was used in this group. The parameters used in this group (static group) include resting PRA (PRA_r), exercise PRA (PRA_e), and the ratio PRA_e/PRA_r. PRA_r was measured on blood samples taken in the morning while the patients were still in bed. In the case of outpatients, the blood sample was withdrawn after 1 hr decubitus. The PRA_e was measured on another blood sample taken in the upright position after a physical exercise. In a third group of 29 patients (dynamic study), PRA was measured in several samples of blood withdrawn before and after the administration per os of a single dose of a dopamine agonist. The first sample of blood was withdrawn before ingestion of the drug while the patients were still in bed. The three other samples were taken 0.5 hr, 1 hr, and 1.5 hr after the administration of the drug, respectively. Out of the 29 parkinsonian patients, 14 patients (9 dyskinetic, 5 stabilized) received 250 mg of L-DOPA–IDC, 10 patients (6 dyskinetic, 4 stabilized) received 7.5 mg of bromocriptine, 5 patients (3 dyskinetic, 2 stabilized) received 50 mg of R.U.24213, a new apomorphine like agent.

Blood pressure was measured under the same conditions as above in the static group of patients. In the dynamic group, blood pressure was measured only in those patients treated with bromocriptine. Blood pressure was also measured during several days and many times a day in a group of 18 dyskinetic parkinsonian patients.

RESULTS

In the first group (the static study), the PRA values are different from one subgroup to the other (Fig. 1, Tables 1 and 2). In the untreated parkinsonians, the PRA_r and PRA_e values are not significantly different from those of the control group. In the treated stabilized parkinsonians, only PRA_e is significantly lower than the value of the control group. PRA_e is lower than the value of the untreated group but it is hardly significant. In the third subgroup (dyskinetic patients), PRA_r and PRA_e are significantly higher than the values in the control group and in the stabilized parkinsonians. Only PRA_e is significantly higher than that of the untreated patients. The ratio is higher in the dyskinetic patients and lower in the stabilized parkinsonians than in the control group of patients. There is a good correlation between the intensity of the dyskinesia and PRA_e as well as PRA_e/PRA_r ratio (Fig. 2).

In the dynamic study (Table 3), the PRA values are modified by the three drugs. After ingestion of 250 mg of L-DOPA–IDC, the PRA is decreased in the five stabilized patients, with a peak half an hour after the drug intake. In the nine dyskinetic patients, the results are scattered. Some patients display a

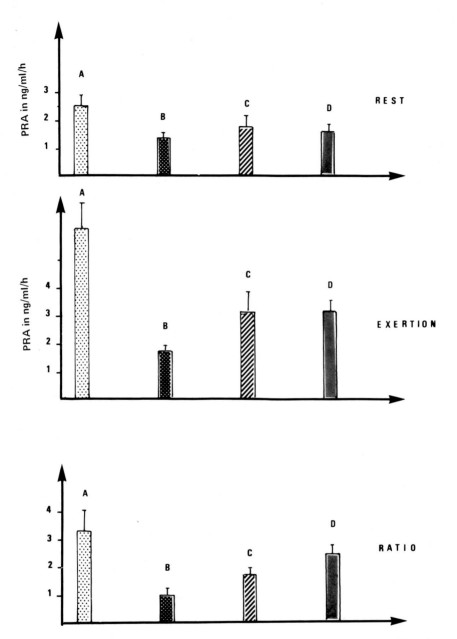

FIG. 1. Results of PRA studies. **A:** dyskinetic parkinsonians. **B:** treated stabilized parkinsonians. **C:** untreated parkinsonians. **D:** controls.

TABLE 1. *Plasmatic renin activity and arterial blood pressure*

Parameters noted	Dyskinetic parkinsons $N=14$	Treated stabilized parkinsons $N=14$	Untreated parkinsons $N=12$	Controls $N=17$	Other patients receiving L-DOPA + IDC
PRA_r	m = 2.552	m = 1.434	m = 1.820	m = 1.545	1.14
	Sm = 0.440	Sm = 0.210	Sm = 0.383	Sm = 0.258	2.58
					4.56
					1.68
					1.38
					1.90
					5.01
PRA_e	m = 6.128	m = 1.748	m = 3.154	m = 3.192	—
	Sm = 0.907	Sm = 0.224	Sm = 0.719	Sm = 0.374	2.63
$R = \dfrac{PRA_e}{PRA_r}$	m = 3.33	m = 1.135	m = 1.667	m = 2.438	1.67
	Sm = 0.732	Sm = 0.157	Sm = 0.232	Sm = 0.279	1.94
Systolic blood pressure					
Rest	m = 12	m = 13.57	m = 14.91		—
	Sm = 0.65	Sm = 0.54	Sm = 0.81		1.90
Exertion	m = 13.28	m = 14.92	m = 15.75		
	Sm = 0.50	Sm = 0.58	Sm = 0.84		

TABLE 2. *Comparison of the PRA figures*

Groups of patients	Dyskinetic parkinsons	Treated stabilized parkinsons	Untreated parkinsons
Treated stabilized	PRA_r[a] $p < 0.05$ PRA_e[a] $p < 0.001$		
Untreated parkinsons	PRA_r[a] ns PRA_e[a] $p < 0.02$	PRA_r ns PRA_e $0.10 < p < 0.05$	
Control	PRA_r[a] $p < 0.05$ PRA_e[a] $p < 0.01$	PRA_r ns PRA_e[a] $p < 0.01$	PRA_r ns PRA_e ns

[a]Student's *t*-test.

decrease of the PRA, but always very slight, whereas the others show an increase of the PRA values, which can be very important especially in the first half hour. After ingestion of 7.5 mg of bromocriptine, the PRA values are homogeneously lowered with a peak 1.5 hr after the drug intake, in the stabilized patients. In the six dyskinetic patients, the values are increased with a still great dispersion. After ingestion of 50 mg RU24213, the PRA is modified. The small number of patients in this subgroup, however, does not permit us to draw firm conclusions or to establish correlations between the PRA values and the state of the patients.

Blood Pressure Study

In the static study, arterial systolic blood pressure is reduced in the parkinsonians treated by L-DOPA–IDC. However, the result is significant only for the dyskinetic group in either supine or upright position (Fig. 3). There is never any correlation between the systolic blood pressure values and the respective values of PRA within each group. The characteristic of the arterial systolic blood pressure in the dyskinetic patients is its instability with sharp hypertensive peaks (Fig. 4). In the dynamic test with bromocriptine, we observe a progressive decrease of systolic and diastolic values significant only for stabilized patients. The lowest values are reached 1.5 hr after drug intake (Fig. 5).

DISCUSSION

In contradistinction to the findings of Barbeau et al. (3) and Michelakis et al. (15), this study does not reveal any decrease in the PRA values in untreated parkinsonians when compared to those of normal subjects. The absence of any marked rise of PRA after exercise in some untreated parkinsonian patients, may be due to the importance of their symptoms. They cannot stand upright for more than a few seconds. The PRA_e values are thus somewhat too low. Treatment of parkinsonians with L-DOPA–IDC results in changes of the PRA values. These changes must be considered as a consequence of the central effect

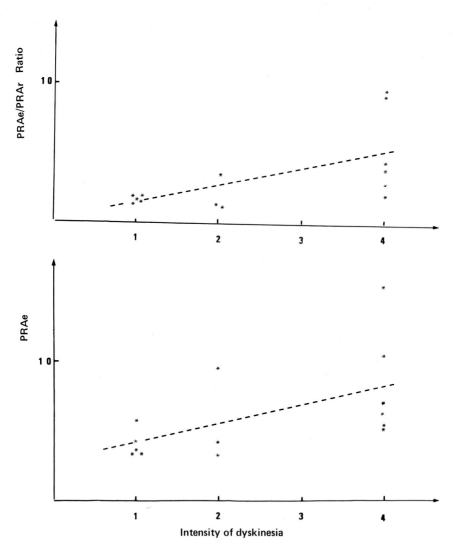

FIG. 2. A: Dyskinesia and Pra_e/PRA_r ratio. $y = 1.27$; $x = 0.15$; $r = 0.65$; and $p < 0.02$. **B:** Dyskinesia and PRA_e ratio. $y = 1.35$; $x = 2.75$; $r = 0.56$; and $p < 0.05$.

of L-DOPA. Similar results obtained with bromocriptine as well as the variations induced by the RU24213 point to a dopaminergic link in these phenomena. We therefore may consider that the PRA reflects the central pharmacological activity of the dopaminergic drugs. In stabilized patients, L-DOPA–IDC lowers the PRA. This result is in accordance with those of Blair et al. (5), Baum et al. (4), and Watanabe et al. (29). The decrease obtained with bromocriptine must be compared with similar results obtained by Nilsson et al. (16) in acromegalics. The results are reversed in dyskinetic patients. In this group the PRA

TABLE 3. *Kinetic values of PRA after drug intake*[a]

Drug/patient	Time after ingestion (hr)		
	0.5	1	1.5
L-DOPA–IDC (250 mg)			
Stabilized	−31.2 ± 7.7	−27.8 ± 6.3	−23 ± 7.2
Dyskinetic	+2.11 ± 11.43	−10 ± 7.9	−5 ± 11.9
Bromocryptine (7.5 mg)			
Stabilized	−35 ± 13.7	−42.8 ± 16	−51.25 ± 20
Dyskinetic	+11.9 ± 9.8	+13.95 ± 18.25	+19.1 ± 29.1
R.U. 24213 (50 mg)			
Stabilized	+0.18	+1.20	+1.26
	−0.18	+0.08	−0.15
Dyskinetic	+0.07	+0.53	+0.97
	+0.06	+0.06	+0.26
	−0.16	−0.13	−0.20

[a] In percent of the initial value ± SE.

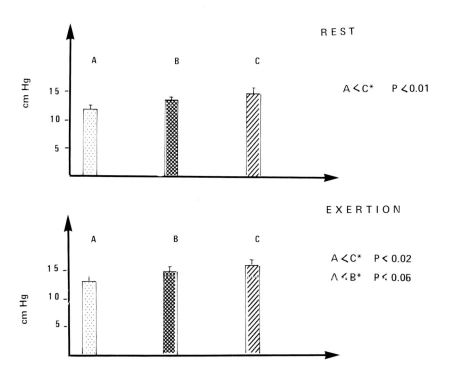

FIG. 3. Systolic arterial pressure in the different groups of parkinsonian patients. **A:** dyskinetic parkinsonians. **B:** treated stabilized parkinsonians. **C:** untreated parkinsonians. All calculations tested by Student's *t*-test.

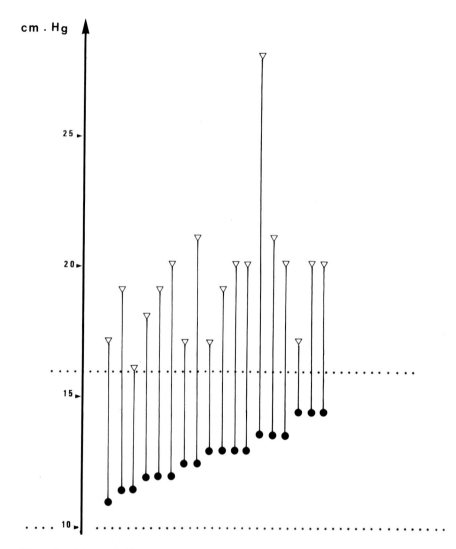

FIG. 4. Arterial systolic blood pressure in dyskinetic parkinsonian patients. *Solid circles:* Mean arterial systolic blood pressure. *Open inverted triangles:* Maximum recorded, at least once. *Asterisks:* superior and inferior limits of basal values. $n = 18$.

values are significantly higher, with a positive correlation between the values of PRA_e or PRA_e/PRA_r and the intensity of dyskinesia. The demonstration of such a difference in physiological response under L-DOPA treatment leads one to reconsider the hypotheses currently proposed to account for L-DOPA-induced dyskinesias. (a) Certain hypotheses state that dyskinetic patients display denervation hypersensitivity (12,26) with hyperreactive receptors. If this was the case, PRA should have been lowered to an even greater extent than in stabilized parkinsonians. Opposite results obtained in this study do not support this hypothesis. (b) The hypothesis of an L-DOPA-induced metabolic deviation characterized by abnormal metabolites (1,14), or topic by-products (19), does not explain why we obtain the same results with bromocriptine and with L-DOPA, unless we suppose that the metabolic error resulting from those two chemical agents is identical. (c) The hypothesis of the preferential stimulation of a second category of dopaminergic receptors (8) would be more logical. Stimulation could take place through the orthosympathetic nerve supply to the kidney, thus increasing the secretion of renin.

The last point to be raised in the discussion concerns the possible effects of

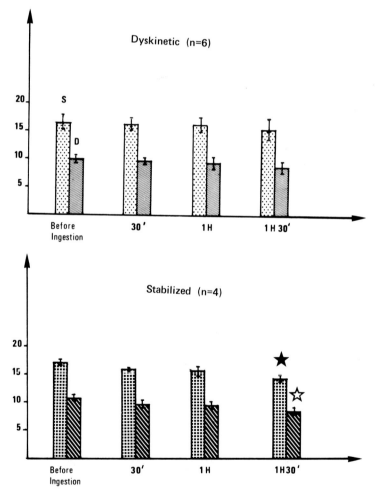

FIG. 5. Blood pressure values after oral intake of bromocryptine (7.5 mg). **S:** Systolic. **D:** diastolic. Significantly lower values; *solid star, $p < 0.01$; open star, $p < 0.05$.*

these variations of PRA in our patients. The excessive PRA of renal origin may have a central action (23) and thus play a role in the L-DOPA-induced dyskinesia. Along this line, it would be of major interest to know whether the abnormalities disclosed in the plasma also occur in the brains of our dyskinetic patients. Under such conditions, the dysfunction underlying dyskinesia may involve, for instance, a peptidergic mechanism. This rather speculative suggestion is supported by the known existence of a brain isorenin angiotensin system (9), its possible role as a modulator of central catecholaminergic transmitters (10), and the established dysfunction of this system in the striatum of choreic patients (2).

The implication of the renin-angiotensin system in the modifications of blood pressure noticed in our patients seems very hypothetical. Our results confirm the preceding reports on the hypotensive action of L-DOPA (7) and of bromocriptine (11,16,28). There is no correlation between the arterial pressure values and those of PRA. Moreover, the dyskinetic parkinsonians whose PRA is high have significantly lower systolic arterial pressure than untreated parkinsonians. PRA in these patients may somehow be related to the corresponding hypertensive variations.

ACKNOWLEDGMENTS

We thank Mrs. Guibert and Mrs. Morin for their technical assistance.

REFERENCES

1. Allain, H. (1977): Etude pharmacologique des stéréotypies induites chez le rat par la L-DOPA associée au Benserazid: Abord comportemental et biochimique. Thèse Médecine, Rennes.
2. Arregui, A., Bennet, J. P., Bird, E. D., Yamamura, H., Iversen, L., and Snyder, S. (1977): Huntington's chorea: selective depletion of activity of angiotensin converting enzyme in the corpus striatum. *Ann. Neurol.,* 2:292–298.
3. Barbeau, A., Gillo-Joffroy L., Boucher, R., Nowaczinski, W., and Genest, J. (1969): Renin-aldosterone system in Parkinson's disease. *Science,* 165:291–292.
4. Baum, T. and Shropshire, A. T. (1973): Reduction of sympathetic outflow by central administration of L-DOPA, dopamine and norepinephrine. *Neuropharmacology,* 12:49–56.
5. Blair, M., Reid, I., and Ganong, W. (1977): Effect of L-DOPA on plasma renin activity with and without inhibition of extracerebral dopa decarboxylase in dogs. *J. Pharmacol. Exp. Ther.,* 202:209–215.
6. Boissier, J., Guidicelli, J., Fichelle, J., Schmitt, H., and Schmitt, H. (1968): Cardiovascular effects of 2-(2,6 dichlorophenylamino-)-2-imidazoline hydrochloride ST 155. I. Peripheral sympathetic system. *Eur. J. Pharmacol.,* 2:333–339.
7. Calne, D. B., and Teychenne, P. F. (1977): L-DOPA effect on blood pressure in man. In: *Progress in Brain Research, Hypertension and Brain Mechanisms, Vol. 47,* edited by W. De Jong, A. Provoost, and A. Shapiro, pp. 331–336. Elsevier Scientific Publishing Co., Amsterdam.
8. Cools, A. R., and Van Rossum, J. M. (1976): Excitation-mediating and inhibition mediating dopamine receptors: a new concept towards a better understanding of electrophysiological, biochemical, pharmacological, functional and clinical data. *Psychopharmacologia,* 45:243–254.
9. Fisher-Ferraro, C., Nahmod, V., Goldstein, D., and Finkielman, S. (1971): Angiotensin and renin in rat and dog brain. *J. Exp. Med.,* 133:353–361.
10. Ganten, D., Fuxe, K., Ganten, U., Hokfelt, T., and Bolme, P. (1977): The brain isorenin-angiotensin system: localization and biological function. In: *Progress in Brain Research, Hypertension and Brain Mechanisms, Vol. 47,* edited by W. De Jong, A. Provoost, and A. Shapiro, pp. 152–159. Elsevier Scientific Publishing Co., Amsterdam.

11. Heise, A. (1976): Hypotensive action by central adrenergic and dopaminergic receptor stimulation. In: *New Antihypertensive Drugs,* edited by A. Scriabine, and C. S. Qweet, pp. 135–145. Spectrum Publications Inc., New York.

12. Klawans, H. L. (1973): The pharmacology of tardive dyskinesia. *Am. J. Psychiatry.,* 130:82–86.

13. Lhermitte, F., Agid, Y., Signoret, J. L., and Studler, J. M. (1977): Les dyskinésies du début et fin de dose provoquées par la L-DOPA. *Rev. Neurol. (Paris),* 133:297–308(b).

14. Lhermitte, F., Rosa, A., and Como, E. (1977): Mouvements anormaux des parkinsoniens traités par la L-DOPA et anomalies du métabolisme de la dopamine. *Rev. Neurol. (Paris),* 133:3–22(a).

15. Michelakis, A., and Robertson, D. (1976): Plasma renin-activity and levodopa in Parkinson's disease. *J.A.M.A.,* 213:83–85.

16. Nilsson, A., and Hokfelt, B. (1978): Effect of the dopamine agonist bromocriptine on blood pressure, catecholamines and renin activity in acromegalies at rest, following exercise and during insulin induced hypoglycemia. *Acta Endocrinol. (Suppl. 216),* 88:83–96.

17. Otsuka, K., Assaykeen, T., Goldfien, A., and Ganong, W. (1970): Effect of hypoglycemia on plasma renin activity in dogs. *Endocrinology,* 87:1306–1317.

18. Passo, S., Assaykeen, T., Otsuka, K., Wise, B., Goldfien, A., and Ganong, W. (1971): Effect of the stimulation of the medulla oblongata on renin secretion in dogs. *Neuroendocrinology,* 7:1–10.

19. Perret, J., Feverstein, Cl., Pellat, J., Serre, F., Gavend, M., and Tanche, M. (1977): Résultats des dosages de la méthoxydopa plasmatique chez les parkinsoniens avec ou sans dyskinésies induites par la L-DOPA. *Rev. Neurol. (Paris),* 133:627–636.

20. Reid, I. A., MacDonald, D. M., Pachnis, B., and Ganong, W. (1975): Studies concerning the mechanism of suppression of renin secretion by clonidine. *J. Pharmacol. Exp. Ther.,* 192:713–721.

21. Richardson, D., Stella, A., Leonetti, G., Bartorelli, A., and Zanchetti, A. (1974): Mechanisms of renal release of renin by electrical stimulation of the brainstem in the cat. *Circ. Res.,* 34:425–434.

22. Schmitt, H., Schmitt, H., and Fenard, S. (1972): New evidence for an adrenergic component in the sympathetic tone by L-DOPA and its antagonism by piperoxane and yohimbine. *Eur. J. Pharmacol.,* 17:293.

23. Severs, W. B., and Daniels-Severs, A. E. (1973): Effect of angiotensin on the central nervous system. *Pharmacol. Rev.,* 25:415–449.

24. Sullivan, J., Nakano, K., and Tyler, R. (1973): Plasma renin-activity during levodopa therapy. *J.A.M.A.,* 224:1726–1729.

25. Ueda, H. (1967): Increased renin release evoked by mesencephalic stimulation in the dog. *Jpn. Heart J.,* 8:498–506.

26. Ungerstedt, U. (1971): Postsynaptic hypersensitivity after 6-hydroxydopamine induced degeneration of the nigro striatal system. *Acta Physiol. Scand. (Suppl.),* 367:79–93.

27. Vander, A. (1965): Effect of catecholamines and the renal nerves on renin secretion in anesthetized dogs. *Am. J. Physiol.,* 209:659–662.

28. Wass, J., Thorner, M., Morris, D., Rees, L., Mason, S., Jones, E., and Besser, G. (1977): Long term treatment of acromegaly with bromocriptine. *Br. Med. J.,* 1:875.

29. Watanabe, A., Judy, W., and Cardon, P. (1974): Effect of L-DOPA on blood pressure and sympathetic nerve activity after decarboxylase inhibition in cats. *J. Pharmacol. Exp. Ther.,* 188:107 113.

30. Zanchetti, A., and Stella, A. (1975): Neural control of renin release. *Clin. Sci. Mol. Med.,* 48:2155–2255.

31. Zehr, J., and Feigl, E. (1923): Suppression of renin activity by hypothalamic stimulation. *Circ. Res.,* 32–33 (Suppl. I), 117–127.

Advances in Neurology, Vol. 24, edited by
L. J. Poirier, T. L. Sourkes, and P. J. Bédard.
Raven Press, New York © 1979.

Parkinsonism and Autoimmunity: Antibody Against Human Sympathetic Ganglion Cells in Parkinson's Disease

Annick Pouplard, Jean Emile, Francois Pouplard,
and Daniel Hurez

*Departments of Immunology and Neurology, Centre Hospitalier Universitaire,
49036 Angers, France*

Dysfunction of autonomic nervous system in Parkinson's disease has been firmly established (1). Pathological lesions may be found over the entire autonomic nervous system including the sympathetic ganglion cells and they also involve brainstem nuclei. The corresponding clinical manifestations are numerous. They include sialorrhea, seborrhea, excessive sweating, postural hypotension (with or without L-DOPA treatment), as well as other vasomotor disturbances.

While searching for islet cell antibody in the serum of a patient who concomitantly suffered from Waldenström macroglobulinemia, diabetes mellitus, and Parkinson's disease, we had the opportunity to observe an unusual positive pattern involving nerves inside the pancreatic section. The serum from this patient stained specifically the α-glucagon cells (known to be of neural crest origin) and reacted strongly with certain structures on a section from the fetal pancreas. The fetal pancreas is richly innervated by sympathetic fibers, which contribute to form the "insulino sympathetic complexes."

Taking into account the known autonomic disturbances of parkinsonism, we applied the indirect immunofluorescence test to the serum of 51 patients with Parkinson's disease. This test, made on sections of human sympathetic ganglia, revealed that the serum of 62.7% of the patients contained an antibody that reacted specifically with the cytoplasm of the nervous cells, in comparison to only 10.4 and 21.4% of positive reactions obtained with the serum from adult blood donors and patients with other diseases, respectively. These results may open new avenues useful for the understanding of the pathogenesis of parkinsonism.

MATERIAL AND METHODS

Patients

The tests were made on serum samples from 51 patients with Parkinson's disease including 32 females and 19 males with a mean age of 61 years. All patients were under drug treatments, most of them receiving L-DOPA with or without a dopamine agonist (piribedil, bromocriptine) and a few receiving amantadine or diprobutine.

In some patients there was an associated disease: diabetes mellitus in two patients, thyrotoxic adenoma in one, rheumatoid arthritis (under steroid treatment) in one, and Waldenström macroglobulinemia in two. Nineteen blood donors and 14 patients with miscellaneous diseases (including 10 neurological diseases) served as controls.

Assays

The technique used was the classic sandwich indirect immunofluorescence made on 5-μm thick and unfixed frozen organ sections (7). Fresh sympathetic ganglia were obtained during abdominal sympathectomy. The specimens were also tested on sections from fresh and unfixed fetal pancreas and adrenal glands, and in 28 cases, we also looked for other antibodies by testing the sera on thyrotoxic thyroid, rat liver, kidney, and stomach. In all cases the sera were tested undiluted and at one-fourth dilution; and, when positive, they were further diluted.

The antisera used in the sandwich technique were fluorescein isothiocyanate (FITC) conjugates of sheep antihuman immunoglobulins and, occasionally, conjugates of specific rabbit anti-IgG, IgA, IgM, and anti-β1C.

RESULTS

Ganglion Cell Immunofluorescence

Out of 51 patients with Parkinson's disease tested, 32 (62.7%) (Table 1) gave a positive granular cytoplasmic fluorescence on the sympathetic ganglion cells, leaving unstained the nucleus and the orange autofluorescent lipofuchsin granules (Fig. 1).

The use of specific antisera applied to the most positive cases suggests that this antibody is exclusively of the IgG class, and of low titer (1/16, 1/32). On the basis of preliminary experiments, it does not seem to fix complement.

In the controls, the sera of 2 of the 19 blood donors (blood bank) and 3 of

TABLE 1. *Incidence of sympathetic ganglion cell antibodies detected by indirect immunofluorescence*

Clinical condition	No. tested	Positive	Negative	%
Parkinson's	51	32	19	62.7
Blood donors	19	2	17	10.5
Mixed cases	14	3	11	21.4

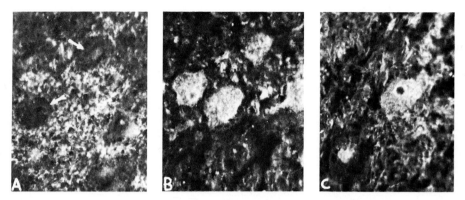

FIG. 1. A: Negative reaction on the sympathetic ganglion cells (*arrows*). B: Positive staining of ganglion cells with the serum from a parkinsonian patient. C: The nucleus is unstained under these conditions.

the 14 patients with various diseases were positive. It is worth mentioning that all 3 patients who reacted positively had a neurological disease, i.e., peripheral facial palsy, vascular accident, and nervous system sarcoidosis, respectively (Table 1).

Immunofluorescence on Fetal Pancreas and Adrenal Glands

All sera that were positive on the nervous cells, cross-reacted with an antigen located in the numerous sympathetic plexuses found in the fetal substrates (Fig. 2A and B, Table 2). In addition, the sera of some patients reacted specifically with the cells within the adrenal medulla (Fig. 2C). In this test, however, we did not find a similar correlation (Table 3) and in addition, two of the controls were positive: one female patient with Huntington's chorea and one male patient with sarcoidosis involving the nervous system.

Twenty-eight patients with Parkinson's disease were tested for other autoimmune abnormalities. Autoantibodies were detected only in a few cases (Table 4) but nine cases (32%) had antireticulin antibodies. This percentage is much higher in the patients than in normal subjects (4%), and the significance of the presence of this antibody is not understood.

COMMENTS

Autoantibodies are known to occur in a number of pathological states or autoimmune disorders being nonorgan specific (SLE) or organ specific (Hashimoto's thyroiditis, myasthenia gravis).

The occurrence of such an antibody in Parkinson's disease can be considered in several ways. (a) Is it only an indirect marker of the undergoing cellular destruction of the autonomic system? In fact, it is generally agreed that an

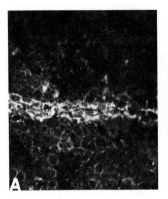 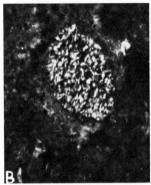 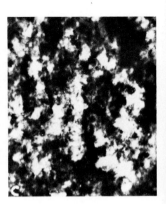

FIG. 2: Fetal pancreas: positive staining of a sympathetic plexus. **A:** Longitudinal section through the plexus. **B:** Cross-section through the plexus. **C:** Positive staining of the unfixed adrenal medulla with the serum from a parkinsonian patient.

alteration of an autologous antigen by a virus or an environmental factor can lead to the synthesis of antibodies against modified "self-antigens": one of the best examples in human pathology being the antibodies occurring after necrosis of the myocardium. In this study, however, two cases of polyneuritis (Guillain–Barré) with dysautonomia were negative. (b) Does it play a direct role in the cellular damage? In recent years, many hypotheses have been put forward in respect to the direct cause of Parkinson's disease. They include virus aging (3), melanin metabolism abnormality (8), and tyrosine hydroxylase deficiency (6). The possible involvement of immunological mechanisms has not yet been taken into consideration.

In most autoimmune diseases the antibody is directed against cytoplasmic "organelles" (microsomal fraction), and in order to cause a direct lesion, the antibody must have access to its antigen *in vivo*. In addition to this hypothesis it is appropriate to take account of the fact that the injection of antibodies specific for certain enzymes can produce the degeneration of noradrenergic fibers in the rat (2). This preliminary study does not permit us to favor either one of these two hypotheses.

Another question may be asked concerning the possible relationship between

TABLE 2. *Indirect immunofluorescence on sympathetic plexuses in 51 cases of Parkinson's disease*

Tissue tested	Positive[a]	Negative	%
Fetal pancreas	32	19	62.7
Fetal adrenal	32	19	62.7

[a] Exact correlation with the positive reaction on sympathetic neuronal cells.

TABLE 3. *Indirect immunofluorescence on human fetal-adrenal medulla in Parkinson's disease*

Serum tested	Positive	Negative
Positive for ganglion cell antibodies 32	16	16
Negative for ganglion cell antibodies 19	6	13
Total tested 51	22 (43%)	29

TABLE 4. *Autoantibodies in 28 cases of Parkinson's disease*

Antibody type	Positive	%
Thyroid	3	10.7
Gastric	2	7.1
ICA (islet cell)	2	7.1
ANA	7	25
Mitochondrial	0	0
SMA (smooth muscle)	6	21.4
"Reticulin"	9	32.1

the presence of these antibodies and the central lesions of parkinsonism. It is interesting to mention that Husby and colleagues (5) found an antibody directed against human caudate nucleus neurons in 33% of Parkinson's cases. Further work including absorption studies is needed to establish whether these antibodies are directed against a common antigen.

In the same way, the positive reaction of the serum on the adrenal medulla in 43% of parkinsonian patients (Table 3) raises the question of whether or not this antibody is directed against an antigen common to all catecholaminergic cells. The discrepancy found in our preliminary results, however, suggests that we may not be dealing with the same antigen, and that there may exist different antibodies in the serum of parkinsonian patients.

In recent years much progress has been made in the understanding of the pathogenesis and in the treatment of Parkinson's disease. The deficiency of the striatal dopaminergic activity is well documented but the exact cause of the disease is still unknown.

Further work is needed to completely understand this disease, but immunological mechanisms are apparently involved, and this fits well with our results concerning the association of HLA antigens with Parkinson's disease (4).

ACKNOWLEDGMENTS

We thank Dr. Chevalier for providing the sympathectomy specimens and M. F. Poron for technical help.

REFERENCES

1. Appenzeller, O., Goss, J. E., and Albuquerque, N. M. (1971): Autonomic deficits in Parkinson's syndrome. *Arch. Neurol.,* 24:50–57.
2. Blessing, W. W., Costa, M., Geffen, L. B., and Rush, R. A. (1977): Immune lesions of noradrenergic neurones in rat central nervous system produced by antibodies to dopamine-β-hydroxylase. *Nature,* 267:368–369.
3. Brown, E. L., and Knox, E. G., (1972): Epidemiological approach to Parkinson's disease. *Lancet,* 1:974–976.
4. Emile, L., Pouplard, A., Truelle, J. L., and Hurez, D. (1977): Association Maladie de Parkinson-Antigènes HLA-B_{17}-HLA-B_{18}, Vol. 6, p. 4144. Nouvelle Presse Med.
5. Husby, G., Li, L., Davis, L. E., Wedege, E., Kokmen, E., and Williams, R. C. (1977): Antibodies to human caudate nucleus neurons in Huntington's chorea. *J. Clin. Invest.,* 59:922–932.
6. Martin, E. W. (1972): Tyrosine hydroxylase deficiency. A unifying concept of parkinsonism. *Lancet,* 1:1050–1051.
7. Roitt, I. M., and Doniach, D. (1969): World Health Organisation manual for autoimmune serology. Geneva.
8. Shuster, S., Thody, A. J., Goolamali, S. K., Burton, J. L., and Plummer, N. (1973): Melanocyte-stimulating hormone and parkinsonism. *Lancet,* 1:463–464.

Advances in Neurology, Vol. 24, edited by
L. J. Poirier, T. L. Sourkes, and P. J. Bédard.
Raven Press, New York © 1979.

The Aging Neuron—Influence on Symptomatology and Therapeutic Response in Parkinson's Syndrome

A.-K. Granérus, A. Carlsson, and A. Svanborg

University of Göteborg, Department of Geriatric and Long-Term Care Medicine, Vasa Hospital, Göteborg, Sweden

Parkinson's syndrome is uncommon at ages below 45 but increases successively at higher ages. Patients with Parkinson's syndrome often have functional changes restricted to the classic parkinsonian symptoms, caused by lesions in the basal ganglia. However, sometimes the syndrome is combined with symptoms indicating a more widespread neuronal disturbance with, e.g., marked lowering of cognitive functions and changes in personality. Recent studies indicate similarities between changes in the neuron transmitters of the brain occurring during physiological aging (1,4) in senile dementia as well as in Parkinson's disease (7,8). Clinical experience also shows that the therapeutic response to L-DOPA is different at different ages. This is also true for the side-effects (9,10).

Since May 1968 a group of patients with Parkinson's syndrome has been followed, and detailed studies have been performed in our institutions. Certain of the observations indicate that the symptomatology of the syndrome, as well as the therapeutic outcome, depend on factors correlated to aging. The aim of this presentation is to discuss age-related variations in the symptomatology and in the outcome of the treatment, as well as the development of side-effects during L-DOPA treatment, against the background of recent findings concerning cerebral neurotransmitter concentrations at higher ages.

MATERIAL AND METHODS

Our material of 134 parkinsonian patients (2,9,10,11), in whom treatment with L-DOPA started between 1968 and 1970, has been analyzed repeatedly concerning age distribution, duration of disease, symptomatic picture, duration of treatment, doses of L-DOPA, and previous neurosurgical treatment, as well as the effect of the L-DOPA treatment on parkinsonian symptoms and the appearance of side-effects. The general motor and activity of daily living (ADL) functions have been scored according to a scale described previously (9,10).

Statistical Analyses

Standard methods were used for the calculation of the mean (M), the standard deviation (SD), the standard error of the mean (SEM), the linear correlation coefficient, and the linear regression. The hypothesis of no differences in the means was tested with Student's t-test or the Wilcoxon-Mann-Whitney Test for ranking of unpaired measurement. The hypothesis of no difference between paired observations in the same subjects was tested with Student's t-test for paired observations. The hypothesis of no difference in proportions between two groups was tested with the chi-square test (5), except for some cases where the exact test of significance by Fisher (6) was used. The correlation between the frequency of later occurring "on–off" symptoms to the age at the onset of Parkinson's syndrome and to the age at the start of L-DOPA treatment, respectively, was tested with Point Biserial Correlation (13).

Differences were considered significant for p values of 0.01 or less if nothing else is mentioned.

RESULTS

The age of the patients at the onset of the symptoms ranged from 32 to 74 years, and at the start of L-DOPA treatment from 39 to 81 years. The duration of the parkinsonian symptoms at the start of L-DOPA treatment varied between 1 and 31 years. In a first follow-up in 1970, the initial improvement in ADL disability was found to be negatively correlated to the age at the start of L-DOPA treatment. The effect of L-DOPA on the physical ability of the patients was thus better in younger than in elderly individuals. Furthermore, the improvement in ADL disability was positively correlated to the occurrence of tremor before treatment, as patients with tremor showed a greater improvement in ADL function than those without tremor. Good effect on ADL functions was also positively correlated to a good effect on tremor. Improvement of tremor was negatively correlated to the duration of the disease, but there was no correlation between the occurrence of tremor and age at the onset of the parkinsonian symptoms. The improvement in ADL disability was also positively correlated to the appearance of involuntary movements during treatment.

During long-term treatment on–off phenomena were found to have appeared in 48 of the 134 patients, and 43 of them had been treated for 5 years or more. Another 42 patients had been treated with L-DOPA for 5 years or more without developing on–off symptoms. Because of this different symptomatology in different patients, the patients were divided in two groups in a second follow-up performed in 1975, one group comprising those who had developed on–off symptoms (the "on–off" group, $n = 43$) and the other group exhibiting a more sustained, unchanging symptomatology (the "even" group, $n = 42$). Thus, all the patients had been treated with L-DOPA, alone or with inhibitor, for 5 years or more. Several differences between these two groups of patients were found.

The patients who were to develop on–off symptoms were found to have been significantly younger (Fig. 1) than those with an even symptomatology, with regard to the onset of the parkinsonian symptoms, at the start of the DOPA treatment and during follow-up. Moreover, the percentage of patients with subsequent on–off symptoms was significantly higher when the patient was younger at the onset of the Parkinson's syndrome (Fig. 2) and at the start of L-DOPA treatment (Fig. 3).

At the start of the present study no patient in the on–off group had symptoms of dementia in contrast to 9 (21%) in the even group ($p < 0.001$). During the treatment with L-DOPA for 5 years or more, 6 patients (14%) in the on–off group and 17 (40%) in the even group had symptoms of dementia ($p < 0.01$). Under the same circumstances the patients with dementia were significantly older (71.8 $\pm$ 1.30 years) than those without dementia (65.7 $\pm$ 1.10 years), but the duration of the disease did not differ between those with and without dementia.

The DOPA dose had been significantly higher throughout the treatment

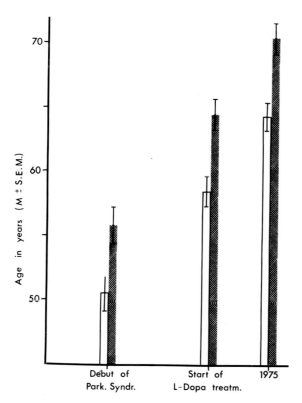

FIG. 1. Age at the beginning of Parkinson's syndrome, at the start of L-DOPA treatment, and at the 1975 follow-up in the patients treated for 5 years or more. □, On–off group ($n = 43$); ■, Even group ($n = 42$).

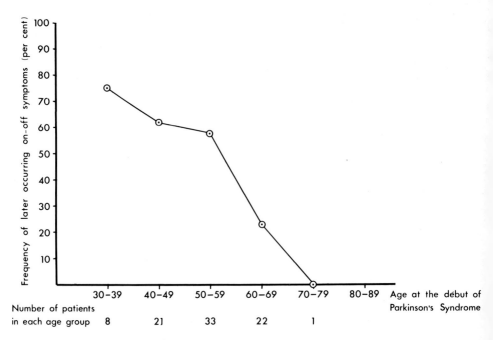

FIG. 2. Percentage of patients with later occurring on–off symptoms in 85 patients treated with L-DOPA for 5 years or more, correlated to age at the beginning of Parkinson's syndrome.

($p < 0.02$, $p < 0.025$, and $p < 0.005$), i.e., at the first optimal dose, during the first and the second period of follow-up, respectively, in the patients who later developed on–off symptoms, in comparison to the even group (Fig. 4). There was no significant correlation between the time when the on–off symptoms began to appear and the magnitude of the DOPA dose, but the patients with the earlier occurrence of on–off symptoms had had the higher DOPA doses, and those with later occurrence of the symptoms received the lower doses.

The initial improvement had been more marked in the patients who later developed on–off symptoms than in the patients who maintained an even symptomatology ($p < 0.05$).

Dyskinesia occurred earlier and was more frequent during L-DOPA treatment in the on–off than in the even group. Taking as a basis half a year of treatment when none of the patients had yet developed the on–off phenomenon, dyskinesia had occurred in 60% of the patients who 5 years later had on–off symptoms, compared to 25% of the patients maintaining an even symptomatology during the same period ($p < 0.005$). The first appearance of dyskinesia was seen within the first year of dopa treatment in more than 90% of the patients who later displayed on–off symptoms, compared to 40% in those who did not show such symptoms ($p < 0.0005$).

Autopsy of the brains of the patients who died was not consistently done. However, it was performed on a patient who died after the second follow-up had been made. This patient initially had responded very well to L-DOPA, but later developed disabling on–off symptoms. Subsequently, less effect of the L-DOPA therapy was seen and symptoms of dementia developed. When the patient died he was severely demented and, for a long time, had been unable to walk, feed himself, or talk. The postmortem study revealed not only the classic signs of Parkinson's disease but also those of Alzheimer's disease.

DISCUSSION

In the present investigation we have distinguished between two groups of parkinsonian patients, although they do not necessarily represent distinct entities. It is perhaps more adequate to speak of two types representing the extremes of a continuum. One type is the patient with an earlier onset and a "clean" parkinsonian symptomatology. The other type begins to show parkinsonian symptoms at an old age, and at the same time symptoms of dementia predominate. The present investigation reveals that the two types of patients respond differently to L-DOPA therapy. The former type shows a good initial response, but tends to have an early onset of dyskinesia and runs a high risk of ending up in an on–off condition. The latter type responds less successfully to L-DOPA but has less disturbing dyskinesia and does not develop on–off phenomena.

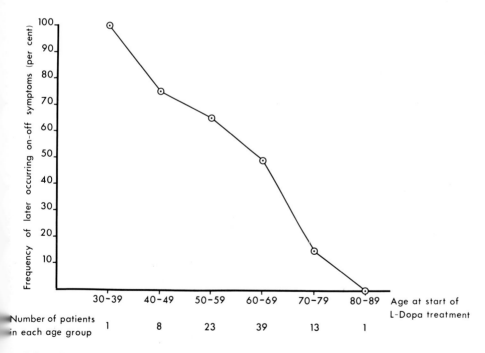

FIG. 3. Percentage of patients with later occurring on–off symptoms in 85 patients treated with L-DOPA for 5 years or more, correlated to age at the start of L-DOPA treatment.

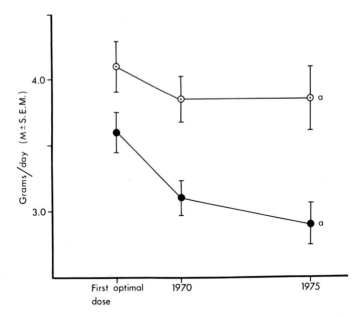

FIG. 4. Maintenance dose of L-DOPA at the first optimal dose level, at the first follow-up (1970) and at the second follow-up (1975) in the patients treated for 5 years or more. *(a)* Adjusted L-DOPA doses, including a fivefold multiplying of the amount of L-DOPA when combined with inhibitor. ○, On-off group (*n* = 43); ●, Even group (*n* = 42).

On the other hand, the progressing dementia of the latter type of patient becomes a problem. The former type tends to be given larger doses of L-DOPA than the latter. The higher incidence or risk of cardiovascular or mental side-effects, for example, may at least to some extent, be correlated with the difference of doses administered to either group. As a consequence of this difference, the lower dose may at least partially explain the weaker therapeutic response and the lower incidence of dyskinesias in the older patients. The difference in dosage may also explain the difference in incidence of the on–off phenomenon. This could in turn be due to the development of receptor subsensitivity or some other adaptive or toxic reaction to L-DOPA. The present data do not permit a definite answer to this question, which is obviously of great theoretical and clinical importance. However, the predominance of the on–off phenomenon in the young parkinsonian with clean symptomatology, where the administration of a dopamine precursor would be expected to more exactly constitute the ideal substitution therapy (see below), is paradoxical. Unless overdosage is involved, one has to infer a more rapid progress of the disease as a causative factor for the earlier appearance of the on–off phenomenon. Although this possibility cannot be excluded at present, the question must be raised whether one should try to keep the dosage of L-DOPA somewhat below that yielding maximal improvement, especially in cases where dyskinesia occurs as a prominent side-effect.

The frequent coexistence of Parkinson's disease and dementia is of considerable interest. Whereas the former disease is predominantly caused by degeneration of nigrostriatal dopaminergic neurons, the latter appears to be due to a more widespread damage, involving several types of neurons (for review, see ref. 4). It is thus logical to suggest that in the light of the present material in parkinsonian patients, the younger patient with a clean parkinsonian symptomatology has a more selective, "mononeuronal type" of damage, restricted in the main to the dopaminergic neurons, whereas the older, demented parkinsonian patient suffers from a more widespread "multineuronal type" of damage. The distinction between the demented parkinsonian and the demented patient of the Alzheimer type without parkinsonian symptoms would thus reside in the more prominent involvement of nigrostriatal dopaminergic neurons in the former type of patient.

The relationship between aging and Parkinson's disease, dementia of Alzheimer type (as distinguished mainly from multiinfarct dementia), and mixed Parkinson–dementia conditions is of great interest. Postmortem examinations of the brains of humans without any known neurological or psychiatric disorder has revealed an age-dependent decrease in the levels of several neurotransmitters and their metabolities and/or their synthetic enzymes. These decreases can be at least partially correlated with a decrease in cell counts of the corresponding neurons (for review, see ref. 3). Moreover, the pattern of neuronal loss in dementia is similar to that occurring in the normal-aged individual, suggesting that in dementia we are dealing with an accelerated neuronal aging. Parkinson's disease could perhaps be considered as a condition with accelerated aging, selectively involving dopaminergic neurons. These neurons, incidentally, show a more rapid age-dependent "normal" decrease than most other types of neuron thus far investigated. It is therefore conceivable that a great proportion of neurogeriatric disorders results from accelerated aging of one or more types of neurons. It should be realized, however, that in some cases we may be dealing with the combined effect of a defect, unrelated to aging, and a normal process of aging, rather than with accelerated aging in the strict sense. Such a defect could be genetic or due to infections, intoxications, etc. during fetal life, postnatally, or at any time later in life.

The recent morphological data of Hakim and Mathiesson (12) may be quoted in favor of the integrated view presented above. Histological features indistinguishable from those of Alzheimer's disease were more frequently observed in cases of Parkinson's disease than in an age-matched control material by these workers. Our case with the simultaneous occurrence of the two diseases as judged from histological data is in line with this view.

It is interesting to note that tremor was a positive prognostic sign insofar as the therapeutic response to L-DOPA is concerned. No explanation can as yet be offered for this phenomenon. Possibly the occurrence of tremor is an indicator of the specificity of the parkinsonian disturbance, i.e., the neuronal damage is restricted to the nigrostriatal dopaminergic system. If this is true, the question may be raised—despite what has been emphasized above concerning the role of high dosage of L-DOPA—whether the occurrence of involuntary movements after L-DOPA treatment could also be a sign of specificity. This may suggest that both tremor and involuntary movements require a high vitality of the nondopaminergic systems involved in the control of motor functions.

REFERENCES

1. Adolfsson, R., Gottfries, C. G., and Winblad, B. (1976): Methodological aspects of postmortem investigations of human brain—with special reference to monoamines and related enzymes. In: *Neuro-Psychopharmacology,* edited by P. Deniker, C. Radouco-Thomas, and A. Villeneuve, pp. 1597–1607. Pergamon Press, New York.
2. Andén, N.-E., Carlsson, A., Kerstell, J., Magnusson, T., Olsson, R., Roos, B.-E., Steen, B., Steg, G., Svanborg, A., Thieme, G., and Werdinius, B. (1970): Oral L-DOPA treatment of parkinsonism. *Acta Med. Scand.,* 187:247–255.
3. Carlsson, A. (1978): The impact of catecholamine research on medical science and practice. *Presented at Fourth International Catecholamine Symposium,* Asilomar, California, *(in press).*
4. Carlsson, A., and Winblad, B. (1976): Influence of age and time interval between death and autopsy on dopamine and 3-methoxytyramine levels in human basal ganglia. *J. Neural Transm.,* 38:271–276.
5. Cochran, W. G. (1954): Some methods for strengthening the common χ^2-test. *Biometrics,* 10:417.
6. Fisher, R. A. (1946): *Statistical Methods for Research Workers,* p. 96. Oliver and Boyd Ltd., Edinburgh.
7. Gottfries, C. G., Gottfries, I., and Roos, B.-E. (1969): The investigation of homovanillic acid in the human brain and its correlation to senile dementia. *Br. J. Psychiatry,* 115:563–574.
8. Gottfries, C. G., Gottfries, I., and Roos, B.-E. (1969): Homovanillic acid and 5-hydroxyindoleacetic acid in the cerebrospinal fluid of patients with senile dementia, presenile dementia and parkinsonism. *J. Neurochem.,* 16:1341–1345.
9. Granérus, A.-K., (1977): L-DOPA treatment in Parkinson's syndrome. Thesis, Gothenburg.
10. Granérus, A.-K., Steg, G., and Svanborg, A. (1972): Clinical analyses of factors influencing L-DOPA treatment of Parkinson's syndrome. *Acta Med. Scand.,* 192:1–11.
11. Granérus, A.-K. (1978): Factors influencing the occurrence of "on–off" symptoms during long term treatment with L-DOPA. *Acta Med. Scand.,* 203:75–85.
12. Hakim, A. M., and Mathieson, G. (1978): Basis of dementia in Parkinson's disease. *Lancet,* 2:729.
13. Kendall, M. G., and Buckland, W. R. (1975): *A Dictionary of Statistical Terms,* 3rd ed. Longman Group Ltd, London.

Advances in Neurology, Vol. 24, edited by
L. J. Poirier, T. L. Sourkes, and P. J. Bédard.
Raven Press, New York © 1979.

Neuropharmacological Investigation and Treatment of Spasmodic Torticollis

S. Lal, K. Hoyte, M. E. Kiely, T. L. Sourkes, D. W. Baxter,
K. Missala, and F. Andermann

Departments of Psychiatry and Neurology, McGill University, Montreal, Quebec, Canada

The etiology and site of pathological lesion in spasmodic torticollis (ST) are unknown and the significance of animal models for this clinical disorder is questioned (55). Biochemical investigations have been few. Kjellin and Stibler (34) found abnormal cerebrospinal fluid (CSF) protein patterns in some patients but not in others. Curzon (19) reported normal mean concentrations of homovanillic acid (HVA) and 5-hydroxyindoleacetic acid (5-HIAA), metabolites of dopamine (DA), and 5-hydroxytryptamine (5-HT), respectively, in lumbar CSF in nine patients, whereas in the single case tabulated by Johansson and Roos (33), there was a considerably lowered value of both acids.

Improvement has been reported following treatment with pipradol (22), amphetamine (45), amantadine (25), L-DOPA (32,49), bromocriptine (40), lithium (16,34), diazepam (6), L-5-hydroxytryptophan (44), quinine (29), anticholinergic agents (23,36,59), tetrabenazine (54), phenothiazines (8,50), haloperidol (14,25,49), and sulpiride (57). However, in other patients some of these same drugs, namely amantadine (7,49), L-DOPA (3,5,49), bromocriptine (40), haloperidol (7,49), and anticholinergic drugs (10), have either had no effect or induce worsening of symptoms. One possible interpretation of the discrepancies in the literature, as well as seemingly contradictory findings that drugs with diametrically opposite pharmacological effects on neurotransmitter function may be of benefit, is that ST is a heterogeneous disorder. Compatible with this view are the findings of Kjellin and Stibler (34) and observations that in a variable number of patients with ST there is a family history of essential tremor, coexisting signs of essential tremor, extranuchal dystonia, and, to a lesser extent, parkinsonism (15).

The present study was undertaken in patients with ST to evaluate (a) the effect of acute administration of various drugs that alter neurotransmitter function or are effective in essential tremor; (b) the response to a single dose of apomorphine, benztropine, or haloperidol as predictor of the response to L-DOPA, benztropine, or pimozide treatment, respectively; and (c) turnover of DA and 5-HT using the probenecid technique. We also wished to correlate the biochemical findings with the pharmacological responses. In view of reports that the growth hormone (GH) response to DA receptor agonists is increased in Huntington's chorea (11) but decreased in Parkinson's disease as well as in a single case of ST (9), we have investigated the GH response to apomorphine in our patients. Finally, some novel data on ventricular CSF monoamine metabolites are presented.

PATIENTS AND METHODS

Data on ventricular CSF monoamine acid catabolites in ST, which have not previously been identified, were taken from the raw data of Papeschi et al. (47). Fifteen other patients (Nos. 1–15, Table 1) with idiopathic ST served as subjects, for the lumbar CSF, pharmacological, and endocrinological studies. None of the patients was of Jewish background or had a history of encephalitis or evidence of hyperthyroidism. Subject 1, however, had been on thyroxine for 14 years for a nodular goiter. Thyroxine was continued during all studies and a euthyroid state was maintained throughout. Except for patient 1 who had received small doses of chlorpromazine for 4 weeks 11 years before the onset of ST, none of the other subjects was known to have been exposed to prior neuroleptic therapy. Apart from patients 4 and 11, none had significant radiological evidence of cervical degenerative disc disease. All subjects were physically well, apart from their neurological findings. Patient 3 had a prior history of carcinoma of the breast but had no evidence of metastases. Although five of the patients had evidence of a neurosis, in none was there evidence of a psychogenic cause of the ST upon psychiatric evaluation. Elimination of phobias in patients 4 and 7 with behavior therapy was not associated with changes in ST. CSF data are also provided on two patients with drug-induced torticollis (Nos. 16 and 17).

The probenecid technique as described by Goodwin et al. (27) was used. Eight milliliters of lumbar CSF was drawn at 9 A.M. on day 1; probenecid, 100 mg/kg in four divided doses, was given at 9 P.M. on day 1, and at 2 A.M., 7 A.M., and 12 P.M. on day 2; and the second lumbar puncture was performed at 3 P.M. on day 2. Only a single tap was done on controls and none received probenecid. Controls consisted of neurological and psychiatric patients undergoing diagnostic lumbar puncture who were on no medication for at least 48 hr, and who were without movement disorder, psychosis, or condition known to affect monoamine metabolism. All punctures were performed only after the subjects had been recumbent for at least 8 hr. 5-HIAA was assayed as described by Young et al. (61), and HVA as reported by Papeschi and McClure (46). Probenecid assays were based on the procedure of Dayton et al. (20).

The GH response to apomorphine HCl (0.75 mg s.c.) (37,38) was performed on subjects 1–8, 14, and 15. Subjects 14 and 15 were on oral contraceptive medication. Each patient was paired with a normal control who was matched for the variables of age, sex, weight, menopausal status, and, in the case of subjects 14 and 15, with birth control medication. None of the subjects was obese. Except as mentioned, subjects had been off all medication for at least 1 week prior to testing.

Apomorphine was used as a short, rapidly acting DA receptor agonist (53) to predict response to L-DOPA, the immediate precursor of DA. A relatively low dose of L-DOPA was used, since there is suggestive evidence that small doses of the drug may be beneficial (32) in contrast to larger doses (3). Haloperidol, a DA receptor blocker (1), which can be given intramuscularly, was used to predict response to the more selective DA receptor blocker, pimozide (1,58), which is not available in injectable form. Benztropine was used as an anticholinergic agent, clonidine as an alpha-receptor agonist (2), propranolol as a beta-blocker, L-tryptophan as a precursor of 5-HT, and methysergide as a putative 5-HT blocker. Other drugs used were diazepam, sodium amytal, and alcohol. The acute pharmacological tests were conducted under videotape recording, except for patients 9 and 10 where direct clinical ratings were made, both before and following drug administration at timed intervals. The position for recording was individualized so as to bring out the disability maximally. Following a 15-min period of adaptation to the test situation, two base-line recordings were made. The doses of drugs used are indicated in Table 6. Vodka, 50 ml, was diluted to a volume of 200 ml with orange juice and ingested over a period of 5 min. The larger dose of vodka, 150 ml, was diluted to 600 ml with orange juice and ingested over 15 min. Sodium amytal and clonidine were injected over a 10-min period. Propranolol was given under electrocardiographic monitoring in a dose of 0.5 mg every 2 min to a miximum total dose of 4 mg. Serial videotape recordings, usually of 1-min duration, were made every 15 or 30 min after drug administration for 60 to 180 min, depending on the drug administered. Except when alcohol or propranolol was administered, the patients were blind as to drug given. Control procedures consisted of saline injections or lactose oral placebos.

The responses to chronic treatment trials were all documented on videotape. Pimozide or L-DOPA were given in a standard placebo-controlled, double-blind crossover design. The placebos were inactive. Pimozide or placebo was given over 3 weeks starting with 2 mg daily and increasing to a maximum dose of 6 mg/day. L-DOPA or placebo were given over a period of 17 weeks. The initial dose of L-DOPA was 250 mg twice a day and this was progressively increased to a maximum of 3 g/day at 6 weeks, which was then maintained for up to 12 weeks. Methysergide was given in a dose of 2 mg four times a day for 5 days in an uncontrolled trial. Benztropine, in an open study, was started at a dose of 0.5 to 1.0 mg twice daily for 1 week and then increased by 0.5 mg/week to a maximum of 8 mg/day, or until side-effects precluded further increases.

Patient 11 was on amitriptyline, 25 mg, and diazepam, 10 mg three times daily, throughout the drug studies. During the acute studies, the drugs were omitted for 12 to 16 hr before testing. Patient 7 was maintained on benztropine,

TABLE 1. *Clinical findings in patients with ST*

Pt.	Sex/Age (yrs)	Neurological findings	Duration of ST (yrs)	Family history of tremor	Comments
1	F/54	Retrocollis; dystonic posturing of outstretched hands; tremor of outstretched hands, especially right hand	2.5	None	Onset of tremor unknown; anxiety neurosis for at least 14 yrs
2	F/47	ST; writer's cramp.	0.25	None	Onset of writer's cramp antedated ST by 2 yrs
3	F/49	ST (mainly tonic); spastic dysphonia	2.0	None	Spastic dysphonia since age 19 yrs; chorioretinal atrophy since age 16; carcinoma of breast
4	F/50	ST (mainly tonic); disturbance of rapid alternating movements of hands	3.0	None	Phobic neurosis for many years
5	F/27	ST	2.0	Father	Tremor of hands and legs and leg cramps when 21 yrs; at 22 yrs developed ST with chin deviated to right; ST lasted 5 mos then disappeared for 3 yrs; ST recurred when 25 yrs with chin deviated to the left; with onset of ST tremor disappeared
6	M/43	ST (mainly tonic); tremor of outstretched hands; irregular movements of soft palate	7.0	Mother	Tremor since a teenager

7	M/32	ST; dystonic posturing of outstretched hands	4.1	Mother, father, maternal and paternal uncle	Tremor of left hand then right antedated ST by 4 yrs; tremor subsided with development of ST; maternal grandmother had a crooked neck; phobic neurosis for 7 yrs
8	M/33	ST; writer's cramp	2.0	Maternal grandmother	Onset of ST associated with tremor of hands and writer's cramp; tremor disappeared with establishment of ST
9	F/47	ST; spastic dysphonia	1.5	None	Spastic dysphonia since the age of 32 yrs; anxiety neurosis for 10 yrs
10	F/35	ST; 7th nerve palsy; tremor on writing	0.75	Father	Writing tremor for 2 yrs; 7th nerve palsy developed 5 yrs before ST
11	M/52	ST; tremor of outstretched hands, especially left hand	14	Mother, maternal grandmother	Tremor of hands antedated ST by 16 yrs; anxiety neurosis for 32 yrs
12	F/50	Retrocollis; hand tremor	5.0	Nephew	Hand tremor for 20 yrs
13	M/28	ST (mainly tonic); tremor of outstretched hands	1.75	None	Tremor as long as able to remember
14	F/23	ST (mainly tonic); tremor of legs and of outstretched hands	10	Father, 2 brothers	Tremor of arms and legs for 6 yrs
15	F/40	ST; tremor of outstretched hands	1.1	None	Head tremor 5 yrs and hand tremor 1 yr before onset of ST

8 mg/day, during the treatment trial with L-DOPA. Apart from patients 1 and 11, subjects were on no medication during the acute studies, which were spaced out depending on the known duration of action of the drugs. Except for occasional diazepam or acetylsalicylic acid, which were not taken for at least 72 hr before videotaping, no other drugs were taken during the treatment trials except as indicated.

Tapes were evaluated without knowledge of the treatment code. Apart from global assessment of change, the frequency of head movements or duration of keeping the head in a given position were noted. Amplitude of movements sometimes decreased markedly despite absence of a change in frequency so that only a semiquantitative assessment of the tapes could be made. The rating scale used is given in Table 6. In addition, in the treatment trials an assessment of daily activities as well as collateral information from relatives was obtained to substantiate changes noted on videotape.

RESULTS

There was no difference in GH concentrations between patients and controls following apomorphine administration at any of the time intervals studied or in the mean individual peak concentration (Table 2).

The concentration of HVA in ventricular CSF in three of the four patients with spasmodic torticollis was low compared with patients with a pain syndrome or obsessive–compulsive neurosis (Table 3). In the single case in which 5-HIAA was estimated, the value was similar to the two patients with an obsessive–compulsive neurosis.

In lumbar CSF basal concentrations of 5-HIAA (but not HVA) were significantly decreased ($p < 0.05$) (Table 4). Following probenecid administration, there was a marked increase in both acid catabolites even in individual patients in whom basal values were very low (Table 5). The magnitude of the increase showed wide variation. The mean HVA concentration increased from 15 ± 6.1 to 166 ± 30.1 ng/ml, and that of 5-HIAA from 14 ± 1.8 to 72 ± 10.3 ng/ml (patients 1–9). CSF probenecid concentration achieved was 13.4 ± 2.6 μg/ml.

Lumbar CSF data in two patients with drug-induced torticollis were within the range of the idiopathic cases.

Results of the response to acute drug administration and to the treatment trials are given in Table 6. Six of the 13 patients showed a clinical change in symptoms following apomorphine; in four there was improvement and in two worsening. The same 6 patients were placed on L-DOPA treatment. Two of the patients who improved with apomorphine improved with L-DOPA and one patient who worsened with apomorphine worsened with L-DOPA. In patient 5, there was almost a complete remission with L-DOPA. However, the improvement was maintained with L-DOPA placebo and continued in the absence of drugs for 2 years at last follow-up.

TABLE 2. *Growth hormone response to apomorphine in ST[a]*

			Serum growth hormone (ng/ml; $\overline{X} \pm$ SEM)						
			Time (min)						
Subjects	Age (yrs)	Wt (kg)	-30	0	30	45	60	Peak
ST (n = 10)	39.8 ± 3.3	59.7 ± 3.0	1.6 ± 0.2	1.4 ± 0.2	5.8 ± 1.4	13.1 ± 2.6	11.9 ± 1.8	14.4 ± 2.4
Controls (n = 10)	40.1 ± 3.3	62.2 ± 3.6	2.0 ± 0.4	2.0 ± 0.2	8.6 ± 2.0	12.8 ± 3.1	12.2 ± 4.1	15.2 ± 3.6
p	ns	ns	ns	ns	ns	ns	ns	ns

[a]Sub ects were administered apomorphine HCl (0.75 mg s.c.) at time 0.

TABLE 3. *HVA and 5-HIAA concentrations in ventricular CSF of patients with ST[a]*

Patients		HVA (ng/ml)	5-HIAA (ng/ml)
Spasmodic torticollis			
Age/Sex	Duration (yrs)		
15/F	5	378	—
63/F	3	178	—
22/F	0.5	203	—
20/M	2	93	45
		213 ± 60 (4)[b]	
Pain syndromes		391 ± 41 (3)	—
Obsessive–Compulsive neurosis		300 ± 16 (3)	37.78

[a] Taken from the raw data of Papeschi et al. (47).
[b] $\bar{X}$ ± SEM; number of cases in parentheses.

Four of the 13 patients showed a clinical change with haloperidol; two improved and two worsened. In only one of these four patients did the direction of change with haloperidol coincide with the direction of change with pimozide; in the other three subjects the response to haloperidol was in an opposite direction to that of pimozide.

Four of the nine patients who received pimozide improved and one worsened. In patient 8, the marked improvement, which was evident under standardized conditions of videotaping where the patient was observed at rest in the sitting position, was not maintained when he was engaged in activity. In patient 5, although there was no improvement at rest, on activity there was a marked decrease in spasmodic movements. Pimozide induced varying degrees of parkinsonism in six of the nine subjects.

Six of the 13 patients improved following benztropine injection and 1 worsened. This improvement was detectable within 15 min to 2 hr of the injection and lasted 2 to 16 hr. Ten of the 13 patients were placed on daily benztropine

TABLE 4. *HVA and 5-HIAA in lumbar CSF of patients with ST[a]*

Group	HVA (ng/ml)	p	5-HIAA (ng/ml)	p	Reference
ST	32 ± 6 (9)	ns	21 ± 4 (9)	ns	Curzon (19)[b]
Controls	37 ± 3 (17)		23 ± 2 (17)		
ST	5 (1)		8 (1)		Johansson and Roos (33)[b]
Controls	31.5 ± 1.2 (24)		28.3 ± 1.4 (35)		
ST	15 ± 6.1 (8)	ns	14 ± 1.8 (8)	< 0.05	Present study[c]
Controls	18 ± 1.9 (10)		23 ± 2.6 (21)		

[a] Data given $\bar{X}$ ± SEM; number of cases in parentheses, ns = $p > 0.05$.
[b] Recumbency requirements prior to lumbar puncture not stated.
[c] Subjects recumbent for at least 8 hr prior to lumbar puncture.

TABLE 5. HVA and 5-HIAA concentrations in lumbar CSF before and after probenecid in ST[a]

Pt.	HVA		5-HIAA		Probenecid	HVA increase[d] Probenecid	HVA[d] Probenecid	5-HIAA increase[d] Probenecid	5-HIAA[d] Probenecid
	before	after	before	after					
1	—	192	14.9	109	5.3	—	36.2	17.8	20.6
2	10.7	245	9.0	79	10.6	22.1	23.1	6.6	7.5
3	11.5	236	15.3	75	12.4	18.1	19.0	4.8	6.1
4	6.6	265	15	70	24.8	10.4	10.7	2.2	2.8
5	55	156	23	106	14.6	6.9	10.7	5.7	7.3
6	12.9	90	12.6	49	13.3	5.8	6.8	2.8	3.7
7	0	124	17.1	68	22.1	5.6	5.6	2.3	3.1
8	4.5	20	6.5	19.4	4	3.9	5.0	3.2	4.9
9	19.4	—	—	—	—	—	—	—	—
16[b]	11.5	—	—	—	—	—	—	—	
17[c]	18.2	198	17.6	97	10.5	17.2	18.9	7.6	9.2

[a] Probenecid test was performed as described in the text. HVA and 5-HIAA are expressed as ng/ml and probenecid as μg/ml. Dash, not available. Subjects 1–9 are cases of idiopathic ST.

[b] 46-year-old male with neuroleptic-induced ST. Neuroleptic originally prescribed for cervical disc pain. CSF study performed 7 weeks following drug withdrawal.

[c] 30-year-old male schizophrenic with neuroleptic-induced truncal dystonia and retrocollis. CSF study performed 9 weeks following drug withdrawal.

[d] Ratio of acid metabolite concentration to probenecid concentration.

TABLE 6. Effect of various drugs on ST[a]

Treatment	Patient number												
	1	2	3	4	5	6	7	8	9	10	11	12	13
Apomorphine (1.5 mg s.c.)	0	1+	0	1+	1.5+	0	2−	2+	0	0	1−	0	0
L-DOPA (2–3 g/day)		1.5+		0	3+[b]		1−	0	0	0	0	0	0
Haloperidol (1 mg i.m.)	2−	0	1.5−	3+	0	0	0	1+	0	0	0	0	0
Pimozide (4–6 mg/day)	3+[c]	1+	1+[c,d]	1.5−[c]	0[c,e]	0[c]	0	3+[c,f]					
Benztropine (2 mg i.v.)	0		1+	3+	1−	0	2+	2+	0	2+	1+		
Benztropine (2–8 mg/day)		2−	3+	3+			3+	3+	1−	1.5+	0	0	0
Clonidine (0.15 mg/i.v.)	0			3+	0	1−	1−	0					
Propranolol (4 mg i.v.)	1+			0	0	2−	2+[g]	2+					
Diazepam (5 mg i.m.)	0	0	2+	2+	0	3−	1+	3+	0	0	0	0	0
Sodium amytal (500 mg i.v.)	1−			3+	3+	3−	3+	3+					
Alcohol (50 ml vodka; 40% v/v)	1−			0	0	1−	2+	0					
Alcohol (150 ml vodka; 40% v/v)	0			0	0	1+	2.5+	1+					
L-Tryptophan (5 g p.o.)	0			0	2−	0	0	1+					
Methysergide (8 mg/day)	0			0	0	0	0	1+					

[a] Response rated under standardized conditions as follows: 0, slight (0–24%) improvement, slight worsening or no change; 1+, modest (25–49%) improvement; 2+, moderate (50–74%) improvement; 3+, marked (75% or more) improvement; 1−, modest worsening; 2−, moderate worsening; 3−, marked worsening. Intermediate values have been given a score of 0.5. Blank space, not done or not completed.
[b] Improvement also maintained with placebo.
[c] Pimozide-induced parkinsonism.
[d] Did not receive pimozide placebo.
[e] Improvement on activity.
[f] No improvement on activity.
[g] Improvement in tonic component but worsening in spasmodic component.

treatment, and of these, 5 showed sustained improvement. All five of these therapeutic successes had improved following intravenous benztropine. Four of the five therapeutic failures on daily benztropine had failed to improve after the single injection of the drug. Patient 11, who improved with the acute dose of benztropine, failed to improve on daily doses of the drug. The onset of improvement with chronic benztropine therapy occurred within 1 to 2 weeks; in patient 8, initial improvement in the first week was lost until the dose received was 4 mg/day. In subjects 3, 4, 7, and 8 the maximum improvement occurred with 6, 4, 8, and 7 mg, respectively; side-effects limited use of greater doses. The duration of sustained improvement to date is 4, 12, 27, and 3 months, respectively. Dose reduction in patient 7 resulted in worsening. In patient 10, who has been followed on benztropine for 1 year, improvement was maximal with 2 mg/day and was sustained at this dose; attempts to exceed this dose or discontinue the drug on three occasions resulted in worsening. In patients 7 and 8, improvement with benztropine was associated with a return of tremor of the hands, which had heralded the disorder, but which had then subsided with establishment of ST. Also, in patient 7, a bobbing motion of the head became apparent with improvement of ST. These emergent symptoms in these two patients could be controlled with a glass of beer or diazepam.

Improvement noted on videotape with L-DOPA, pimozide (except for patient 8), or benztropine therapy closely reflected improvement in the range and capacity for day-to-day and recreational activities and this was further confirmed by informants.

Of the six patients receiving clonidine, one improved and two worsened. After propranolol, two out of six improved and one worsened. In patient 7, the propranolol improved the tonic component, which was more troublesome to the patient, but worsened the frequency of spasmodic movements. Four of 13 patients improved with diazepam and one worsened. After sodium amytal four of six patients improved and two worsened; the response to amytal paralleled that of diazepam in four of the patients. With the smaller dose of alcohol one of six patients improved and two worsened, whereas with the larger dose, three of the six patients improved. The beneficial effect occurred within 15 to 30 min of commencing ingestion of alcohol and lasted only 15 to 30 min or less. Following the improvement in two of the subjects, there was a trend toward worsening. In each subject, improvement was associated with mild intoxication.

Tryptophan, which was administered to six patients, resulted in worsening in one patient and improvement in another. Methysergide had no effect in four patients.

The three patients with the highest turnover of DA on the probenecid test as well as the patient with the lowest turnover of DA improved with pimozide, although in the latter patient improvement was restricted to the resting state. No pattern emerged when CSF 5-HIAA findings were compared with response to a single dose of tryptophan or methysergide treatment, or when apomorphine, pimozide, or benztropine were compared with one another, or when the response to propranolol was compared with alcohol.

DISCUSSION

The associated neurological findings in our patients with ST is in keeping with observations in the literature that describe spasmodic movements of the palate (48), family history of essential tremor, features of essential tremor, and extranuchal dystonia coexisting with ST (15), writer's cramp (41,42), spastic dysphonia (18,31), and seventh-nerve paresis (48). Neurotic symptoms have been described in patients with ST (30,48), although the significance of these findings for the etiology of ST, as in the present cases, is questioned (12).

In the present study the GH response to apomorphine was no different from well-matched controls. The failure of the patient reported by Brown et al. (9) to respond to apomorphine, may be related to the lower dose of apomorphine they used or to the fact that normal women may show no GH response to apomorphine (21).

The low ventricular CSF HVA in three of four patients suggests that in some patients DA turnover may be diminished, and this may account for improvement that is reported in the literature following DA receptor activation (40,49).

In lumbar CSF the mean basal HVA was similar to controls. Postprobenecid control values were not available. On rank ordering of the postprobenecid HVA concentrations, there was a seven-fold difference between the lowest and the highest value. The three with the highest values improved with the selective DA receptor blocker, pimozide. This might suggest that in some patients with ST there is an increase in DA turnover, and hence, might account for the improvement with haloperidol therapy (14,25) and worsening with L-DOPA (3). However, the patient with the lowest turnover of DA also improved with pimozide. Also, although patient 2 had a large accumulation of HVA, improvement occurred not only with pimozide but also with L-DOPA.

In the present study lumbar CSF 5-HIAA was significantly decreased. A lowered 5-HIAA might explain the improvement with L5-hydroxytryptophan reported by Mori et al. (44). However, if 5-HT turnover is reduced, one might have expected improvement with L-tryptophan or worsening with methysergide. Only one patient improved with L-tryptophan, and none of the four patients receiving methysergide clearly worsened. The patient with the highest 5-HIAA accumulation after probenecid did not improve with methysergide.

Improvement with a single intravenous dose of benztropine predicted a therapeutic response to chronic benztropine therapy. The one exception was a patient who was under regular treatment with amitriptyline, which is known to be a potent central anticholinergic agent (4). Thus, the patient may have already benefited maximally from anticholinergic treatment. When tested acutely, the patient had been off amitriptyline for 14 hr. Foltz et al. (23) noted improvement in two out of five patients with anticholinergic agents. Isolated cases have also been reported by others to improve with anticholinergic drugs administered in conjunction with other agents (36,45,48,59). Bunts (10), however, states, without providing data, that anticholinergic drugs are disappointing. Gilbert (25) reported mild relief with benztropine in one patient but, apart from this incidental comment, reports with benztropine are not available. It is possible that benztropine differs from other anticholinergics. In this regard, Foltz et al. (23) reported a differential response with different combinations of anticholinergics. It is possible that improvement noted with phenothiazines (8,50) is in part related to the anticholinergic effects which these drugs are known to possess (52), rather than, or in addition to, their DA receptor-blocking properties (51). It is important to realize that benztropine also has antihistaminic properties (24) and, in addition, decreases reuptake of DA at nerve endings (more potently than trihexyphenidyl) (17), releases DA from dendrites of cell bodies in the substantia nigra, and decreases the release of DA in the caudate nucleus (26). Thus, the mode of action of benztropine is complex and the exact mechanism by which it improves some patients with ST is unclear. The present results suggest that some patients with ST improve with benztropine treatment, and that this group of patients can be readily identified by observing the effects of a single intravenous dose of the drug. Also, in some patients there may be a therapeutic dose range above which worsening may occur.

Tolosa (56) reported improvement with apomorphine in two out of seven patients with ST. In the present study 4 out of 13 improved with this DA receptor agonist. Changes with apomorphine showed a trend toward predicting responses to L-DOPA. A greater elasticity of dose ranges of the two drugs may be necessary before a correlation can be established. In patient 5 the maintenance of improvement with placebo and also after discontinuation of all drugs might suggest a spontaneous improvement. However, spontaneous improvement is unusual after the first year of affliction with torticollis (43). Chronic activation of DA receptors may alter receptor function (35), so it is possible that in patient 5, L-DOPA had a similar mode of action. Interestingly, six of the nine patients receiving pimozide developed parkinsonian symptoms despite the small doses used; this was marked in patient 5. Whether this points to diminished DA receptor function in some patients with ST is unclear, but of note is that three of the four patients who improved with apomorphine developed pimozide-induced parkinsonism.

Changes in response to a single dose of haloperidol, if anything, showed an inverse relationship with response to daily pimozide treatment. Of note is that the only 2 of the 13 patients who improved with a single dose of haloperidol, improved with apomorphine.

The model of parkinsonism in which response to anticholinergic drugs parallels response to dopaminergic activation does not seem to pertain to ST. It was possible for improvement to occur with benztropine and pimozide, or improvement with benztropine and worsening with L-DOPA. Further, it was possible for improvement to occur with L-DOPA or apomorphine as well as with pimozide.

Both alcohol (28) and propranolol (60) are effective in essential tremor. It has been stated that alcohol improves ST (15,48) but details have not been published. In the present study, improvement occurred in some patients with alcohol and propranolol but not necessarily in the same patient. The response to alcohol depended on the dose of alcohol. Improvement, when it did occur, was transient and associated with mild intoxication.

Improvement has been reported to occur following diazepam (6). In the present study 4 of the 13 patients showed improvement. Diazepam enhances GABA-ergic mechanisms (13), but whether this mode of action is pertinent to its beneficial effects in ST is unknown. Amytal improved four of six patients; in general, changes with amytal paralleled changes with diazepam. Both drugs have a sedative action, but it is unlikely that a nonspecific sedative effect accounted for their ameliorative action, as clonidine, which is a potent sedative in the dose used (39), improved only one of the six subjects.

ACKNOWLEDGMENTS

This work was supported in part by the Fund for Research in the Fields of Dyskinesia and Torticollis and the Medical Research Council (Canada). The authors thank F. Feldmuller for assistance with the CSF measurements, Dr. H. Guyda for performing the GH assays, and Drs. M. Rasminsky and G. Bertrand for referring patients for the study. The authors also thank Hoffmann-La Roche Ltd., Montreal, for providing L-DOPA and placebos and McNeil Laboratories, (Canada) Ltd., Don Mills, Ontario, for providing pimozide and placebos.

REFERENCES

1. Andén, N.-E., Butcher, S. G., Corrodi, H., Fuxe, K., and Ungerstedt, U. (1970): Receptor activity and turnover of dopamine and noradrenaline after neuroleptics. *Eur. J. Pharmacol.,* 11:303–314.
2. Andén, N.-E., Corrodi, H., Fuxe, K., Hokfelt, B., Hökfelt, T., Rydin, C., and Svensson, T. (1970): Evidence for a central noradrenaline receptor stimulation by clonidine. *Life Sci.,* 9:513–523.
3. Ansari, K. A., Webster, D., and Manning, N. (1972): Spasmodic torticollis and L-DOPA. *Neurology (Minneap.),* 22:670–674.
4. Aquilonius, S. M. (1978): Physostigmine in the treatment of drug overdose. In: *Cholinergic Mechanisms and Psychopharmacology,* edited by J. Jenden, pp. 817–825. Plenum Press, New York.
5. Barrett, R. E., Yahr, M. D., and Duvoisin, R. C. (1970): Torsion dystonia and spasmodic torticollis—results of treatment with L-DOPA. *Neurology (Minneap.),* 20:107–113.
6. Bianchine, J. R., and Bianchine, J. W. (1971): Treatment of spasmodic torticollis with diazepam. *South Med. J.,* 64:893–894.
7. Bigwood, G. F. (1972): Treatment of spasmodic torticollis. *N. Engl. J. Med.,* 286:1161.
8. Blom, S., and Ekbom, K. A. (1961): Comparison between akathisia developing in treatment with phenothiazine derivatives and the restless legs syndrome. *Acta Med. Scand.,* 170:689–694.

9. Brown, W. A., Van Woert, M. H., and Ambani, L. M. (1973): Effect of apomorphine on growth hormone release in humans. *J. Clin. Endocrinol. Metab.,* 37:463–465.
10. Bunts, A. T. (1960): The surgical treatment of spasmodic torticollis. *Am. Surg.,* 26:560–563.
11. Caraceni, T., Panerai, A. E., Parati, E. A., Cocchi, D., and Muller, E. E. (1977): Altered growth hormone and prolactin responses to dopaminergic stimulation in Huntington's chorea. *J. Clin. Endocrinol. Metab.,* 44:870–875.
12. Cockburn, J. J. (1971): Spasmodic torticollis. A psychogenic condition? *J. Psychosom. Res.,* 15:471–477.
13. Costa, E., Guidotti, A., Mao, C. C., and Suria, A. (1975): New concepts on the mechanism of action of benzodiazepines. *Life Sci.,* 17:167–186.
14. Couch, J. R. (1976): General discussion on drug therapy in dystonia. *Adv. Neurol.,* 14:417–422.
15. Couch, J. R. (1976): Dystonia and tremor in spasmodic torticollis. *Adv. Neurol.,* 14:245–258.
16. Couper-Smartt, J. (1973): Lithium in spasmodic torticollis. *Lancet,* 2:741–742.
17. Coyle, J. T., and Snyder, S. H. (1969): Antiparkinsonian drugs: inhibition of dopamine uptake in the corpus striatum as a possible mechanism of action. *Science,* 166:899–901.
18. Critchley, M. (1939): Spastic dysphonia ("inspiratory speech"). *Brain,* 62:96–103.
19. Curzon, G. (1973): Involuntary movements other than parkinsonism: biochemical aspects. *Proc. R. Soc. Med.,* 66:873–876.
20. Dayton, P. G., Yu, T. F., Chen, W., Berger, L., West, L. A., and Gutman, A. B. (1963): The physiological disposition of probenecid, including renal clearance in man, studied by an improved method for its estimation in biological material. *J. Pharmacol. Exp. Ther.,* 140:278–286.
21. Ettigi, P., Lal, S., Martin, J. B., and Friesen, H. G. (1975): Effect of sex, oral contraceptives and glucose loading on apomorphine-induced growth hormone secretion. *J. Clin. Endocrinol. Metab.,* 40:1094–1098.
22. Fabing, H. D. (1954): Alpha-(2-piperidyl) benzhydrol hydrochloride, a new central stimulant in the treatment of blepharospasm, spasmodic torticollis and narcolepsy. Preliminary report. *Trans. Am. Neurol. Assoc.,* 79:159–163.
23. Foltz, E. L., Knopp, L. M., and Ward, A. A. (1959): Experimental spasmodic torticollis. *J. Neurosurg.,* 16:55–72.
24. Franz, D. N. (1975): Drugs for Parkinson's disease; centrally acting muscle relaxants. In: *The Pharmacological Basis of Therapeutics,* edited by L. S. Goodman and A. Gilman, 5th ed., pp. 186–191. Macmillan Co. Inc., New York.
25. Gilbert, G. J., (1972): The medical treatment of spasmodic torticollis. *Arch. Neurol.,* 27:503–506.
26. Glowinski, J. (1978): Dendriatic release of dopamine: its role in the control of nigrostriatal dopaminergic neurons. *Fourth International Catecholamine Symposium,* Pacific Grove, California, September 17–22.
27. Goodwin, F. K., Post, R. M., Dunner, D. L., and Gordon, E. K. (1973): Cerebrospinal fluid amine metabolites in affective illness: the probenecid technique. *Am. J. Psychiatry,* 130:73–79.
28. Growdon, J. H., Shahani, B. T., and Young, R. R. (1975): The effect of alcohol on essential tremor. *Ne:rology (Minneap.),* 25:259–262.
29. Hassin, G. B. (1939): Quinine and dystonia musculorum deformans. *J.A.M.A.,* 113:12–14.
30. Herz, E., and Glazer, G. H. (1949): Spasmodic torticollis II. Clinical evaluation. *Arch. Neurol. Psychiatry,* 61:227–239.
31. Heuyer, M, G., Vogt, C., and Mme. Boudinesco (1934): Spasmes toniques du cou avec troubles spasmodiques de la parole entraînant l'aphonie. *Rev Neurol. (Paris),* 2:570–574.
32. Hirschmann, J., and Mayer, K. (1964): Zur Beeinflussung der Akinese und anderer extrapyramidal-motorischer Störungen mit L-DOPA (L-Dihydroxyphenylalanin) *Dtsch. Med. Wochenschr.,* 89:1877–1880.
33. Johansson, B., and Roos, B-E. (1974): 5-Hydroxyindoleacetic acid and homovanillic acid in cerebrospinal fluid of patients with neurological disease. *Eur. Neurol.,* 11:37–45.
34. Kjellin, K. G., and Stibler, H. (1975): Cerebrospinal fluid protein patterns in spasmodic torticollis. *Eur. Neurol.,* 13:461–475.
35. Klawans, H. L., Margolin, D. I., Dana, N., and Crosset, P. (1975): Supersensitivity to *d*-amphetamine- and apomorphine-induced stereotyped behaviour induced by chronic *d*-amphetamine administration. *J. Neurol. Sci.,* 25:283–289.

36. Krebs, M. E. (1939): Note sur le traitement pratique dans un cas de torticolis spasmodique. *Rev. Neurol. (Paris),* 71:423–424.
37. Lal, S., de la Vega, C. E., Sourkes, T. L., and Friesen, H. G. (1972): Effect of apomorphine on human growth hormone. *Lancet,* 2:661.
38. Lal, S., de la Vega, C. E., Sourkes, T. L., and Friesen, H. G. (1973): Effect of apomorphine on growth hormone, prolactin, luteinizing hormone and follicle stimulating hormone levels in human serum. *J. Clin. Endocrinol. Metab.,* 37:719–724.
39. Lal, S., Tolis, G., Martin, J. B., Brown, G. M., and Guyda, H. (1975): Effect of clonidine on growth hormone, prolactin luteinizing hormone, follicle stimulating hormone and thyroid stimulating hormone in the serum of normal men. *J. Clin. Endocrinol. Metab.,* 41:827–832.
40. Lees, A., Shaw, K. M., and Stern, G. M. (1976): Bromocriptine and spasmodic torticollis. *Br. Med. J.,* 1:1343.
41. Marsden, C. D. (1976): The problem of adult-onset idiopathic torsion dystonia and other isolated dyskinesias in adult life (including blepharospasm, oromandibular dystonia, dystonic writer's cramp, and torticollis or axial dystonia). *Adv. Neurol.,* 14:259–276.
42. Meares, R. (1971). An association of spasmodic torticollis and writer's cramp. *Br. J. Psychiatry,* 119:441–442.
43. Meares, R. (1971): Natural history of spasmodic torticollis, and effect of surgery. *Lancet,* 2:149–151.
44. Mori, K., Fujita, Y., Shimabukuro, H., Ito, M., and Handa, H. (1975): Some considerations for the treatment of spasmodic torticollis. Clinical and experimental studies. *Confin. Neurol.,* 37:265–269.
45. Myerson, A., and Loman, J. (1942): Amphetamine sulfate in the treatment of spasmodic torticollis. Report of two cases. *Arch. Neurol. Psychiatry,* 48:823–828.
46. Papeschi, R., and McClure, D. J. (1971): Homovanillic and 5-hydroxyindoleacetic acids in cerebrospinal fluid of depressed patients. *Arch. Gen. Psychiatry,* 25:354–358.
47. Papeschi, R., Molina-Negro, P., Sourkes, T. L., and Erba, G. (1972): The concentration of homovanillic acid and 5-hydroxyindoleacetic acids in ventricular and lumbar CSF. *Neurology (Minneap.),* 22:1151–1159.
48. Patterson, R. M., and Little, S. C. (1943). Spasmodic torticollis. *J. Nerv. Ment. Dis.,* 98:571–599.
49. Shaw, K. M., Hunter, K. R., and Stern, G. M. (1972). Medical treatment of spasmodic torticollis. *Lancet,* 1:1399.
50. Sigwald, J., Bouthier, D., Mme. Caille, and Ginestet, D. (1959): Deux cas de syndrome dystonique et dyskinétique cervico-céphalique (torticolis spasmodique, retrocolis) transformés par le 2-bis méthane sulfonate de diméthysulfamido-3 [(méthyl-4(piperazinyl)]-3' propyl]-10 phenothiazine (7843 RP). *Rev. Neurol. (Paris),* 100:778–780.
51. Snyder, S. H., Banerjee, S. P., Yamamura, H. I., and Greenberg, D. (1974): Drugs, neurotransmitters and schizophrenia. *Science,* 184:1243–1253.
52. Snyder, S., Greenberg, D., and Yamamura, H. I. (1974): Antischizophrenic drugs and brain cholinergic receptors. *Arch. Gen. Psychiatry,* 31:58–61.
53. Sourkes, T. L., and Lal, S. (1975): Apomorphine and its relation to dopamine in the nervous system. *Adv. Neurochem.,* 1:247–299.
54. Swash, M., Roberts, A. H., Zakko, H., and Heathfield, K. W. G. (1972): Treatment of involuntary movement disorders with tetrabenazine. *J. Neurol. Neurosurg. Psychiatry,* 35:186–191.
55. Tarlov, E. (1970): On the problem of the pathology of spasmodic torticollis. *J. Neurol. Neurosurg. Psychiatry,* 33:457–463.
56. Tolosa, E. S. (1978): Modification of tardive dyskinesia and spasmodic torticollis by apomorphine. *Arch. Neurol.,* 35:459–462.
57. Trillet, M., Joyeux, O., and Masson, R. (1977): Tiapride et mouvements anormaux. *Sem. Hôp. Paris,* 53:21–27.
58. Tsang, D., and Lal, S. (1977): Effect of monoamine receptor agonists and antagonists on cyclic AMP accumulation in human cerebral cortex slices. *Can. J. Physiol. Pharmacol.,* 55:1263–1269.
59. Urechia, C. I., and Mme. Retezeanu (1937): Parkinsonisme avec torticolis spasmodique ou avec tics buccaux. *Arch. Neurol.,* 56:491–494.

60. Winkler, G. F., and Young, R. R. (1974): Efficacy of chronic propranolol therapy in action tremors of the familial, senile or essential varieties. *New Engl. J. Med.*, 290:984–988.
61. Young, S. N., Lal, S., Sourkes, T. L., Feldmuller, F., Aronoff, A., and Martin, J. B. (1975): Relationships between tryptophan in the serum and CSF and 5-hydroxyindoleacetic acid in the CSF of man; the effect of cirrhosis of the liver and probenecid administration. *J. Neurol. Neurosurg. Psychiatry*, 38:322–330.

Advances in Neurology, Vol. 24, edited by
L. J. Poirier, T. L. Sourkes, and P. J. Bédard.
Raven Press, New York © 1979.

Comparative Study of Spinal Reflexes in L-DOPA-Induced Dyskinesia and Dystonia

N. Bathien, S. Toma, and P. Rondot

Service de Neurologie, Centre Hospitalier Sainte-Anne, Paris, France

Whatever may be the variety of abnormal movements observed in extrapyramidal disorders, they all have a "common final pathway," namely the motoneuron. Therefore, it seemed interesting to test and compare motoneuron excitability in several extrapyramidal disorders (parkinsonism, dystonia), through mono- and polysynaptic reflexes.

Certain patterns being thus established they could be more easily ascribed to a biochemical disorder. Although it has been difficult until recently to establish such correlations in the above-mentioned disorders, it is now possible to establish them in models of abnormal movements induced by stimulation of dopaminergic receptors in parkinsonian patients treated with L-DOPA. Such a study has been undertaken and the results of these tests will be compared with those obtained in untreated patients with parkinsonian rigidity and patients with dystonia and athetosis.

METHODS

The tests were performed on 11 parkinsonian patients with L-DOPA dyskinesia in the extremities and 6 patients with dystonia. Stimulation and recording techniques of spinal reflexes in man were performed as published in detail elsewhere (1,2,5). The H reflex technique, standardized by Hugon and reported at the International Congress in Brussels (1973) (4), was also employed. The tibial nerve was stimulated in the popliteal fossa by rectangular electric pulses of 1-msec duration at frequency of 0.3/sec. The activity of the soleus muscle (Sol) was recorded by surface electrodes placed on the midline at the lower and middle third of the calf. Polysynaptic reflex responses were obtained by stimulation of the sural nerve at the ankle and by recording the activity of the biceps femoris muscle (Bi) and the tibialis anterior muscle (Ta). Shortening reaction was recorded from Ta. Passive movement of the ankle was monitored by a goniometer giving a linear deflection throughout the movement. Dyskinesia was recorded by surface electrodes at the level of the extensor digitorum muscle (Ext dig) and flexor digitorum muscle (Fl dig). All these tests were recorded during the same session. For parkinsonian patients, records from the rigid phase and the hyperkinetic phase were obtained on the same day during the fluctuations due to the therapeutic effects.

RESULTS

L-DOPA Dyskinesia

Abnormal Movements

Figure 1 shows two types of EMG activity in the 11 parkinsonian patients presenting dyskinesia of the extremities after prolonged treatment with L-DOPA. The first type consists of short busts of arrhythmic activity that are irregular in amplitude and frequency. The activities recorded at the level of the finger flexors (Fl dig) and extensors (Ext dig) are not coordinated. This type of EMG activity corresponds to the choreiform pattern (Ch P).

The second type of activity is characterized by a grouping of the discharges in longer bursts, about 500 msec. These activities are recorded simultaneously in both antagonistic muscles (Fl dig and Ext dig). They are more rhythmical, their average frequency being 1 to 2 c/sec and are therefore termed the *rhythmic pattern* (Rh P). Out of the 11 patients observed, the Ch P was recorded seven times, the Rh P once, and three cases showed fluctuations between both patterns of activity (Table 1). We see that in two patients presenting dyskinesias of the diphasic type (start and end of dose), the Ch P pattern is found in one, and both the Ch P and Rh P in the other.

Figure 2 shows that an intravenous injection of 3 mg piribedil transforms the Ch P in Rh P in the same patient: at the 5th min a grouping of discharges is observed. The secondary effects (nausea, vomiting) have disappeared. At the 10th min the bursts become rhythmical and synchronous in both Ta and Sol muscles. The bursts begin to desynchronize at the 15th min and the dyskinesias resume completely. The Ch P pattern reappeared at about the 30th min. The same effects were obtained with apomorphine. These results show that these

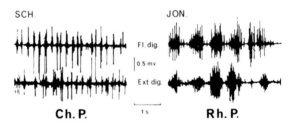

FIG. 1. Two EMG types of L-DOPA dyskinesia. The recordings were made at the level of the upper limb flexor digitorum (Fl dig) and extensor digitorum (Ext dig) muscles. Note that the choreiform pattern (Ch P) consists of uncoordinated bursts of irregular frequency, and that the second type, rhythmical pattern (Rh P), is more regular while the Ext Fl bursts are synchronous.

TABLE 1. *Clinical and neurophysiological parameters in L-DOPA induced dyskinesia*[a]

Patient	Clinical types	EMG patterns	H/M ratio (% of control)	Polys. noc. reflex	Shortening reaction
1	M	Ch	150	N	0
2	M	Rh	300	+	0
3	M	Rh + Ch	170	+	0
4	M	Ch	130	+	0
5	M	Ch	130	+	0
6	D	Ch	130	+	0
7	M	Rh + Ch	170	+	0
8	M	Ch	150	+	0
9	D	Rh + Ch	150	+	0
10	M	Ch	160	+	0
11	M	Ch	140	+	0
Summary	2D 9M	10 Ch 4 Rh	H/M ratio increased	facilitated	abolished

[a] Abbreviations: M, monophasic; Ch, choreiform; N, normal; D, diphasic; Rh, rhythmical; +, facilitated.

dyskinesias are intensified by a DA agonist and that the Ch P and the Rh P pattern correspond to different degrees of stimulation of the dopaminergic receptor.

Spinal Reflexes

We have previously shown that in patients with parkinsonian rigidity, the monosynaptic excitability of the extensor motoneurons tested by the H reflex (H/Sol) is lowered (2).

The H/M ratio average of the group tested is 12.5 ± 4.0%. It is significantly lower than in normal individuals. Figure 3A2 illustrates the results in a patient whose H/M is 0.10 during a rigid phase. During the hyperkinetic phase it rises up to 0.40 in all patients. Compared with the rigid phase, increases of 61.8 ± 5.1% are recorded. H/M, although not normalized as in the case shown in Fig. 3, is significantly improved.

The polysynaptic excitability of motoneurons is shown in Fig. 3A3. We see that the stimulation of the sural nerve in the ankle produces a nociceptive reflex response (1) at the level of the femoral biceps in the normal subject. At a stimulation level that results in a preliminary nociceptive response in the femoral biceps (Bi), no reflex activity of the same latency is recorded in the Ta during the rigid phase. During L-DOPA dyskinesias, the same intensity of stimulation causes a nociceptive response in Ta and Bi. This phenomenon corresponds to an increase of excitability of the nociceptive polysynaptic system. It was observed in 10 out of the 11 cases tested.

During passive movement a shortening reaction is generally recorded in the wrist extensor and the Ta (5). Figure 3A4 shows tonic activity of the Ta muscle

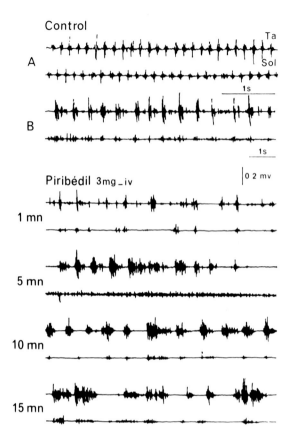

FIG. 2. Effect of piribedil on L-DOPA dyskinesia. **A:** EMG recording of the parkinsonian tremor in the tibialis anterior muscle (Ta) and the soleus muscle (Sol) during the rigid phase. It is a well-organized and coordinated 5–6-c/sec tremor. **B:** same recording in the same patient during the hyperkinetic phase. Note that the dyskinesia is of the choreiform type (Ch P). Under the influence of piribedil (3 mg i.v.), the EMG activity becomes more rhythmical and synchronous. The Rh P is recorded 10 min after the injection.

during passive dorsal flexion of the ankle. This tonic shortening reaction is superseded by a phasic reaction in connection with the flexion movement during the L-DOPA dyskinesia. This phenomenon was observed in all 11 patients observed.

Dystonia

The muscular activity produced by passive mobilization is the prevailing disorder recorded in athetosis and dystonias. We tried to determine the characteristics of the passive movement which cause this phenomenon in 6 dystonic patients. Figure 4 shows that the shortening reaction (SR) appears only with a certain amplitude of movement which corresponds to a true stimulation level. In the case shown in Fig. 4 it appears after flexion of 18° of the ankle joint. The average in the six patients is an angle of 15.0 ± 2.0°.

Figure 5 sums up the results of 31 measurements. A significant correlation can be noted between the ankle angulation and the SR amplitude ($r = 0.92$). The correlation coefficient is of 0.25 (ns) for the movement speed.

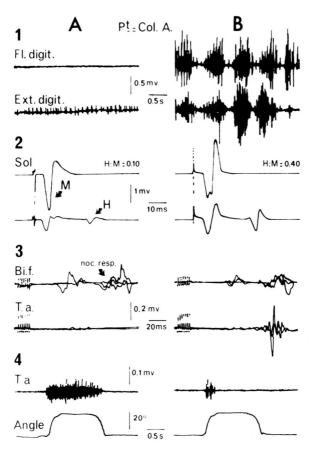

FIG. 3. Changes in spinal reflexes during L-DOPA dyskinocia. **A:** The recordings were made on the same patient during the rigid phase with tremor confined to the extremities, and **B:** during the hyperkinetic phase with abnormal movements of the Rh P type. **1:** EMG recording of the upper limb dyskinesia at the level of the flexor digitorum muscle (Fl dig) and of the extensor digitorum muscle (Ext dig). *A1,* 6–7-c/sec tremor in Ext dig; *B1,* L-DOPA dyskinesia of the Rh P type at the level of Fl dig and Ext dig. **2:** H soleus reflex (Sol). The M max (M) and H max (H) responses are shown in *A2* and *B2.* Note that the H/M ratio is increased in *B2.* **3:** Polysynaptic reflex of lower limb. The reflex responses of the biceps femoris muscle (Bi f) and of the tibialis anterior muscle (Ta) are induced by stimulation of the sural nerve at the ankle. **4:** SR is tonic in *A4,* the EMG activity is recorded during the whole lapse of shortening. SR is phasic in *B4.*

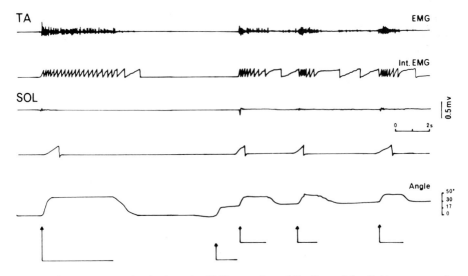

FIG. 4. Shortening reaction in dystonia: EMG recording of the Ta and the Sol in response to the angulation of the ankle *(angle)*. It may be observed that there exists an angle level at which SR is induced.

The H/M ratio of the dystonic patient is slightly increased compared with normal subjects; it is 0.50–0.70 (Table 2). It has a significantly higher amplitude in comparison to the amplitude recorded in parkinsonian rigidity.

The polysynaptic excitability tested through the nociceptive polysynaptic reflex of the lower limb is increased. When applying stimulation which causes a nociceptive preliminary response in Bi f, a reflex discharge of identical latency is recorded in the Ta.

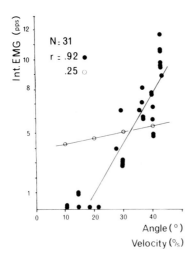

FIG. 5. Relation between the EMG activity of the SR and the passive movement of the ankle. Ordinates: integrated EMG activity (int. EMG). Abscissa: Angulation of ankle *(angle)* and rate of movement. Note a significant correlation between the angulation and EMG int. ($r = 0.92$), while the correlation between rate and int. EMG ($r = 0.25$) is not significant. ●, experimental values; O, statistical values of the correlation curve.

TABLE 2. *Neurophysiologic parameters in patients with dystonia*

Patient	H/M ratio	Polys. noc. reflex	Shortening reaction
1	0.70	Facilitated	Tonic
2	0.50	Normal	Tonic
3	0.60	Facilitated	Tonic
4	0.70	Facilitated	Tonic
5	0.65	Facilitated	Tonic
6	0.60	Facilitated	Tonic

The abnormal movements recorded are associated with grouped discharges of long duration and of an average frequency of 1 c/sec.

DISCUSSION

The present study shows that abnormal movements provoked by L-DOPA involve a state of monosynaptic excitability that is close to normal. It also involves hyperexcitability to the polysynaptic test responsible for the facilitation of the nociceptive system. There does not exist a difference of nature but of intensity between the two types of abnormal movements provoked by L-DOPA (choreiform pattern or rhythmic pattern), whether they appear during the middle of the administered dose or in a biphasic way.

The tendency of the monosynaptic test to be normal may be considered as being due to the disappearance of rigidity. The latter is correspondingly associated with a decrease of the H/M ratio, which results from the inhibition produced by the antagonists on the agonistic motoneurons (2). The hyperexcitability of the nociceptive system appears as a quite particular phenomenon which may be compared to the inhibition of the opiate receptors caused by L-DOPA (3).

The occurrence of a low frequency rhythmical activity, which consists of long-lasting bursts associated with an almost normal monosynaptic excitability and an hyperexcitability of the nociceptive system, may be considered characteristic of the stimulation of the dopaminergic receptors. The question arises of whether the presence of a phasic shortening reflex should be added to these elements, or if it should be considered as a step toward normality of the exaggerated shortening reflex observed in the parkinsonian patient. We would be inclined to favor the latter view, the SR being phasic in the normal subject (5).

In dystonia, several of the former elements are present together. As with L-DOPA dyskinesia, the nociceptive reflexes are exaggerated and the monosynaptic reflex is normal or slightly increased. There is also a SR but it is of the tonic type (7). Moreover, the spontaneous activity is not grouped in bursts which tend to be rhythmical, as revealed in the EMG. Therefore, these two types of movement disorders must be clearly separated, the second one representing an hyperactivity of the dopaminergic receptors.

Another element may be derived from this study: the difference of nature between the mechanisms causing the nociceptive reflex and those responsible for the SR. Indeed, we have noted that in parkinsonian rigidity the nociceptive reflex is normal, while the SR is exaggerated (6) and becomes tonic. On the contrary, during L-DOPA dyskinesias, while the nociceptive reflex is increased, the SR tends to be normal. These two types of reactions must therefore be differentiated. The study of SR during passive movement leads us to consider the articular or cutaneous tactile fibers as being an important part of the mechanism involved in this reaction.

SUMMARY

Neurophysiological investigations were performed in 11 parkinsonian patients with L-DOPA dyskinesia and in 6 patients with dystonia. EMG activity during abnormal movements, monosynaptic, nociceptive polysynaptic reflex responses of the lower limb and muscular response to passive movement (shortening and myotatic reaction) were recorded. During L-DOPA dyskinesia, EMG activities can be classified in two types: (a) the choreiform pattern (Ch P), which is irregular in amplitude and frequency, and is not coordinated in EMG flexor and extensor activity; and (b) the rhythmic pattern (Rh P), which includes bursts of 500-msec duration with a frequency of 1 to 2 c/sec. They are synchronous with EMG activity in antagonist muscles. Dopaminergic drugs (apomorphine and piribedil) injected intravenously change Ch P to Rh P.

In comparison to the rigid phase, H/M ratio is increased, the nociceptive polysynaptic reflex enhanced and the shortening reaction abolished. During dystonia, the spontaneous activity frequency is lower. Shortening reaction was recorded in all the six cases. Monosynaptic excitability tested by H/M ratio is within normal range or slightly increased. Polysynaptic nociceptive reflex is increased in every case. The mechanisms responsible for the changes in motoneuron excitability in these extrapyramidal disorders are discussed.

REFERENCES

1. Bathien, N., and Bourdarias, H. (1972): Lower limb cutaneous reflexes in hemiplegia. *Brain,* 95:447–456.
2. Bathien, N., and Rondot, P. (1977): Reciprocal continuous inhibition in rigidity of parkinsonism. *J. Neurol. Neurosurg. Psychiatry,* 40:20–24.
3. Cuello, A. C. (1978): Enkephalin and substance P containing neurones in the trigeminal and extrapyramidal systems. In: *Advances in Biochemical Psychopharmacology,* Vol. 18, edited by E. Costa and M. Trabucchi, 111–123. Raven Press, New York.
4. Hugon, M. (1973): Methodology of the Hoffmann reflex in man. In: *New Developments in Electromyography and Clinical Neurophysiology,* Vol. 3, edited by J. E. Desmedt, pp. 277–293. Karger, Basel.
5. Katz, R., and Rondot, P. (1978): Reaction to muscle passive shortening in normal man. *EEG Clin. Neurophysiol.,* 45:90–99.
6. Rondot, P., and Metral, S. (1973): Analysis of the shortening reaction in man. In: *New Developments in Electromyography and Clinical Neurophysiology,* Vol. 3, edited by J. E. Desmedt, pp. 629–634. Karger, Basel.
7. Rondot, P., and Scherrer, J. (1966): Contraction réflexe provoquée par le raccourcissement passif du muscle dans l'athétose et les dystonies d'attitude. *Rev. Neurol. (Paris),* 114:329–337.

Advances in Neurology, Vol. 24, edited by
L. J. Poirier, T. L. Sourkes, and P. J. Bédard.
Raven Press, New York © 1979.

Analysis of Two Factors Influencing Involuntary Movement: Psychological Stress Effect and Motor Effect

H. Narabayashi, T. Chida, and T. Kondo

Department of Neurology, Juntendo Medical School, Tokyo, Japan

Various types of involuntary movements are known to be influenced by voluntary movements. Intention tremor, which appears only during active movements of the limbs, is a typical example. Postural tremor, which occurs in certain postures of the limbs, may be considered as occurring during the static and voluntary contractions of the muscles. Even the jerky and irregular involuntary movements (choreic) seen in Huntington's disease (HD) are möre conspicuous and they are worsened when the patient tries to perform movements such as standing, walking, or complex coordination (11,12,29).

For the severely handicapped patients, however, the voluntary movements or the maintenance of certain postures are not as easily or smoothly performed as in normal persons, and they might involve, at least, two factors. The first is obviously the movement or muscular tension itself, which usually involves the integration of the activities of several muscles, and the second is the psychological tension associated with the effort to accurately perform a difficult task. It may easily be imagined that psychological tension is great when the patient with coarse intention or postural tremor due to cerebellar disease attempts to perform the finger–nose test, or else, when the severely choreic patients try to walk or to write.

METHOD OF ANALYSIS

The purpose of this study is to differentiate and evaluate separately the effect of each of these two factors, i.e., the influence of motor performance itself and of psychological effort on the importance and the amount of involuntary movements, by applying the simple clinical maneuvers described below (Fig. 1).

At first the patient is placed in the supine position under complete psychological and motor relaxation (no loading, situation 1). Then he is asked to keep the arm flexed at elbow at 90° in a relaxing posture, which means slight contraction of the biceps brachii muscle only (motor loading, situation 2). In some

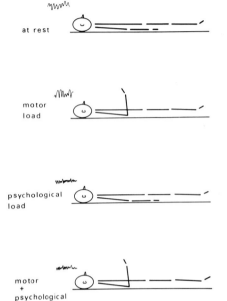

at rest

motor
load

FIG. 1. Four situations of loading test (see text). EEG waves on the *left* indicate the degree of attention.

psychological
load

motor
+
psychological
load

instances a slightly greater task was tested, such as holding the arm straight up in a relaxed manner, at right angle to the body-axis at the shoulder.

The third situation consists in asking the patient to perform (without any motor activity) some psychological tasks, such as mentally counting back serial numbers from one hundred, or mental calculation (psychological loading, situation 3).

In the fourth situation, the above two tasks, motor and psychological, are applied together (motor and psychological loading, situation 4), the patient being in the supine position.

These four situations were applied to patients with involuntary movements of different types. The changes in the amount and in the pattern of involuntary movements were examined clinically and recorded on 16-mm film. Multichannel surface EMG recording of the muscles involved in the involuntary movements was done.

RESULTS

Cases displaying the various involuntary movements were examined under four test situations.

Case 1. The choreic abnormal movements in Huntington's disease, characterized by the abrupt and irregular muscle contractions involving different muscular groups of the face, trunk and extremities, are already present in situation 1

(Fig. 2). The particular case recorded was a 50-year-old male patient (with a typical family history) who began to show abnormal choreic movements 4 years earlier. The choreic movements occurring a little more often in the left arm and the right leg were seen even in the completely relaxed supine position.

The choreic movements did not increase significantly when the motor loading test was applied, even though occasional minimum changes cannot be ruled out. In Fig. 2, tonic contractions of the biceps brachii and of the forearm flexor muscles are noticeable on EMG, which corresponds to elbow flexed posture. Compared with the marked increase of choreic twitches under psychological load, the minimum increase under motor loading is almost negligible. Under psychological loading, involuntary movements markedly increase and spread all over the body, i.e., face, trunk, and extremities.

A 68-year-old female patient with hemiballism due to thrombosis presented similar features, i.e., the left-sided ballistic movements being similar at rest and under motor loading. These movements were violent and flinging even when the patient was in the supine resting position and they were almost the same under motor loading. However, they were markedly increased by psychological loading.

Perioral dyskinesia in the adult patient and DOPA-induced dyskinesia in parkinsonism also displayed the same characteristics in choreic movements. They were worsened and of greater amplitude under psychological loading but not under motor loading.

All types of involuntary movements had similar features in that they were present even during complete rest and did not increase much under motor loading. However, they were noticeably increased under psychological loading, though the original pattern of each involuntary movement was unchanged.

Case 2. Parkinsonian tremor reacted similarly to the above four conditions in its response to the loading tests (Fig. 3). In the 58-year-old male patient, the regular rhythmic tremor of the arm of about 5.5 Hz was already present in the resting and supine position, therefore, was named "tremor at rest." It tended to disappear when the arm was active or passively moved to an elbow-flexed position, and soon started again when the arm remained in the new position, corresponding to the phenomenon well known as "resetting of tremor." The moderate amount of rhythmic tremor was similar at rest and under motor loading as illustrated in Fig. 3, although the right extensor muscles showed some increased activity. However, the remarkable increase under psychological load in all triceps, forearm flexor, and extensor muscles greatly contrasts with the slight increase caused by motor loading.

Combined motor and psychological loading resulted in the maximally increased tremor of all four muscles.

Case 3. Postural tremor and intention tremor are characterized by the fact that they are not present "at rest," thus providing the diagnostic basis of the original disease. In this way, they are different from the rest tremor in parkinsonism. Figure 4 illustrates the coarse postural tremor of the right arm due to a

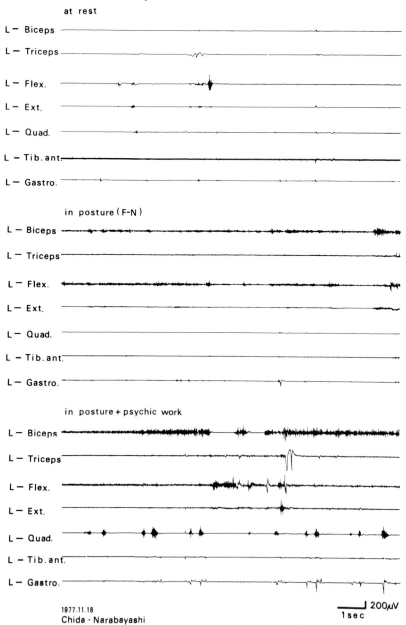

Case S.Y. 50y. male. H.D.

FIG. 2. Choreic movements in Huntington's disease (see text).

Case K.S. 58 y. male. Parkinson

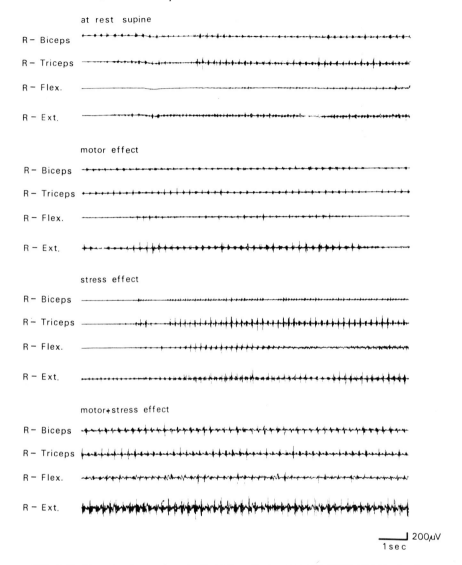

FIG. 3. Parkinsonian tremor (see text). *Motor effect* means the effect of motor loading.

vascular lesion at the upper midbrain level in a 71-year-old female patient. It is not present at all at rest (supine position) but it becomes very marked during posture such as finger touching the nose (FN). Under this condition, there is marked grouping of discharges in the finger extensors and flexors and the biceps muscles. Tight finger grasping also results in marked and rhythmic tremor,

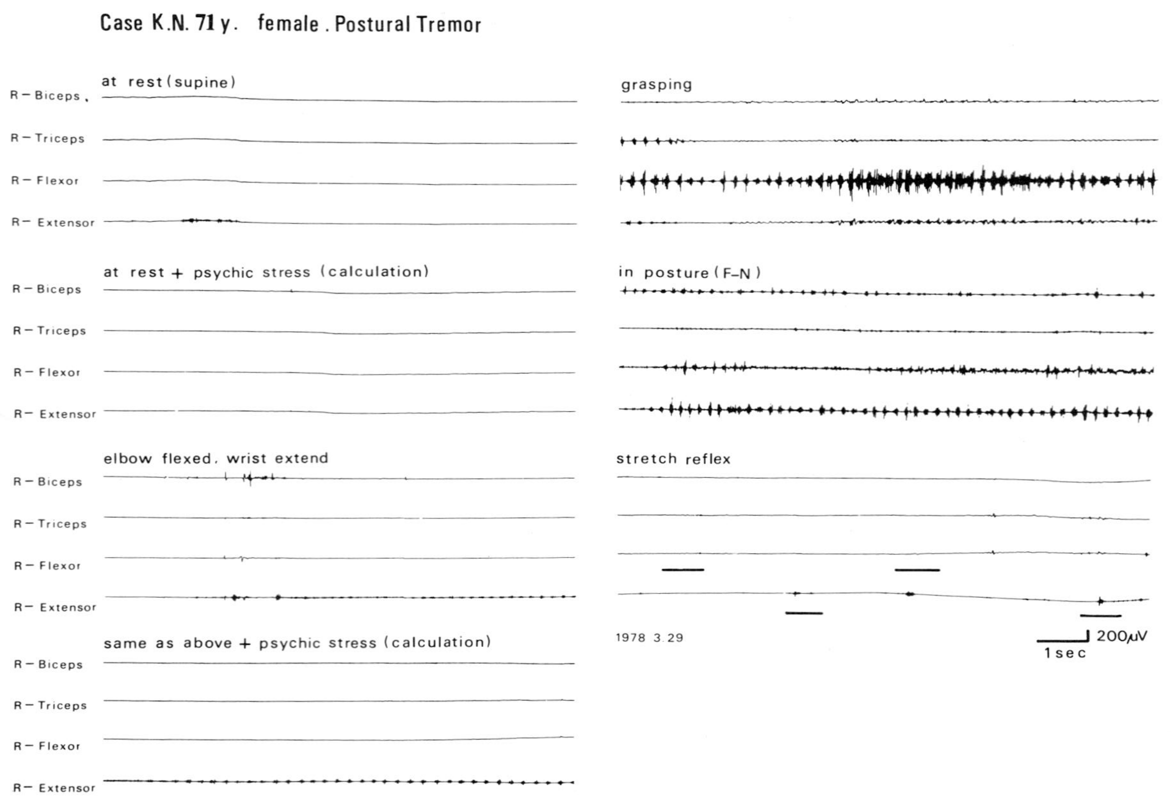

Case K.N. 71 y. female. Postural Tremor

at rest (supine)   grasping

R − Biceps.
R − Triceps
R − Flexor
R − Extensor

at rest + psychic stress (calculation)   in posture (F−N)

R − Biceps
R − Triceps
R − Flexor
R − Extensor

elbow flexed. wrist extend   stretch reflex

R − Biceps
R − Triceps
R − Flexor
R − Extensor

same as above + psychic stress (calculation)   1978 3. 29

R − Biceps
R − Triceps
R − Flexor
R − Extensor

200 μV
1 sec

FIG. 4. Postural tremor (see text). *Stress* means psychological loading.

especially in the finger flexors as seen on the EMG. There is no increase of tone at rest, as shown by the absence of passive stretch reflexes, and moreover, the muscles were relatively hypotonic.

In this patient, no tremulous movements were obtained in response to psychological loading (calculation), but motor loading, produced by flexing the elbow and extending the wrist, caused slight tremor of the biceps and forearm extensor muscles; they gradually tended to increase. When the psychological loading is added to motor loading, the tremorous discharges and movements are greater and more sustained.

DISCUSSION AND COMMENTS

From these results involving very simple maneuvers, it is obvious that there are two groups of involuntary movements. The first group includes the abnormal movements that are already present and obvious even in complete rest. Choreic movements in HD, hemiballism, peroral dyskinesia, DOPA-induced dyskinesia, and the parkinsonian tremor belong to this group. They are exaggerated and worsened by psychological loading but not by motor loading.

The second group of symptoms do not appear during complete rest but they tend to start and are easily observed under motor loading. The typical example is the postural or intention tremor. This group of involuntary movements is little influenced by psychological loading alone.

The different reaction of each symptom to loading test might be due to the difference in the underlying pathophysiology. They have been regarded as "positive symptoms" in contrast to the "negative symptoms" in the sense of loss of function. Such difference is thought to be related to the difference in the nature and site of the pathological changes. Therefore, we should now consider the site of the pathology for each symptom.

In Huntington's chorea, the choreic movements are thought to result from pathology in the striatum (2,12,26). The small nerve cells are selectively degenerated in the caudate nucleus and putamen. This is considered as the main pathological change responsible for choreic movements in this disease, whereas the frontal atrophy is responsible for the mental symptoms.

Hemiballism (3,13,27,28) is well recognized as being due to lesions in the subthalamic nucleus. The subthalamic nucleus receives afferents from the external segment of the globus pallidus (GP) and heavily projects to the internal segment of the pallidum. The nucleus is therefore closely linked with the GP.

The pathology responsible for peroral dykinesia in eight aged patients has been reported by Kameyama et al. (9). They found that small vascular lesions in or near the head of the caudate nucleus were the common finding. This is also the case in our patient *(unpublished data)*.

The three above-mentioned abnormal movements belong to the same category, in view of the fact that the symptom-generating mechanism is in the basal ganglia. This, in turn, acts through the pallidal efferent pathways mostly on the base of the thalamus.

Parkinsonian motor symptoms are now regarded as resulting from pharmacodynamic changes in the striatum secondary to nigral or nigrostriatal pathology. The latter finding has been known for several decades, but recent knowledge concerning the role of striatal dopamine opened new avenues for the understanding of the parkinsonian symptoms. Although the neuronal mechanisms, and the question of whether synaptic dopamine has an inhibitory or facilitatory effect on the striatal neurons, are still not well explained, it is generally agreed that the active mechanisms responsible for the symptoms, especially rigidity and akinesia, can be assumed to be located in the striopallidum and not in the nigra.

The author has slightly different views concerning tremor-generating mechanisms as opposed to those responsible for rigidity, as reported elsewhere (14–16,21,24,25). According to the author's investigation of the neuronal activities of the thalamic subnuclei during the procedure of stereotaxic thalamotomy, tremor-generating mechanisms appear to be located in, or at least closely linked (through pathways), with the ventralis intermedius nucleus (Vim) of the thalamus.

At any rate, what is important for discussion in this chapter is that neither rigidity nor tremor may be considered any longer as a direct consequence of nigral pathology, for the active physiological loci responsible for these positive symptoms are situated in the basal ganglia for rigidity, and in the thalamic subnuclei for tremor, respectively.

Therefore, the pathophysiological mechanisms responsible for all five symptoms constituting the first group are located in the basal ganglia or diencephalon.

Symptoms of the second group differ from those of the first group by the fact that the underlying pathology is more specific. They are associated with structural changes of the cerebellocerebral efferent pathways, as well as with lesions in the basal ganglia or diencephalon. The postural or intention tremor, the dentato-rubro-pallido-Luysian atrophy (DRPLA) (10) and posticteric athetosis (7) seem to belong to this group. For the sake of clarity, the DRPLA and athetosis will not be considered since their pathology varies so much from case to case. They would require another chapter.

Postural or intention tremor is abolished and well modified by stereotaxic thalamotomy (4,13). The target of the surgical lesion for alleviation of this type of tremor is radiologically and physiologically identical to the target aimed at in thalamotomy for parkinsonian tremor. In cases with either postural or parkinsonian tremor, the microrecording from neurons within the Vim reveals the existence of bursts of unit discharges, which are synchronous in phase with the peripheral tremor. Such bursts are thought to be due to deafferentation from the cerebellar input in cases of tremor of cerebellar origin (1,18). Electrical microstimulation of these cells suppresses or modifies the tremorous movements, and a small surgical destruction promptly abolishes tremor. From these observations it may be postulated that the subnuclei of the thalamus contain a tremorogenic mechanism common to the three different types of tremor.

In postural or intention tremor as opposed to parkinsonian tremor, the existence of pathology of the cerebellar efferents to the thalamus is obvious. The difference in clinical features between rest tremor and postural or intention tremor may reasonably be assumed to relate to the absence or existence of this pathology.

From these studies, deficit of the cerebellar inflow to the thalamus might explain why involuntary movements, such as postural or intention tremor, are not obvious in resting posture. The cerebellothalamic projections are facilitatory in nature (5). In the clinical sense they might provide the driving impulses to the pathophysiological mechanism occurring in the basal ganglia and diencephalon and causing the involuntary movements (19,20,22,23).

The pattern of each type of involuntary movement, such as choreic, ballistic, athetoid, or tremulous movement, is related to the pathology or pathophysiological disturbance within the basal ganglia and diencephalon. They usually appear in the resting state. When the interruption or deficit of the cerebellar efferent system is superimposed, these involuntary movements tend to disappear in the resting state. They will appear only under motor loading.

Psychological loading using mental calculation or counting back serial numbers is an easy test that may be routinely applied to induce or facilitate involuntary movements at bedside, especially parkinsonian tremor. At this time, the mechanisms by which loading influences movements are not explained. This represents one of the key problems in psychophysiology of movement. Göpfert et al. (6) reported that the psychological task, using Kraepelin's continuous adding test, resulted in a very slight increase of muscle tone. It must be remembered that psychological loading alone is not sufficient to induce abnormal movements when tremor is absent at rest, such as in intention or postural tremor. However, it may increase already existing involuntary movements. Tremor, intentional or postural, which already appears under motor loading, becomes severe when psychological loading is further superimposed.

The disclosure that the cerebellar output to the cerebrum is probably providing the tonic, facilitatory activity sustaining the involuntary movements that originate in the cerebrum, may contribute to the definition of the role played by the cerebellum even in normal physiology. This observation may help to understand why cerebellar symptoms are absent at rest, when the patient is making no movement, and are present only during movement or posture (Fig. 5).

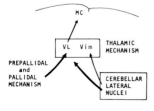

FIG. 5. Cerebellar driving *(thick line)* acting on the motor mechanisms of the basal ganglia (prepallidal mechanism) and the thalamus. The latter two structures constitute together a prethalamic mechanism. The degeneration of the small cerebellar efferents projecting to the Vim is thought to cause tremor bursts.

On the other hand, the interrelationship between the basal ganglia–diencephalic mechanism and those of the cerebellum might be an important feature to consider in understanding the degeneration which involves more than one nervous structure such as DRPLA (10), strionigral degeneration (SND), or olivopontocerebellar atrophy (OPCA) (8).

Many clinical pictures may result from the combined impairment of both systems, each being involved to a different degree. However, the general rule derived from the typical cases described in this short paper could not be directly applied. But the general rule of differentiating between the influence of motor loading and of psychological loading provides the basis of analyzing such complex clinical pictures. The important role of movement or posture in modifying the involuntary movements must be acknowledged (17).

Other abnormal motor activities, such as dystonia and myoclonic movements, need further discussion, and observations on athetosis and DRPLA will be reported elsewhere. In addition, the manner in which motor loading induces the involuntary movements that are absent at rest must be investigated. The latter movements are associated with pathology of the cerebellar efferent system. In this regard, it could be of key importance to determine the role played by muscle tone, and especially, the amount of muscle afferents involved at rest, in posture, or in action.

SUMMARY

1. Simple clinical maneuvers, motor loading and psychological loading tests, are useful to differentiate two groups of involuntary movements.

REFERENCES

1. Bates, J. A. V. (1971): The pathophysiology of parkinsonism. In: *Bel Air Symposium, IV,* pp. 269–274. Masson, Paris.
2. Bruyn, G. W. (1968): Huntington's chorea. Historical, clinical and laboratory synapsis. In: *Handbook of Clinical Neurology, Vol. 6: Disease of the Basal Ganglia,* edited by P. J. Vinken and G. W. Bruyn, pp. 298–378. North-Holland, Amsterdam.
3. Carpenter, M. B. (1955): Ballism associated with partial destruction of the subthalamic nucleus of Luys. *Neurology (Minneap.),* 5:479–489.
4. Cooper, I. S. (1969): Intention tremor. In: *Involuntary Movement Disorders,* Chap. 3, pp. 95–130. Harper & Row, New York.
5. Eccles, J. C., Ito, M., and Szentagothai, J. (1967): *The Cerebellum as a Neuronal Machine,* pp. 270–272. Springer, Berlin.
6. Göpfert, H., Bernsmeier, A., and Stufler, R. (1953): Über die steigerungen des Energiestoffwechsels und der Muskelinnervation bei geistiger Arbeit. *Pflugers Arch.,* 256:304–320.
7. Haymaker, W., Margoles, C., Pentschew, A., Jacob, H., Lindenberg, R., Arroyo, L. S., Stochdorph, O., and Stowens, D. (1961): Pathology of kernicterus and posticteric encephalopathy. In: *Kernicterus and Its Importance in Cerebral Palsy* (Conference presented by the American Academy for Cerebral Palsy), pp. 21–229. Charles C Thomas, Springfield, Ill.
8. Hirayama, K. (1977): Symptoms due to combined lesions in cerebellar and extrapyramidal structures. *Rinshyo Shinkeigaku (Clinical Neurology),* 17:832–835 (in Japanese).
9. Kameyama, M., Yamanouchi, H., Suda, E., Togi, H., and Inoue, S. (1974): Oral dyskinesia in the aged. *Saishin Igaku (Modern Medicine),* 29:290–298 (in Japanese).

10. Kosaka, K., Oyanagi, S. Matsushita, M., Hori, A., Iwase, S. (1977): Multiple system degeneration involving thalamus, reticular degeneration, pallidonigral, pallido-Luysian and dentate-rubral systems. A case report. *Acta Neuropathol.,* 39:89–95.
11. Mayer, C., and Reisch, O. (1925): Zur Symptomatologie der Huntingtonschen Chorea. *Arch. Psychiatr. Nervenkr.,* 74:795.
12. Merritt, H. H. (1955): *A Textbook of Neurology,* pp. 428–432. Lea & Febiger, Philadelphia.
13. Mundinger, F., Riechert, T., and Disselhoff, J. (1970): Long-term results of stereotaxic operations on extrapyramidal hyperkinesia (excluding parkinsonism). *Confin. Neurol.,* 32:71–78.
14. Narabayashi, H. (1968): Functional differentiation in and around the ventrolateral nucleus of the thalamus based on experience in human stereoencephalotomy. *Johns Hopkins Med. J.,* 122:295–300.
15. Narabayashi, H. (1968): Tremor localization within the thalamus. *Shinkei Kenkyu no Shinpo (Advances in Neurological Sciences),* 12:933–937 (in Japanese).
16. Narabayashi, H. (1969): Muscle tone conducting system and tremor concerned structures. In: *Third Symposium on Parkinson's Disease,* edited by F. J. Gillingham and I. M. L. Donaldson, pp. 246–251. Livingstone, Edinburgh.
17. Narabayashi, H. (1973): Importance of muscle tone in production or modification of tremorous movements. In: *Parkinson's Disease,* edited by J. Siegfried, pp. 27–36. Hans Huber, Bern.
18. Narabayashi, H. (1974): Possible role of cerebellar circuits in parkinsonian symptoms. *Confin. Neurol.,* 36:292–301.
19. Narabayashi, H. (1977): Influence of cerebellar pathology on clinical pictures of extrapyramidal symptoms—hypothesis. *Shinkei Kenkyu no Shinpo (Advances in Neurological Sciences),* 21:86–90 (in Japanese).
20. Narabayashi, H. (1978): Involuntary movements. Its new understanding from experiences of stereoencephalotomy. *Neurol. Med. Chir. (Tokyo),* 18(2):355–360 (in Japanese).
21. Narabayashi, H.: Tremor mechanism. In: *Textbook of Stereotaxy of the Human Brain,* 2nd ed., edited by G. Schaltenbrand and E. Walker. Georg Thieme, Stuttgart *(in press).*
22. Narabayashi, H.: Cerebellar modification of involuntary movements. In: *Integrative Control Functions of the Brain,* publication by the Research Committee on "Integrative Control Function of the Brain" supported by grant of Ministry of Education, Japan *(in press).*
23. Narabayashi, H., Goto, A., Miyazaki, S., and Kosaka, K. (1974): Importance of the cerebellar hemisphere in production of tremulous movement or choreodystonic movement in monkeys. *Acta Neurochir. (Suppl.),* 21:35–38.
24. Narabayashi, H., and Ohye, Ch. (1978): Parkinsonian tremor and nucleus ventralis intermedius (Vim) of human thalamus. In: *Progress in Clinical Neurophysiology,* Vol. 5, edited by J. E. Desmedt, 165–172. Karger, Basel.
25. Ohye, Ch., Saito, Y., Fukamachi, A., and Narabayashi, H. (1974): An analysis of the spontaneous rhythmic and non-rhythmic burst discharges in the human thalamus. *J. Neurol. Sci.,* 22:245–259.
26. Spiegel, E. A., and Wycis, H. T. (1952): Thalamotomy and pallidotomy for treatment of choreic movements. *Acts Neurochir.,* 2:417–422.
27. Tsubokawa, T., and Moriyasu, N. (1975): Lateral pallidotomy for relief of ballistic movement. Its basic evidences and clinical application. *Confin. Neurol.,* 37:10–15.
28. Tsubokawa, T., Moriyasu, N., and Sutin, J. (1973): Functions of the pallidosubthalamic fiber. *Neurosurgery,* 1:225–233.
29. Yanagisawa, N., Tsukagoshi, H., Toyokura, Y., and Narabayashi, H. (1975): Huntington's chorea. Analysis of motor disorders with electromyography. *Shinkei Naika (Neurological Medicine),* 2:259–471 (in Japanese).

Advances in Neurology, Vol. 24, edited by
L. J. Poirier, T. L. Sourkes, and P. J. Bédard.
Raven Press, New York © 1979.

Essential Tremor and Dystonic Syndromes

D. W. Baxter and S. Lal

*Division of Neurology, Departments of Medicine and Psychiatry, Montreal General Hospital,
Montreal, Quebec, Canada*

The clinical features of essential tremor are well known to most clinicians. It is a postural tremor that may persist through action, is frequently familial, and characteristically restricted in distribution to the hands and the facial–nuchal–vocal musculature. The tremor may remain confined to one or other of these regions for long periods or even indefinitely. Many find their tremor influenced by alcohol, and in almost all the tremor is worsened by excitement, anxiety, and fatigue. Perhaps the majority of persons with essential tremor attribute their symptoms to nervousness and never consult a physician because of it. In others, the tremor is a source of considerable anxiety or embarrassment, while for a few it results in serious social or occupational disability. Late in life, some patients with prominent essential tremor may develop other mild extrapyramidal signs, in that the tremor assumes more cerebellar-type characteristics; there may be some loss of facial expressivity and gait may become mildly uncertain. It is, however, distinctly unusual for manifestations of overt parkinsonism or cerebellar ataxia to develop in such patients.

A possible relationship between the dystonic syndromes and essential tremor has been suggested in papers which have appeared sporadically over the past 100 years. Nevertheless, for the majority of contemporary clinicians, essential tremor remains a monosymptomatic disorder unlikely to become associated with other neurologic symptoms or signs. Conversely, it is more generally accepted that head and/or hand tremors are not uncommonly associated symptoms in patients with overt spasmodic torticollis.

METHODS

The diagnoses on consecutive alphabetically filed office charts were reviewed until 100 patients had been identified who had consulted a physician because of tremor, and in whom a diagnosis of essential tremor, familial tremor, or senile tremor had been made. A retrospective search for recorded dystonic symptoms or signs was carried out. Documentation was good in the majority, poor in a few, and the appropriateness of the diagnosis questionable in two.

RESULTS

Fifty-two of our patients were male and 48 female. They presented in every decade of life with the average age of presentation being 57 years. A family history was recorded in 47 (Table 1). Twenty-nine felt that alcohol influenced their tremor and nine were considered to be misusing alcohol. Dystonic symptoms or signs were recorded in 12 patients. The diagnosis at the time of presentation was considered inappropriate in 2 (Table 2). The severity of the dystonic features recorded ranged from incapacitating to asymptomatic. The dystonia involved neck muscles in eight patients and when dystonia of limb or trunk muscles was described, it was usually in association with more severe neck dystonia. In this group of patients, head tremor almost invariably was a more prominent symptom than hand tremor and had predated the development of dystonia for as long as 27 years. Six of these 10 patients gave a family history of tremor.

TABLE 1. *Age of presentation*[a]

Age group (yrs)	Total	Essential	Familial	Senile
< 20	4	4	—	—
20–30	9	8	1	—
30–40	6	1	5	—
40–50	12	4	8	—
50–60	22	7	15	—
60–70	22	11	9	2
70–80	19	4	6	9
> 80	6	0	2	4
Total	100	38	47	15

[a] Essential: onset of tremor under the age of 65 in patients without a positive family history. Familial: onset of tremor in any age group with a positive family history. Senile: onset of tremor over the age of 65 with a negative family history.

CASE REPORTS

Mr. H. C. first noted head tremor at age 30. This gradually increased in prominence and could be partially alleviated by alcohol. He was first seen at age 43 because of fear of developing parkinsonism. In addition to his head tremor, examination revealed a mild bilateral postural finger tremor and slight dystonic posturing of the neck. He was next seen at age 47 when his principal complaint was spasmodic pulling of his chin toward the left shoulder and lateral flexion of his head to the right. A postural finger tremor was again evident and in addition there was dystonic posturing of the left wrist such that it was difficult for him to hold objects in that hand. Alcohol would still alleviate his symptoms to an appreciable degree. He had also found that he could lessen his spasmodic torticollis for periods up to 30 min by vigorous painful massage over the left mastoid area.

Mr. A. G. first consulted a physician at the age of 21 years because of a hand tremor severe enough to interfere with his handwriting. This tremor was lessened by alcohol and by the 30 mg of diazepam, which he used each working day. At age 26 he developed a head tremor and shortly thereafter a recurrent tendency for his head to pull toward his left shoulder. By age 28 he had gross spasmodic torticollis with some spread of dystonia to his limb and paraspinal muscles.

Ms. M. C. presented at 67 years with spasmodic torticollis and a head tremor evident only when she tried to maintain her head in a neutral position. She denied any family history of tremor or dystonia. However, 2 years later her sister presented with a head, hand, and voice tremor. She stated that Mrs. M. C. had had a prominent head tremor through most of her adult life. Beginning in her mid-50s her head began to rotate toward her left shoulder under conditions of stress. As years passed, the head tremor became less apparent as the torticollis increased in severity. Two brothers had prominent head tremors but no torticollis.

Mr. B. B. was seen at age 41 because of generalized body and limb tremulousness with a recurrent tendency for his chin to rotate, and for his head to flex, toward the left shoulder. Facial and tongue muscles were constantly tremulous and his limbs were in constant motion while sitting. Any attempt at examination markedly accentuated his tremulousness and evoked hyperhydrosis. These symptoms had first developed at age 15 years and had become increasingly prominent. His mother had a mild bilateral postural hand tremor. It was felt that this man's tremor was of such a distribution and degree that the original diagnosis of essential tremor could be doubted.

Mr. H. G. was 67 years old when he presented with deterioration of his handwriting and mild uncertainty on his feet. A side-to-side tremor had been present for at least 27 years. This could be partially controlled by alcohol or a combination of Nembutal and amphetamines, which he had used regularly during his working years. On retirement at age 60, he had gradually discontinued the Nembutal and amphetamines but had replaced them by increasing amounts of alcohol. At about the same time he developed spasmodic torticollis which became increasingly more prominent over a year and then stabilized. At age 65, a bilateral hand tremor developed and gradually came to overshadow all other symptoms. Shortly before presentation he had noted mild uncertainty on his feet.

Ms. F. B. presented at age 42 with a head tremor which had increased in prominence over the previous 12 years. The tremor was most prominent when sitting or standing or attempting to hold her head in a neutral position. There were occasional spasmodic movements with the head flexing toward the right shoulder. Her handwriting was tremulous. Her mother had developed a head tremor in her mid-40s which had become very marked with advancing age.

Ms. E. F. developed a head tremor at age 41 which gradually increased in prominence until she was seen at age 48 because of her concern about parkinsonism. She was unable to write letters because on attempting to do so "her right upper extremity seems to stiffen and become tremulous." On examination her head was tilted toward her right shoulder with the chin rotated to the left. The right sternomastoid muscle was hypertrophied and repetitive muscle contractions were palpable in this muscle and in the left splenius muscles. Details of family history were not available.

Mr. J. L. was 57 when he presented with a head tremor and recurrent tendency for his head to tilt to the left of 1 year's duration. His habitual posture was to hold his chin with his right hand while sitting or standing. There was no hand tremor. A family history was not recorded.

Ms. L. D. presented at age 22 with a mild tremor of both hands and her head of 4 years duration. Her hand tremor and a "tendency for her hand to become cramped and clumsy" interfered with her ability to write. Her father and a sister have hand tremors. This patient's symptoms did not progress over the subsequent 7 years.

Mr. W. J. was seen at age 22 with a hand tremor of such severity that it seriously interfered with his handwriting and embarrassed him socially. Examination revealed a coarse, bilateral hand tremor, a low-amplitude side-to-side head tremor, dystonic posturing of the outstretched arms, and sudden involuntary movements about the neck and

TABLE 2. *Patients with dystonic syndromes associated with essential tremor*

Patient	Age/Sex	Tremor site	Dystonia			Tic	Duration of tremor	Family history
			Neck	Limb	Trunk			
H.G.	47/M	Head	+++	++	0	0	17 yrs.	No
A.G.	28/M	Hands Head	+++	++	++	0	8 yrs.	Yes
M.C.	66/F	Head	+++	0	0	0	10 yrs.	Yes
B.B.[a]	41/M	Head Hands	+++	+	+	+	24 yrs.	Yes
H.G.	67/M	Head Hands	++	0	0	0	27 yrs.	Yes
F.B.	42/F	Head	+++	0	0	0	12 yrs.	Yes
E.F.	48/F	Head	+++	++	0	0	7 yrs.	?
J.L.[a]	57/M	Head	++	0	0	0	1 yr.	?
W.J.	23/M	Hands Head	0	++	0	++	6 yrs.	No
L.D.	22/F	Hands Head	0	+	0	0	4 yrs.	Yes
M.B.	43/F	Head Hands	+	0	0	0	20 yrs.	Yes
B.I.	19/F	Head Hands	+	0	0	0	6 yrs.	?

[a] Clinical criteria for diagnosis of essential tremor considered inadequate.

wrist. When seen 2 years later because of the development of seizures, these motor abnormalities had not changed.

Ms. M. B. was seen at age 43 with a 20-year history of head tremor and a more recent hand tremor when tense or tired. She was described as having "a slight tilt of her head to the left with a constant mild titubating head tremor." Her mother and one sister have head tremors.

Ms. B. I. developed a head tremor at age 13 which was worse when tired or upset. When seen at age 19, she had a hand tremor severe enough to interfere with her writing, a side-to-side head tremor and "some posturing of the neck suggestive of an early tremulous form of torticollis." There was no definite family history and the patient faced major psychological and environmental problems.

DISCUSSION

The risk of dystonic syndromes developing in patients with essential tremor must be extremely small. In 1949, MacDonald Critchley (3) summarized the extensive European literature on essential tremor. He refers to several individual case reports and certain remarkable families in which torticollis was associated with essential tremor. In 1960, Larsen and Sjögren (4) surveyed an isolated inland Scandinavian parish and estimated that 210 of the 7,449 inhabitants had an essential tremor. Eighty-one of these 210 patients were examined and no patients with dystonic features were found. They did, however, describe two elderly patients, one of whom had chronic twitchings of facial muscles with continuous opening and closing movements of the jaw, while a second showed occasional twitchings of the eyebrows. Their conclusion, based on these and other findings, was that essential tremor "cannot generally be labelled monosymptomatic." Edmund Critchley (2) reported 42 patients whose essential tremor was associated with other neurological deficits, including one patient with limb dystonia. Postural hand tremors have frequently been reported in patients with spasmodic torticollis and dystonia musculorum deformans. The most striking of these reports is that of Couch (1) in 1976 who described a postural hand tremor in 26 of 30 patients with spasmodic torticollis, and a family history of tremor in 16.

Our retrospectively acquired data suggest that patients with long-standing head tremor of increasing prominence are at risk of developing dystonic symptomatology, and particularly, spasmodic torticollis. Further, such patients not infrequently present for neurological assessment of their tremor several years before the dystonic features develop. Under these circumstances the physical characteristics, distribution, and behavior of the tremor often fulfill the diagnostic criteria for essential tremor.

REFERENCES

1. Couch, J. R. (1976): Dystonia and tremor in spasmodic torticollis. *Adv. Neurol.* 14:245–258.
2. Critchley, E. (1972): Clinical manifestations of essential tremor. *J. Neurol. Neurosurg. Psychiatry,* 35:365–372.
3. Critchley, M. (1949): Observations on essential (heredofamilial) tremor. *Brain,* 72:113–139.
4. Larson, T., and Sjögren, T. (1960): Essential tremor: a genetic and population study. *Acta Psychiatr. Neurol. Scand. (Suppl.),* 36:144.

Advances in Neurology, Vol. 24, edited by
L. J. Poirier, T. L. Sourkes, and P. J. Bédard.
Raven Press, New York © 1979.

Dopamine and GABA Agonists in the Treatment of Hyperkinetic Extrapyramidal Disorders

*Thomas N. Chase, and **Carol A. Tamminga

*Experimental Therapeutics Branch, National Institute of Neurological and
Communicative Disorders and Stroke and **Adult Psychiatry Branch, National Institute
of Mental Health, Bethesda, Maryland 20205*

Dyskinesias constitute one of the major complications of L-DOPA treatment of Parkinson's disease. Typically, these abnormal involuntary movements arise as a dose-dependent reaction and presumably would occur in all parkinsonian patients given a sufficient amount of L-DOPA. In some patients, a vigorous therapeutic response cannot be obtained without the simultaneous occurrence of dyskinesias. Clinical observations suggest that individuals with Parkinson's disease may be more sensitive to L-DOPA-induced dyskinesias than individuals who are free of dopamine (DA) system damage of a type leading to parkinsonian symptoms (7). Hyperfunction of certain dopaminergic pathways, due to denervation supersensitivity of postsynaptic DA receptors, undoubtedly contributes to the appearance of these abnormal movements.

L-DOPA-induced dyskinesias can be reduced by DA receptor blocking agents such as the antipsychotic phenothiazine and butyrophenone derivatives. Typically, however, these drugs suppress dyskinesias only at doses that also block the antiparkinsonian action of L-DOPA. In theory, other drug classes, which act directly or indirectly to diminish the effects of DA system hyperfunction, should also be expected to ameliorate L-DOPA dyskinesias. In this regard, several DA and γ-aminobutyric acid (GABA) agonists warrant consideration.

Tardive dyskinesias that develop during long-term antipsychotic drug therapy (1,12,16) often resemble the dyskinesias that complicate the administration of L-DOPA. Moreover, abnormal movements in tardive dyskinesia patients characteristically diminish during treatment with DA receptor blocking agents and increase with L-DOPA or potent DA agonists (6,41). DA system hyperfunction is generally assumed to play a role in the pathophysiology of this disorder. Indeed, clinical (19,28,41) as well as preclinical observations (31,36,40,43) suggest that DA receptors chronically subjected to pharmacologic blockade may develop increased sensitivity to the natural transmitter as well as to DA agonists. In view of apparent parallels between tardive dyskinesia and L-DOPA-induced dyskinesia, studies of drug effects on patients with the former disorder may have relevance to the ability of these agents to ameliorate the latter state.

DOPAMINE RECEPTOR AGONISTS

Many DA agonists possess antiparkinsonian activity and at higher dose levels can induce dyskinesias, presumably through stimulation of central postsynaptic DA receptors. On the other hand, under certain conditions, some DA agents appear able to attenuate rather than exacerbate hyperkinetic extrapyramidal disorders. Although plausible explanations for these seemingly anomalous results can be advanced, the underlying pharmacologic mechanisms remain uncertain.

Apomorphine

This tetracyclic alkaloid directly stimulates central postsynaptic DA receptors to induce hyperkinetic stereotyped behaviors, antagonize reserpine-induced depression (23), stimulate DA-sensitive adenylyl cyclase in various animal species (27), and to ameliorate symptoms in parkinsonian patients (11). Paradoxically, quite the opposite effects of apomorphine have been noted in certain circumstances. For example, apomorphine acts to decrease striatal DA synthesis (49,50). This inhibition continues despite interruption of feedback pathways from striatum to substantia nigra, thus identifying the mechanism as a locally mediated phenomenon rather than one involving an interneuronal feedback loop (50). At low doses, apomorphine has also be found to inhibit DA-dependent turning behavior in rats, although it stimulates turning at higher doses (4). These findings could indicate a low-dose inhibitory effect of apomorphine at presynaptic DA receptors and a high-dose stimulatory effect at postsynaptic sites. Clinical evidence suggesting therapeutic activity of apomorphine in putative hyperdopaminergic syndromes is also available. Apomorphine has been reported to benefit motor function in patients with Huntington's chorea and tardive dyskinesia (5,9,46,47).

In a recent study apomorphine was administered to six drug-free tardive dyskinesia patients (41). Each received 0.5 to 6 mg by subcutaneous injection in daily increasing doses. Movements were evaluated by blind raters from direct observation and videotapes. A substantial decrease in dyskinesia ratings 20 and 40 min following apomorphine injection occurred in most patients; remaining individuals evidenced little or no change.

Ergot Derivatives

The view that ergot derivatives such as bromocriptine and CF 25,397 stimulate DA receptors derives from their ability to diminish cerebral DA turnover (8) and induce contralateral rotation in rats with unilateral striatal lesions (18). In man, bromocriptine, but not CF 25,397, evidences potent antiparkinsonian activity (3,44). The effects of ergot drugs on the DA system appear to differ from those of apomorphine, since their behavioral action can be partially blocked with alpha-methylparatyrosine or reserpine (8,18,24). Moreover, most ergots do not stimulate DA-sensitive adenylyl cyclase (48). These observations suggest that in addition to direct receptor agonist activity, some ergot derivatives exert their effect through presynaptic mechanisms involving catecholamine synthesis and storage. Published accounts of these drugs in human hyperkinetic extrapyramidal disorders have thus far been limited to studies of bromocriptine in patients with Huntington's disease. Although one report noted improvement, the other did not (17,25); doses used in patients who benefited tended to be lower than in those where no change was observed.

Bromocriptine was administered to six patients with tardive dyskinesia in a double-blind, placebo-controlled crossover study. All subjects were free of neuroleptic medications. Periods of bromocriptine (10 mg daily) or placebo treatment each lasted 2 weeks. Tardive dyskinesia ratings were performed twice weekly (41). No consistent change in dyskinesia scores was observed during or immediately after bromocriptine therapy (Table 1).

CF 25,397, an ergoline which, as already noted, possesses some characteristics of DA agonist drugs but has no therapeutic activity in Parkinson's disease (44), was also given to six patients with tardive dyskinesia. Two weeks of treatment at a daily dose of 60 mg produced no significant alteration in involuntary movements (Table 1). The effect of CF 25,397 in three patients also receiving haloperidol did not differ from that observed in three otherwise untreated individuals.

The present results indicate that while a nonergot DA agonist, apomorphine, tends to alleviate abnormal movements in patients with tardive dyskinesia, two ergot DA agonists, bromocriptine and CF 25,397, have no apparent antidyskinetic activity. A comparison of pharmacologic characteristics of these three drugs suggests that stimulation of DA-sensitive adenylyl cyclase and regulation of tyrosine activity may be two biochemical properties which predict antidyskinetic efficacy. In view of the relatively potent ability of apomorphine to influence tyrosine hydroxylase (51), and because the presynaptic DA receptor contributes to the regulation of this enzyme (21), it is tempting to speculate that apomorphine's clinical activity in suspected hyperdopaminergic disorders may relate

TABLE 1. *Effect of DA or GABA agonists on motor function in patients with tardive dyskinesia*

Drug	No. of pts	Placebo	Treatment	p
Bromocriptine	6	5.7 ± 1.1	5.7 ± 1.6	ns
CF 25,397	6	4.9 ± 1.4	3.7 ± 1.5	ns
Muscimol	6	6.8 ± 1.6	3.5 ± .84	< 0.001

Patients were evaluated during subacute oral treatment with bromocriptine (10 mg/day) or CF 25,397 (60 mg/day) or 2 hr after a single oral dose of muscimol (7–9 mg). Values are mean ± SEM dyskinesia scores, based on double-blind evaluations of 26 aspects of motor function, each rated on a scale of 0 (absent or normal) to 4 (very severe or abnormal).

to presynaptic DA receptor activation. Ergot derivatives, on the other hand, appear to have relatively little influence on tyrosine hydroxylase activity (22,26), and, therefore, may have relatively low potency at the presynaptic DA receptor. Biochemical studies consistent with this interpretation suggest that ergot derivatives act primarily as postsynaptic DA receptor agonists or as mixed receptor agonist–antagonists (20,22).

GABA RECEPTOR AGONISTS

Recent advances in our understanding of GABA system function suggest that pharmacologic manipulation of certain GABA pathways may provide another approach to the symptomatic relief of some hyperkinetic extrapyramidal disorders. GABA-containing cells serve as interneurons within the corpus striatum and nucleus accumbens, comprise fibers in the striatonigral tract, and contribute to efferents from pallidum and accumbens to the thalamus and elsewhere. Naturally occurring or drug-induced alterations in GABA neuron activity at any of these sites might be expected to influence extrapyramidal motor function. In rodents, unilateral GABA elevations in the zona reticulata of substantia nigra produce ipsilateral rotation in amphetamine-pretreated animals (14), and contralateral turning in the absence of DA agonist pretreatment (29). Contralateral turning following the unilateral injection of GABA or the GABA agonist, muscimol, into the zona reticulata can be inhibited by the GABA-blocking agent, picrotoxin (34,35,37). Systemically administered GABA transaminase inhibitors (10) or muscimol, when applied to the nucleus accumbens of rats, inhibit DA agonist-induced hyperactivity, but potentiate DA agonist-induced stereotypy (39). The various effects of GABA-active drugs on rodent motor behavior appear at least partially independent of the functional state of the DA system (10,35,37,38).

In man, recent biochemical observations indicate that GABA levels may be diminished in the cerebrospinal fluid of tardive dyskinesia patients (33). This decrease is not specific to tardive dyskinesia and it has yet to be verified by direct biochemical measurements in postmortem tissues. Nevertheless, findings suggestive of an alteration in GABA-mediated neural transmission in tardive dyskinesia are not unexpected in view of observations in the experimental animal, and indicate that pharmacologic attempts to augment GABA-mediated neuronal activity might benefit patients with this syndrome.

Muscimol

As a test of this possibility, muscimol was given to six patients who manifested the typical signs of tardive dyskinesia in a double-blind, placebo-controlled study. In the experimental animal, muscimol (3-hydroxy-5-amino-methylisoxazole) manifests many of the properties of a potent GABA agonist (2,13,32). The drug or an active metabolite can penetrate the blood–brain barrier, since oral muscimol administration is associated with alterations in behavioral state and various centrally regulated physiologic functions (42,45,52). All study subjects were free of neuroleptic drugs for at least 5 days prior to testing. Muscimol was given once daily in oral doses beginning at 3 mg and increasing in 2-mg increments to 9 mg or the highest tolerated dose. A significant diminution in dyskinesias was observed 2 and 4 hr following muscimol administration in doses ranging from to 7 to 9 mg (Table 1). A concomitant exacerbation in resting tremor was observed in two of three individuals who manifested this parkinsonian sign. Although muscimol tended to sedate some patients, reductions in involuntary movements occurred either before or in the absence of this effect. Diffuse myoclonic twitching and a worsening of psychotic behavior commonly attended high-dose muscimol treatment.

Clearly, muscimol's toxicity precludes general clinical usefulness. On the other hand, available results, including those arising from the treatment of tardive dyskinesia with the GABA transaminase inhibitor, valproate (30), suggest that other drugs which augment GABA-mediated synaptic function might be usefully explored in patients with hyperkinetic extrapyramidal disorders.

CONCLUDING REMARKS

The foregoing clinical data indicate that apomorphine tends to suppress abnormal movements in patients with tardive dyskinesia, whereas bromocriptine and CF 25,397 lack this activity. Perhaps the most conservative interpretation of these results is that stimulation of presynaptic DA receptors reduces DA-mediated neuronal transmission; however, other interpretations exist. For example, either a partial agonist effect at postsynaptic DA receptors or an action on some other neurohumoral system could explain the observed results. An alternative approach to the symptomatic relief of certain hyperkinetic disorders is suggested by the apparent ability of muscimol to benefit tardive dyskinesia patients, an effect which may reflect stimulation of efferent GABA pathways from the basal ganglia. Whatever the pharmacologic mechanisms, available evidence indicates that the involuntary movements that characterize tardive dyskinesia may be benefited by the administration of certain drugs with DA or GABA agonist properties. Efforts to further explore this possibility may be of value not only for patients with tardive dyskinesia, but also for individuals with other neurologic or psychiatric syndromes which reflect DA hyperfunction. In view of the similarities between the pathophysiology of tardive dyskinesia and L-DOPA-induced dyskinesia, it is possible that drugs of this type might in the future prove useful as an adjunct in the clinical management of Parkinson's disease. Some clinical observations in support of the possibility are already available (15).

REFERENCES

1. American College of Neuropsychopharmacology—Food and Drug Administration Task Force (1973): Neurological syndromes associated with antipsychotic drug use. A special report. *Arch. Gen. Psychiatry,* 28:463–467.

2. Beaumont, K., Chilton, W., Yamamura, H. I., and Enna, S. J. (1977): Specific ^{3}H muscimol binding to synaptic GABA receptors. *Neurosci. Abstr.,* 3:1442.
3. Calne, D. B. (1977): Developments in the pharmacology and therapeutics of parkinsonism. *Neurology (Minneap.),* 1:111–119.
4. Carlsson, A. (1975): Some aspects of dopamine in the basal ganglia. In: *Basal Ganglia,* edited by M. O. Yahr, pp. 181–189. Raven Press, New York.
5. Carroll, B. J., Curtis, G. C., and Kokmen, E. (1977): Paradoxical responses to dopamine agonists in tardive dyskinesia. *Am. J. Psychiatry,* 134:785–789.
6. Chase, T. N. (1972): Drug-induced extrapyramidal disorders. *Res. Publ., Assoc. Nerv. Ment. Dis.,* 50:448–471.
7. Chase, T. N., Holden, E. M., and Brody, J. A. (1973): Levodopa-induced dyskinesias: comparison in parkinsonism-dementia and amyotrophic lateral sclerosis. *Arch. Neurol.,* 29:328–330.
8. Corrodi, H., Fuxe, K., Hökfelt, T., Lindbrink, P., and Ungerstedt, U. (1973): Effects of ergot drugs on central catecholamine neurons: evidence for a stimulation of central dopamine neurons. *J. Pharm. Pharmacol.,* 25:409–412.
9. Corsini, G. U., Onali, P. L., Masala, C., Cianchetti, C., Mangoni, A., and Gesse, G. L. (1978): Apomorphine hydrochloride-induced improvement in Huntington's chorea. *Arch. Neurol.,* 35:27–30.
10. Cott, J., and Engel, J. (1977): Suppression by GABAergic drugs of the locomotor stimulation induced by morphine, amphetamine, and apomorphine: evidence for both pre- and post-synaptic inhibition of catecholamine systems. *J. Neurol. Transm.,* 40:253–268.
11. Cotzias, G. C., Papavasiliou, P. S., Fehling, C., Kaufman, B., and Mean, I. (1970): Similarities between neurologic effects of L-DOPA and of apomorphine. *N. Engl. J. Med.,* 282:31–33.
12. Crane, G. E. (1974): Factors predisposing to drug-induced neurologic effects. *Adv. Biochem. Psychopharmacol.,* 9:269–279.
13. Curtis, D. R., Duggan, A. W., Felix, D., and Johnston, G. A. R. (1971): Bicuculline, an antagonist of GABA and synaptic inhibition in the spinal cord of the cat. *Brain Res.,* 32:69–96.
14. Dray, A., and Straughan, D. W. (1976): Synaptic mechanisms in the substantia nigra. *J. Pharm. Pharmacol.,* 28:400–405.
15. Duby, S. E., Cotzias, G. C., Papavasilious, P. S., and Lawrence, W. H. (1972): Injected apomorphine and orally administered levodopa in parkinsonism. *Arch. Neurol.,* 27:474–480.
16. Fann, W. E., Davis, J. M., and Janowsky, D. S. (1972): The prevalence of tardive dyskinesias in mental hospital patients. *Dis. Nerv. Syst.,* 30:182–186.
17. Frattola, L., Albizzati, M. G., Spano, P. F., and Trabucchi, M. (1977): Treatment of Huntington's chorea with bromocriptine. *Acta. Neurol. Scand.,* 56:37–45.
18. Fuxe, K., Corrodi, H., Hökfelt, T., Lindbrink, P., Ungerstedt, U. (1974): Ergocormine and 2-Br-ergocryptine: evidence for prolonged dopamine receptor stimulation. *Med. Biol.,* 52:121–132.
19. Gerlach, J., Reisby, N., and Randrup, A. (1974): Dopaminergic hypersensitivity and cholinergic hypofunction in the pathophysiology of tardive dyskinesia. *Psychopharmacologia,* 34:21–35.
20. Goldstein, M., Battista, A. F., Matsumoto, Y., Bronaugh, R. L., Lew, J. Y., Fuxe, K., and Hökfelt, T. (1976): Pre- and postsynaptic effects of dopaminergic agonists. Antiparkinsonian efficacy and effects on DA synthesis. In: *Advances in Parkinsonism,* edited by W. Birkmayer and O. Hornykiewicz, pp. 236–243. Editiones (Roche), Basel.
21. Goldstein, M., Bronaugh, R. L., Lew, J. Y., Ohashi, T., Drummond, G. S., and Fuxe, K. (1977): Effect of dopaminephilic agents and cAMP on tyrosine hydroxylase activity. *Adv. Biochem. Psychopharmacol.,* 16:447–453.
22. Goldstein, M., Lew, J. Y., Nakamura, S., Battista, A. F., Lieberman, A., and Fuxe, K. (1978): Dopaminephilic properties of ergot alkaloids. *Fed. Proc.,* 37:2202–2206.
23. Haefely, W., Bartholini, G., Pletscher, A. (1976): Monoaminergic drugs: general pharmacology. *Pharmacol. Ther. B,* 2:185–218.
24. Johnson, A. M., Loew, D. M., and Vigouret, J. M. (1976): Stimulant properties of bromocriptine on central dopamine receptors in comparison to apomorphine, (+)-amphetamine and L-DOPA. *Br. J. Pharmacol.,* 56:59–68.
25. Kartzinel, R., Hunt, R. B., and Calne, D. B., (1976): Bromocriptine in Huntington's chorea. *Arch. Neurol.,* 33:517–518.
26. Kebabian, J. W., and Kebabian, P. R. (1978): Lergotrile and lisuride: in vivo dopaminergic

agonists which do not stimulate the presynaptic dopamine autoreceptor. *Life Sci.,* 23:2199–2204.

27. Kebabian, J. W., Petzold, G. L., and Greengard, P. (1972): Dopamine-sensitive adenylate cyclase in caudate nucleus of rat brain, and its similarity to the "dopamine receptor." *Proc. Natl. Acad. Sci. U.S.A.,* 69:2145–2149.

28. Klawans, H. L. (1973): The pharmacology of tardive dyskinesia. *Am. J. Psychiatry,* 130:82–85.

29. Koob, G., Del Fiacco, M., and Iversen, S. D. (1976): The behavioural effects of EOS induced changes in substantia nigra GABA levels. *Br. J. Pharmacol.,* 58:454P.

30. Linnoila, M., Viukari, M., Hietala, O. (1974): Effect of sodium valproate on tardive dyskinesia. *Br. J. Psychiatry,* 129:114–119.

31. Moore, K. E., and Thornberg, J. E. (1975): Drug-induced dopaminergic supersensitivity. In: *Advances in Neurology, Vol. 9: Dopaminergic Mechanisms,* edited by D. Calne, T. N. Chase, and A. Barbeau, pp. 250–257. Raven Press, New York.

32. Naik, S. R., Guidotti, A., and Costa, E. (1976): Central GABA receptor agonists: comparison of muscimol and baclofen, *Neuropharmacology,* 15:479–484.

33. Neophytides, A. N., Suria, A., Waniewski, R. A., and Chase, T. N. (1978): Cerebrospinal fluid GABA in neurologic disease. *Neurology (in press).*

34. Oberlander, C., Dumont, C., and Boissier, J. R. (1977): Rotational behavior after unilateral intranigral injection of muscimol in rats. *Eur. J. Pharmacol.,* 43:389–390.

35. Olpe, H. R., Schellenberg, H., and Koella, W. P. (1977): Rotational behavior induced in rats by intranigral application of GABA-related drugs and GABA antagonists. *Eur. J. Pharmacol.,* 45:251–294.

36. Rubovits, R., and Klawans, H. L. (1973): Implications for amphetamine-induced stereotyped behavior as a model for tardive dyskinesia. *Arch. Gen. Psychiatry,* 27:502–507.

37. Scheel-Krüger, J., Arnt, J., and Magelund, G. (1977): Behavioral stimulation induced by muscimol and other GABA agonists infected into the substantia nigra. *Neurosci. Lett.,* 4:351–356.

38. Scheel-Krüger, J., Christensen, A. V., and Arnt, J. (1978): Muscimol differentially facilitates stereotypy but antagonizes motility induced by dopaminergic drugs: a complex GABA–dopamine interaction. *Life Sci.,* 22:75–84.

39. Scheel-Krüger, J., Cools, A. R., and van Wel, P. M. (1977): Muscimol, a GABA-agonist injected into the nucleus accumbens increases apomorphine stereotypy and decreases the motility. *Life Sci.,* 21:1697–1702.

40. Smith, R. C., and Davis, J. M. (1976): Behavioral evidence for supersensitivity after chronic administration of haloperidol, clozapine, and thioridazine. *Life Sci.,* 19:725–732.

41. Smith, R. C., Tamminga, C. A., Haraszti, J., Pandey, G. N., and Davis, J. M. (1977): Effects of dopamine agonists in tardive dyskinesia. *Am. J. Psychiatry,* 134:763–768.

42. Tamminga, C. A., Crayton, J. W., and Chase, T. N. (1978): Muscimol: GABA agonist therapy in schizophrenia. *Am. J. Psychiatry,* 135:746–747.

43. Tarsy, D., and Baldessarini, R. J. (1974): Behavioral supersensitivity to apomorphine following chronic treatment with drugs which interfere with the synaptic function of catecholamines. *Neuropharmacology,* 13:927–940.

44. Teychenne, P. F., Pfeiffer, R., Bern, S. M., and Calne, D. B. (1977): Experiences with a new ergoline (CF 25,397) in parkinsonism. *Neurology (Minneap.),* 27:1140–1143.

45. Theobald, W., Buch, O., Kunz, A. A., Krupp, P., Stenger, E. G., and Heimann, H. (1968): Pharmacological and experimental psychologic studies on two components of the toadstool *(Amanita muscaria). Arzneim. Forsch.,* 18:311–315.

46. Tolosa, E. S. (1978): Modification of tardive dyskinesia and spasmodic torticollis by apomorphine. *Arch. Neurol.,* 35:459–462.

47. Tolosa, E. S., and Sparker, S. B. (1974): Apomorphine in Huntington's chorea: clinical observations and theoretical considerations. *Life Sci.,* 15:1371–1380.

48. Trabucchi, M., Spano, P. F., Tonon, G. C., and Frattola, L. (1976): Effects of bromocriptine on central dopaminergic receptors. *Life Sci.,* 19:225–232.

49. Walters, J. R., Bunney, B. S., and Roth, R. H. (1975): Piribedil and apomorphine: pre- and postsynaptic effects of dopamine synthesis and neuronal activity. In: *Advances in Neurology, Vol. 9: Dopaminergic Mechanisms,* edited by D. Calne, T. N. Chase, and A. Barbeau, pp. 273–284. Raven Press, New York.

50. Walters, J. R., and Roth, R. H. (1974): Dopaminergic neurons: Drug-induced antagonism of

the increase in tyrosine hydroxylase activity produced by cessation of impulse flow. *J. Pharmacol. Exp. Ther.*, 191:82–91.

51. Walters, J. R., and Roth, R. H. (1976): Dopaminergic neurons: an in vivo system for measuring drug interaction with presynaptic receptors. *Naunyn Schmiedebergs Arch. Pharmacol.*, 296:5–14.

52. Waser, P. G. (1967): The pharmacology of *Amanita muscaris*. In: *Ethnopharmacologic Search for Psycho-active Drugs,* edited by D. H. Efron, B. Holmstedt, and N. S. Kline, pp. 419–439. U.S. Public Health Service Publication No. 1645.

Advances in Neurology, Vol. 24, edited by
L. J. Poirier, T. L. Sourkes, and P. J. Bédard.
Raven Press, New York © 1979.

Choline, Lecithin, and Tardive Dyskinesia

John H. Growdon

Tufts–New England Medical Center, Boston, Massachusetts 02111

This chapter describes the relationship between choline and brain acetylcholine levels, and shows that the administration of choline—either as choline chloride or phosphatidylcholine (lecithin)—exerts a major influence on the rate of acetylcholine synthesis, and on the amount of acetylcholine released when a neuron is depolarized. This chapter also describes the biochemical and clinical effects of choline chloride and lecithin administration to patients with tardive dyskinesia and "senile" chorea.

BACKGROUND

Acetylcholine is synthesized from choline and acetyl coenzyme A in a reaction catalyzed by the enzyme choline acetyltransferase (CAT):

$$\text{Choline} + \text{acetyl coenzyme A} \xrightarrow{\text{CAT}} \text{acetylcholine}$$

The brain is apparently unable to synthesize choline *de novo,* and therefore must obtain it from the systemic circulation by low-affinity uptake mechanism at the blood–brain barrier (1,20). Blood choline derives from two sources: some is synthesized in the liver by a stepwise methylation of ethanolamines to form phosphatidyl choline (2,3), and some is obtained from dietary sources (22). Cohen and Wurtman first showed that the systemic administration of choline by injection (8) or by dietary supplementation (9) produced sequential elevation in blood choline, brain choline, and brain acetylcholine levels in rats (Fig. 1). Haubrich et al. obtained similar results from experiments in which choline was administered by intracarotid (25), intraventricular (25), or intraperitoneal injections (24). Choline administration increased acetylcholine levels in all brain regions examined, including the cortex, caudate nucleus, and in the cholinergic nerve terminals of the hippocampus (26). Phosphatidylcholine, or lecithin, is the predominant source of choline in the diet; it contains choline bound to a glycerol molecule with two fatty acid moieties (Fig. 2). Choline ingested as lecithin also increased brain acetylcholine levels in rats (27), and was far more effective in elevating plasma choline levels in humans (42) than choline chloride. Following absorption, choline circulates as the free base, in the form of lecithin,

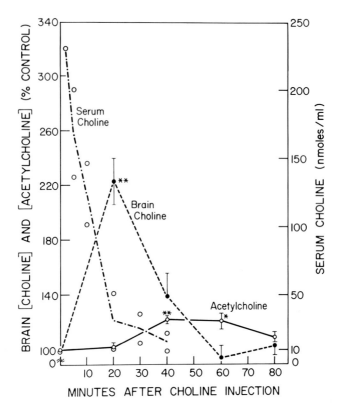

FIG. 1: Time-course of the response of serum Ch, brain Ch, and brain ACh to Ch administered by injection. Groups of five to nine 150–200-g male rats received Ch chloride (60 mg/kg, i. p.) in saline (0.9% NaCl) or the diluent alone. The animals were killed at various intervals after the injection by microwave irradiation of the head and whole brain Ch and ACh concentrations were measured. Data for brain Ch and ACh levels are expressed as percents of control means. *Bars,* SEM. Groups of 2 or 3 rats were injected as described above and killed by decapitation at various intervals after injection. Blood was collected from the cervical wound and serum Ch levels are expressed as nanomoles per milliliter. *Open circles,* range of values for serum Ch levels at each point; *$p < 0.01$, **$p < 0.001$, differs from corresponding concentrations in rats injected with saline alone. (From Wurtman et al., ref. 41, with permission.)

or as lysolecithin bound to albumin. Free choline is transported into the brain by a low-affinity uptake system at the blood–brain barrier that is highly unsaturated (34); thus, any significant variation in plasma choline levels should generate corresponding changes in brain choline uptake, and eventually in brain choline and acetylcholine levels. The low-affinity system is distinct from the high-affinity choline uptake system that has been observed in synaptosomes prepared from cholinergic terminals (32,43); this latter mechanism functions to allow neurons to recapture and reutilize the choline formed by the hydrolysis of acetylcholine after the transmitter has been released into synapses. The increases in brain acetylcholine levels that are induced by choline administration apparently result

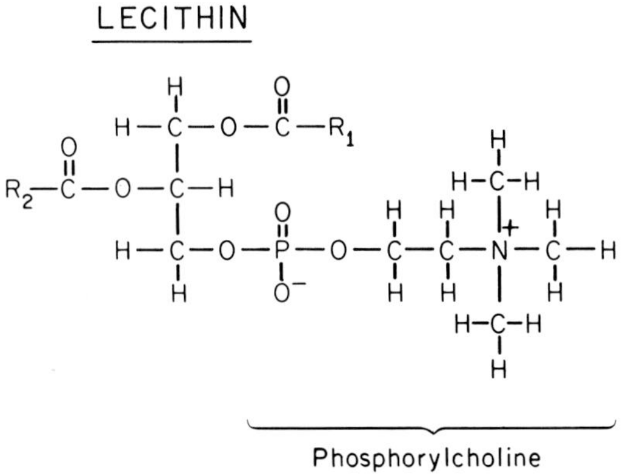

LECITHIN

Phosphorylcholine

FIG. 2. Phosphatidylcholine (lecithin) molecule. R_1 and R_2 indicate fatty acid side chains that are unsaturated in soya lecithin and more saturated in egg lecithin.

from increased synthesis and not from slowed degradation. Thus, Cohen and Wurtman (9) gave physostigmine, a cholinesterase inhibitor which is active in the central nervous system, to rats in conjunction with choline injections and found that the resulting increase in brain acetylcholine content was equal to the sum of the effects of either agent alone. The increase in acetylcholine synthesis and levels induced by choline probably causes a corresponding increase in the amount of acetylcholine that is released as well. Ulus et al. (39,40) reported indirect evidence that choline administration increased cholinergic neurotransmission, since they found biochemical changes in dopaminergic cells (in the caudate nucleus) and in chromaffin cells (in the adrenal medulla) that are postsynaptic to cholinergic neurons. They reported that choline administration increased acetylcholine levels in these tissues, and also increased tyrosine hydroxylase activity. This effect was dose-dependent and, in the caudate, was blocked by pretreatment with atropine, an anticholinergic drug. Choline administration also caused a parallel acceleration in the accumulation of DOPA, the product of this enzyme, in animals treated with an inhibitor of DOPA decarboxylase. These observations all indicate that choline administration accelerates acetylcholine synthesis, increases acetylcholine levels, and probably stimulates acetylcholine release as well. These data provide the scientific basis for administering choline or lecithin to patients with diseases, such as tardive dyskinesia, in which there may be deficient cholinergic tone.

CHOLINE AND LECITHIN ADMINISTRATION TO PATIENTS WITH TARDIVE DYSKINESIA

Tardive dyskinesia is a choreiform disorder characterized by involuntary movements of the eyelids, lips, tongue, or jaw; the extremities may be involved as well (11). Similar movements can arise spontaneously, especially in older people ("senile" chorea) but they generally occur in association with the chronic ingestion of neuroleptic drugs (phenothiazines, butyrophenones) (19). It is generally believed that tardive dyskinesia may result from an imbalance in the postulated reciprocal relationship between dopamine and acetylcholine in the basal ganglia, in which dopaminergic neurotransmission is increased at the expense of cholinergic transmission (14,30). The precise mechanism whereby this occurs remains unknown; neuroleptics block intrasynaptic dopamine receptors and may cause tardive dyskinesia as a result of increased dopamine turnover (5), denervation supersensitivity (37), or increased dopamine receptor density (4). Because of the emphasis on dopaminergic mechanisms, drugs used to treat tardive dyskinesia have included those that block catecholamine synthesis, such as α-methyl-p-tyrosine (7,21), deplete the brain of biogenic amines, such as reserpine, tetrabenazine (28), or antagonize dopamine's action on synaptic receptors, such as the neuroleptics (29). These attempts, however, have not been universally effective and have serious limitations: for example, α-methyl-p-tyrosine and reserpine produce a rigid parkinsonian syndrome (17) and neuroleptic administration is counterproductive since these drugs initially caused the syndrome. An alternate strategy would be to increase cholinergic tone at the synapse distal to the one employing dopamine. Thus, intravenously administered physostigmine reportedly decreased choreic movements temporarily in some patients with tardive dyskinesia, whereas the anticholinergic drug scopolamine worsened it (13,31). The choline precursor deanol apparently produced some benefit in a few instances (6,15,18), but not in most (10,16,38); its ability to increase brain acetylcholine levels remains controversial (44). With the demonstration that exogenous choline elevates blood choline, brain choline, and brain acetylcholine levels in rats, it became possible for the first time to test the long-term clinical effects of increasing cholinergic tone in patients with tardive dyskinesia. Shortly after the initial publication of the animal data, Davis et al. (12) reported that choline chloride could suppress tardive dyskinesia; Growdon et al. (23) then reported a double-blind crossover study in which choline suppressed tardive dyskinesia in 9 of 20 patients. The present study confirms choline's efficacy, and demonstrates that lecithin is equally effective.

PROTOCOL

Twelve patients with facial and limb dyskinetic movements took choline and/or lecithin according to a single drug nonblind protocol. All patients gave informed consent; nine had an associated history of antipsychotic medication (tardive dyskinesia) and three did not ("senile" chorea). The nine patients with tardive dyskinesia met the following criteria: (a) oral, facial, or limb dyskinetic movements that had been stable for at least 6 months; and (b) well-documented onset of movements while taking antipsychotic drugs, or within 4 weeks after their discontinuation. Four of the patients continued to take antipsychotic medication during choline or lecithin ingestion, while these drugs had been discontinued in the other 5. Psychiatric diagnoses were schizophrenia in two, bipolar affective illness in one, unipolar affective illness in one, chronic anxiety in three, and severe obsessive–compulsive disorder in two. Three additional patients had similar movements but did not have a prior history of psychiatric illness and had not taken neuroleptic medication. Six of the nine patients with tardive dyskinesia, and all three patients with spontaneous dyskinesia, took 150 to 200 mg/kg/day of choline chloride. Choline was supplied as a white salt which patients mixed in sweetened beverages and drank in three daily divided doses. Seven patients with tardive dyskinesia took equimolar doses of choline as lecithin, supplied either as granules (15% phosphatidylcholine) or lumps (80% phosphatidylcholine) mixed with food and ingested in three daily divided doses. Dyskinetic movements were rated weekly according to the NIMH Abnormal Involuntary Movement Scale (AIMS); additional clinical evaluation included counting the number of movements observed over 30 sec, and reviewing films and videotapes taken before and during treatment. Serum choline levels before and during choline and lecithin administration were measured by a radioenzymatic method (35).

RESULTS

Before treatment, plasma choline levels ranged between 7.1 and 18.6 nmoles/ml (13.2 $\pm$ 1.1, mean $\pm$SEM). During the final week of choline administration (200 mg/kg/day) plasma choline levels in blood obtained 1 hr after the last choline dose increased in all patients with a mean of 35.1 $\pm$ 4.5 nmoles/ml ($p < 0.01$). During the final weeks of lecithin administration, mean plasma choline levels in blood obtained 1 to 4 hr after a lecithin dose were 32.9 $\pm$ 3.5 nmoles/ml ($p < 0.01$) (Fig. 3). Mean plasma choline levels before and during treatment in patients who improved did not differ significantly from the mean of those who did not.

The number of involuntary movements decreased by more than 25% in five of six patients with tardive dyskinesia during choline ingestion and were unchanged in one patient. Four of the patients who took choline discontinued it, and, along with three additional patients who had not received choline, took oral doses of lecithin. Lecithin administration suppressed dyskinetic movements in three patients who had improved with choline and in two of the three additional patients; lecithin did not suppress the movements in the one patient who had not improved during choline ingestion. Thus, five of six patients with tardive dyskinesia improved during choline administration, and five of seven patients improved with lecithin administration. In contrast, choline administration did not suppress oral–buccal–lingual movements in the three patients with "senile" chorea.

CONCLUSION

Choline is the physiologic precursor of the neurotransmitter acetylcholine; its administration increases blood choline, brain choline, and brain acetylcholine

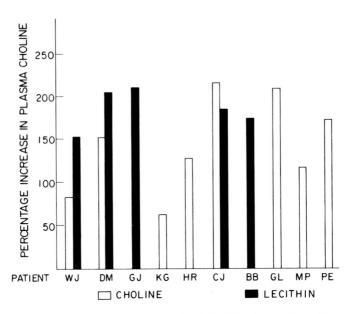

FIG. 3: Percentage increase in plasma choline levels in 10 patients with oral–buccal–lingual or limb dyskinetic movements. Plasma choline levels increased in all patients 1 hr after a maximal dose of choline or 1–4 hr after a dose of lecithin. Patients GL, MP, and PE had "senile" chorea; the other patients had tardive dyskinesia. Patients WJ, DM, GJ, KG, and HR improved during treatment; CJ, BB, GL, MP, and PE did not.

levels in rats, and blood and CSF choline levels in humans. Lecithin is the naturally occurring dietary source of choline; its administration elevates brain acetylcholine levels in rats, and produces greater and more prolonged elevations in plasma choline levels in humans than choline chloride. Choline has already been used successfully to treat patients with tardive dyskinesia; the present study demonstrates that lecithin can suppress tardive dyskinesia as well. The ability of choline and lecithin to suppress tardive dyskinesia illustrates a new mode of medical therapy, in which a naturally occurring dietary substance (choline) that is a precursor for a neurotransmitter (acetylcholine) may be used to treat a nonnutritional brain disease (tardive dyskinesia) in which physicians may wish to enhance central cholinergic tone. The finding that choline did not suppress oral–buccal–lingual movements that occurred spontaneously, suggests that cholinergic mechanisms may not be significantly involved in the production of "senile" chorea.

Dyskinetic movements also occur in some parkinsonian patients during L-DOPA administration; they may result from increased dopamine turnover (5) or from L-DOPA-induced supersensitivity (36). Cholinergic mechanisms may be involved as well, since nigral dopaminergic neurons normally inhibit some cholinergic interneurons in the striatum (33), and further increases in dopaminergic tone might be expected to impair acetylcholine release even more.

Choline or lecithin administration would restore cholinergic tone and, in combination with L-DOPA, may suppress the dyskinetic movements without worsening other aspects of parkinsonism.

BIBLIOGRAPHY

1. Ansell, G. B., and Spanner, S. (1975): The origin and metabolism of brain choline. In: *Cholinergic Mechanisms,* edited by P. G. Waser, pp. 92–149. Raven Press, New York.
2. Bremer, J., and Greenberg, D. M. (1960): Biosynthesis of choline in vitro. *Biochem. Biophys. Acta,* 37:173–175.
3. Bremer, J., and Greenberg, D. M. (1961): Methyl transferring enzyme system in the biosynthesis of lecithin (phosphatidylcholine). *Biochem. Biophys. Acta,* 46:205–211.
4. Burt, D. R., Creese, I., and Snyder, S. (1977): Antischizophrenic drugs: chronic treatment elevates dopamine receptor binding in the brain. *Science,* 196:326–328.
5. Carlsson, A. (1976): Some aspects of dopamine in the basal ganglia. *Res. Publ. Assoc. Res. Nerv. Ment. Dis.,* 55:181–189.
6. Casey, D. E., Denny, D. (1975): Deanol in the treatment of tardive dyskinesia. *Am. J. Psychiatry,* 132:864–867.
7. Chase, T. N. (1972): Drug-induced extrapyramidal disorder. *Res. Pub. Assoc. Res. Nerv. Ment. Dis.,* 50:448–471.
8. Cohen, E. L., and Wurtman, R. J. (1975): Brain acetylcholine: increase after systemic choline administration. *Life Sci.,* 16:1095–1102.
9. Cohen, E. L., and Wurtman, R. J. (1976): Brain acetylcholine: control by dietary choline. *Science,* 191:561–562.
10. Crane, G. E. (1975): Deanol for tardive dyskinesia. *N. Engl. J. Med.,* 292:926.
11. Crane, G. E. (1968): Tardive dyskinesia in patients treated with major neuroleptics: a review of the literature. *Am. J. Psychiatry Suppl.,* 124(8):40–54.
12. Davis, K. L., Berger, P. A., and Hollister, L. E. (1975): Choline for tardive dyskinesia. *N. Engl. J. Med.,* 293:152.
13. Davis, K. L., Hollister, L. E., Barchas, J. D., and Berger, P. A. (1976): Choline in tardive dyskinesia and Huntington's disease. *Life Sci.,* 19:1507–1516.
14. Davis, K. L., Hollister, L. E., Berger, P. A., and Barchas, J. D. (1975): Cholinergic imbalance hypotheses of psychoses and movement disorders: strategies for evaluation. *Psychopharmacol. Commun.,* 1:533–543.
15. DeSilva, L., and Huang, C. Y. (1975): Deanol in tardive dyskinesia. *Br. Med. J.,* 3:466.
16. Escobar, J. I., and Kemp, K. F. (1975): Dimethylaminoethanol for tardive dyskinesia. *N. Engl. J. Med.,* 292:317–318.
17. Fahn, S. (1978): Treatment of tardive dyskinesia with combined reserpine and alpha-methyltyrosine. *Ann. Neurol.,* 4:169.
18. Fann, W. E., Sullivan, J. L. III., Miller, R. D., and McKenzie, G. M. (1975): Deanol in tardive dyskinesia: a preliminary report. *Psychopharmacologia,* 42:135–137.
19. Food and Drug Administration Task Force, American College of Neuropsychopharmacology (1973): Neurological syndromes associated with antipsychotic drug use: a special report. *Arch. Gen. Psychiatry,* 28:463–467.
20. Freeman, J. J., Choi, R. L., and Jenden, D. J. (1975): Plasma choline: its turnover and exchange with brain choline. *J. Neurochem.,* 24:729–734.
21. Gerlach, J., Reisby, N., and Randrup, A. (1974): Dopaminergic hypersensitivity and cholinergic hypofunction in the pathophysiology of tardive dyskinesia. *Psychopharmacologia,* 34:21–35.
22. Goodhart, R. S., and Shils, M. E. (1975): *Modern Nutrition in Health and Disease,* 5th ed. Lea & Febiger, Philadelphia.
23. Growdon, J. H., Hirsch, M. J., Wurtman, R. J., and Wiener, W. (1977): Oral choline administration to patients with tardive dyskinesia. *N. Engl. J. Med.,* 297:524–527.
24. Haubrich, D. R., Wang, P. F. L., Clody, D. E., and Wedeking, P. W. (1975): Increases in rat brain acetylcholine induced by choline or deanol. *Life Sci.,* 17:975–980.
25. Haubrich, D. R., Wang, P. F. L., Wedeking, P. (1974): Role of choline in biosynthesis of acetylcholine. *Fed. Proc.,* 33:477.

26. Hirsch, M. J., Growdon, J. H., and Wurtman, R. J. (1977): Increase in hippocampal acetycholine after choline administration. *Brain Res.,* 332:383–385.

27. Hirsch, M. J., and Wurtman, R. J. (1978): Lecithin consumption elevates acetylcholine concentrations in rat brain and adrenal gland. *Science,* 202:223–225.

28. Kazamatsuri, H., Chien, C., and Cole, J. O. (1972): Treatment of tardive dyskinesia. I. Clinical efficacy of a dopamine-depleting agent, tetrabenazine. *Arch. Gen. Psychiatry,* 27:95–99.

29. Kazamutsuri, H., Chien, C., and Cole, J. O. (1972): Treatment of tardive dyskinesia. II. Short-term efficacy of dopamine-blocking agents, haloperidol and thiopropazate. *Arch. Gen. Psychiatry,* 27:100–103.

30. Klawans, H. L., Jr. (1973): The pharmacology of tardive dyskinesia. *Am. J. Psychiatry,* 130:82–86.

31. Klawans, H. L., Jr., and Rubovits, R. (1974): Effects of cholinergic and anticholinergic agents on tardive dyskinesia. *J. Neurol. Neurosurg. Psychiatry,* 27:941–947.

32. Kuhar, M. J., Sethy, V. H., Roth, R. H., and Aghajanian, G. K. (1973): Choline: selective accumulation by central cholinergic neurons. *J. Neurochem.,* 20:581–593.

33. McGeer, P. L., Grewaal, D. S., and McGeer, E. G. (1974): Influence of noncholinergic drugs on rat striatal acetylcholine levels. *Brain Res.,* 80:211–217.

34. Pardridge, W. M., and Oldendorf, W. H. (1977): Transport of metabolic substrates through the blood–brain barrier. *J. Neurochem.,* 28:5–12.

35. Shea, P. A., and Aprison, M. H. (1973): An enzymatic method for measuring picomole quantities of acetylcholine in CNS tissue. *Anal. Biochem.,* 56:165–177.

36. Tang, L. C., and Cotzias, G. C. (1977): L-3,4-Dihydroxyphenylalanine-induced hypersensitivity simulating features of denervation. *Proc. Natl. Acad. Sci. U.S.A.,* 74:2126–2129.

37. Tarsy, D., and Baldessarini, R. J. (1974): Behavioral supersensitivity to apomorphine following chronic treatment with drugs which interfere with the synaptic function of catecholamines. *Neuropharmacology,* 13:927–940.

38. Tarsy, D., and Bralower, M. (1977): Deanol acetamidobenzoate treatment in choreiform movement disorders. *Arch. Neurol.,* 34:756–758.

39. Ulus, I. H., Hirsch, M. J., and Wurtman, R. J. (1977): Trans-synaptic induction of adrenomedullary tyrosine hydroxlase activity by choline: evidence that choline administration increases cholinergic transmission. *Proc. Natl. Acad. Sci. U.S.A.,* 74:798–800.

40. Ulus, I. H., and Wurtman, R. J. (1976): Choline administration: activation of tyrosine hydroxylase in dopaminergic neurons of rat brain. *Science,* 194:1060–1061.

41. Wurtman, R. J., Cohen, E. L., and Fernstrom, J. D. (1977): Control of brain neurotransmitter synthesis by precursor availability and food consumption. In: *Neuro-regulator and Psychiatric Disorders,* edited by E. Usdin, D. A. Hamburg, and J. D. Barchas. ch. 12, pp. 103–121. Oxford University Press, New York.

42. Wurtman, R. J., Hirsch, M. J., and Growdon, J. H. (1977): Lecithin consumption elevates serum-free choline levels. *Lancet,* 2:68–69.

43. Yamamura, H. I., and Snyder, S. H. (1973): High affinity transport of choline into synaptosomes of rat brain. *J. Neurochem.,* 21:1355–1374.

44. Zahniser, N. R., Chou, D., and Hanin, I. (1977): Is 2-dimethylaminoethanol (deanol) indeed a precursor of brain acetylcholine? A gas chromatographic evaluation. *J. Pharmacol. Exp. Ther.,* 200:545–559.

Advances in Neurology, Vol. 24, edited by
L. J. Poirier, T. L. Sourkes, and P. J. Bédard.
Raven Press, New York © 1979.

Stereotactic Targets for Dystonias and Dyskinesias: Relationship to Corticobulbar Fibers and Other Adjoining Structures

C. Bertrand, P. Molina-Negro, and S. N. Martinez

*Division of Neurosurgery, Hôpital Notre-Dame and Université de Montréal
Montréal, P. Q., Canada*

Stereotactic surgery offers a unique opportunity to map out the relationship of certain basal structures of the human brain when precise points of reference are associated with electrophysiological means of localization. At the *Third International Symposium on Parkinson's Disease* in Edinburgh in 1968, we (4) reported on the localization of the target for the abolition of tremor. In spite of individual variations, Velasco et al. (12) in 1970, plotting the trajectories of our stimulating electrodes, found that the points which produced arrest of tremor were all grouped together immediately below the thalamus within the prelemniscal radiations, that is, between the 8th and 9th segments when using proportional measurements obtained simply by dividing the anterior commissure–posterior commissure (AC-PC) line in 10 equal segments: that would be 20 to 22 mm behind the anterior commissure for an AC-PC line of 25 mm. Under those circumstances, these points, grouped at the junction of the 5th and 6th segments laterally, lie 12 to 14 mm from the midline and they are 2 to 4 mm below the AC-PC line; they are situated 6 to 8 mm medial to the motor fibers and are anterior to the sensory fibers coursing in the lemniscus.

MATERIAL AND METHODS

Penetration of the target for dystonias is identified by the abolition of the increment in the electromyographic discharge, which appears in these cases on lateral gaze (2). This target lies in posterior VOI which has been identified by Hassler and Hess (9) as part of the vestibulo–interstitio–thalamo–cortical circuit. In a coronal plane, it is located at or just behind the midpoint of the intercommissural line, immediately above it, that is 12.5 to 14 mm behind the anterior commissure (AC), and four segments lateral, that is 10 mm lateral to the midline for an AC-PC line of 25 mm. At that level, the internal capsule is much closer to the wedge-shaped thalamus. As mentioned previously (7), an analysis of 625 consecutive cases of stereotactic surgery for involuntary move-

ments revealed that disturbances associated with the involvement of corticobulbar
fibers in the form of dysarthria, occasionally dysphagia, slowness of movements
with a tendency to pronation, occurred after operation in 12 instances, that is
2%. A composite picture of these lesions (Fig. 1) demonstrates that the fibers
responsible for this syndrome lie in the internal capsule, at the level of the
midpoint between the anterior and posterior commissure and laterally at the
junction of the 5th and 6th segments. They are located at least 5 mm anterior
and medial to the classic motor corticospinal fibers.

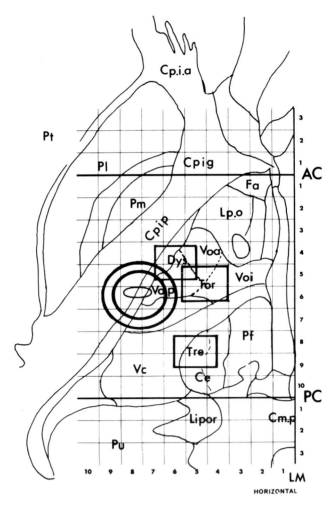

FIG. 1. Targets for dystonias and corticobulbar fibers. Composite drawing in the horizontal
plane of the AC-PC line showing lesions which caused a corticobulbar syndrome. All lesions
encroached upon the internal capsule. They are in the coronal plane of VOI and near the
midpoint of the AC-PC line.

COMMENTS

The presence of dysarthria only in some cases and of slowness and difficulty in opening the hand without dysarthria in others, suggests that the fibers are segmentally distributed within the involved fiber bundles. The clinical manifestations indicate that the responsible fibers are corticobulbar and possibly adjoining corticospinal fibers. However, frontopontine fibers among others are also known to travel in that portion of the internal capsule. The slow awkward movements observed suggest that a lesion of the corticobulbar fibers combined with a subthalamic lesion might mimic choreoathetosis. The latter motor disturbance has been difficult to produce experimentally. In the above-mentioned series of patients, bilateral lesions had been used in all cases except one, indicating that partial lesions of the target area were usually well tolerated.

In order to render this procedure quite safe, in the past 3 years unilateral lesions have been used exclusively, and whenever required, they were combined with selective peripheral denervation. The results were satisfactory (3) as shown in Table 1.

The importance of recording and stimulation and of producing oriented quadrantic lesions was further demonstrated by the fact that there were no motor or sensory deficits and not a single case of hemiballismus, although the lesion for dystonias lies 2 to 4 mm above the subthalamic nucleus. Evidently the lower border of the thalamus and the upper limit of the subthalamic nucleus are easily identified as large spikes, and 12/sec slow waves are recorded on penetrating the corpus Luysii (5).

There is strong evidence against the presence of any primary motor fibers anterior to the coronal plane, passing through the midpoint of the AC-PC line: of all the pallidal lesions that have been made, many of them involving the adjoining part of the internal capsule at or behind the genu, none has produced any motor disturbance. The motor corticospinal tract, well localized by the studies of Marion Smith (11), Brion et al. (8), and Bertrand et al., (5), is situated more posteriorly and laterally than the fibers responsible for the corticobulbar

TABLE 1. *Unilateral stereotactic surgery and/or peripheral denervation in 19 consecutive cases of late dystonia*

Surgical procedures	Results
17 unilateral stereotactic procedures	
10 without peripheral denervation	4 excellent
	4 good
	2 fair
7 with peripheral denervation	1 excellent
	6 good
2 peripheral denervation alone	1 excellent
	1 good

syndrome. Many other corticospinal fibers most likely are injured when large hemorrhagic lesions in the posterior limb of the internal capsule result in marked spasticity. The selectivity of the various corticospinal pathways was shown in a case reported previously (6). This patient with bilateral metastases destroying most of area 4 on each side of the brain developed over a period of a few months total flaccid quadriplegia and hypotonia. It was associated with marked wasting and slightly pendular tendon reflexes. Since that report, the myotatic reflexes of two patients with similar disturbances have been studied. They showed a marked diminution in the excitability of the alpha motor neurones. Pre- and postoperative examination of the myotatic reflexes helped to confirm the site of the lesion and the structures involved. After a well-localized and effective lesion resulting in contralateral hypotonia as assessed clinically, a definite hypoexcitability of the gamma motor neurones is recorded (10). On the other hand, when localization and clinical signs suggest that corticobulbar and adjoining corticospinal fibers are involved by the lesion, hyperexcitability of the alpha motor neurones is obvious and to a lesser degree there is also some hyperactivity of the gamma motor neurones.

SUMMARY AND CONCLUSION

Penetration of the target for dystonia is signaled on the electromyogram during operation by the abolition of the increment in the discharge of affected muscles which occurs in these cases on lateral gaze. This target area, which is not as precisely circumscribed as the target for the abolition of tremor is situated in posterior VOI. The lesion probably interrupts the vestibulo–interstitio–thalamo–cortical circuit at the level of VOI. The fibers which, as a result of their interruption, produce the corticobulbar syndrome lie in the internal capsule close to the thalamus, in a coronal plane passing through VOI, at least 5 mm medial and anterior to the motor corticospinal fibers. A study of the myotactic reflexes demonstrates a hypoexcitability of the gamma motor neurones after a well-localized lesion associated with contralateral hypotonia. By contrast, interruption of the corticobulbar and adjoining corticospinal fibers is accompanied by hyperexcitability of the alpha motor neurones. For maximum safety, when using posterior VOI lesions with or without ipsilateral pallidotomy, these lesions were only made unilaterally for the past 3 years. They were combined with selective peripheral denervation whenever required with satisfactory results.

REFERENCES

1. Bertrand, C. (1966): Localization of lesions. *J. Neurosurg. (Suppl.),* 24 (2):446–452.
2. Bertrand, C. (1976): The treatment of spasmodic torticollis with particular reference to thalamotomy. In: *Current Controversies in Neurosurgery,* edited by T. P. Morley, pp. 455–459. Saunders, Philadelphia.
3. Bertrand, C. (1978): *Torticollis Revisited.* First William Cone Memorial Lecture. III Foundation Lectures, Montreal Neurological Institute, Montreal *(in press).*

4. Bertrand, C., Hardy, J., Molina-Negro, P., and Martinez, S. N. (1969): Optimum physiological target for the arrest of tremor. In: *Third Symposium on Parkinson's Disease,* edited by J. Gillingham and I. M. L. Donaldson, pp. 251–259. E. and S. Livingstone, Edinburgh and London.
5. Bertrand, C., Martinez, S. N., Hardy, J., Molina-Negro, P., and F. Velasco (1973): Stereotactic surgery for parkinsonism. Microelectrode recording, stimulation and oriented sections with a leucotome. *Prog. Neurol. Surg.,* 5:79–122.
6. Bertrand, C., Martinez, S. N., Robert, F., Bouvier, G., and Mathieu, J. P. (1972): L'origine des fibres cortico-spinales motrices: A propos d'un cas de quadriplégie flasque par lésion corticale bilatérale. *Rev. Can. Biol.,* 31:263–271.
7. Bertrand, C., Molina-Negro, P., and Martinez, S. N. (1978): Combined stereotactic and peripheral surgical approach for spasmodic torticollis. *Appl. Neurophysiol.,* 41:122–133.
8. Brion, S., and Guiot, G. (1964): Topographie des faisceaux de projection du cortex dans la capsule interne et dans le pédoncule cérébral. Etude des dégénérescences secondaires dans la sclérose latérale amyotrophique et la maladie de Pick. *Rev. Neurol. (Paris),* 110:123–144.
9. Hassler, R., and Hess, W. R. (1954): Experimentell und anatomische befunde über die Drehbewegungen und ihre nervösen Apparate. *Arch. Psychiatr. Nervenkr.,* 192:488–526.
10. Molina-Negro, P.: The role of the vestibular system in relation to the muscle tone and postural reflexes in man. *Acta Otorhinolaryngol. (in press).*
11. Smith, M. C. (1960): Nerve fibre degeneration in the brain in amyotrophic lateral sclerosis. *J. Neurol. Neurosurg. Psychiatry,* 23:269–282.
12. Velasco, F., Molina-Negro, P. Bertrand, C., and Hardy, J. (1972): Further definition of the sub-thalamic target for the arrest of tremor. *J. Neurosurg.,* 36:184–191.

Advances in Neurology, Vol. 24, edited by
L. J. Poirier, T. L. Sourkes, and P. J. Bédard.
Raven Press, New York © 1979.

Clinical, Pharmacological, and Biochemical Approach of "Onset- and End-of-Dose" Dyskinesias

Yves Agid, Anne-Marie Bonnet, Jean-Louis Signoret,
and François Lhermitte

Clinique de Neurologie et Neuropsychologie, Hôpital de la Salpêtrière, Paris, France

Abnormal involuntary movements are among the most disabling complications of long term L-DOPA therapy in Parkinson's disease. These dyskinesias have been classified according to their clinical features (choreic, athetosic, dystonic, myoclonic, ballic) or their localization, mainly in the orofacial area (5,22,23). More recently these abnormal involuntary movements have been differentiated according to their chronology after administration of L-DOPA (13,14,18). Most patients have mild choreoathetoid movements occurring at the time of maximum therapeutic response. These monophasic dyskinesias have been called "interdose" dyskinesias (14) or "improvement–dystonia–improvement" sequence (18). A smaller number of patients develop dystonic and ballic involuntary movements mainly characterized by their occurrence at the beginning and end of the period of clinical alleviation after administration of L-DOPA. These biphasic dyskinesias which include end-of-dose dyskinesias (3), have been extensively described (13–15,18) and also observed by several authors (12,26). They have been called "onset- and end-of-dose" dyskinesias or "dystonia–improvement–dystonia" response (18).

The purposes of this chapter are: (a) to give new clinical data on 24 patients exhibiting onset- and end-of-dose abnormal movements under long-term L-DOPA therapy, with special reference to the clinical features of Parkinson's disease; and (b) to suggest, on the basis of previous pharmacological and biochemical reports, that dyskinesias presumably result from the modification of central dopamine transmission at the level of the postsynaptic receptor.

CLINICAL ASPECT

One hundred and eighty-eight parkinsonian patients who received a long-term therapeutic trial of L-DOPA in combination with a peripheral decarboxylase inhibitor (PDI: benserazide or carbidopa) were divided into three groups: 76 patients (40%) with no dyskinesias, 88 patients (47%) with pure interdose dys-

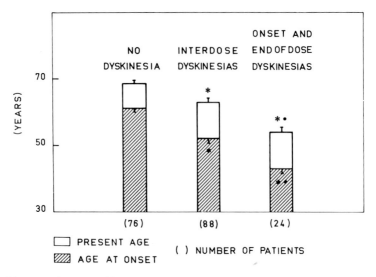

FIG. 1. Mean age in 188 parkinsonian patients treated with L-DOPA + PDI. *: $p \leq .05$ when compared to "no dyskinesia." •: $p \leq .05$ when compared to "interdose dyskinesia."

kinesias, and 24 patients (13%) with onset- and end-of-dose dyskinesias. Six other dyskinetic patients were not included in this study because the abnormal involuntary movements could not be clearly classified. Several patients were also taking anticholinergic medication.

Present age and age at onset of the disease are presented in Fig. 1 and will be discussed later. There was an equal number of men and women in each group, except in the group of patients with interdose dyskinesias, in which there were 55 men and 33 women. A unilateral thalamotomy had been performed in 13 patients with involuntary movements, including three patients with onset- and end-of-dose dyskinesias. A history of encephalitis could be found only in 4 patients with interdose dyskinesias. Interestingly, only one patient in the group with onset- and end-of-dose dyskinesias had a family history of parkinsonism, as opposed to 16 patients in the two other groups (no dyskinesias: 7 patients; interdose dyskinesias: 9 patients).

Parkinsonian motor disability was estimated by measuring the following signs: gait, posture, postural stability, speech, facial appearance, bradykinesia, rigidity and tremor of neck and upper and lower extremities, alternate motion rate of fingers, forearms, and feet. Each of these features was graded on a scale from 0 (normal) to 4 (maximal severity). A total disability score was calculated; the highest theoretical disability score was 88.

Clinical improvement was calculated by comparing the score of parkinsonian syndrome before and after administration of one dose of L-DOPA + PDI. For this purpose, L-DOPA treatment was held at least 12 hr before administration of L-DOPA + PDI.

Description of Onset- and End-of-Dose Dyskinesias

The delay between the start of onset- and end-of-dose dyskinesias and the beginning of L-DOPA treatment in patients was 17 months (interdose dyskinesias: 16 months). All patients had a consistent and a reproducible response to L-DOPA characterized by a biphasic pattern of abnormal movements. Following administration of a single dose of L-DOPA, the first burst of abnormal movements (onset-of-dose dyskinesias) occurred after 15 to 60 min and lasted from a few seconds to 30 min. During this phase, the patients were in a clinical "in between" state and had progressive relief of akinesia alternating with abrupt reinforcement of parkinsonism during the paroxyms of dyskinesia. Each paroxysm consisted of repeated extremely violent and stereotyped ballic and dystonic movements beginning in the legs with twisting movements of the trunk. These movements became generalized in half of the cases. Most of the patients displayed severe anxiety, profuse perspiration, and tachycardia. This brief phase of hyperkinesia was suddenly followed by a prolonged reduction in parkinsonian disability, the duration of which was directly related to the amount of the dose of L-DOPA + PDI. Mild choreoathetoid movements were noted during the hypotonic phase in 8 patients. These interdose dyskinesias were observed in the face, neck, and upper limbs, areas which were usually more affected by the disease and not affected by onset- and end-of-dose dyskinesias. Dysphonia, dysphagia, and blepharospasm were present in 5 patients. A second set of involuntary movements (end-of-dose dyskinesias) similar to those seen during the first phase but generally longer and less severe occurred at the end of the period of clinical improvement.

Description of Underlying Parkinsonism

Patients with onset- and end-of-dose dyskinesias appeared to be younger, more disabled, mainly affected by rigidity and akinesia, and had a good response to L-DOPA therapy.

As shown in Fig. 1, mean age of onset of the disease and present age (43 and 54 years, respectively) were significantly lower in patients with onset- and end-of-dose dyskinesias than in the other two groups of patients. Patients with interdose abnormal movements were also significantly younger (onset: 52 years; present age: 63 years) than those free of dyskinesias (onset: 61 years; present age: 66 years). Although the duration of the disease was the same (11 years) in patients with interdose and onset- and end-of-dose dyskinesias, the disease was already far advanced in the latter group (Table 1). Akinesia and rigidity were more severe in patients with biphasic abnormal movements, but this difference was not statistically significant for tremor (Fig. 2). In patients with interdose dyskinesias, as compared to parkinsonians with no involuntary movements, only akinesia was significantly more disabling. Rigidity and/or akinesia were the initial symptoms in 54% of patients with onset- and end-of-dose dyskinesias,

TABLE 1. *Stage of parkinsonism*

No dyskinesias (74)	2.8 ± 0.2
Interdose dyskinesias (87)	3.3 ± 0.1
Onset- and end-of-dose dyskinesias (24)	3.8 ± 0.3

Number of patients in parentheses.

in 55% of those with interdose dyskinesias, and in 43% of patients without dyskinesias. In all other patients, tremor was present at the beginning of the disease.

The reduction in parkinsonian motor disability following administration of a single dose of L-DOPA + PDI differed between the three groups (onset- and end-of-dose dyskinesias > interdose dyskinesias > no dyskinesia) (Fig. 3). There was no positive correlation between percentage of the L-DOPA-induced overall improvement and the dose of L-DOPA + PDI. However, higher daily doses of L-DOPA + PDI were required in those patients with onset- and end-of-dose dyskinesias in order to obtain improvement of abnormal involuntary movements (15) and sustained alleviation of the parkinsonian signs (Table 2).

The frequency of occurrence of other L-DOPA-induced adverse reactions, such as hypotension and confusion, was the same in both groups of dyskinetic patients. However on–off phenomena were observed in all 24 patients with onset- and end-of-dose dyskinesias and in only 32 out of 88 patients with interdose dyskinesias.

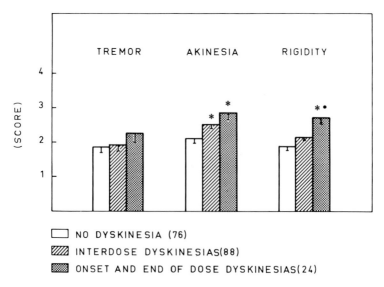

FIG. 2. Cardinal symptoms in 188 parkinsonian patients with L-DOPA-induced abnormal movements. *:$p \leqslant .05$ when compared to "no dyskinesia." ●: $p \leqslant .05$ when compared to "interdose dyskinesia."

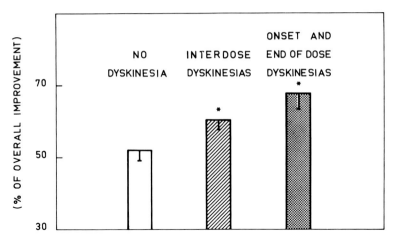

FIG. 3. Effect of L-DOPA + PDI in 188 parkinsonian patients. *: $p < .05$ when compared to "no dyskinesia."

PHARMACOLOGICAL AND BIOCHEMICAL APPROACH

Previous detailed pharmacological and biochemical data have shown that onset- and end-of-dose dyskinesias differ dramatically from interdose dyskinesias. To examine these differences, acute studies were carried out in parkinsonian patients who had a high incidence of biphasic abnormal movement; these studies consisted of determinations of disability score within five hours after administration of a single dose of L-DOPA + PDI.

First, an attempt was made to modify the clinical pattern of these movements with drugs known to interact with various central neurotransmissions (13). Thus the two phases of dyskinesias could be triggered by different dopamine agonists, such as apomorphine, bromocriptine, or L-DOPA ± PDI. In contrast, permanent abnormal movements could be induced by ingestion of low doses of L-DOPA or by the concomitant administration of dopaminergic antagonist drugs such as haloperidol or tiapride (17). On the other hand, high doses of haloperidol have been shown to reduce the intensity of dystonia and to cause an immediate and generalized worsening of Parkinson's disease (18). In contrast to what would be expected in patients with classic interdose dyskinesias, increasing the dose of L-DOPA + PDI tends to reduce the duration of the first phase

TABLE 2. *Dosage of L-DOPA therapy*

No dyskinesias (74)	494 ± 26
Interdose dyskinesias (86)	591 ± 29
Onset- and end-of-dose dyskinesias (23)	887 ± 82

Number of patients in parentheses.

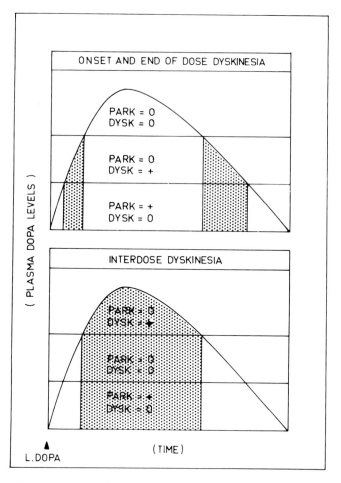

FIG. 4. Schematic representation of the correlation between occurrence of abnormal involuntary movements and DOPA concentrations in the plasma after administration of a single dose of L-DOPA ± PDI.

of onset- and end-of-dose dyskinesias. The modifications in intensity and duration of these biphasic dyskinesias by dopaminergic agonists and antagonists suggest that their mechanism is essentially dependent on the modification of the dopaminergic transmission at central synaptic sites. This is further confirmed by the fact that the dyskinesias were not improved by other drugs (propanolol, baclofen, methysergide, 5-hydroxytryptophan, physostigmine). However, in one patient the second phase of abnormal movements was most favorably improved by the previous administration of an anticholinergic drug (21); furthermore, diazepam and phenobarbital were shown to be effective in reducing the severity of both phases of dyskinesias.

In another series of observations performed on patients with both types of abnormal movements, the sequence of clinical events after administration of L-DOPA + PDI was correlated with the pattern of DOPA concentrations in plasma, taken as an index of brain dopamine levels. As reported by many authors (8,19,20,27), interdose dyskinesias and improvement of parkinsonism were shown to occur during the peak of DOPA plasma levels (Fig. 4). Consequently treatment of these patients requires a gradual and slow reduction in the L-DOPA daily dosage (4) or the addition of dopamine blocking agents (11,25) with considerable risk of increasing the severity of the parkinsonian state. During the course of parkinsonism, however, the period during which the patients are devoid both of parkinsonian signs and abnormal movements (Fig. 4) is progressively reduced so that after a certain period of time, clinical improvement appears to be optimal only if there is some dystonia.

A distinctly different response pattern was obtained in patients with onset- and end-of-dose dyskinesias (13). These striking abnormal movements appeared neither when DOPA concentrations in the plasma were high, i.e., at the time of clinical efficacy, nor when they were low, i.e., when the patients were in an akinetic state. They occurred during the increase and the decrease phases of DOPA blood levels, i.e., at the onset and at the end of action of L-DOPA. Thus it appeared possible to delay the occurrence of the second phase of dyskinesias by maintaining high and constant levels of L-DOPA + PDI. These observations, similar to those reported by Muenter et al. (18), led us to increase the frequency of administration and the daily doses of L-DOPA + PDI. A reduction by 46% of the duration of the phases of hyperkinesia was obtained by increasing the daily doses of L-DOPA by 41% (15). However, caution must be taken when using this therapeutic approach on a long-term basis, because severe L-DOPA side-effects frequently result. The occurrence of onset- and end-of-dose dyskinesias when the plasma DOPA levels reach a critical level might suggest that their incidence depends on a transient disturbance in the central dopaminergic transmission (Fig. 4).

DISCUSSION

Neither the pathogenesis nor pathophysiology of L-DOPA-induced abnormal movements in patients with parkinsonism is well understood. On the basis of pharmacological data, several investigators have suggested that the development of these dyskinesias (namely interdose dyskinesias) are related to supersensitivity of the striatal dopamine receptor sites caused by prolonged denervation (2,10,28). This relationship, however, is not widely accepted (6). Evidence favoring the participation of a deviation in the degradation of dopamine toward abnormal metabolites remains another possibility. Thus o-methyldopa might effectively play a role in inducing such dyskinesias, since patients treated with L-DOPA + PDI have high plasma o-methyldopa levels compared to those who have no dyskinesias (9). Biochemical analysis of the urinary degradation products

TABLE 3. *Main characteristics of "interdose" and "onset- and end-of-dose" dyskinesias*

	Interdose dyskinesias	Onset- and end-of-dose dyskinesias
Aspect	Choreoathetoid	Dystonic and/or ballic
Timing	During the period of L-DOPA-induced clinical improvement	At the beginning and at the end of the period of L-DOPA-induced clinical improvement
Correlation with DOPA concentrations in plasma	During the peak of DOPA blood levels	During the increase and decrease of DOPA blood levels
Parkinsonism		Younger and more disabled patients with severe akinesia and rigidity
Treatment	Reduction and fractionation of the daily doses of L-DOPA	Possible improvement by increasing and fractionating the daily doses of L-DOPA

of L-DOPA revealed the presence of a deviation in the catabolism of dopamine leading to 4-*o*-methylated derivatives (13). Nevertheless, the function of these metabolites in the genesis of abnormal involuntary movements must be rigorously documented. Finally, interdose dyskinesias may be attributed to the modification of many other neurotransmitter systems.

As summarized in Table 3, onset- and end-of-dose dyskinesias have opposite patterns as compared to interdose dyskinesias, suggesting that they are different in nature and that their mechanism is also different. The present results, based on clinical observation together with pharmacological and biochemical analysis in parkinsonian patients, suggest that these biphasic hyperkinesias are to some extent related to the modification of central dopaminergic transmission: (a) They were present in patients with the most clinically advanced disease mainly characterized by an akinetic state, which presumably indicates the profound loss of nigrostriatal dopaminergic neurons; (b) they were observed in patients who had the greatest degree of response to L-DOPA; (c) they were produced only by dopamine agonists and were dramatically modified by drugs known to increase or reduce dopaminergic transmission; and (d) they occurred when the concentrations of DOPA in the plasma reached a critical level. Muenter et al. (18) postulated that they might result from a depolarization blockade due to supraximal stimulation of the postsynaptic receptors of a specific neuronal system. In the light of recent hypotheses suggesting the existence of two kinds of dopamine postsynaptic receptors (7, and Calne, *this volume*), the development of mono- or biphasic dyskinesias could be mediated through the stimulation of type 1 and 2 striatal dopamine receptors, respectively. After administration of L-DOPA, stimulation of type 1 dopamine receptors would induce the first phase of onset- and end-of-dose abnormal movements. While concentration of L-DOPA, and thus of dopamine, progressively increases at receptor sites, excitation of type 2 dopamine receptors might trigger the alleviation of parkinsonian signs. The first phase of abnormal movements would disappear as a result of intrinsic interaction between postsynaptic neurons which seem to be mainly cholinergic (1,24). Interdose dyskinesias would develop in some patients as a consequence of overactivity of striatal neurons mediated through type 2 dopamine receptors. The second phase of the biphasic abnormal movements would occur at the reappearance of akinesia during the decrease of DOPA concentrations in the plasma in response to reduced stimulation of type 2 receptors while stimulation of type 1 receptors is still present.

SUMMARY

Abnormal movements produced by L-DOPA were observed in 112 of 188 patients with Parkinson's disease. The patients were divided in two groups. Eighty-eight patients experienced "interdose dyskinesias" occurring at the maximum therapeutic effect. Twenty-four patients exhibited "onset- and end-of-dose" dyskinesias characterized by four essential features: (a) the nature of the underlying parkinsonism, i.e., young age at onset of disease, severity of the akinetorigid state, and quality of response to L-DOPA; (b) the ballic and dystonic features of the involuntary movements producing an extreme disability; (c) occurrence of dyskinesias at the beginning and end of the period of effectiveness of a dose of L-DOPA, coinciding with rise and fall in plasma levels of DOPA; and (d) aggravation of dyskinesias by dopamine-blocking agents, and reduction of dyskinesias by an increase and fractionation of the daily dose of L-DOPA.

ACKNOWLEDGMENT

We wish to thank F. Javoy-Agid and Robert O'Hara for reviewing the manuscript.

REFERENCES

1. Agid, Y., Guyenet, P., Glowinski, J., Beaujouan, J. C., and Javoy, F. (1975): Inhibitory influence of the nigrostriatal dopamine system on the striatal cholinergic neurons in the rat. *Brain Res.,* 86:488–492.
2. Andén, N. E. (1970): Pharmacological and anatomical implications of induced abnormal movements with L-DOPA. In: *L-DOPA and Parkinsonism,* edited by A. Barbeau and F. H. MacDowell, pp. 132–143. Davis, Philadelphia.
3. Barbeau, A. (1975): Diphasic dyskinesias during levodopa therapy. *Lancet,* 1:756.
4. Barbeau, A. (1976): Neurological and psychiatric side effects of L-DOPA. In: *Pharmacology and Therapeutics,* Vol. 1, pp. 475–494. Pergamon Press, Elmsford, New York.
5. Barbeau, A., Mars, H., Gillo-Joffroy, L., and Arsenault, A. (1970): A proposed classification of DOPA-induced dyskinesias. In: *L-DOPA and Parkinsonism,* edited by A. Barbeau and F. H. MacDowell. pp. 118–120. Davis, Philadelphia.
6. Chase, T. N., Holden, E. M., and Brody, J. A. (1973): Levodopa induced dyskinesias. Comparison in parkinsonism—Dementia and amyotrophic lateral sclerosis. *Arch. Neurol.,* 29:328–330.
7. Cools, A. R., and Van Rossum, J. M. (1976): Excitation-mediating and inhibition-mediating dopamine receptors: A new concept towards a better understanding of electrophysiological, biochemical, pharmacological, functional and clinical data. *Psychopharmacologia,* 45:243–254.
8. Fahn, S. (1974): "On-off" phenomenon with levodopa therapy in parkinsonism: Clinical and

pharmacological correlations and the effect of intramuscular pyridoxine. *Neurology,* 24:431–441.

9. Feuerstein, C., Tanche, M., Serre, F., Gavend, M., Pellat, J. and Perret, J. (1977): Does *o*-methyl-DOPA play a role in levodopa-induced dyskinesias? *Acta Neurol. Scand.,* 56:79–82.
10. Klawans, H. L., Ilahi, M. M., and Shenker, D. (1970): Theoretical implications of the use of L-DOPA in parkinsonism. *Acta. Neurol. Scand.,* 46:409–411.
11. Klawans, H. L., and Weiner, W. J. (1974): Attempted use of haloperidol in the treatment of L-DOPA-induced dyskinesias. *J. Neurol. Neurosurg. Psychiatry,* 37:427–430.
12. Lees, A., Shaw, K. M., and Stern, G. M. (1977): "Off period" dystonia and "on period" choreoathetosis in levodopa-treated patients with Parkinson's disease. *Lancet,* 12:1034.
13. Lhermitte, F., Agid, Y., Feuerstein, C., Serre, F., Signoret, J. L., Studler, J. M., and Bonnet, A. M. (1977): Mouvements anormaux provoqués par la L-DOPA dans la maladie de Parkinson: Correlations avec les concentrations plasmatiques de DOPA et de *o*-methyl-DOPA. *Rev. Neurol.,* 133:445–454.
14. Lhermitte, F., Agid, Y., Signoret, J. L., and Studler, J. M. (1977): Les dyskinesies de "début et fin de dose" provoquées par la L-DOPA. *Rev. Neurol.* 133:297–308.
15. Lhermitte, F., Agid, Y., and Signoret, J. L. (1978): Onset and end of dose levodopa-induced dyskinesias. Possible treatment by increasing the daily doses of levodopa. *Arch. Neurol.,* 35:261–263.
16. Lhermitte, F., Rosa, A., and Comoy, E. (1977): Mouvements anormaux des parkinsoniens traités par la L-DOPA et anomalies du métabolisme de la dopamine. *Rev. Neurol.,* 133:3–11.
17. Lhermitte, F., Signoret, J. L., and Agid, Y. (1977): Etude des effets d'une molécule originale, le tiapride, dans le traitement des mouvements anormaux d'origine extrapyramidale. *Sem. Hop. Paris,* 53:9–15.
18. Muenter, M. D., Sharpless, N. S., Tyce, G. M., and Darley, F. L. (1977): Patterns of dystonia ("I.D.I" and "D.I.D") in response to L-DOPA therapy for Parkinson's disease. *Mayo Clin. Proc.,* 52:163–174.
19. Muenter, M. D., and Tyce, G. M. (1971): L-DOPA therapy of Parkinson's disease: Plasma L-DOPA concentration, therapeutic response and side effects. *Mayo Clin. Proc.,* 46:231–239.
20. Peaston, M. J. T., and Bianchine, J. R. (1970): Metabolic studies and clinical observations during L-DOPA treatment of Parkinson's disease. *Br. Med. J.,* 1:400–403.
21. Pollak, P., (1978): Les mouvements anormaux involontaires provoqués par la L-DOPA dans la maladie de Parkinson, *thèse de médecine,* Paris.
22. Rondot, P., and Ribadeau-Dumas, J. L. (1972): Dopamine et mouvements anormaux. *Rev. Neurol.,* 127:99–113.
23. Sigwald, J., and Raymondeau, C. (1970): Les mouvements anormaux observés au cours du traitement de la maladie de Parkinson par la L-DOPA. *Rev. Neurol.,* 112:103–112.
24. Stadler, H., Lloyd, K. G., Gadea-Ciria, M., and Bartholini, G. (1973): Enhanced striatal release by chlorpromazine and its reversal by apomorphine. *Brain Res.,* 55:476–480.
25. Tarsy, D., Parkes, J. D., and Marsden, C. D. (1975): Metoclopramide and Pimozide in Parkinson's disease and levodopa-induced dyskinesias. *J. Neurol. Neurosurg. Psychiatry,* 38:331–335.
26. Tolosa, E. S., Martin, W. E., and Cohen, H. P. (1975): Dyskinesias during levodopa therapy. *Lancet,* 2:1381–1382.
27. Tolosa, E. S., Martin, W. E., Cohen, H. P., and Jacobson, R. L. (1975): Patterns of clinical response and plasma dopa levels in Parkinson's disease. *Neurology,* 25:177–183.
28. Ungerstedt, U. (1971): Postsynaptic supersensitivity after 6-hydroxydopamine induced degeneration of the nigro-striatal dopamine system. *Acta Physiol. Scand. (Suppl.),* 367:69–93.

Advances in Neurology, Vol. 24, edited by
L. J. Poirier, T. L. Sourkes, and P. J. Bédard.
Raven Press, New York © 1979.

Estrogens, Progesterone, and the Extrapyramidal System

*P. J. Bédard, **P. Langelier, *J. Dankova, †A. Villeneuve, ‡T. Di Paolo, ‡N. Barden, ‡F. Labrie, §J. R. Boissier, and §C. Euvrard

*Departments of *Anatomy, **Obstetrics–Gynecology, and †Psychiatry, Faculty of Medicine, Laval University, Quebec, Canada; ‡MRC Group in Molecular Endocrinology, Le Centre Hospitalier de l'Université Laval, Quebec G1V 4G2, Canada; and §Centre de Recherches Roussel-UCLAF, Romainville 93230, France*

The interaction between monoamines and peripheral hormones is well recognized at the level of the hypothalamopituitary axis. Dopamine, for example, inhibits the release of prolactin (3,17–19), while estrogens have the opposite effect (10,17,21). Estrogens exert their stimulatory effect on prolactin secretion by direct action at the anterior pituitary level (17). We report here a similar antidopaminergic action of estrogens in other brain areas rich in dopamine receptors, especially the basal ganglia. Such an effect of estrogens was suggested by the following observations: Tardive dyskinesias was, according to earlier reports (4), more frequent in postmenopausal women than in men of comparable age. Moreover, estrogens administered to young women taking neuroleptic drugs for psychosis can sometimes precipitate a parkinsonian syndrome (13), thus suggesting that estrogens can also exert an inhibitory effect on dopamine receptors in the human. It should be added that pregnancy and oral contraceptive therapy are sometimes associated with chorea (11), thus suggesting that progesterone or some combinations of sex steroid hormones can lead to increased sensitivity of dopaminergic receptors.

CLINICAL STUDIES

L-DOPA-Induced Dyskinesias

Patient 1

This patient was a 64-year-old woman in whom Parkinson's disease had been diagnosed at age 50, 1 year after menopause. At first, she was treated with anticholinergics, but was placed on L-DOPA at age 57. Initially, the therapeutic response was satisfactory, but within a few months, she developed generalized dyskinesias, expecially at the peak of the effect of L-DOPA. The dyskinetic

TABLE 1. *Influence of estrogens on parkinsonian disability and L-DOPA-induced dyskinesias in 1 patient (No. 1). Average of scores obtained during a 4-month trial*

	L-DOPA 4.5 g/day + placebo mean ± SEM	L-DOPA 4.5 g/day + conjugated estrogens 0.625 mg/day mean ± SEM
Dyskinesia score (Max 21)	6.77 ± 1.26 (15)	0.55 ± 0.20[a] (20)
Parkinson disability score (Max 123)	26.6 ± 6.7 (15)	34.4 ± 4.9 (20)

Number of examinations in parentheses.
[a] $p < 0.001$ by the student's *t*-test.

periods became progressively longer, and any attempt to decrease the dose of L-DOPA was followed by a return of rigidity and bradykinesia. Her usual dosage of L-DOPA was 4.5 g/day associated with ethopropazine, 100 mg/day. In the hospital, she was examined several times and scored for dyskinesia (0–21) and parkinsonian disability (0–123), according to the King's College rating scale. With her informed consent, she was given conjugated estrogens (Premarin®), 0.625 mg/day, for periods of up to 3 weeks, alternating with periods of 1 week during which she was given a placebo. Conjugated estrogens had a striking effect on the dyskinesias (see Table 1), which reappeared during placebo treatment. Our clinical impression was that the parkinsonian disability increased, but the difference in scores was not significant (Table 1).

Patient 2

A 63-year-old woman, who had suffered from Parkinson's disease for 7 years, was taking L-DOPA (250 mg) and carbidopa (25 mg, Sinemet®) q.i.d. She had almost constant dyskinesias during the day. Conjugated estrogens, added to her usual medication, at a dose of 0.625 mg/day reduced her dyskinesia score by 50% during 3 months without any increase of her parkinsonian disability score.

Patient 3

A 74-year-old woman, with severe Parkinson's disease diagnosed 3 years before, was taking levodopa/carbidopa (Sinemet®) 125 mg q.i.d., and had dyskinesias of moderate intensity. Conjugated estrogens, 0.625 mg/day, given in two separate 2-week periods, resulted in total disappearance of her dyskinesias during the test periods. Surprisingly, her rigidity score also improved.

Additional Patients

In 4 additional patients (3 men ages 44, 55, and 66 and one woman aged 80), conjugated estrogens (Premarin®) was tested double-blind for 1 week and compared with an identical-looking placebo for another week. Patients were instructed not to change their usual medication. Dyskinesia and disability scores were assessed 3 times each Friday afternoon during 3 successive weeks: before therapy, at the end of the estrogen therapy, and at the end of the placebo treatment.

In the woman, there was a complete disappearance of the dyskinesias during estrogen treatment, but not during administration of the placebo. Her disability score did, however, increase with estrogen treatment. One man (age 66) reported no effect, and his scores were unchanged. In the two other men, no change could be detected in the actual scores, but one had increased his dose of DOPA by 50%, while the other reported that his "on" period lasted 3 hr instead of 4. In both cases, this deterioration of parkinsonian symptoms occurred only during estrogen therapy and disappeared with use of the placebo.

Summary

In summary, 4 of 7 patients showed subjective and objective improvement of their dyskinesias with estrogen treatment. Interestingly, all were women. In 4 patients (including two men), a deterioration of the parkinsonian symptoms occurred. In 6 of 7 patients, therefore, the change was suggestive of a decrease in dopaminergic activity in the striatum.

Tardive Dyskinesia

Initial Case

A 51-year-old woman, when first seen in consultation, stated that she had noticed about two years earlier an involuntary movement of her mouth after taking neuroleptic drugs. This progressed to a severe buccolinguomasticatory dyskinesia which responded moderately to a combination of reserpine and deanol. It was noted, however, that the greatest improvement coincided with a 4-month period of amenorrhea. Thereafter, a striking relationship between the dyskinesia and the menstrual period was noticed. Improvement generally coincided with amenorrhea and worsened with menstruation (27). When her gynecologist prescribed a progestogen (norethindrone), a marked aggravation occurred. Conjugated estrogens (Premarin®), given in increasing doses of 0.625, 1.25, and 2.50 mg/day for several weeks, resulted in a striking improvement which persisted for almost a month after cessation of therapy. A mild tremor of the right hand was also noticed in conjunction with the highest dose of the estrogens.

Additional Patients

A group of 20 institutionalized psychiatric male patients were selected. All exhibited some form of tardive dyskinesia resulting from prolonged administration of neuroleptics, and only one was completely without neuroleptic medication. The patients were divided into four equivalent groups of five, taking into account age and dosage of conjugated estrogens (Premarin®). The dyskinetic movements were evaluated before the study according to the Villeneuve rating scale (28) and weekly thereafter. Conjugated estrogens were then given orally for 6 weeks, 10 patients taking 1.25 mg/day and 10 receiving 2.50 mg/day. In each group (Table 2), 4 of 5 patients (16 of 20) improved in various degrees ($p < 0.006$). No clear trend was observed in the parkinsonian disability scores (29).

Pharmacological Studies

To confirm our clinical impression, we have studied the effect of female sex steroid hormones in two animal models which, in some way, reflect dopaminergic activity in the basal ganglia: apomorphine-induced circling and motility in rats having a unilateral lesion of the entopeduncular nucleus (5,6). This lesion was selected because it inactivates one of the main outflows of the striopallidal system. We have found circling rates after such lesions to be quite stable even after several months (1,6). Apomorphine was chosen because it is generally considered to be a direct dopamine agonist, and any interference with its effect can be presumed to occur from inhibition at the receptor site or beyond (9).

In a group of female rats weighting 200 g each, a radiofrequency lesion was performed stereotactically in the left entopeduncular nucleus. After recovery, the effect of apomorphine (0.5 mg/kg, s.c.) on circling and motility was tested three times. Circling was estimated by counting the maximal number of turns per minute during the first hour following apomorphine injection, while motility was measured in Automex® motility boxes (Columbus Instruments) and counts

TABLE 2. *Effect of various daily doses of conjugated estrogens on tardive dyskinesia in 20 male psychiatric patients[a]*

Group (N = 5 in each group)	Oral daily doses of conjugated estrogens	Number of patients improved[b] after 6 weeks[c]
1. Ages ≤ 51	1.25 mg	4
2. Ages < 51	2.50 mg	4
3. Ages ≥ 52	1.25 mg	4
4. Ages ≥ 52	2.50 mg	4

[a] From ref. 29.
[b] In varying degrees.
[c] $p < 0.006$, Fisher sign test.

recorded automatically every 10 min during the first hour following apomorphine. Only the 20 rats showing stable circling and motility rates were used in these experiments. They were then divided into four groups of five, each group being given one of the following treatments twice a day for 15 days:

1. The vehicle: 1% agar in 0.9% NaCl (V)
2. 17β-estradiol benzoate, 5 μg s.c. (E_2)
3. R5020, a potent progestin (22), 200 μg, s.c.
4. A combination of estradiol benzoate and R5020 (E_2 + R5020)

During the second week of treatment, circling and motility were measured three times. As shown in Fig. 1, while the circling rate remained constant in the vehicle-treated animals, it decreased in the three hormone-treated groups, the effect of estradiol and R5020 being partially additive. The rates of circling of the hormone-treated groups are significantly different ($p < 0.05$) from the rates measured in the same groups before treatment and also from the vehicle-treated group. There was however no significant effect of sex steroid treatment on the motility counts.

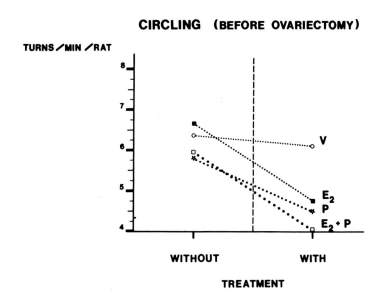

CIRCLING (BEFORE OVARIECTOMY)

FIG. 1. Effect of estradiol benzoate (E_2), R5020 (P), a combined treatment with estradiol and R5020 (E_2 + P), or the vehicle alone (V) on apomorphine-induced circling in female rats having a lesion of the left entopeduncular nucleus. These different treatments were given twice a day (see text) for 2 weeks. Circling was measured three times before and three times during the second week of treatment. Note the clear drop in circling rates in all steroid-treated groups. The following differences are significant ($p < 0.05$): circling rates in the three hormone-treated groups compared to the vehicle-treated animals, and the circling rates of the same three groups compared to the circling rates obtained before hormonal treatment.

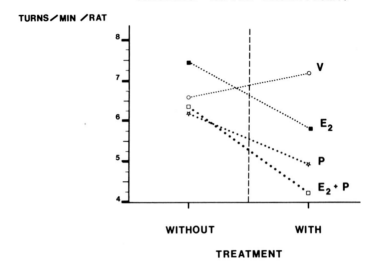

FIG. 2. Effect of estradiol benzoate (E₂), R5020 (P), a combination of E₂ and R5020 (E₂ +P), or the vehicle alone (V) on circling in ovariectomized rats. The experiment was performed as described in Fig. 1. Note that the effects and differences observed are the same.

A month later, all animals were ovariectomized and the same treatments were repeated under the same conditions. The effect of hormone treatment on circling was essentially the same (Fig. 2). There was, however, a 50% ($p <$ 0.05) reduction in the motility counts after estradiol administration.

Biochemical Studies

Effect on Dopamine-Sensitive Adenyl Cyclase

Since the above results suggest an effect of sex steroids on striatal dopaminergic mechanism, we then studied the effect of estrogen treatment on the stimulation of the dopamine-sensitive adenyl cyclase in the rat striatum.

Five male rats weighing 200 g each were treated for 10 days with 17β-estradiol benzoate (5 μg, b.i.d.). On the 10th day, they were decapitated, the brain rapidly dissected out over ice, and the striatum and limbic structures (nucleus accumbens, septal area, and tuberculum olfactorium) were isolated. Dopamine-sensitive adenyl cyclase was assayed according to the method of Salomon et al. (24). As shown in Fig. 3, the dose-response curves of dopamine (DA)-stimulated adenyl cyclase activity in the striatum were essentially the same in hormone- and vehicle-treated groups. Similar results were obtained in mesolimbic structures.

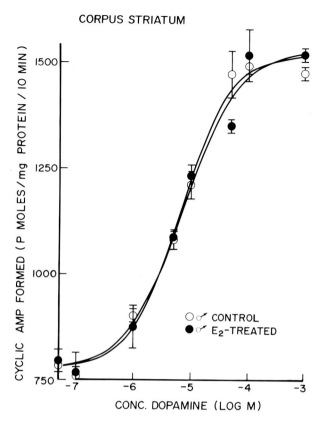

FIG. 3. Effects of increasing concentrations of dopamine on adenyl cyclase activity of the corpus striatum obtained from intact and estrogen-treated adult male rats. Animals were treated with 17β-estradiol (10 μg, twice a day) for 10 days or the vehicle alone (0.1% gelatin). Incubation of total homogenate was performed for 10 min at 30°C and cyclic AMP formation measured as described (22). Results shown are means $\pm$ SEM of three experiments.

Effect on Striatal Levels of Acetyl Choline

As demonstrated by anatomical, electrophysiological, and biochemical studies, the nigrostriatal dopaminergic pathway exerts a direct inhibitory control on striatal cholinergic neurons (15). Therefore, stimulation or blockade of dopaminergic receptors induced by dopaminergic agonists or antagonists can induce marked changes in the activity of striatal cholinergic neurons. Besides determinations of striatal acetylcholine (ACh) release (25) and turnover (26), measurements of striatal ACh levels (14) are a good index of dopaminergic influences on striatal cholinergic neurons.

In order to test the possibility of an antidopaminergic action of estrogens at the striatal level, we have studied the effect of the potent synthetic estrogen

TABLE 3. *Effect of estrogen pretreatment on changes in striatal ACh levels induced by dopaminergic drugs*

Pretreatment	Treatment			
	Saline	Apomorphine (2.5 mg/kg, i.p.)	Bromocryptine (5 mg/kg, i.p.)	Haloperidol (0.05 mg/kg, i.p.)
Saline	39.5 ± 1.8	68.2 ± 4.9[b]	70.6 ± 3.6[b]	33.9 ± 1.3[a]
	100%	174%	180%	86%
Moxestrol, 20 μg/kg	38.7 ± 2.1	52.1 ± 3.3[b]	55.2 ± 2.6[b]	23.5 ± 0.9[b]
s.c. for 5 days	98%	133%	142%	60%
Effect of pretreatment	NS	−55%[b]	−48%[b]	+185%[b]

Intact male rats were injected daily for 5 days with moxestrol (20 μg/kg, s.c.) or saline. Twenty-four hours after the last estrogen administration, animals received saline or the mentioned DA drug i.p. and were killed 45 min later. The striatum was dissected over ice and ACh levels determined. Values are expressed as nanomoles ACh/g fresh weight and are the mean ±SEM of results obtained with groups of eight rats. Statistical significance was evaluated by an analysis of variance and indicated by [a]when $p < 0.05$ and [b]when $p < 0.01$. NS = not significant.

moxestrol (11β-methoxy-17-ethinyl-1,3,5' (23) estratène 3,17β-diol) on the changes in striatal ACh levels induced by various dopaminergic drugs.

As shown in Table 3, while no change of basal striatal ACh levels was observed after repeated administration of moxestrol (20 μg/kg, s.c., q.d. for 5 days), this estrogen pretreatment did significantly reduce the stimulation of ACh accumulation in the striatum induced by the dopaminergic agonists apomorphine (2.5 mg/kg, i.p.) and bromocriptine (5 mg/kg, i.p.). In contrast, the same pretreatment with moxestrol led to a marked potentiation of the slight decrease in striatal ACh levels produced by a low dose of haloperidol (0.05 mg/kg, i.p.). These results clearly demonstrate an antidopaminergic action of estrogens at the striatal level, since estrogen pretreatment not only reduces the stimulatory effect of a dopaminergic agonist, but also potentiates the inhibitory effect of a dopaminergic antagonist on the activity of striatal cholinergic neurons.

As demonstrated by using rats with a unilateral lesion of the nigrostriatal dopaminergic pathway, the antidopaminergic activity of estrogens at the striatal level is independent from the integrity of the nigrostriatal dopaminergic neurons. In fact, after moxestrol pretreatment, the same inhibition of the striatal ACh increase induced by apomorphine (2.5 mg/kg, i.p.) was found in striata on both sides (Table 4). In agreement with these results was the finding that estrogens did not induce any change in dopamine turnover in the rat striatum (8).

Receptor-Binding Studies

Since hypersensitivity of the response to DA agonists in both man and experimental animals has been found to be associated with increased [³H]haloperidol binding in the striatum (2,18), we examined the possibility of an effect of estrogen treatment on the binding of [³H]spiroperidol in the rat striatum, nucleus accum-

TABLE 4. *Effect of striatal ACh increase induced by apomorphine in rats with a unilateral degeneration of the nigrostriatal dopaminergic pathway*

	Treatment			
	Intact side		Lesioned side	
Pretreatment	Saline	Apomorphine (2.5 mg/kg, i.p.)	Saline	Apomorphine (2.5 mg/kg, i.p.)
Saline	38.8 ± 1.9 100%	60.6 ± 2.4 [b] 156%	39.4 ± 2.0 100%	75.2 ± 4.7 [b] 190%
Moxestrol, 20 µg/kg s.c. for 5 days	39.1 ± 2.3 101%	49.6 ± 2.6 [a] 127%	40.6 ± 1.8 103%	57.5 ± 3.1 [b] 141%
Effect of pretreatment	NS	−52% [b]		−54% [b]

Intact adult male rats with a unilateral lesion of the nigrostriatal dopaminergic pathway induced by a microinjection of 6-OH-DA (8 µg/4 µl) into the right substantia nigra, were injected daily for 5 days with moxestrol (20 µg/kg, s.c.) or saline. Twenty-four hours after the last estrogen administration, animals received saline or apomorphine and were killed 45 min later. Both striata were dissected over ice and their ACh and DA contents measured. Striatal DA levels in the lesioned side were reduced to undetectable levels (DA levels in nmol/g fresh weight in the intact side were 65 ± 3.5). Values are expressed as nanomoles ACh/g fresh weight and are the mean ± SEM of results obtained with groups of 8 rats. Statistical significance was evaluated by an analysis of variance and indicated by [a]when $p < 0.05$ and [b]when $p < 0.01$. NS = not significant.

bens + olfactive tubercle, frontal cortex, and anterior pituitary gland. In order to detect possible changes of agonist and antagonist states of the DA receptor, specificity of binding was examined with a series of unlabeled DA agonists and antagonists.

Adult female Sprague-Dawley rats weighing 200–300 g were used throughout these experiments. Ten days after bilateral ovariectomy under ether anesthesia, the animals (60/group) were injected either with 17β-estradiol (10 µg b.i.d., s.c.) or with the vehicle alone (0.5 ml of 1% gelatin–0.9% NaCl b.i.d., s.c.) for 7 days. The animals were decapitated the morning following the last injection.

The striatum, nucleus accumbens + olfactive tubercle, frontal cortex, and anterior pituitary gland were immediately removed and homogenized in ice-cold 30 vol (wt/vol) of 0.25 M sucrose, 25 mM Tris-HCl, 2 mM $MgCl_2$ (pH 7.4 at 4°C) using a motor-driven glass-Teflon® homogenizer. Binding was measured according to the technique described (3).

Contrary to the expected findings, treatment of castrated (10 days previously) rats with 17β-estradiol (10 µg b.i.d. for 7 days) led to a slight increase of [^{3}H]spiroperidol binding in striatal, nucleus accumbens + olfactive tubercle, and frontal cortex homogenate. That the increased binding is due to an increased number of binding sites and not to higher affinity is indicated by the absence of effect of estrogen treatment on the K_I values of spiroperidol, RU24213, apomorphine, and dihydroergocryptine (DHEC) for displacement of labeled ligand (data not shown).

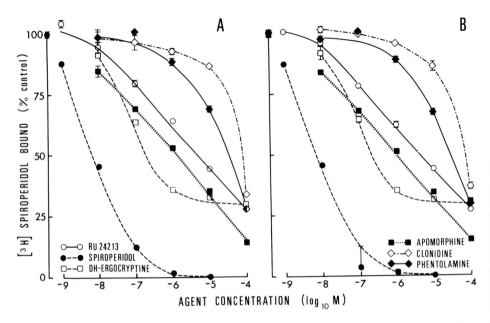

FIG. 4. Effect of 17β-estradiol treatment on the competition by increasing concentrations of unlabeled RU24213, spiroperidol, dihydroergocryptine, apomorphine, clonidine, or phentolamine for [³H]spiroperidol binding to rat striatal homogenate in **A:** castrated control animals, and **B:** castrated animals treated with estrogens.

Figure 4 shows that the order of potency to compete for [³H]spiroperidol binding in the rat striatum was: spiroperidol, DHEC, apomorphine, RU24213, phentolamine, clonidine, and that superimposable displacement curves were found in control and estrogen-treated animals.

Therefore, the potent antidopaminergic action of estrogen treatment at the anterior pituitary (17) and striatal (10) levels cannot be explained by a decreased level of DA receptors nor a change of their specificity for at least one DA antagonist (spiroperidol).

DISCUSSION

The present results, both clinical and experimental, demonstrate an effect of female sex steroid hormones on motor behavior especially in relation to the extrapyramidal system. This effect could already be suspected from earlier clinical observations (11,13). However, the exact site of the action of sex steroids is not clear. Circling and motility induced by apomorphine are generally regarded as indexes of dopaminergic activity (5) in telencephalic structures (striatum and mesolimbic area). Both, however, involve numerous other mechanisms (12), and an effect on cholinergic or GABAergic mechanisms cannot be ruled out. In fact, estradiol can modify the metabolism of GABA (7).

Estradiol did not alter the stimulation of adenyl cyclase in response to dopamine in those telencephalic structures. However, this experiment was performed in intact male rats, and it is possible that the results might be different in castrated female animals. Indeed, we observed a difference in the clinical response to estrogens in our patients with DOPA-induced dyskinesias. None of our three male patients was improved.

Considering the known balance between dopaminergic and cholinergic influences in diseases of the extrapyramidal system, the clear effect of estrogen treatment on the modifications of ACh levels in the striatum produced by dopaminergic agonists and antagonists becomes especially interesting and confirms biochemically our pharmacological results on circling behavior.

Since no effect of estrogen treatment was seen in ACh levels in the absence of drugs affecting the dopamine receptor, at least part of the effect of estradiol must be sought in the dopamine–acetylcholine coupling. The absence of modification of the dopamine-sensitive adenyl cyclase and of the number and affinity of the [^{3}H]spiroperidol binding sites suggests that the effect of estradiol is mediated beyond the receptor–cyclic AMP complex or through another mechanism.

Although much remains to be done in order to elucidate the precise mode of action of sex steroid hormones, the present data open new possibilities of interrelationships between endocrine changes and neuronal mechanisms outside the hypothalamopituitary axis. Such interactions may have interesting clinical applications not only in diseases of the extrapyramidal system but probably also in other fields of neurology.

ACKNOWLEDGMENTS

P. B. and P. L. are scholars of the Canadian Life Insurance Association and Conseil de la Recherche en Santé du Québec, respectively, while F. L. is an Associate of the Medical Research Council of Canada (MRC).

REFERENCES

1. Bedard, P., Dankova, J., Boucher, R., and Langelier, P. (1978): Effects of estrogens on apomorphine-induced circling behavior in the rat. *Can. J. Physiol. Pharmacol.,* 56:538–541.
2. Burt, D. R., Creese, I., and Snyder, S. H. (1977): Antischizophrenic drugs: Chronic treatment elevates dopamine receptor binding in brain. *Science,* 196:326–338.
3. Caron, M. G., Beaulieu, M., Raymond, V., Gagné, B., Drouin, J., Lefkowitz, R. J., and Labrie, F. (1978): Dopaminergic receptors in the anterior pituitary gland, correlation of [^{3}H] dihydroergocryptine binding with the dopaminergic control of prolactin release. *J. Biol. Chem.,* 253:2244–2253.
4. Crane, G. E. (1968): Tardive dyskinesia in patients treated with major neuroleptics. A review of the literature. *Am. J. Psychiatry (Suppl.),* 124:40–48.
5. Dankova, J., Bedard, P., Langelier, P., and Poirier, L. J. (1978): Dopaminergic agents and circling behavior. *Gen. Pharmacol.,* 9:295–302.
6. Dankova, J., Boucher, R., and Poirier, L. J. (1975): Role of the striopallidal system and motor cortex in induced circus movements in rats and cats. *Expl. Neurol.,* 47:135–149.
7. Early, C. J., and Leonard, B. E. (1978): GABA and gonadal hormones. *Brain Res.,* 155:27–34.
8. Eikenburg, D. C., Ravits, A. J., Gudelsky, G. A., and Moore, K. E. (1977): Effect of estrogen on prolactin and tuberoinfundibular dopaminergic neurons. *J. Neural Transm.,* 40:235–244.

9. Ernst, A., and Smelik, P. G. (1966): Site of action of dopamine and apomorphine on compulsive gnawing behaviour in rats. *Experientia,* 22:837.
10. Ferland, L., Labrie, F., Euvrard, C., and Raynaud, J. P. (1978): Antidopaminergic activity of estrogens on prolactin release at the anterior pituitary level *in vivo. J. Mol. Cell. Endocrinol. (in press).*
11. Fernando, S. J. M. (1966): An attack of chorea complicating oral contraceptive therapy. *Practitioner,* 197:210–211.
12. Glick, S. D., Jerussi, T. P., and Fleisher, L. N. (1976): Turning in circles: The neuropharmacology of rotation. *Life Sci.,* 18:889–896.
13. Gratton, L. (1960) Neuroleptiques, parkinsonisme et schizophrénie. *Union Med. Can.,* 89:681–694.
14. Guyenet, P. G., Agid, Y., Javoy, F., Beaujouan, J. C., Rossier, J., and Glowinsky, J. (1975): Effects of dopaminergic receptor agonists and antagonists on the activity of the neostriatal cholinergic system. *Brain Res.,* 84:227–244.
15. Guyenet, P. G., Javoy, F., Agid, Y., Beaujouan, J. C., and Glowinsky, J. (1975): Dopamine receptors and cholinergic neurons in the rat neostriatum. In: *Advances in Neurology, Vol. 9,* edited by D. B. Calne, pp. 43–51. Raven Press, New York.
16. Hwang, P., Guyda, H., and Friesen, H. G. (1971): A radioimmunoassay for human prolactin. *Proc. Natl. Acad. Sci. USA,* 68:1902–1906.
17. Labrie, F., Beaulieu, M., Caron, M., and Raymond, V. (1978): The adenohypophyseal dopamine receptors, specificity and modulation of its activity by estradiol. In: *Proceedings of the International Symposium on Prolactin,* edited by C. Robyn and M. Harter, pp. 121–136. Elsevier/North-Holland, Biomedical Press, New York.
18. Lee, T., Seeman, P., Rajput, A., Farley, I. J., and Hornykiewicz, O. (1978): Receptor basis for doapminergic supersensitivity in Parkinson's disease. *Nature,* 273:59–61.
19. Maanen, J. H. van, and Smelik, P. G. (1968): Induction of pseudopregnancy in rats following local depletion of monoamines in the median eminence of rats. *Neuroendocrinology,* 3:177–186.
20. Maj, J., Grabowska, M., and Gajda, M. (1972): Effect of apomorphine on motility in rats. *Eur. J. Pharmacol.,* 17:208–214.
21. Raymond, V., Beaulieu, M., Labrie, F., and Boissier, J. R. (1978): Potent antidopaminergic activity of estradiol at the pituitary level on prolactin release. *Science,* 200:1173–1175.
22. Raynaud, J. P. (1977): R5020, A tag for the progestin receptor. In: *Progesterone Receptors in Normal and Neoplastic Tissues,* edited by W. L. McGuire, J. P. Raynaud, and E. E. Baulieu, pp. 9–21. Raven Press, New York.
23. Raynaud, J. P., Ojasoo, T., Delarue, J. C., Magdelenat, H., Martin, P., and Philibert, D. (1977): Estrogen and progestin receptors in human breast cancer. In: *Progesterone Receptors in Normal and Neoplastic Tissues,* edited by W. L. McGuire, J. P. Raynaud, and E. E. Baulieu, pp. 171–191. Raven Press, New York.
24. Salomon, Y., Londos, C., and Rodbell, M. (1974): A highly sensitive adenylate cyclase assay. *Anal. Biochem.,* 58:541–548.
25. Stadler, H., Lloyd, K. G., Gadea-Ciria, M., and Bartholini, G. (1973): Enhanced striatal acetylcholine release by chlorpromazine and its reversal by apomorphine. *Brain Res.,* 55:476–480.
26. Trabucchi, M., Cheney, D. L., Racagni, G., and Costa, E. (1975): In vivo inhibition of striatal ACh turnover by L-DOPA, apomorphine and (+) amphetamine. *Brain Res.,* 85:130–134.
27. Villeneuve, A., Langelier, P., and Bédard, P. (1978): Estrogens, dopamine and dyskinesias. *Can. Psychiatr. Assoc. J.,* 23:68–70.
28. Villeneuve, A., Lavallée, J. C., and Lemieux, L. H. (1969): Dyskinésie tardive post-neuroleptique. *Laval Med.,* 40:832–837.
29. Villeneuve, A., Cazejust, T., and Côté, M. (1978): Estrogens in tardive dyskinesia in male psychiatric patients Neuropsychobiology *(in press).*

Advances in Neurology, Vol. 24, edited by
L. J. Poirier, T. L. Sourkes, and P. J. Bédard.
Raven Press, New York © 1979.

Is There Evidence for Different Classes of Cerebral Dopamine Receptors in Man?

P. Price, A. Debono, P. Jenner, J. D. Parkes, and C. D. Marsden

University Department of Neurology, Institute of Psychiatry and King's College Hospital Medical School, Denmark Hill, London SE5, U.K.

At present, there is considerable interest in whether more than one type of dopamine receptor exists in the brain. Of course, there are dopamine receptors in different parts of the brain (i.e., in the area postrema, hypothalamus, striatum, mesolimbic areas, and mesocortical areas). In addition to postsynaptic dopamine receptors, there are presynaptic dopamine receptors (both autoreceptors on dopamine neurons, and presynaptic dopamine receptors on other nerve terminals). But the point of debate is whether all these dopamine receptors are of similar character as regards agonist/antagonist specificity and biochemical effector mechanism, or whether there are differences. If there are differences, the opportunity arises to manipulate selectively some dopamine mechanisms while sparing others.

Many workers have suggested the existence of two classes of cerebral dopamine receptors. Thus, on the basis of behavioral and biochemical data, Cools and Van Rossum (1; excitation-mediating and inhibition-mediating dopamine receptors) and Costall and Naylor (2) have postulated a "double dopamine receptor hypothesis" in one form or another, as had Klawans (9) and Marsden (10) earlier on the basis of clinical evidence.

Recently, Kebabian (8) has elaborated another "double dopamine receptor hypothesis," based on involvement of dopamine-sensitive adenylate cyclase. He states:

Two classes of dopamine receptor mechanism are defined according to their association with, or independence from, a dopamine-sensitive adenylyl cyclase. Dopamine receptors unrelated to adenylyl cyclase are designated type alpha. Dopamine receptors linked to adenylyl cyclase are designated type beta. Drugs discriminate between the two receptor mechanisms. The dopamine ergots (lisuride, lergotrile and CB 154) and their antagonists (such as metoclopramide) are relatively specific for the alpha-dopaminergic receptor in the anterior pituitary. Other agonists (e.g. apomorphine and dopamine) and antagonists (e.g. antipsychotic phenothiazines and butyrophenones) affect both classes of receptor.

This concept was based on two key observations. First, metoclopramide and a range of other substituted benzamides, while exhibiting behavioral and biochemical features of dopamine receptor antagonists, do not inhibit dopamine-sensitive adenylate cyclase *in vitro* (6,7,12). Second, dopaminergic ergot alkaloids such as bromocriptine do not stimulate striatal dopamine-sensitive adenylate cyclase *in vitro* (4,14) [although others have found ergots to stimulate retinal dopamine-sensitive adenylate cyclase (13)].

This chapter investigates whether there is evidence for the Kebabian hypothesis in man. We have tested the proposal in two ways. First, we compare the effects of L-DOPA and bromocriptine in Parkinson's disease. Dopamine formed from L-DOPA should stimulate both α- and β-dopamine receptors in the brain, while, according to Kebabian, bromocriptine should preferentially stimulate α-receptors. Second, we compare the effects of metoclopramide (an α-dopamine antagonist) with pimozide (a classic neuroleptic antagonizing both α- and β-dopamine receptors) on the effect of L-DOPA in Parkinson's disease.

We have examined the response to large single doses of carbidopa + L-DOPA (Sinemet®), with or without metoclopramide and pimozide, and a range of doses of bromocriptine on Parkinsonian disability, dyskinesias, and plasma growth hormone.

METHODS

Patients

Thirty-two patients, 18 men and 14 women, ages 36–69, with idiopathic Parkinson's disease of minor to moderate severity and of 2 to 20 years' duration, were studied. All these patients were on long-term treatment with antiparkinsonian drugs, including L-DOPA, Sinemet, bromocriptine, amantadine, and anticholinergics, and were selected for this study by their ability to tolerate treatment without severe nausea or vomiting or symptomatic postural hypotension.

Drugs Investigated

The acute actions of the following drugs (given orally as a single dose at 9:30 A.M. after an overnight fast) were investigated:

1. $Sinemet_{275}$. One tablet (L-DOPA 250 mg with 1-alphamethyldopa hydrazine 25 mg);
2. Bromocriptine 25, 50, and 100 mg.

The same subjects were given on separate occasions $Sinemet_{275}$ preceded by

1. Metoclopramide 60 mg, 30 min prior to a single dose of $Sinemet_{275}$ or bromocriptine 50 mg;
2. Pimozide 6 mg, 2 hr prior to $Sinemet_{275}$.

All previous antiparkinsonian treatment was discontinued 24 hr before the above drugs or drug combinations were given.

Assessment

The following determinations were made:

1. Plasma L-DOPA or bromocriptine level as appropriate. Peak plasma levels were determined for each drug and also, by extrapolation, plasma levels at 80 min for L-DOPA and 100 min for bromocriptine, these being the mean times at which peak levels of each individual drug occurred.
2. Percentage increase or decrease in parkinsonian disability score. The mean pretreatment disability score at −60 and −30 min was compared with that 90 min after Sinemet or 130 min after bromocriptine.
3. Dyskinesia scores at 60, 90, 120, and 150 min following administration of each drug; no subjects had dyskinesias before drug administration.
4. Increase in plasma growth hormone level (ng ml^{-1}), compared with pretreatment level, at 90 min following Sinemet and 170 min after bromocriptine.

RESULTS

L-DOPA

Sinemet$_{275}$, 1 tablet, containing L-DOPA 250 mg, caused improvement in akinesia, tremor, and rigidity in all subjects for periods lasting between 2 and 3 hr with maximal improvement at 90 min following oral dosage (Fig. 1). There was a statistically significant correlation between the degree of improvement in parkinsonism and the plasma DOPA levels occurring 10 min previously ($N = 18$; $r = 0.69$, $p < 0.001$).

Dyskinesias occurred in 9 of 18 subjects given Sinemet (Fig. 2), but the severity and duration of these involuntary movements were unrelated to plasma DOPA levels at 80 min following oral dosage.

Sinemet caused a rise in the plasma growth hormone level > 3 ng ml^{-1} in 20 of 26 subjects (Fig. 3). There was a significant correlation between the plasma growth hormone level at 90 min and plasma DOPA levels at 80 min following Sinemet$_{275}$ ($N = 26$; $r = 0.49$, $p < 0.01$).

Bromocriptine

Bromocriptine caused a dose-dependent improvement in tremor, rigidity, and akinesia lasting up to 8 hours, with maximal effect at 120 to 130 min after oral dosage. This improvement was not preceded by a short-lived period of deterioration in any symptom. In comparison to a single tablet of Sinemet$_{275}$, a 25-mg dose of bromocriptine was, on average, less potent, a 50-mg dose a little less potent, and a 100-mg dose about equipotent (Fig. 1).

The degree of improvement in the symptoms of parkinsonism was on the whole greater in subjects with high plasma bromocriptine levels than in subjects with low levels ($N = 26$; $r = 0.461$, $p < 0.05$). However, in three subjects,

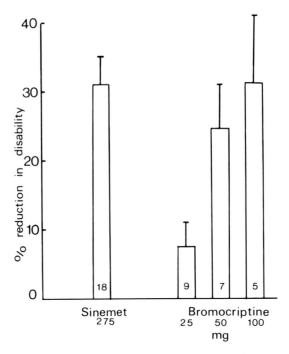

FIG. 1. Therapeutic action of L-DOPA (250 mg) plus α-methyldopa-hydrazine (25 mg) (as 1 tablet of Sinemet$_{275}$) given 90 min earlier, and bromocriptine (25, 50, and 100 mg) given 130 min earlier. The change in disability score, compared with pretreatment values, is shown as the percentage of reduction in disability. (The numbers in each column refer to the number of patients studied. Means $\pm$ 1 SEM are shown.)

the clinical responses accompanying very high plasma bromocriptine levels (15, 17, and 22 ng ml^{-1}) were lower than those achieved in the same subjects on separate occasions accompanying lower plasma bromocriptine levels (6, 9, and 12 ng ml^{-1}, respectively).

Dyskinesias occurred in 10 of 21 subjects given bromocriptine. The severity of dyskinesias was greatest between 90 and 210 min following oral dosage. Dyskinesias due to bromocriptine were similar in severity and nature to those caused by Sinemet$_{275}$ in the same subjects (Fig. 2).

Bromocriptine caused a rise in plasma growth hormone concentration > 3 ng ml^{-1} in 10 of 21 subjects (Fig. 3). The magnitude of this rise was unrelated to the dosage of bromocriptine and also unrelated to peak plasma bromocriptine levels achieved ($N = 23$; $r = -0.1$, NS). The mean peak rise in plasma growth hormone level following bromocriptine was significantly less than that following Sinemet ($t = 4.84$, $p < 0.001$ Student's t-test).

Sinemet and Dopamine Antagonists (Fig. 4)

Plasma levodopa levels 80 min after one tablet of Sinemet$_{275}$ averaged 4.5 $\pm$ 1.0 μmol/l. Pretreatment with metoclopramide (60 mg 30 min prior to Si-

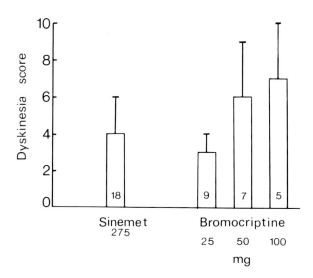

FIG. 2. Dyskinesias caused by L-DOPA (as Sinemet$_{275}$) and bromocriptine, administered as described in Fig. 1. Severity of dyskinesias was assessed in arbitrary units, a high score indicating severe and widespread abnormal involuntary movements.

nemet) slightly increased plasma L-DOPA levels to 5.1 ± 1.0 μmol/liter, but these changes did not reach statistical significance. Pretreatment with pimozide (6 mg 2 hr prior to Sinemet) had no effect on plasma L-DOPA levels (4.4 ± 1.0 μmol/liter).

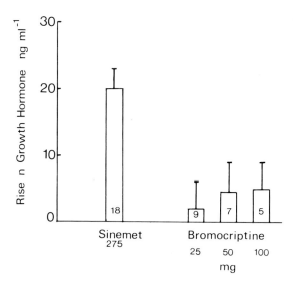

FIG. 3. Rise in plasma growth hormone produced by L-DOPA (as Sinemet$_{275}$) and bromocriptine, administered as described in Fig. 1. Plasma growth hormone was measured prior to and 90 min after Sinemet, or 170 min after bromocriptine. (Means $\pm$ 1 SEM are shown.)

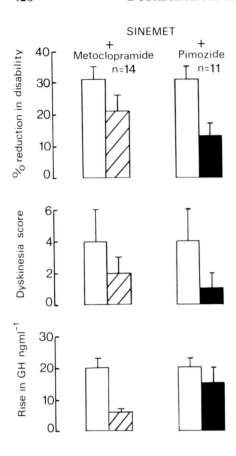

FIG. 4. Effect of metoclopramide (60 mg 30 min earlier) and pimozide (6 mg 120 min earlier) on therapeutic effect, dyskinesias, and plasma growth hormone rise caused by $Sinemet_{275}$ (1 tablet). The open columns indicate effects of $Sinemet_{275}$ alone, the shaded columns show the effect of, on the left, metoclopramide before $Sinemet_{275}$ and, on the right, pimozide before $Sinemet_{275}$. (Means ± 1 SEM are shown.)

Metoclopramide (60 mg) reduced the antiparkinsonian effect of $Sinemet_{275}$ by some 32%, although these changes did not reach statistical significance. Pimozide (6 mg) reduced the antiparkinsonian effect of Sinemet by some 58% ($p < 0.01$).

Metoclopramide (60 mg) and pimozide (6 mg) reduced dyskinesias provoked by $Sinemet_{275}$ by 50 and 75%, respectively.

Metoclopramide (60 mg) reduced the rise in plasma growth hormone 90 min after $Sinemet_{275}$ by 70% ($p < 0.01$). Pimozide only reduced the growth hormone rise by 25% ($p > 0.05$).

Bromocriptine and Metoclopramide (Fig. 5)

Metoclopramide (60 mg), 30 min prior to bromocriptine (50 mg), in 5 patients reduced the antiparkinsonian effect of bromocriptine by some 72% ($p < 0.01$), abolished dyskinesias, and virtually abolished the rise in plasma growth hormone provoked by bromocriptine.

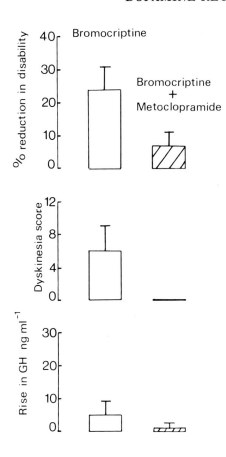

FIG. 5. Effect of metoclopramide (60 mg 30 min earlier) on therapeutic action, dyskinesias, and rise in growth hormone produced by bromocriptine (50 mg). Open columns show effect of bromocriptine alone, hatched columns show effect of metoclopramide plus bromocriptine. (Means $\pm$ 1 SEM are shown; $N = 5$.)

DISCUSSION

Metoclopramide, an antagonist not acting on adenylate cyclase, certainly inhibited the effects of bromocriptine, an agonist not usually found to stimulate dopamine-sensitive adenylate cyclase in the brain. Thus metoclopramide reduced both the therapeutic effect and the dyskinesias caused by bromocriptine, and virtually abolished the latter's modest effect on plasma growth hormone.

Metoclopramide had a less dramatic effect on the actions of Sinemet. In therapeutic terms, Sinemet$_{275}$ (1 tablet) and bromocriptine (50 mg) were approximately equipotent. Metoclopramide (60 mg) prior to Sinemet$_{275}$ caused over a 32% reduction in therapeutic action and a 50% reduction in dyskinesias. In contrast, metoclopramide reduced bromocriptine's therapeutic effect by 72% and abolished dyskinesias. These data could be taken to indicate that a proportion of the actions of Sinemet, or rather of the dopamine formed from its L-DOPA, are not sensitive to metoclopramide, i.e., they might be acting via the postulated

β-dopamine receptor. Dopamine is held to stimulate both α- and β-receptors, although it acts in lower concentrations on α- than on β-receptors (8).

If the actions of dopamine formed from L-DOPA were mediated by stimulation of both α- and β-dopamine receptors, then conventional neuroleptics, which block both receptors, should have greater antagonistic effect than metoclopramide, a relatively poor β-dopamine antagonist. To some extent, our data support this hypothesis, for pimozide was slightly more potent than metoclopramide in reducing Sinemet's therapeutic action and preventing dyskinesias. But it is a much more potent drug. For example, it is some 400 times more potent than metoclopramide in displacing ^{3}H-haloperidol from striatal binding sites (5), yet we gave pimozide in only one-tenth of the dose of metoclopramide. So quantitative comparison between the effects of both drugs on the response to L-DOPA is not justified. In qualitative terms, both metoclopramide and pimozide had similar effects on the therapeutic actions and dyskinesias of Si-nemet. Also, in qualitative terms, L-DOPA (as Sinemet) and bromocriptine had similar therapeutic actions and produced similar dyskinesias. This can be taken to indicate either that both therapeutic action and dyskinesias are due to stimulation of α-receptors alone or that α- and β-dopamine receptors as conceived do not exist.

The only real difference between, on the one hand L-DOPA (as Sinemet) and bromocriptine, and on the other hand, metoclopramide and pimozide, was the effect on plasma growth hormone.

Bromocriptine in doses known to have similar antiparkinsonian and dyskinetic actions had much less effect on plasma growth hormone than did Sinemet. This may reflect the role of norepinephrine as well as dopamine in growth hormone control (11). L-DOPA increases both norepinephrine and dopamine turnover in the brain, whereas bromocriptine, if anything, appears to antagonize cerebral norepinephrine mechanisms (3).

With regard to antagonists, metoclopramide had greater effect than pimozide on the rise in plasma growth hormone produced by Sinemet. There is no convincing explanation for this observation, but perhaps it reflects differences in penetration of the two drugs into the brain, or differences in pharmacokinetics. Alternatively, it could indicate that the dopamine receptors concerned with growth hormone release are of the α type, and thus are more strongly inhibited by metoclopramide.

In conclusion, our data do not decisively indicate whether α- and β-dopamine receptors exist in the human brain. The findings are compatible with such a hypothesis if one assumes that the antiparkinsonian and dyskinetic actions of L-DOPA are due mainly to stimulation of the hypothetical α-dopamine receptors. If this were the case, it would be postulated that β-dopamine antagonists would (a) not cause drug-induced parkinsonism, and (b) not antagonize the actions of L-DOPA in Parkinson's disease. Unfortunately, selective β-dopamine agonists and antagonists are not yet available for clinical use.

REFERENCES

1. Cools, A. R., and Van Rossum, J. M. (1976): Excitation-mediating and inhibition-mediating dopamine-receptors: A new concept towards a better understanding of electrophysiological, biochemical, pharmacological, functional and clinical data. *Psychopharmacologia,* 45:243–254.
2. Costall, B., and Naylor, R. J. (1975): Neuroleptic antagonism of dyskinetic phenomena. *Eur. J. Pharmacol.,* 33:301–312.
3. Dolphin, A. C., Jenner, P., Sawaya, M. C. B., Marsden, C. D., and Testa, B. (1977): The effect of bromocriptine on locomotor activity and cerebral catecholamines in rodents. *J. Pharm. Pharmacol.,* 29:727–734.
4. Govoni, S., Iuliano, E., Spano, P. F., and Trabucchi, M. (1977): Effect of ergotamine and dihydroergotamine on dopamine-stimulated adenylate-cyclase in rat caudate nucleus. *J. Pharm. Pharmacol.,* 29:45–47.
5. Hyttel, J. (1978): Effects of neuroleptics on ³H-haloperidol and ³H-*cis*(Z)-flupenthixol binding and on adenylate cyclase activity in vitro. *Life Sci.,* 23:551–556.
6. Jenner, P., Clow, A., Reavill, C., Theodorou, A., and Marsden, C. D. (1978): A behavioural and biochemical comparison of dopamine receptor blockade produced by haloperidol with that produced by substituted benzamide drugs. *Life Sci.,* 23:545–550.
7. Jenner, P., Elliott, P. N. C., Clow, A., Reavill, C. and Marsden, C. D. (1978): A comparison of *in vitro* and *in vivo* dopamine receptor antagonism by substituted benzamide drugs. *J. Pharm. Pharmacol.,* 30:46–48.
8. Kebabian, J. W. (1978): Multiple classes of dopamine receptors in mammalian central nervous system: The involvement of dopamine-sensitive adenylyl cyclase. *Life Sci.,* 23:479–484.
9. Klawans, H. L. (1973): *The Pharmacology of Extrapyramidal Movement Disorders.* Karger, Basel.
10. Marsden, C. D. (1975): The neuropharmacology of abnormal involuntary movement disorders (the dyskinesias). In: *Modern Trends in Neurology, Vol. 6,* edited by D. Williams, pp. 141–166. Butterworths, London.
11. Martin, J. B., Reichlin, S., and Brown, G. M. (1977): *Contemporary Neurology Series, Vol. 14: Clinical Neuroendocrinology,* edited by F. Plum and F. H. McDowell. F. A. Davis & Co., Philadelphia.
12. Perringer, E., Jenner, P., Donaldson, I. M., Marsden, C. D., and Miller, R. (1976): Metoclopramide and dopamine receptor blockade. *Neuropharmacology,* 15:463–469.
13. Schorderet, M. (1976): Direct evidence for the stimulation of rabbit retina dopamine receptors by ergot alkaloids. *Neurosci. Lett.,* 2:87–91.
14. Trabucchi, M., Spano, P. F., Tonon, G. C., and Frattola, L. (1976): Effect of bromocriptine on central dopamine receptors. *Life Sci.,* 19:225–232.

NOTE ADDED IN PROOF: Since the preparation of this chapter, Kebabian and Calne (1979: Multiple receptors for dopamine. *Nature,* 277:93–96), have elaborated Kebabian's hypothesis and have altered their terminology. They now call the α-dopamine receptor a type D-2 dopamine receptor, and the β-dopamine receptor a type D-1 dopamine receptor.

Advances in Neurology, Vol. 24, edited by
L. J. Poirier, T. L. Sourkes, and P. J. Bédard.
Raven Press, New York © 1979.

Newer Therapeutic Approaches in Parkinson's Disease

A. Barbeau, M. Roy, M. Gonce, and R. Labrecque

*Department of Neurobiology, Clinical Research Institute of Montreal,
Montreal, Quebec, Canada H2W 1R7*

Levodopa therapy for Parkinson's disease was introduced 18 years ago (3,22). This therapeutical procedure, as modified and codified by Cotzias and collaborators (43), is now the undisputed standard mode of treatment against this chronic neurological disorder (5,41,107). Long-term results with high-dosage levodopa show that continued positive effects are obtained in the majority of cases even after 10 years, but a decline of efficacy is also observed in a significant number of cases (9,95).

In the earlier years, the main problems were complications of intolerance (nausea, vomiting) and central (abnormal involuntary movements) or peripheral (cardiac arrhythmias) side-effects caused by interaction with already supersensitive receptors (16,69,70), while more recently decreases in the sensitivity of these same receptors, possibly as a consequence of the long-term effect of high doses of levodopa, are characterized by a large variety of oscillations in performance and even total unresponsiveness (7,9,10,50,83,87).

Most peripheral side-effects have been controlled by the introduction of peripheral DOPA-decarboxylase inhibitors in combination with levodopa (14,17,23). Two such inhibitors, benserazide (Ro4-4602) and carbidopa (MK-486), have been used successfully in practice, with the advantages of fewer peripheral side-effects and faster onset of response; however, the central and long-term side-effects have been as frequent and severe as before (17,95). We more and more frequently see patients in whom each dose of levodopa (plus inhibitor) has a markedly reduced duration of action (from the former 4 to 4½ hr to a more frequent 2 to 2½ hr) or patients who experience long periods during which levodopa does not seem to be active.

In order to correct these severe inconveniences, researchers and drug companies have explored new avenues and new formulas. In the absence of effective slow-release levodopa combinations, and to avoid the presumed complications due to other DOPA metabolites, three main paths have been followed:

1. Use of dopamine receptor agonists;
2. Use of drugs that potentiate the action of dopamine;

3. Use of drugs that modify the functional balance between dopamine and other neurotransmitters.

The present chapter will review our personal experience with each of these approaches, and indicate some promising leads for future investigation.

DOPAMINE RECEPTOR STIMULATION

Apomorphine and Aporphines

The first attempt to reproduce the more complex action of levodopa through stimulation of dopamine receptors involved the use of apomorphine intravenously or orally (Fig. 1) (29,42,47). Although clinical effects were obtained in man as they are in animals, with stimulation of motility and even production of stereotyped movements, the short duration of action of apomorphine proved to be a major drawback. Oral use of the drug was also beneficial, but was unfortunately accompanied by prerenal azotemia (42). The distribution and turnover of apomorphine in the brain is not exactly what could have been predicted

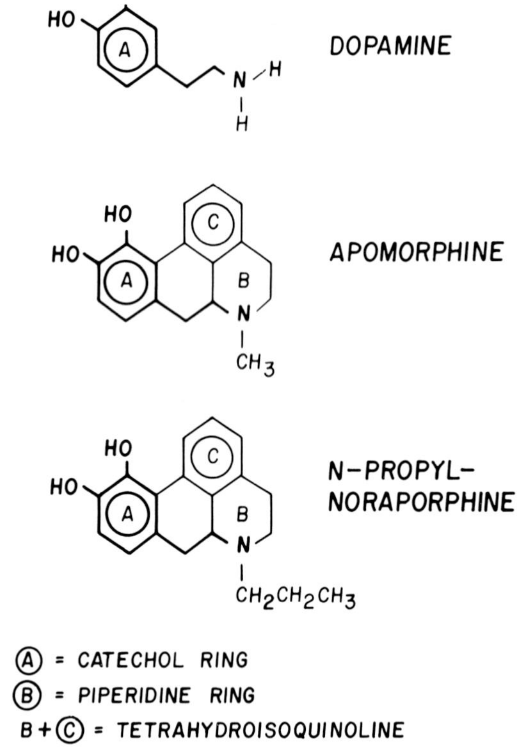

FIG. 1. Dopamine, apomorphine, and *N*-propyl-noraporphine.

from clinical effects. In fact, the striatum, possibly because it already contains large amounts of dopamine to compete with apomorphine at the same sites, accumulates much less of the drug than other regions of the brain (26). More recently the same group (42) has studied N-propyl-noraporphine (NPA) with promising results.

Piribedil

Piribedil (ET 495) (Fig. 2) is 1-(3,4-methylene-dioxybenzyl)-4-(2-pyrimidyl)piperazine. It was first shown to be active as a peripheral vasodilator and later as a stimulator of brain dopamine receptors in rats with unilateral 6-hydroxydopamine-induced degeneration of the nigroneostriatal dopamine pathway (38). The direct dopamine activity was later confirmed by Poignant et al. (94) and Costall and Naylor (40), who investigated the production of stereotypy. The influence of piribedil on various components of locomotor activity was further studied by Jenner and Marsden (65) and by Butterworth et al. (28). The compound was also shown to decrease dopamine turnover (36), striatal homovanillic acid levels (66), and firing in substantia nigra neurons (105). However, it appears that piribedil does not stimulate the dopamine-sensitive adenylate cyclase system

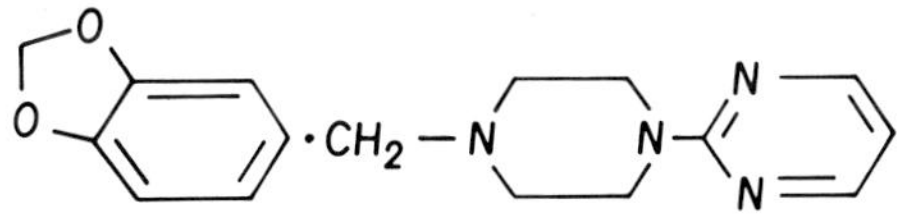

FIG. 2. Piribedil (ET-495).

in the rat striatum (84), nor does it produce contralateral turning when injected directly into one striatum of reserpine-treated rats. Thus it has been suggested that the action of piribedil is through an active metabolite. Antiparkinson activity of piribedil has indeed been demonstrated in monkeys by Goldstein et al. (56). This led to clinical trials using this drug in treating Parkinson's disease and to initial encouraging results (79,103).

Our own experience with piribedil in Parkinson's disease is summarized in Table 1. It can be seen that this drug possesses definite antiparkinsonian activity, mainly on tremor and less so on akinesia and rigidity. The extent of this efficacy

TABLE 1. *Piribedil in Parkinson's disease. Summary of our experience*

No. patients	20
Motor performance score	
initial	374 ± 38
final (6 months)	434 ± 27
Symptom evaluation	
tremor	−22%
rigidity	−12%
akinesia	−15%

is not, however, very great, and when higher doses are reached a number of central side-effects, such as hallucinations and confusion, are observed. Nausea and vomiting are not uncommon. In accordance with Feigenson et al. (51) and with Truelle et al. (103) we find this drug to be somewhat useful when combined to other antiparkinsonian medication, particularly when the tremor is not alleviated by levodopa, and against end-of-dose akinetic episodes. Our own experience with piribedil alone does not indicate any advantage of this compound over existing medication.

Nomifensine

Nomifensine (Hoe 984) (Fig. 3) (8-amino-2-methyl-4-phenyl-1,2,3,4,-tetrahydroisoquinoline hydrogenmaleate) is a new antidepressant with a pharmacological profile somewhat different from the classic tricyclic antidepressants. It has been shown to increase motor activity in rats (53), to be a potent stereotypic agent (39), and to block the uptake mechanism of catecholamines, particularly dopamine (53,63,97). These properties led Costall and collaborators (39) to propose that this agent may have antiparkinsonian activity in addition to its antidepressive effects.

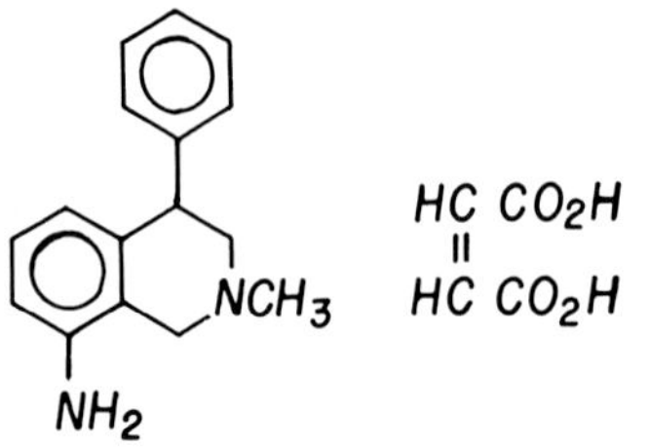

FIG. 3. Nomifensine (HOE-984).

Our own results with this compound are given in Table 2. As can be seen, we investigated this drug alone and in combination with levodopa. In our experience, nomifensine is not an antiparkinsonian drug to any *clinically* significant degree. The drug is well tolerated by patients, except when the stage of the disease is so advanced that nightmares, visual hallucinations, and dizzy spells are frequent. These symptoms appear to be exacerbated by nomifensine. In less advanced cases, nomifensine appears to relieve certain situational depressions in some patients, and through increased motivation on a background of improved mood, it may contribute to initial improvement in physical performance. However this effect does not appear to last. In levodopa-treated patients, stimulation may result in an increase in the symptoms of parkinsonism, particularly tremor. Although our sample is relatively small, we conclude that, in our opinion, nomifensine does not provide a useful addition to the pharmacological treatment of Parkinson's disease. Our results are in conflict with those of Teychenne et al. (102), who used much higher dosages, but they agree with those of Bédard et al. (20) at identical doses.

TABLE 2. *Nomifensine in Parkinson's disease*

	1st Study (No DOPA)	2nd Study (With DOPA)
No. patients	17	10
Age	63.2 ± 2.0 yr	58.3 ± 3.8 yr
Duration of illness	6.5 ± 0.9 yr	12.8 ± 1.6 yr
Duration of study	6 months	6 months
Duration of DOPA therapy	—	5.4 ± 0.8 yr
Dosage range (die)	25–150 mg	25–150 mg
Motor performance		
initial	585.5 ± 60.1	564.3 ± 37.6
final	623.3 ± 72.4	543.4 ± 40.1
Patient's subjective evaluation		
improved	8 patients	6 patients
worsened	3 patients	3 patients
no change	6 patients	1 patient

Lergotrile Mesylate

Lergotrile mesylate (compound 83636) (Fig. 4) is an ergot derivative that has been shown to produce a potent inhibitory effect on prolactin secretion (75) and therefore to have a direct-acting dopamine agonist activity. Clinical studies with lergotrile in parkinsonism have demonstrated antiparkinsonian activity in some patients, particularly in conjunction with levodopa (76,78), but also alone (71). The drug has also been effective in relieving some complications of long-term levodopa therapy. Lergotrile was more effective in alleviating "on–off" problems than in restoring loss of levodopa efficacy. Side-effects of lergotrile include exacerbation of hallucinations, dyskinesias, hypotension, and alterations in liver function tests (71). The latter complication is of such amplitude as to make it improbable that lergotrile will reach the marketing stage. Unfortunately we have no personal experience with lergotrile in Parkinson's disease.

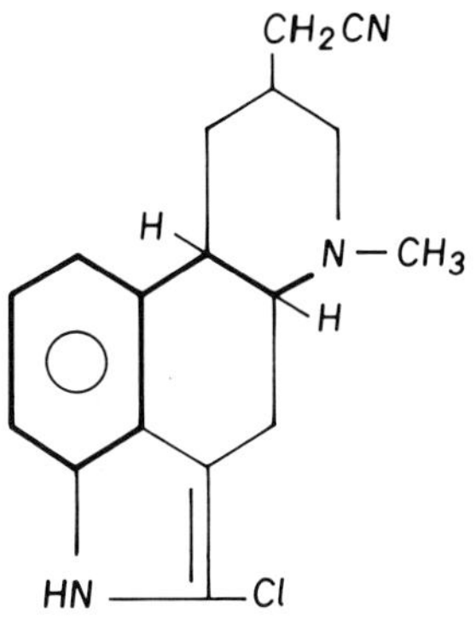

FIG. 4. Lergotrile.

Bromocriptine

Bromocriptine (CB-154) (Fig. 5) (2-bromo-α-ergocriptine) was the first of the ergot derivatives to be recognized as possessing direct dopamine receptor agonist activity, mainly evident through its effect on prolactin (37,90). In monkeys it shows antitremor effects (86). Calne and collaborators (30) first demonstrated its antiparkinsonian activity in man. Almost every study has confirmed this benefit at low doses (54,58,77,91). Some authors claim that at higher doses, bromocriptine is equal to levodopa in antiparkinsonian action (67,101).

Our own uncontrolled studies are in accordance with most other published investigations, particularly those of longer duration (73,92,98). There is no doubt that bromocriptine possesses antiparkinsonian activity in man, particularly in the earlier (non-levodopa-treated) period of the disease. In these cases, objective improvement of functional tests averages 40 to 50% in about half the cases, which in our experience is significantly lower than the 70% of patients who improve by more than 50% with levodopa (5). The main improvement is on tremor and to a lesser extent on akinesia. One apparent advantage is that there is little if any "on–off" effect with bromocriptine when used alone, at least for the period of observation of 1 to 2 years. In our experience, and that of Lees et al. (73), some loss of benefit occurs after 2 years. Contrary to early claims (67), we do not find activity of bromocriptine in patients who previously were unresponsive to levodopa (so-called levodopa failures), nor do we find any real advantage in the levodopa late "failures" or in "on–off" effects. Thus, in our experience, bromocriptine does not offer additional benefits to *properly monitored* levodopa-treated parkinsonian patients. In accordance with Shaw et al. (98), the high incidence of side-effects, particularly in the mental sphere (confusion, hallucinations, and even frank psychoses), in addition to the prohibitive cost of the drug, make bromocriptine no more than a useful but limited early therapy for a minority of idiopathic parkinsonians with mild disabilities of recent onset. To date this conclusion appears to apply to all the putative

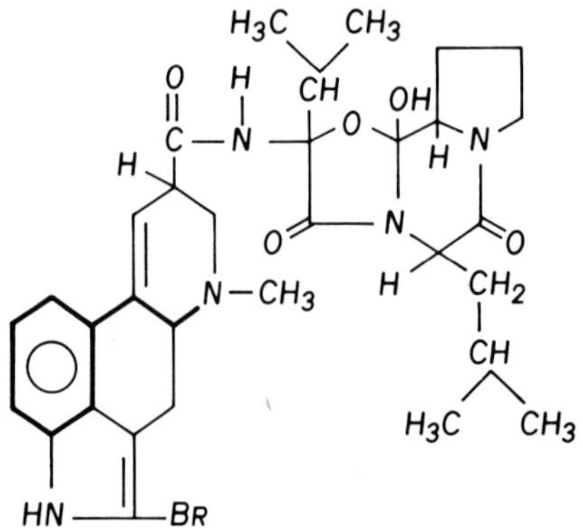

FIG. 5. Bromocriptine (CB-154).

dopamine agonists that have been studied in Parkinson's disease, or on animal models of hypokinesia (27).

DOPAMINE POTENTIATION

Other approaches to the control of the action of dopamine have been to attempt blockage of its metabolism, or to modulate the response of dopamine receptors. Dopamine is metabolized by catecholamine-*o*-methyl-transferase (COMT) and monoamine oxidase (MAO) eventually into homovanillic acid, and by dopamine β-hydroxylase into norepinephrine. Blockage of each of the following enzymes has been attempted.

Dopamine Potentiation Through Enzyme Inhibition

In the early days of levodopa therapy, MAO inhibition was attempted, but the production of severe hypertensive reactions (4) forced abandonment of this approach. No nontoxic COMT inhibitor has yet received proper clinical evaluation in Parkinson's disease, although we have evidence (R. F. Butterworth, and A. Barbeau, *unpublished observations*) that the DOPA-decarboxylase inhibitor Ro4-4602 (benserazide) also has some COMT-inhibiting properties, which could explain some of its potentiation of dopamine action. Finally the studies of fusaric acid, an inhibitor of dopamine β-hydroxylase, have been essentially negative in Parkinson's disease.

In 1970, Collins et al. (35) demonstrated the existence of multiple forms of monoamine oxidase (MAO) in the human brain. In fact, two main forms exist: *MAO-A,* which by oxidation deaminates serotonin, norepinephrine, octopamine, tyramine, and to a lesser extent dopamine, and which is sensitive to clorgyline and harmaline; *MAO-B,* which oxidizes phenylethylamine, tyramine, dopamine, and benzylamine, and is sensitive to deprenil (96). MAO-B plays an important role in the intraneuronal metabolism of dopamine in the human brain. In 1975, Birkmayer et al. (24) demonstrated that L-deprenyl potentiated the antiparkinsonian effect of levodopa and decreased the "on–off" phenomena. This was also true in association with the levodopa–benserazide combination. Results were less obvious in the series reported by Lees et al. (74), who could find only minimal potentiation of the levodopa effect. Unfortunately, we do not yet have experience with this drug in the treatment of Parkinson's disease.

Dopamine Potentiation Through Peptide-Induced Receptor Modulation

In 1971, Nair et al. (88) synthesized a tripeptide, L-prolyl-L-leucyl-glycine amide (Pro-Leu-Gly-NH$_2$; PLG), which they claimed had melanocyte-stimulating hormone (MSH)-release-inhibitory (MIF) properties (Fig. 6). They called this peptide MIF-I, but we would now prefer to use the initials PLG, because subsequent studies by some authors have failed to confirm the hormonal activity.

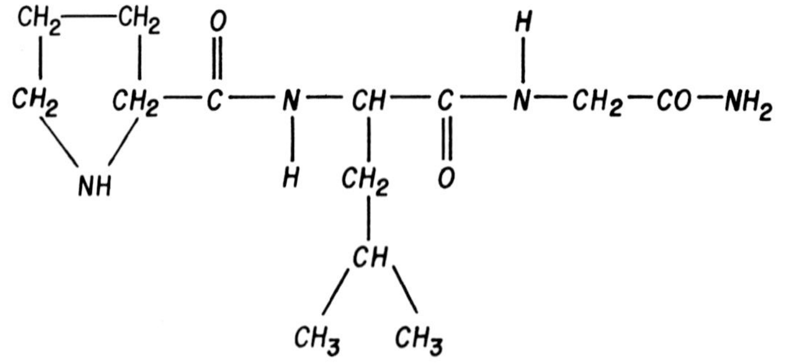

FIG. 6. Pro-Leu-Gly-NH₂ [PLG on MIF-I (MSH release inhibiting factor)].

However animal experiments soon revealed that this substance was neurologically active in that it potentiated the actions of levodopa and oxotremorine in both intact and hypophysectomized animals (93).

Preliminary studies (68) with *intravenous* slow infusions of PLG (20–40 mg) in 8 parkinsonian patients did reveal objective improvement in motor performance tests in an acute experiment. These results were partially confirmed by Chase et al. (32) and Fischer and collaborators (52). The latter authors observed simultaneous mood brightening and positive effects on motivation. Unfortunately a double-blind study with *oral* PLG in 20 parkinsonian patients revealed only a significant downward trend in rigidity and tremor scores (20 and 40% decreases, respectively) without significant improvement in the overall performance score (18). A single bolus injection of 200 mg PLG in an additional eight patients (15) again demonstrated the efficacy of this compound, with persistence of the effect for nearly 6 hr.

Animal studies by Plotnikoff and Kastin (93) and by Barbeau and Kastin (15) had shown that PLG potentiates the levodopa-induced effect on motility. In a further series of experiments (8), we were able to show the same type of potentiation in human parkinsonian subjects. Two hundred milligrams of PLG given intravenously produced a 44% improvement in performance scores, which lasted for at least 4 hr. In four of the six patients, and for the first time since the very onset of treatment with levodopa, performance scores within the normal range were obtained. All patients also noted a marked amelioration in the clarity of their thinking. Similar results were recently obtained by Gerstenbrand and collaborators (55).

In more recent studies, Gonce and Barbeau (57) were able to investigate the acute and semichronic effects of PLG, administered intravenously in doses of 400 mg per day, in nine parkinsonian patients. As shown in Table 3, acute PLG produced a significant increase in motor performance scores, which is in inverse relationship to the akinesia score. The latter symptom significantly decreased over the 4-hr period of observation. Control patients without PLG modified their score, through "apprentissage," by levels never exceeding 5% over

TABLE 3. *Acute intravenous injections of PLG in Parkinson's disease*
(N = 9 patients)

Time	Motor performance score	Dexterity score	Akinesia score
−30 hr	539 ± 36	26 ± 3	204 ± 28
+60 hr	566 ± 41	27 ± 3	191 ± 34
+120 hr	611 ± 36	29 ± 2.5	176 ± 28
+180 hr	628 ± 36	29 ± 3	163 ± 30
+240 hr	669 ± 40	31 ± 4	130 ± 31

the same period and with the same frequency of tests. Semichronic daily injections of 400 mg in three patients over a period of 9 days also produced improvement of akinesia (25%), dexterity (12%), tremor (18%), rigidity (6%), and overall performance (32%) in the already levodopa-treated patients who had been stabilized at their optimal levels.

In our studies, PLG was ineffective in modifying brain levels, turnover, or distribution of catecholamines (15). Neither could we demonstrate inhibition of MAO or COMT activity by PLG. Furthermore there was no evidence that PLG acted on the reuptake mechanism or facilitated the release of catecholamines in an amphetamine-like fashion. Therefore a presynaptic or metabolic mode of action is unlikely. PLG is still active in animals after hypophysectomy, indicating that the effect on the brain is probably not through peripheral hormones. Finally, we have demonstrated that PLG potentiates the action of apomorphine in reversing the akinesia produced by a bilateral hypothalamic lesion with 6-hydroxydopamine in the rat. This would favor a postsynaptic site of action for PLG, probably through modulation of the receptor. Indeed Mishra and Makman (85) found an interaction between PLG and dopamine receptor-linked adenylate cyclase.

Recently, in association with Ayerst Laboratories, we have started the investigation of pareptide (AY-24,856) (Fig. 7), a compound that is a modification of PLG and whose chemical name is L-prolyl-N-methyl-D-leucylglycinamide hemisulfate. This compound is active, even when taken orally, in producing rotational behavior and in reversing some types of akinesia in rats with 6-hydroxydopamine-induced lesions. Its intravenous activity is of the same order as that of PLG. Unfortunately, it is too early to report the clinical results of the pilot study

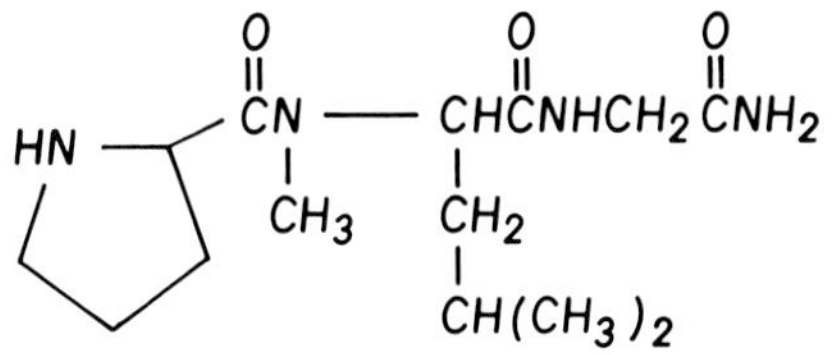

FIG. 7. Pareptide (L-propyl-N-methyl-D-leucylglycin amide).

OTHER APPROACHES—MECHANISM STILL UNCERTAIN

A number of other approaches based on mechanisms not involving dopamine have also been investigated for the control of Parkinson's disease. We have personal experience with two such approaches.

Diprobutine

Diprobutine (LCG-21.519) (Fig. 8) is tripropylmethylamine. It was prepared as a possible analog of amantadine, a drug with clear antiparkinson activity. In experimental animals, this drug inhibits catatonia produced by reserpine or neuroleptics; it occasionally induces stereotyped movements of its own and potentiates stereotypies produced by amphetamine and apomorphine. On the other hand, it does not possess anticholinergic activity and therefore does not antagonize tremorine or oxotremorine effects. Alone it does not cause rotational behavior in unilateral nigrostriatal lesioned rats, but it can potentiate the rotation induced by apomorphine or amphetamine. Curiously, it has only slight effects on the brain concentrations of monoamines, but may increase dopamine turnover, as demonstrated by increased striatal homovanillic acid levels and slight decreases in norepinephrine and serotonin in the hypothalamus (25). Thus the drug possesses antiparkinson activity in animals and deserves a trial in man. A number of studies using this compound have been undertaken in France and the Benelux countries in 1977, but they have not yet been published.

Our own pilot investigations cover a period of 4 months (mean duration 8.2 weeks) in an open trial in 17 patients, and reveal that although the overall results do not indicate significant improvement in motor performance (from a mean of 574.2 ± 34.9 to 589.8 ± 41.8) and only a slight decrease in the functional impairment scores (from a mean of 22.4 ± 3.0 to 21.5 ± 3.1), there is no doubt that in the patients who tolerate the drug, there is a clear improvement of akinesia and tremor. The most striking finding is that the effect of a single dose of levodopa is markedly prolonged (by an average of 1 hr) without an increase in dyskinesias. The margin between efficacy and toxicity (dizziness, confusion, hallucinations, and vomiting) is, however, relatively small. We observed that increased doses of diprobutine were associated with toxic side-effects and resulted in a reappearance of most parkinsonian symptoms, particularly the akinesia and rigidity. In the light of these preliminary results, we believe that diprobutine does possess antiparkinson activity in man and deserves a more thorough controlled study.

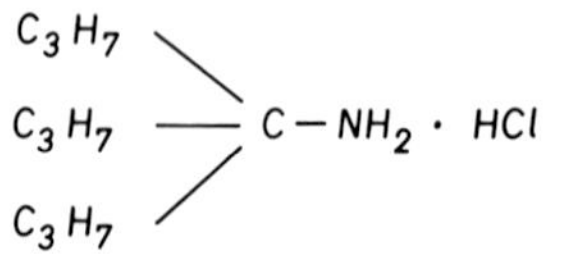

$$
\begin{array}{c}
C_3H_7 \\
C_3H_7 \longrightarrow C-NH_2 \cdot HCl \\
C_3H_7
\end{array}
$$

FIG. 8. Diprobutine.

Naloxone

It is now well known that the central nervous system of mammals contains opiate-like peptides (endorphins) and specific receptors for these endogenous substances. These peptides, probably stored in neurons, are widely distributed throughout the nervous system, particularly the striatum. Recently Cuello and Paxinos (45) presented evidence for a long leu-enkephalin striopallidal pathway in the rat brain. An injection of β-endorphin into the cisterna magna, the periaqueductal gray, or the lateral ventricle in rats has been demonstrated to produce catalepsy or akinesia in addition to analgesia. This behavior was fully reversed by naloxone (a specific antagonist for opiates), levodopa with a peripheral decarboxylase inhibitor, or apomorphine. Levodopa or apomorphine did not reverse the analgesia, while naloxone at least partially reversed both analgesia and akinesia (64).

The observation that naloxone could reverse the akinesia–catatonia signs produced in animals by the intraventricular injection of β-endorphin prompted studies of the use of this compound in human Parkinson's disease. We investigated the effect of a single i.v. naloxone injection (0.4 mg naloxone chlorhydrate) on a battery of motor performance tests in 20 akinetic parkinsonian patients and 10 age-matched normal controls. There were no significant changes in tremor, rigidity, akinesia, or total motor performance scores at 30, 60, or 90 min postinjection. The parkinsonian state did not improve objectively, but subjectively, most patients stated that some of the tests (particularly the puzzle) were carried out with less difficulty. We subsequently pursued this observation by studying the performance of a colored and of a black and white puzzle (both representing an identical shape of a duck and consisting of 10 pieces) by 10 parkinsonian patients, 10 subjects with essential tremor, and 10 normal controls. The puzzle test was carried out at 0, 30, and 90 min. In normal subjects and essential tremor patients, there is a significant apprentissage from the first to the third test with the colored puzzle test, but not with the black and white puzzle. Parkinsonian patients are unable to improve this score with either puzzle. However, only the parkinsonian patients significantly improved their performance with the colored puzzle after i.v. injection of naloxone (0.4 mg). We are investigating further this interesting improvement in apprentissage with naloxone in parkinsonian subjects.

MODIFICATIONS OF THE DOPAMINE/ACETYLCHOLINE BALANCE

Early in the investigation of the pharmacology of Parkinson's disease it became evident that the metabolism of dopamine was closely linked to that of acetylcholine (4,80). This observation has been repeatedly made and confirmed since. Thus anticholinergic medication was the standard therapeutic approach until levodopa came into use. Based on the "balance hypothesis," it was proposed that hyperkinetic movements, such as chorea and tics, could be due to hyperactivity at striatal dopamine receptors and that, in fact, in such disorders there could be a relative cholinergic hypoactivity (6,72). In Huntington's chorea, low levels of choline acetyltransferase, the enzyme that catalyzes the combination of choline and acetylcoenzyme A to form acetylcholine, have been clearly demonstrated (21,81,99). Muscarinic cholinergic receptor binding was also found to be decreased in brain of patients with Huntington's chorea (49). Similar evidence indicates that there may also be a cholinergic deficit in tardive dyskinesia, the syndrome complex observed after long-term treatment with phenothiazines (44). In both these entities, the hyperkinesia is attributed to the combination of dopamine receptor hypersensitivity and relative cholinergic deficiencies. Thus these hyperkinetic disorders are candidates for replacement therapy of acetylcholine.

Such an approach has been proposed recently. As mentioned above, brain acetylcholine is synthesized from choline and acetylcoenzyme A by choline acetyltransferase. It is metabolized by acetylcholinesterase. The metabolism of acetylcholine could be blocked to increase its concentration. Physostigmine has been shown to function in this way (48), and we recently demonstrated that thiamine and choline can also inhibit acetylcholinesterase (89). Physostigmine was found to be useful, for short periods, in choreiform and dyskinetic movements (2,72,100).

The precursor *choline* cannot be made in the brain and must come from synthesis in the liver or from the diet. An adequate supply of choline is critical for cholinergic nerve function. This necessitates functional transport mechanisms for choline in the brain. Both low- and high-affinity transport systems were demonstrated in brain synaptosomes by Yamamura and Snyder (108), and regional differences were identified (31). Uptake is not saturated even at very high concentrations of choline in plasma (19). There is also good evidence that the concentration of free choline in tissues may be important in regulating the rate of synthesis of acetylcholine and possibly also of tyrosine hydroxylase in dopaminergic neurons (104). The brain contains fair concentrations of free choline (82), and these can be increased by systemic injection or oral administration of choline in rats (33,34,61). The administration of choline chloride causes a sequential increase in serum choline, brain choline, and brain acetylcholine levels. The increase in acetylcholine occurs within presynaptic terminals (62) and is followed by biochemical changes within postsynaptic cells that have a cholinergic innervation (104). Choline probably increases the release of acetylcholine into the synapses.

Such experimental background was sufficient to justify the use of choline in man. It was shown that choline consumption caused dose-related increases in the choline levels of serum and cerebrospinal fluid (1,59). Choline, given orally in doses up to 20 g per day, was found to be active against the choreiform and dyskinetic movements of some patients with Huntington's chorea and tardive dyskinesia (1,46,59). Our own experience (12) with choline chloride given orally in daily doses up to 10 g in hyperkinesis, is limited to observations in 9 patients (4 with Huntington's chorea, 3 with Gilles de la Tourette, and 2 with tardive

TABLE 4. *Lecithin in hyperkinetic disorders*

	N	Mean duration of treatment (weeks)	Average dose (mg/day)	Mean max. improvement	Mean final improvement
(1) Huntington's chorea	3	19.6	7,200 (3,600–10,000)[a]	29%	25%
(2) Tardive dyskinesia	2	10.0	33,000	52%	52%
(3) Gilles de la Tourette	1	3.0	22,000	30%	30%

[a] Range.

dyskinesia). There was objective improvement in 2 patients with chorea, in 1 with tics, and in 1 with tardive dyskinesia. However nausea and bad odors made this approach difficult, and a search for better drugs is mandatory.

Recently, Wurtman and his collaborators (106) have shown that oral lecithin (phosphatidylcholine, the bound form of choline) is more effective in raising human serum choline levels than the equivalent quantity of choline chloride (265 to 86% above control levels, respectively). This rise persists much longer after lecithin administration (12 to 4 hr, respectively). In our own studies (13), lecithin was given in doses of 3 to 33 g/day in 6 patients with hyperkinesia (Table 4). Lecithin proved to have only moderate, but real, effects upon the dyskinesias. The most clear-cut improvement was seen in tardive dyskinesia where one patient went from a dyskinesia score of 72 to 32 and another from 58 to 31. None however, were cured of their abnormal movements.

These preliminary results indicated that lecithin, or choline, could possibly have useful effects on the abnormal movements induced by overdosage of levodopa or the "on–off" phenomena from supersensitivity of the dopamine receptors (10). We therefore carried out a pilot study in 8 parkinsonian patients, all of whom had severe periods of abnormal involuntary movements, accompanied by end-of-dose akinesia (five cases) or akinesia paradoxica (3 cases). Lecithin was given in daily doses of 30 g/day. As seen in Table 5, no patient was improved from the "on–off" phenomena. However of the 8 patients, 7 noted a measurable decrease in their involuntary movements without loss of antiparkinsonian activ-

TABLE 5. *Lecithin in Parkinson's disease*
(30 g/day)

Effect on "on–off" phenomenon
   end-of-dose akinesia—improvement: 0/5 cases
   akinesia paradoxica—improvement: 0/3 cases
Effect on abnormal involuntary movements
   marked decrease: 3/8 cases
   moderate decrease: 4/8 cases
   no change: 1/8 cases

ity. All 8 patients had been receiving levodopa with a DOPA-decarboxylase inhibitor for at least 4 years.

CONCLUSIONS

Although levodopa, and more so the combination levodopa–inhibitor of DOPA decarboxylase, is still by far the best available treatment for Parkinson's disease, it is becoming obvious that the passage of time is accompanied by progressive loss of efficacy, return of parkinsonian symptoms, and even in some rarer cases complete unresponsiveness. The complications of oscillations in performance, of abnormal involuntary movements and of intellectual deterioration also cry out for trials of newer therapeutic approaches. In this present chapter we have reviewed, and illustrated with our own results, a number of current new paths currently followed by researchers in order to replace, or improve, levodopa therapy. Although most of these results are preliminary and still fragmentary, optimism for the future is justified.

ACKNOWLEDGMENTS

The various studies from the authors, laboratory reported in this chapter were supported in part through grants from the Medical Research Council of Canada and the United Parkinson Foundation. The authors would like to thank the various drug companies (Hoffmann La Roche, Montreal; Merk Sharpe and Dohme, Montreal; Servier, France; Hoechst, Montreal; Sandoz Company, Montreal; Abbott Company, Ltd., Chicago; Ayerst McKenna and Harrisson, Montreal; Labbaz, France), who contributed drugs and some financial support.

REFERENCES

1. Aquilonius, S. M., and Eckernäs, S. A. (1975): Plasma concentration of free choline in patients with Huntington's chorea on high doses of choline chloride. *New Engl. J. Med.,* 293:1105–1106.
2. Aquilonius, S. M., and Sjostrom, R. (1971): Cholinergic and dopaminergic mechanisms in Huntington's chorea. *Life Sci.,* 10:405–414.
3. Barbeau, A. (1961): Biochemistry of Parkinson's disease. *Excerpta Medica, Int. Congr. Ser.,* 38:152–153.
4. Barbeau, A. (1962): The pathogenesis of Parkinson's disease: A new hypothesis. *Can. Med. Assoc. J.,* 87:1242–1243.
5. Barbeau, A. (1969): L-DOPA therapy in Parkinson's disease—A critical review of nine years' experience. *Can. Med. Assoc. J.,* 101:791–800.
6. Barbeau, A. (1973): Biochemistry of Huntington's chorea. In: *Advances in Neurology, Vol. 1,* edited by A. Barbeau, T. N. Chase, and G. W. Paulson, pp. 473–516. Raven Press, New York.
7. Barbeau, A. (1974): The clinical physiology of side-effects in long-term L-DOPA therapy. In: *Advances in Neurology, Vol. 5,* edited by F. H. McDowell and A. Barbeau, pp. 347–365. Raven Press, New York.
8. Barbeau, A. (1975): Potentiation of L-DOPA effect by intravenous L-prolyl-L-leucyl-glycine amide in man. *Lancet,* 2:683.
9. Barbeau, A. (1976): Six years of high-level levodopa therapy in severely akinetic parkinsonian patients. *Arch. Neurol.,* 33:333–338.

10. Barbeau, A. (1976): Neurological and psychiatric side-effects of L-DOPA. In: *Pharmacology and Therapeutics, Part C, Vol. 1,* edited by O. Hornykiewicz, pp. 475–494. Pergammon, Oxford.
11. Barbeau, A. (1976): Pathophysiology of the oscillations in performance after long-term therapy with L-DOPA. In: *Advances in Parkinsonism,* edited by W. Birkmayer and O. Hornykiewicz, pp. 424–434. Editiones Roche, Basel.
12. Barbeau, A. (1978): Emerging treatments: Replacement therapy with choline or lecithin in neurological diseases. *Can. J. Neurol. Sci.,* 5:157–160.
13. Barbeau, A. (1978): Phosphatidyl choline (lecithin) in neurological disorders. *Neurology,* 28:358.
14. Barbeau, A., Gillo-Joffroy, L., and Mars, H. (1971): Treatment of Parkinson's disease with levodopa and Ro4–4602. *Clin. Pharmacol. Ther.,* 2:353–359.
15. Barbeau, A., and Kastin, A. J. (1976): Polypeptide therapy in Parkinson's disease—A new approach. In: *Advances in Parkinsonism,* edited by W. Birkmayer and O. Hornykiewicz, pp. 483–487. Editiones Roche, Basel.
16. Barbeau, A., Mars, H., and Gillo-Joffroy, L. (1971): Adverse clinical side effects of levodopa therapy. In: *Recent Advances in Parkinson's Disease,* edited by F. H. McDowell and C. H. Markham, pp. 203–237. Davis, Philadelphia.
17. Barbeau, A., and Roy, M. (1976): Six-year results of treatment with levodopa plus benzerazide in Parkinson's disease. *Neurology,* 26:399–404.
18. Barbeau, A., Roy, M., and Kastin, A. J. (1976): Double-blind evaluation of oral L-prolyl-L-leucyl-glycine amide in Parkinson's disease. *Can. Med. Assoc. J.,* 114:120–122.
19. Barker, L. A., and Mittag, T. W. (1975): Comparative studies of substrates and inhibitors of choline transport and choline acetyltransferase. *J. Pharmacol. Exp. Ther.,* 192:86–94.
20. Bédard, P., Parkes, J. D., and Marsden, C. D. (1977): Nomifensine in Parkinson's disease. *Br. J. Clin. Pharmacol.,* 4:1875–1905.
21. Bird, E. D., and Iversen, L. L. (1974): Huntington's chorea. Post-mortem measurement of glutamic acid decarboxylase, choline acetyl transferase and dopamine in basal ganglia. *Brain,* 97:457–472.
22. Birkmayer, W., and Hornykiewicz, O. (1961): Der L-Dioxyphenylalanin-(= DOPA)—Effekt bei der Parkinson-akinese. *Wien. Klin. Wochenschr.,* 73:787–788.
23. Birkmayer, W., and Mentasti, M. (1967): Weitere expenmentelle untersuchungen über den catecholamin—stoffwechsel bei extrᴜpyramidalen erkrankungen (Parkinson and chorea syndrome). *Arch. Psychiatr. Nervenkr.,* 210:29–35.
24. Birkmayer, W., Riederer, P., Youdim, M. B. H., and Linauer, W. (1975): The potentiation of the anti-akinetic effect after L-DOPA treatment by an inhibitor of MAO-B, Deprenil. *J. Neural Transm.,* 36:303–326.
25. Broll, M., Eymard, P., Ferrandes, B., and Werbenec, J. P. (1977): Pharmacologie d'un nouvel anti-parkinsonien, la diprobutine (LCG 21519). *J. Pharmacol.,* 8:524–525.
26. Butterworth, R. F., and Barbeau, A. (1975): Apomorphine: Stereotyped behaviour and regional distribution in rat brain. *Can. J. Biochem.,* 53:308–311.
27. Butterworth, R. F., Bélanger, F., and Barbeau, A. (1978): Hypokinesia produced by antero-lateral hypothalamic 6-hydroxydopamine lesions and its reversal by some antiparkinson drugs. *Pharm. Biochem. Behav.,* 8:41–45.
28. Butterworth, R. F., Poignant, J. C., and Barbeau, A. (1975): Apomorphine and Piribedil in rats: Biochemical and pharmacologic studies. In: *Advances in Neurology, Vol. 9,* edited by D. B. Calne, T. N. Chase, and A. Barbeau, pp. 307–327. Raven Press, New York.
29. Calne, D. B., Chase, T. N., and Barbeau, A. (eds.) (1975): Dopaminergic mechanisms. In: *Advances in Neurology, Vol. 9,* edited by D. B. Calne, T. N. Chase, and A. Barbeau, pp. 1–427. Raven Press, New York.
30. Calne, D. B., Leigh, P. N., Teychenne, P. F., Bamji, A. N., and Greenacre, J. K. (1974): Bromocriptine in parkinsonism. *Br. Med. J.,* 4:442–444.
31. Carroll, P. T., and Buterbaugh, G. G. (1975): Regional differences in high affinity choline transport velocity in guinea-pig brain. *J. Neurochem.,* 24:229–232.
32. Chase, T. N., Woods, A. C., Lipton, M. A., and Morris, C. E. (1974): Hypothalamic releasing factors and Parkinson's disease. *Arch. Neurol.,* 31:55–56.
33. Cohen, E. L., and Wurtman, R. J. (1975): Brain acetylcholine; increase after systemic choline administration. *Life Sci.,* 16:1095–1102.
34. Cohen, E. L., and Wurtman, R. J. (1976): Brain acetyl choline: Control by dietary choline. *Science,* 191:561–562.

35. Collins, G. G. S., Sandler, M., Williams, E. D., and Youdim, M. B. H. (1970): Multiple forms of human brain mitochondrial monoamine oxidase. *Nature,* 225:817–820.
36. Corrodi, H., Farnebo, L., Fuxe, K., Hamberger, B., and Ungerstedt, U. (1972): ET 495 and brain catecholamine mechanisms: Evidence for stimulation of dopamine receptors. *Eur. J. Pharmacol.,* 20:195–199.
37. Corrodi, H., Fuxe, K., Hökfelt, T., Lidbrink, P., and Ungerstedt, U. (1973): Effect of ergot drugs on central catecholamine neurons. Evidence for a stimulation of central dopamine neurons. *J. Pharm. Pharmacol.,* 25:409–412.
38. Corrodi, H., Fuxe, K., and Ungerstedt, U. (1971): Evidence for a new type of dopamine receptor stimulating agent. *J. Pharm. Pharmacol.,* 23:989–991.
39. Costall, B., Kelly, D. M., and Naylor, R. J. (1975): Nomifensine: A potent dopaminergic agonist of antiparkinsonian potential. *Psychopharmacologia,* 41:153–164.
40. Costall, B., and Naylor, R. J. (1973): The site and mode of action of ET 495 for the mediation of stereotyped behaviour in the rat. *Naunyn Schmiedebergs Arch. Pharmakol.,* 278:117–121.
41. Cotzias, G. C., Papavasiliou, P. S., and Gellene, R. (1969): Modification of parkinsonism: Chronic treatment with L-DOPA. *N. Engl. J. Med.,* 280:337–345.
42. Cotzias, G. C., Papavasiliou, P. S., Tolosa, E. S., Mendez, J. S., and Bell-Midura, M. (1976): Treatment of Parkinson's disease with aporphines—Possible role of growth hormone. *N. Engl. J. Med.,* 294:567–572.
43. Cotzias, G. C., Van Woert, M. H., and Schiffer, L. M. (1967): Aromatic amino acids and modification of parkinsonism. *N. Engl. J. Med.,* 276:374–380.
44. Crane, G. E. (1973): Is tardive dyskinesia a drug effect? *Am. J. Psychiatr.,* 130:1043.
45. Cuello, A. C., and Paxinos, G. (1978): Evidence for a long leu-enkephalin striopallidal pathway in rat brain. *Nature,* 271:178–180.
46. Davis, K. L., Berger, P. A., and Hollister, L. E. (1975): Choline for tardive dyskinesia. *N. Engl. J. Med.,* 293:152.
47. Duby, S. E., Cotzias, G. C., and Papavasiliou, P. (1972): Injected apomorphine and orally administered levodopa in parkinsonism. *Arch. Neurol.,* 27:474–480.
48. Duvoisin, R. C., and Katz, R. (1968): Reversal of central anticholinergic syndrome in man by physostigmine. *J. Am. Med. Assoc.,* 206:1963–1965.
49. Enna, S. J., Bird, E. D., Bennett, J. P., Bylund, D. B., Yamamura, H. I., Iversen, L. L., and Snyder, S. H. (1976): Huntington's chorea. Changes in neurotransmitter receptors in the brain. *N. Engl. J. Med.,* 294:1305–1309.
50. Fahn, S. (1974): 'On-off' phenomenon with levodopa therapy in parkinsonism—Clinical and pharmacologic correlations and the effect of intramuscular pyridoxone. *Neurology,* 24:431–441.
51. Feigenson, J. S., Sweet, R. D., and McDowell, F. H. (1976): Piribedil: Its synergistic effect in multidrug regimens for parkinsonism. *Neurology,* 26:430–433.
52. Fischer, P. A., Schneider, E., Jacobi, P., and Maxion, H. (1974): Effect of melanocyte-stimulating hormone-release inhibiting factor (MIF) in Parkinson's syndrome. *Eur. Neurol.,* 12:360–368.
53. Gerhards, H. J., Carenzi, A., and Costa, E. (1974): Effect of Nomifensine on motor activity, dopamine turnover rate and cyclic $3',5'$-adenosine monophosphate concentrations of rat striatum. *Naunyn Schmiedebergs Arch. Pathol. Pharmakol.,* 286:49–63.
54. Gerlach, J. (1976): Effect of CB154 (2-bromo-alpha-ergocryptine) on paralysis agitans compared with Madopar in a double-blind, cross-over trial. *Acta Neurol. Scand.,* 53:189–200.
55. Gerstenbrand, F., Binder, H., Grünberger, J., Kozma, C., Push, S., and Reisner, T. (1976): Infusion therapy with MIF (melanocyte inhibiting factor) in Parkinson. In: *Advances in Parkinsonism,* edited by W. Birkmayer and O. Hornykiewicz, pp. 456–461. Editiones Roche, Basel.
56. Goldstein, M., Battista, A. F., Ohmoto, T., Anagnoste, B., and Fuxe, K. (1973): Tremor and involuntary movement in monkeys: Effect of L-Dopa and of a dopamine receptor stimulating agent. *Science,* 179:816–817.
57. Gonce, M., and Barbeau, A. (1978): Expériences thérapeutiques avec le propyl-leucyl-glycine amide dans la maladie de Parkinson. *Rev. Neurol.,* 134:141–150.
58. Gron, U. (1977): Bromocriptine versus placebo in levodopa-treated patients with Parkinson's disease. *Acta Neurol. Scand.,* 56:269–273.
59. Growdon, J. H., Cohen, E. L., and Wurtman, R. J. (1977): Effects of oral choline administration on serum and CSF choline levels in patients with Huntington's disease. *J. Neurochem.,* 28:229–231.

60. Growdon, J. H., Gelenberg, A. J., Doller, J., and Wurtman, R. J. (1978): Lecithin can suppress tardive dyskinesia. *N. Engl. J. Med.,* 298:1029–1030.
61. Haubrich, D. R., Wang, P. F. L., Chippendale, T., and Proctor, E. (1976): Choline and acetyl choline in rats: Effect of dietary choline. *J. Neurochem.,* 27:1305–1313.
62. Hirsch, M. J., Growdon, J., and Wurtman, R. J. (1977): Increase in hippocampal acetyl choline after choline administration. *Brain Res.,* 125:383–385.
63. Hunt, P., Kannengiesser, M. H., and Raynaud, J. P. (1974): Nomifensine: A new potent inhibitor of dopamine uptake into synaptosomes from rat brain corpus striatum. *J. Pharm. Pharmacol.,* 26:370–371.
64. Izumi, K., Motomatsu, T., Chrétien, M., Butterworth, R. J., Lis, M., Seidah, N., and Barbeau, A. (1977): β-endorphin induced akinesia in rats: Effect of apomorphine and α-methyl-p-tyrosine and related modifications of dopamine turnover in the basal ganglia. *Life Sci.,* 20:1149–1156.
65. Jenner, P., and Marsden, C. D. (1975): The influence of piribedil (ET-495) on components of locomotor activity. *Eur. J. Pharmacol.,* 33:211–215.
66. Jori, A., Cecchetti, G., Dolfini, E., Monti, E., and Garattini, S. (1974): Effect of piribedil and one of its metabolites on the concentration of homovanillic acid in the rat brain. *Eur. J. Pharmacol.,* 27:245–250.
67. Kartzinel, R., Perlow, M., Teychenne, P. F., Gielen, A. C., Gillespie, M. M., Sadowsky, D. A., and Calne, D. B. (1976): Bromocriptine and levodopa (with or without carbidopa) in parkinsonism. *Lancet,* 2:272–275.
68. Kastin, A. J., and Barbeau, A. (1972): Preliminary clinical studies with L-prolyl-L-leucyl-glycine amide in Parkinson's disease. *Can. Med. Assoc. J.,* 107:1079–1081.
69. Klawans, H. L. (1973): *The Pharmacology of Extrapyramidal Movement Disorders.* S. Karger, Basel.
70. Klawans, H. L., Goetz, C., Nausieda, P. A., and Weiner, W. J. (1977): Levodopa-induced dopamine receptor hypersensitivity. *Ann. Neurol.,* 2:125–129.
71. Klawans, H. L., Goetz, C. G., Volkman, P., Nausieda, P. A., and Weiner, W. J. (1978): Lergotrile in the treatment of parkinsonism. *Neurology,* 28:699–702.
72. Klawans, H. L., and Rubovits, R. (1972): Central cholinergic-anticholinergic antagonism in Huntington's chorea. *Neurology,* 22:107–116.
73. Lees, A. J., Haddad, S., Shaw, K. M., Kohout, L. J., and Stern, G. M. (1978): Bromocriptine in parkinsonism—A long term study. *Arch. Neurol.,* 35:503–505.
74. Lees, A. J., Kohout, L. J., Shaw, K. M., Stern, G. M., Elsworth, J. D., Sandler, M., and Youdim, M. B. H. (1977): Deprenyl in Parkinson's disease. *Lancet,* 2:791–795.
75. Lemberger, L., Crabtree, R., Clemens, J., Dyke, R. W., and Woodburn, R. T. (1974): The inhibitory effect of an ergoline derivative (Lergotrile, compound 83636) on prolactin secretion in man. *J. Clin. Endocrinol. Metab.,* 39:579–584.
76. Liebermann, A. N., Estey, E., Kupersmith, M., Gopinatham, G., and Goldstein, M. (1977): Treatment of Parkinson's disease with lergotrile mesylate. *Neurology,* 27:390.
77. Liebermann, A., Kupersmith, K., Estey, E., and Goldstein, M. (1976): Treatment of Parkinson's disease with bromocriptine. *N. Engl. J. Med.* 25:1400–1404.
78. Liebermann, A. N., Miyamoto, T., Battista, A. F., and Goldstein, M. (1975): Studies on the antiparkinsonian efficacy of lergotrile. *Neurology,* 25:459–462.
79. McDellan, D. L., Chalmers, R. J., and Johnson, R. H. (1975): Clinical and pharmacological evaluation of the effects of Piribedil in patients with parkinsonism. *Acta Neurol. Scand.,* 51:74–82.
80. McGeer, P. L., Boulding, J. E., Gibson, W. C., and Foulkes, R. G. (1961): Drug-induced extrapyramidal reactions. Treatment with diphenhydramine hydrochloride and dihydroxyphe-nylalanine. *J. Am. Med. Assoc.,* 177:665–670.
81. McGeer, P. L., McGeer, E. G., and Fibiger, H. C. (1973): Choline acetylase and glutamic acid decarboxylase in Huntington's chorea. *Neurology,* 23:912–917.
82. Mann, S. P., and Hebb, C. (1977): Free choline in the brain of the rat. *J. Neurochem.,* 28:241–244.
83. Marsden, C. D., and Parkes, J. D. (1976): "On-off" effects in patients with Parkinson's disease on chronic levodopa therapy. *Lancet,* 1:292–296.
84. Miller, R. J., and Iversen, L. L. (1974): Stimulation of a dopamine-sensitive adenylate cyclase in homogenates of rat striatum by a metabolite of piribedil (ET 495). *Naunyn Schmiedebergs Arch. Pharmakol.,* 282:213–215.

85. Mishra, R. K., and Makman, M. H. (1975): Interaction of L-prolyl-L-leucyl-glycine amide, a hypothalamic factor, with adenylate cyclase associated with dopamine receptor in rat striatum and monkey striatum and retina. *Pharmacologist,* 17:195.
86. Miyamoto, T., Battista, A., and Goldstein, M. (1974): Long lasting anti-tremor activity induced by 2-Br-alpha-ergocryptine in monkeys. *J. Pharm. Pharmacol.,* 26:452–454.
87. Muenter, M. D., Sharpless, N. S., Tyce, G. M., and Darley, F. L. (1977): Patterns of dystonia ("I-D-I" and "D-I-D") in response to L-DOPA therapy for Parkinson's disease. *Mayo Clin. Proc.,* 52:163–174.
88. Nair, R. M. G., Kastin, A. J., and Schally, A. V. (1971): Isolation and structure of hypothalamic MSH release-inhibiting hormone. *Biochem. Biophys. Res. Commun.,* 43:1376–1381.
89. Ngo, T. T., Tunnicliff, G., Yam, C. F., Charbonneau, M., and Barbeau, A. (1978): The inhibition of human plasma acetyl cholinesterase by some naturally occurring compounds. *Gen. Pharmacol.,* 9:21–24.
90. Parkes, J. D. (1977): Bromocriptine. *Adv. Drug Res.,* 12:247–344.
91. Parkes, J. D., Debono, A. G., and Marsden, C. D. (1976): Bromocriptine in parkinsonism: Long-term treatment, dose response and comparison with levodopa. *J. Neurol. Neurosurg. Psychiatr.,* 39:1101–1108.
92. Pearce, I., and Pearce, J. M. S. (1978): Bromocriptine in parkinsonism. *Br. Med. J.,* 8:1402–1404.
93. Plotnikoff, N. P., and Kastin, A. J. (1974): Pharmacological studies with a tripeptide, prolyl-leucyl-glycine amide. *Arch. Int. Pharmacodyn. Ther.,* 211:211–224.
94. Poignant, J. C., Lejeune, F., Malecot, E., Petijean, M., Regnier, G., and Canevari, R. (1974): Effets comparés du piribedil et de trois de ses métabolites sur le système extrapyramidal du rat. *Experientia,* 30:70.
95. Rinne, V. K. (1978): Recent advances in research on parkinsonism. *Acta Neurol. Scand.* [*Suppl. 67*], 57:77–113.
96. Sandler, M., and Youdim, M. B. H. (1974): Monoamine oxidase: The present status. *Int. Pharmacopsychiatr.,* 9:27–34.
97. Schacht, U., and Heptner, W. (1974): Effect of Nomifensine (HOE 984), a new antidepressant, on uptake of noradrenaline and serotonin and on release of noradrenaline in rat brain synaptosomes. *Biochem. Pharmacol.,* 23:3413–3422.
98. Shaw, K. M., Lees, A. J., and Stern, G. M. (1978): Bromocriptine in Parkinson's disease. *Lancet,* 1:1255.
99. Stahl, W. L., and Swanson, P. D. (1974): Biochemical abnormalities in Huntington's chorea brains. *Neurology,* 24:813–819.
100. Tarsy, D., Leopold, N., and Sax, D. S. (1974): Physostigmine in choreiform movement disorders. *Neurology,* 24:28–33.
101. Teychenne, P. F., Calne, D. B., Leigh, P. N., Greenacre, J. K., Reid, J. L., Petrie, A., and Bamji, A. N. (1975): Idiopathic parkinsonism treated with bromocriptine. *Lancet,* 2:473–476.
102. Teychenne, P. F., Park, D. M., Findley, L. J., Rose, F. C., and Calne, D. B. (1976): Nomifensine in parkinsonism. *J. Neurol. Neurosurg. Psychiatry,* 39:1219–1221.
103. Truelle, J. L., Chanelet, J., Bastard, J., Six, P., and Emile, J. (1977): Etude clinique et électrophysiologique prolongée, chez 54 parkinsoniens, d'un nouvel agoniste dopaminergique. *Sem. Hop. Ther. (Paris),* 53:453–456.
104. Ulus, I., and Wurtman, R. J. (1976): Choline administration: Activation of tyrosine hydroxylase in dopaminergic neurons of rat brain. *Science,* 194:1060–1061.
105. Walters, J. R., Bunney, B. S., and Roth, R. H. (1975): Piribedil and apomorphine: Pre- and post-synaptic effects on dopamine synthesis and neuronal activity. In: *Advances in Neurology, Vol. 9,* edited by D. B. Calne, T. N. Chase, and A. Barbeau, pp. 273–284. Raven Press, New York.
106. Wurtman, R. J., Hirsch, M. J., and Growdon, J. H. (1977): Lecithin consumption raises serum-free choline levels. *Lancet,* 2:68–69.
107. Yahr, M. D., Duvoisin, R. C., Shear, M. J., Barrett, R. E., and Hoehn, M. M. (1969): Treatment of parkinsonism with levodopa. *Arch. Neurol.,* 21:343–354.
108. Yamamura, H. I., and Snyder, S. H. (1973): High affinity transport of choline into synaptosomes of rat brain. *J. Neurochem.,* 21:1355–1374.

Advances in Neurology, Vol. 24, edited by
L. J. Poirier, T. L. Sourkes, and P. J. Bédard.
Raven Press, New York © 1979.

Increase of Parkinsonian Symptoms as a Manifestation of Levodopa Toxicity

Stanley Fahn and Robert E. Barrett

Department of Neurology, Columbia University College of Physicians and Surgeons, New York, New York, 10032; and The Neurological Institute of New York, New York, New York 10032

The CNS complications of levodopa therapy in the treatment of parkinsonism are the major limitations in providing maximum amelioration of symptoms in most patients. The most common CNS adverse effect seen in a recent survey of the residual symptoms of parkinsonism and of the adverse effects induced by levodopa was the development of abnormal involuntary movements (16). Mental side-effects, sleep disturbances, autonomic dysfunction, and clinical fluctuations are other commonly encountered problems with levodopa therapy (Table 1). These adverse reactions are well recognized as a problem related to the drug itself and usually present no difficulty in their being diagnosed as such. Perhaps the only exception is the development of dystonic movements and spasms, since dystonic posturing (e.g., ulnar-deviated hands, stooped posture) and sustained flexion contractions of the feet and toes (striatal foot) are features of parkinsonism that were seen prior to the initiation of levodopa therapy (8). The sustained muscular contractions of dystonia that occur with levodopa therapy may resemble severe rigidity in some patients and can lead the clinician to uncertainty as to whether this symptom represents undertreatment with levodopa or excessive treatment (10). We have encountered five patients who had moderate to marked improvement in their parkinsonian symptoms with levodopa therapy, but when given higher doses in an attempt to obtain further improve-

TABLE I. *CNS manifestations of levodopa-induced adverse reactions*

Abnormal involuntary movements: Chorea, dystonia
Mental: Hallucinations, delusions, agitation, mania, depression, negativism, compulsiveness, hypersexuality, confusion, dementia
Sleep disturbances: Hypersomnia, insomnia, altered sleep cycle
Postural hypotension and autonomic dysfunction
Diaphoresis
Clinical fluctuations: "On–off" effect, wearing-off effect, sudden transient freezing, start–hesitation

451

ment, they showed an increase of certain parkinsonian symptoms. These symptoms lessened with the reduction of levodopa dosage. Recognition of this form of toxic reaction to levodopa is important to clinicians because the tendency might be to further increase the dosage of levodopa on the assumption that the disease process rather than the medication was responsible for the increase in symptoms.

CASE REPORTS

Case 1

This man was 69 years of age when he developed increased parkinsonism from levodopa. The onset of Parkinson's disease had occurred 9 years earlier with stooped posture, bradykinesia, rigidity, and deterioration of handwriting. Tremor was never present throughout the course of his illness. Levodopa was begun 4 years after onset of the disease and produced modest benefit. Nevertheless, symptoms progressed and he also developed impairment of balance. He was switched to combination levodopa with carbidopa (Sinemet®) in 1976 (age 69) with some improvement at a dose of 25/250 mg q.i.d. Supplemental levodopa was added and was gradually increased to 250 mg q.i.d. This resulted in increased rigidity, bradykinesia, and postural imbalance. He did not develop tremor, and there were never signs of abnormal involuntary movements. Removal of the supplemental DOPA led to improvement, as did reduction of Sinemet to 20/200 mg q.i.d. A subsequent trial of bromocriptine caused postural hypotension at a dose of 5 mg/day, and this was discontinued.

Case 2

This woman developed increased parkinsonism from levodopa at the age of 67. She had the onset of Parkinson's disease at age 60, with slowing down of her gait and stooped posture. With time there was progressive balance difficulty, bradykinesia of the hands, action tremor, cogwheel rigidity, and difficulty in rising from a chair. Sinemet was begun at age 62, but a dose of 20/200 mg q.i.d. resulted in postural hypotension. The dosage was reduced, and she did best with mild improvement on a dose of 10/100 mg q.i.d. A trial of bromocriptine in 1977 (age 67) caused confusion and disorientation at a dose of 20 mg/day. Bromocriptine was discontinued. She was then placed on supplemental levodopa up to 250 mg q.i.d., which resulted in deterioration of her balance, increased rigidity, increased bradykinesia, confusion, and disorientation. The dosage of supplemental levodopa was reduced to 50 mg q.i.d., which led to the disappearance of all these adverse symptoms. At no time did abnormal involuntary movements develop.

Case 3

This man was 63 years of age when he developed increased parkinsonian symptoms with levodopa. The onset of Parkinson's disease had occurred 4 years earlier with shuffling gait. Gradually, there was progressive bradykinesia, stooped posture, and balance difficulty. Amantadine was started and improved the symptoms for 6 months, and then it lost its effect. Levodopa was begun at the age of 60, and resulted in virtually complete control of symptoms. This caused some intermittent mild facial and nuchal chorea. After 2 years of excellent response, he began to have increasing signs of parkinsonism. There was increasing rigidity, clumsiness of the hands, and shuffling gait. The dosage of levodopa was gradually increased, reaching 11 g/day. It was noted that with each increase of dosage, there was increasing rigidity and bradykinesia. Discontinuation of levodopa resulted in marked clinical improvement, which lasted 2 weeks, and then increasing signs of parkinsonism began to occur. He was placed on Sinemet, and a dose of 25/250 mg q.i.d. led to moderate improvement. He was then given supplemental levodopa, which resulted in shuffling gait, bradykinesia, and frequent sighing movements. The supplementary levodopa was discontinued, and he improved. Over the next couple of years he became more depressed, and this led to his suicide at the age of 65. Pathologic examination revealed classic characteristics of Parkinson's disease.

Case 4

This woman developed increased parkinsonism from levodopa at age 41. The onset of Parkinson's disease had occurred 7 years earlier with tremor of the left foot. Treatment with amantadine relieved this symptom for 9 months. Gradually, tremor developed in the left hand and rigidity on the left side of the body. A pneumoencephalogram done elsewhere was normal. Levodopa therapy was begun in 1971 (age 36). A dosage of 5 g/day resulted in marked clinical improvement. She developed choreic movements which necessitated constant adjustment of the dosage. After 3 years of levodopa therapy, dystonic movements were noted. In 1975, Sinemet was substituted for levodopa; a dose of 10/100 mg q.i.d. provided considerable benefit. She began to develop intermittent episodes of tremor and bradykinesia ("on–off" effect). Supplemental levodopa at a dosage of 350 mg q.i.d. relieved the parkinsonian symptoms ("off" phenomenon) but caused choreic movements. Levodopa was increased to 500 mg q.i.d., which resulted in increased rigidity of the lower extremities and the axial musculature, loss of facial expression, Myerson's sign, and profound bradykinesia. She could not stand or walk without help. Sinemet and levodopa were discontinued, and for the next 48 hr her symptoms reversed through a stage of chorea and then to classical parkinsonism with tremor and rigidity. Resumption of Sinemet 10/100 mg q.i.d., and then supplemental bromocriptine 5 mg q.i.d., led to marked improvement.

Case 5

This man developed increasing gait difficulty secondary to levodopa at the age of 33. He had the onset of Parkinson's disease at age 27 with tremor of the right hand. Gradually there was progressive bradykinesia on the right side of his body and dragging of the right leg. Carotid arteriography done elsewhere was normal. Levodopa was begun at the age of 30 and led to mild reduction of his symptoms. The dosage was limited to 2 g/day because of gastrointestinal side effects. The following year, sexual impotency and autonomic dysfunction of the bladder and bowel developed. At the age of 32, parkinsonian tremor and brady-kinesia of the right extremities were severe, and Sinemet was substituted for levodopa, with considerable benefit. The effectiveness of Sinemet would not last through the night, and he had considerable parkinsonism when he awakened in the mornings. At the age of 33 while on Sinemet 175/1750 mg/day, he developed postural hypotension and gait imbalance which led to falling. A reduction of the dose resulted in wearing-off effects. During the "off" state, his blood pressure was normal, but there was considerable bradykinesia and rigidity, right side greater than left, with right-sided tremor. There were many adjustments of the dosage of Sinemet over the next 3 years. It was repeatedly observed that a dosage > 15/150 mg every 2½ hr resulted in autonomic dysfunction and increasing difficulty with his balance and gait, with a tendency to fall. At this dosage, his parkinsonian symptoms were moderately well controlled with only mild to moderate wearing-off effects.

DISCUSSION

The salient features in the five patients reported are presented in Table 2. Four of the patients had, at one time or another, other CNS toxic reactions to levodopa. Two (cases 3 and 4) had abnormal involuntary movements which disappeared when the dosage of levodopa was further increased to the point of producing increased parkinsonism. Two patients had other manifestations of CNS toxicity occurring simultaneously with the parkinsonian toxic state. Case 3 had mental confusion and disorientation, and case 5 had increased autonomic dysfunction including postural hypotension. With these two exceptions the increased parkinsonian state was not associated with other symptoms usually recognized as toxicity to levodopa. When confronted with increasing parkinsonism, the clinician might tend to further increase the dosage of levodopa. In contrast, a reduction of dosage led to clinical improvement in our patients. Therefore, the clinician must be aware of this form of toxic reaction to the medication when he treats patients with this drug. Increasing gait difficulty was probably the most sensitive indicator of toxicity in our five patients. There was an increase of imbalance, loss of postural stability, and falling. Bradykinesia and rigidity were also frequently seen. Whereas rigidity could be confused with

TABLE 2. Characteristics of patients with increased parkinsonian signs as a toxic effect from levodopa

Case	Sex	Age	Age at onset	Tremor	Improved with levodopa	Years on DOPA	Toxic signs from levodopa		DOPA
							Classic	Parkinsonian	
1	M	69	60	−	mild	5	none[a]	PI, B,R,F	S + LD
2	F	67	60	action	mild	5	postural hypotension	PI, B,R,F,	S + LD
3	M	63	58	−	marked	3	mild chorea	B,R, shuffling, sighing	LD; S + LD
4	F	41	34	+	marked	5	chorea, dystonia (on-off)	PI, B,R,F	S + LD
5	M	33	27	+	moderate	3	dysautonomia (wearing-off)	PI, F	S

[a] Postural hypotension with supplemental bromocriptine.
PI, postural instability; B, bradykinesia; R, rigidity; F, falling; S, Sinemet; LD, levodopa.

dystonia and therefore suspect as a feature of levodopa toxicity, the presence of bradykinesia is virtually pathognomonic for the syndrome of parkinsonism regardless of etiology (11). If the clinician is not aware that increased bradykinesia can be due to levodopa itself, a further increase of levodopa might be implemented with resulting failure to obtain clinical improvement.

All five of our patients had received levodopa in combination with carbidopa. One of them (case 2) did have some increased parkinsonian state on levodopa alone, but this became more severe when he received levodopa/carbidopa. Four of our patients were receiving supplementary levodopa in addition to the commercially available preparation of levodopa/carbidopa (Sinemet®). In calculating the equivalent effective dose of supplementary levodopa, the presence of carbidopa in the therapeutic regimen from levodopa/carbidopa would amplify the potency of supplementary levodopa approximately fourfold. It was probably the presence of such total high dosage levodopa that made us aware of the increased parkinsonian state that can be obtained with levodopa. Many patients on chronic levodopa therapy have increasing parkinsonian symptoms that are considered to be due to loss of efficacy of levodopa with time (7,21). We wonder if the increased parkinsonian state in some of these patients might, in fact, be due to excess dosage of levodopa; if so, such patients would benefit from a reduction of dosage. This would be an important point to check on these patients. Our observations suggest that the clinician must determine constantly the effectiveness and toxicity of levodopa.

The mechanism by which excess levodopa can produce symptoms of parkinsonism is unknown. We can speculate that it might depend not only on dosage but also on the duration of therapy. Our five patients had been receiving levodopa for more than 3 years, and three of them for more than 5 years, before this problem was encountered. The dopaminergic nigrostriatal pathway and its receptors in the striatum appear to have some special properties that lead to adverse effects with chronic therapy with drugs that interfere with or augment dopaminergic transmission. Neurologists are all aware of the "on–off" effect with chronic high dosage levodopa therapy. Such a rapid transition from an improved to a parkinsonian state and back again seems to be unique in therapeutic pharmacology. The hypothesis that the striatal dopaminergic receptors become desensitized with constant bombardment of high dosage dopamine (9) has been proposed as a factor in explaining this unusual clinical phenomenon. It is possible that a related mechanism occurs in patients who become increasingly parkinsonian with excess levodopa, as in our five patients. Instead of developing a flip-flop receptor response, the receptor might simply be constantly desensitized leading to a state of steady parkinsonism rather than sudden and transient parkinsonism. In such a situation, reducing the dosage of levodopa would restore the receptor and allow for therapeutic response to levodopa.

Another possible mechanism relates to the fact that dopamine exerts both excitatory and inhibitory responses in the striatum (1,5,13,14,17–19). Perhaps at therapeutic doses of levodopa, one of these responses predominates, leading to therapeutic results. With higher doses, the opposite type of receptor may be affected, leading to increased parkinsonism. A third possibility is that exogenous dopamine from levodopa therapy inhibits the presynaptic nigrostriatal neuron at either the presynaptic site in the striatum (autoreceptors) (3) or at dendritic sites in the substantia nigra (2,12). This third hypothesis does not seem plausible to us because the striatonigral neurons are heavily degenerated in parkinsonism, and dopamine supplied to the brain should be bypassing these neurons and affecting the downstream target, the striatal postsynaptic receptors. Consequently, it would matter little if the presynaptic neuron is further inhibited by exogenously supplied dopamine.

Not only in the therapy of parkinsonism does the clinician affect the dopaminergic transmitter system; antipsychotic medications which are predominantly dopamine receptor blockers (4) also produce an unusual constellation of neurologic syndromes. It is commonly assumed that simple overdosage of these antipsychotic drugs leads to a state of parkinsonism, which is analogous to the state of chorea produced by simple overdosage of levodopa. However, with more chronic use of the antipsychotic drugs, the choreatic state of tardive dyskinesia may develop (6). Tardive dyskinesia might be due to the development of hypersensitivity of the dopamine receptors (15), which would be analogous to a development of desensitivity with chronic levodopa therapy and which could lead to the parkinsonian state reported here. However, there are problems with this analogy since tardive dyskinesia can usually be suppressed for awhile by increased dosage of the antipsychotic medication, and it can be enhanced by discontinuing these drugs.

An increase of parkinsonian symptoms, especially tremor, does occasionally occur when initiating levodopa therapy, but with further increase of dosage and the passage of time, the parkinsonian symptoms begin to be controlled. An explanation for this phenomenon might be that the presynaptic dopamine receptor (autoreceptor) has a lower threshold than the postsynaptic receptor (3), which would lead to inhibition of presynaptic dopamine release. Recently, Weiner et al (20) described a patient who developed increased parkinsonian signs with levodopa, Sinemet, or lergotrile mesylate, a direct-acting dopamine receptor agonist, without deriving any beneficial therapeutic response. This patient, therefore, differs from the five patients reported here who all had definite improvement of their parkinsonian state with levodopa. Weiner and his colleagues speculated that their patient might have had some dysfunction of the postsynaptic dopamine receptor. Whereas their patient had an increase of parkinsonism that was more severe than the native state, it is not clear from our five patients whether excess levodopa would have actually produced a parkinsonian state that was more severe than the natural state if the patients had not responded to levodopa or were without the drug. Their parkinsonian state with excess levodopa might be merely a partial expression of their natural disease due to partial lack of response of the dopamine receptor, perhaps by one of the mechanisms postulated above.

SUMMARY

Five patients with parkinsonism who obtained partial or marked improvement with levodopa therapy showed increased symptoms of parkinsonism when the dosage of levodopa was increased. The "toxic" parkinsonian symptoms with levodopa overdosage were primarily an increase of bradykinesia, rigidity, and postural instability, which led to difficulty walking and to falling. Tremor was not encountered. These toxic symptoms disappeared when the dosage of levodopa was reduced. The development of parkinsonian symptoms from an overdosage of levodopa is not only of interest in terms of the pharmacology of dopamine receptors in the striatum, but also raises new considerations in the management of patients with parkinsonism.

REFERENCES

1. Bloom, F. E., Costa, E., and Salmoiraghi, G. C. (1965): Anesthesia and the responsiveness of individual neurons of the caudate nucleus of the cat to acetylcholine, norepinephrine and dopamine administered by microelectrophoresis. *J. Pharm. Exp. Ther.,* 150:244–252.
2. Bunney, B. S., and Aghajanian, G. K. (1976): Feedback control of central dopaminergic activity: Neurophysiological and neuropharmacological evidence. In: *Advances in Parkinsonism,* edited by W. Birkmayer and O. Hornykiewicz, pp. 82–92. Editiones Roche, Basel.
3. Carlsson, A. (1976): Some aspects of dopamine in the basal ganglia. *Res. Publ. Assoc. Res. Nerv. Ment. Dis.,* 55:101–109.
4. Carlsson, A. (1978): Mechanism of action of neuroleptic drugs. In: *Psychopharmacology: A Generation of Progress,* edited by M. A. Lipton, A. DiMascio, and K. F. Killam, pp. 1057–1070. Raven Press, New York.
5. Connor, J. D. (1970): Caudate nucleus neurones: Correlation of the effects of substantia nigra stimulation with iontophoretic dopamine. *J. Physiol.,* 208:691–703.
6. Crane, G. E. (1970): High doses of trifluperazine and tardive dyskinesia. *Arch. Neurol.,* 22:176–180.
7. Diamond, S. G., Markham, C. H., and Treciokas, L. J. (1976): Long-term experience with L-dopa: efficacy, progression and mortality. In: *Advances in Parkinsonism,* edited by W. Birkmayer and O. Hornykiewicz, pp. 444–455. Editiones Roche, Basel.
8. Duvoisin, R. C., Yahr, M. D., Lieberman, J., Antunes, J., and Rhee, S. (1972): The striatal foot. *Trans. Am. Neurol. Assoc.,* 92:267.
9. Fahn, S. (1974): "On–off" phenomenon with levodopa therapy in parkinsonism. *Neurology,* 24:431–441.
10. Fahn, S. (1976): Medical treatment of movement disorders. In: *Neurological Reviews 1976,* pp. 72–106. American Academy of Neurology, Minneapolis.
11. Fahn, S. (1977): Secondary Parkinsonism. In: *Scientific Approaches to Clinical Neurology,* edited by E. S. Goldensohn and S. H. Appel, pp. 1159–1189. Lea & Febiger, Philadelphia.
12. Groves, P. M., Wilson, C. J., Young, S. J., and Rebec, G. V. (1975): Self-inhibition by dopaminergic neurons: An alternative to the "neuronal feedback loop" hypothesis for the mode of action of certain psychotropic drugs. *Science,* 190:522–527.
13. Herz, A., and Zieglgaensberger, W. (1966): Synaptic excitation in the corpus striatum inhibited by microelectrophoretically administered dopamine. *Experientia,* 22:839–840.
14. Kitai, S. T., Sugimori, M., and Kocsis, J. D. (1976): Excitatory nature of dopamine in the nigro-caudate pathway. *Exp. Brain Res.,* 24:351–363.
15. Klawans, H. L. (1973): The pharmacology of tardive dyskinesias. *Am. J. Psychiatry,* 130:82–86.
16. Lesser, R. P., Fahn, S., Snider, S. R., Cote, L. J., Barrett, R. E., and Isgreen, W. P. (1978): Analysis of the clinical problem in parkinsonism and of the complications of long-term levodopa therapy. *Neurology,* 28:342.

17. McLennan, H., and York, D. H. (1967): The action of dopamine on neurones of the caudate nucleus. *J. Physiol.,* 189:393–402.
18. Purpura, D. P. (1976): Physiological organization of the basal ganglia. *Res. Publ. Assoc. Res. Nerv. Ment. Dis.,* 55:91–114.
19. Siggins, G. R., Hoffer, B. J., Bloom, F. E., and Ungerstedt, U. (1976): Cytochemical and electrophysiological studies of dopamine in the caudate nucleus. *Res. Publ. Assoc. Res. Nerv. Ment. Dis.,* 55:227–247.
20. Weiner, W. J., Kramer, J., Nausieda, P. A., and Klawans, H. L. (1978): Paradoxical response to dopaminergic agents in parkinsonism. *Arch. Neurol.,* 35:453–455.
21. Yahr, M. D. (1976): Evaluation of long-term therapy in Parkinson's disease: Mortality and therapeutic efficacy. In: *Advances in Parkinsonism,* edited by W. Birkmayer and O. Hornykiewicz, pp. 435–443. Editiones Roche, Basel.

Advances in Neurology, Vol. 24, edited by
L. J. Poirier, T. L. Sourkes, and P. J. Bédard.
Raven Press, New York © 1979.

Bromocriptine and Lergotrile: Comparative Efficacy in Parkinson Disease

A. N. Lieberman, M. Kupersmith, I. Casson, R. Durso, S. H. Foo, M. Khayali, T. Tartaro, and M. Goldstein

New York University School of Medicine, New York, New York 10016

INTRODUCTION

It is apparent that despite the use of levodopa, alone or with a peripheral decarboxylase inhibitor, many patients with Parkinson disease (PD) become severely disabled after 2 to 5 years of treatment (14,17,27,34,39). This problem arises because PD is characterized by a dopamine deficiency resulting from degeneration of the nigrostriatal neurons (2,8,10,33). Initially, the administration of levodopa compensates for the deficiency through an increased conversion of DOPA to dopamine by the remaining neurons. Later, levodopa no longer compensates for the deficiency, because among other things, the remaining neurons may be too few in number to generate sufficient dopamine (6,28,29). Theoretically, these patients should benefit from drugs that stimulate the striatum directly (3,26). Two of these drugs, bromocriptine and lergotrile, have been effective in many such patients (3,4,9,16,18,20–22,24–26,31,37,38). Because of the growing interest in such dopamine agonists, we thought it pertinent to compare our experience with bromocriptine and lergotrile.

METHODS

Between 1974 and 1977, 81 patients with advanced PD were treated with bromocriptine or lergotrile. Sixty-six of these 81 patients were treated with bromocriptine (24). Forty-eight of them had, at one time, improved at least one stage on levodopa (Table 1). Fifty-three of the 81 patients were treated with lergotrile (21). Thirty-nine of the 53 patients had, at one time, improved at least one stage on levodopa (Table 1).

At the time of the study, most patients were increasingly disabled despite optimal treatment with levodopa (alone or with a peripheral decarboxylase inhibitor). Attempts to increase levodopa resulted in adverse reactions [involuntary movements (IMs), mental changes]; and attempts to decrease levodopa resulted in worsening parkinsonism. All patients had previously been treated with amantadine or an anticholinergic agent, and 15 of the 66 patients receiving bromocriptine

TABLE 1. *Results of prior treatment with levodopa*

	No. of patients	Age (years)	Duration PD (years)	Duration of treatment with levodopa (years)	Dose levodopa/ carbidopa (mg levodopa)	Severity PD prior to treatment with levodopa[a]	Severity PD at time of peak effect levodopa	Severity PD prior to treatment with ergot alkaloid
Bromocriptine								
mean (±SEM)	66	62.3 ± 1.5	10.0 ± 1.4	5.6 ± 0.7	1170 ± 73	2.7 ± 0.1	1.6 ± 0.1	3.7 ± 0.1
range		(45–80)	(2–48)	(0–9)	(150–2000)	(2–4)	(0–3)	(2–5)
Lergotrile								
mean (±SEM)	53	62.2 ± 1.5	9.9 ± 1.3	6.3 ± 0.8	1075 ± 101	2.6 ± 0.1	1.5 ± 0.2	3.2 ± 0.2
range		(45–85)	(2–48)	(0–9)	(150–2000)	(2–4)	(0–3)	(2–5)

[a] Scale of Hoehn and Yahr (13).

and 18 of the 53 patients receiving lergotrile were still receiving amantadine or anticholinergics. Patients with moderate dementia were excluded, but patients with mild dementia were included.

After complete physical, neurological, and laboratory evaluation, and informed consent, bromocriptine or lergotrile was begun at a dose of 5 to 10 mg/day. It was increased by 5 to 10 mg/day each week until toxicity ensued or to an arbitrary maximum of 100 mg/day for bromocriptine or 150 mg/day for lergotrile was achieved. Selection of patients to treatment first with bromocriptine or lergotrile was arbitrary. Initially, no attempt was made to decrease the amount of levodopa. However, additive toxic effects (IMs, orthostatic hypotension, mental changes) in time led to a decrease in the dose of levodopa. Other antiparkinsonian medications were not changed. Patients who experienced adverse effects on one agonist or who failed to improve at least one stage on at least 25 mg/day of bromocriptine or 20 mg/day of lergotrile were changed to the other agonist. Thirty-eight patients were, at different times, treated with both bromocriptine and lergotrile (19). At regular intervals an observer, unaware of the medications the patients were receiving, assessed the cardinal signs of the disease—rigidity, tremor, bradykinesia and gait disturbance—using a detailed graded examination with "0" representing no disability, and "100%" representing maximal disability. A total score was obtained by adding the scores for each sign. Patients were also assessed by the method of Hoehn and Yahr (13). Involuntary movements were assessed separately. Patients with diurnal oscillations in performance, "on–off" phenomena, were evaluated each time they were in an "on" and an "off" period by an observer. "On–off" phenomena were also evaluated by having the patient keep a daily log of medication and the number of "on–off" periods (15,23). The patient's self-evaluations were periodically verified by a trained observer. From the log, the following items were determined: the number of hours between doses of medication, the number of "on" and "off" periods, the mean duration of "on" and "off" periods, and the total number of hours spent in "on" and "off" periods. Statistical analyses were performed, using the Wilcoxon matched pair signed rank test at the 5% level of significance.

RESULTS

Among the 66 patients (Table 2), 45 were able to tolerate at least 25 mg of bromocriptine (adequately treated), and only in these patients was therapeutic efficacy analyzed. However, data on adverse effects were analyzed in all 66 patients. Among the 45 adequately treated patients, the mean dose of bromocriptine was 45 mg (range 25 to 100 mg), and mean duration of treatment was 7 months (range 2 to 24 months). The dose of levodopa was reduced by 10% in the group and eliminated in 7 patients. There was a significant reduction in rigidity, tremor, bradykinesia, gait disturbance, total score, stage, and a significant increase in IMs among the 45 patients. Twenty-five patients showed at

TABLE 2. Results of treatment in patients able to tolerate at least 25 mg of bromocriptine or 20 mg of lergotrile

	Rigidity	Tremor	Bradykinesia	Gait	Total	Stage	IMs
Bromocriptine:							
Mean dose 45 mg							
before	28.3 ± 4.5	10.0 ± 2.6	40.0 ± 3.4	46.8 ± 4.4	34.3 ± 2.7	3.2 ± 0.2	15 ± 3.7
after	20.4 ± 3.9	4.0 ± 1.4	30.2 ± 3.3	36.8 ± 4.1	25.9 ± 2.1	2.5 ± 0.1	29 ± 5.3
change	−28%	−60%	−25%	−21%	−24%	−19%	+93%
	$p < 0.01$	$p < 0.01$	$p < 0.01$	$p < 0.01$	$p < 0.01$	$p < 0.01$	$p < 0.01$
Lergotrile:							
Mean dose 49 mg							
before	33.3 ± 3.5	11.0 ± 2.3	44.9 ± 3.9	35.2 ± 2.3	33.4 ± 2.5	2.9 ± 0.2	17.8 ± 3.5
after	23.8 ± 3.2	6.0 ± 1.2	32.3 ± 2.9	30.1 ± 2.2	27.3 ± 2.4	2.2 ± 0.1	20.4 ± 3.5
change	−29%	−45%	−28%	−14%	−18%	−24%	+15%
	$p < 0.01$	$p < 0.01$	$p < 0.01$	$p < 0.01$	$p < 0.01$	$p < 0.01$	NS

All values are mean ± SEM.
IMs, involuntary movements; NS, not significant.

TABLE 3. *Results of treatment in patients with "on-off" phenomena*

Bromocriptine	Total score "Off"	Total score "On"	Stage "Off"	Stage "On"
Bromocriptine				
before	57 ± 4.2	32 ± 2.4	4.1 ± 0.2	2.9 ± 0.2
after	46 ± 3.9	22 ± 2.1	3.6 ± 0.2	2.2 ± 0.1
change	−19%	−31%	−12%	−24%
	$p < 0.01$	$p < 0.01$	$p < 0.05$	$p < 0.01$
Lergotrile				
before	58.2 ± 4.1	25.4 ± 2.4	4.1 ± 0.2	2.8 ± 0.2
after	56.0 ± 4.1	21.6 ± 1.9	4.0 ± 0.2	2.2 ± 0.1
change	−4%	−15%	−2%	−21%
	NS	$p < 0.01$	NS	$p < 0.01$

All values are mean ± SEM.
NS, not significant.

least one-stage improvement. Twelve patients were treated with bromocriptine for at least 1 year, and in eight there was no decrease in efficacy.

Among the 53 patients (Table 2), 39 were able to tolerate at least 20 mg of lergotrile (adequately treated), and only in these patients was therapeutic efficacy analyzed. Data on adverse effects were analyzed for all 53 patients. Among the 39 adequately treated patients, the mean dose of lergotrile was 49 mg (range 20 to 150 mg), and mean duration of treatment was 6 months (range 2 to 19 months). The dose of levodopa was reduced by 10% in the group and eliminated in 2 patients. There was a significant reduction in rigidity, tremor, bradykinesia, gait disturbance, total score, and stage among the 39 patients. Twenty-one patients showed at least a one stage improvement. Five patients were treated with lergotrile for at least 1 year, and in four there was a decrease in efficacy.

Among the 45 patients who were adequately treated with bromocriptine, 27 had "on–off" phenomena. There was a significant reduction in total score and stage in both "on" and "off" periods for the group of 27 patients as a whole. Nineteen of the 27 patients improved at least one stage. Among the 39 patients who were adequately treated with lergotrile, 23 had "on–off" phenomena. There was a significant reduction in total score and stage in the "on" periods but not in the "off" periods. Thirteen of the 23 patients improved at least one stage (Table 3). Patients on bromocriptine and lergotrile experienced an increase in the number of "on" periods, a decrease in the number of "off" periods, an increase in the mean length of "on" periods, and a decrease in the length of "off" periods. Total time spent in "off" periods decreased, and total time spent in "on" periods increased. Only the last change was significant. "On–off" phenomena disappeared in five patients on bromocriptine and one on lergotrile (Table 4).

Twenty-four of the 38 patients treated with both bromocriptine and lergotrile were able to tolerate, at different times, at least 25 mg/day of bromocriptine and at least 20 mg/day of lergotrile. In these 24 patients, there was a significant

TABLE 4. Results of treatment on the number and duration of "on-off" periods

		No. "on" periods	Mean duration "on" periods (hr.)	Total time "on" (hr.)	No. "off" periods	Mean duration "off" periods (hr.)	Total time "off" (hr.)
Bromocriptine							
before	Mean	3.2	2.1	6.0	4.6	2.6	10.0
	Range	(1–6)	(0.5–6)	(4–12)	(2–9)	(0.5–9)	(5–13)
after	Mean	4.5	3.8	11.1	3.2	1.7	4.9
	Range	(2–9)	(2–16)	(7–16)	(0–7)	(0–5)	(3–8)
change (%)		40	80	85 $p < 0.05$	–30	–35	–51
Lergotrile							
before	Mean	3.3	2.0	6.1	4.5	2.4	9.9
	Range	(1–6)	(0.5–6)	(4–11)	(2–9)	(1–8)	(5–13)
after	Mean	4.3	3.8	10.9	3.3	1.8	5.1
	Range	(2–8)	(2–16)	(6–16)	(0–8)	(0–5)	(3–9)
change (%)		30	90	79 $p < 0.05$	–27	–25	–45

SEM ± 5–11%.

decrease in rigidity, bradykinesia, total score, and stage on both drugs (Table 5). Eleven patients responded equally to both drugs, three responded better to bromocriptine, and two responded better to lergotrile. Eight patients responded to neither drug. Best results were obtained when bromocriptine or lergotrile was combined with levodopa.

Bromocriptine and lergotrile differed principally with regard to adverse effects. For the group as a whole, bromocriptine resulted in a significant increase in IMs, while lergotrile did not; bromocriptine had to be discontinued in 9 of 66 patients (14%) because of IMs, whereas lergotrile was discontinued in only one patient because of IMs. Eleven patients on lergotrile developed elevations in serum transaminase, and one patient became jaundiced. Abnormalities occurred 3 months after initiation of lergotrile at a mean dose of 48 mg (range 30 to 70 mg). Only one patient developed elevations in serum transaminase and became jaundiced on bromocriptine. All abnormalities disappeared within 1.5 months of discontinuing the drugs. Eight patients on lergotrile experienced orthostatic hypotension, five with syncope. Only four patients on bromocriptine experienced orthostatic hypotension, one with syncope. Mental changes were similar with use of the two drugs (35) and were similar to those experienced on levodopa (5,36) (Table 6).

DISCUSSION

Bromocriptine and lergotrile are useful drugs in the management of patients with advanced PD who are no longer satisfactorily responding to levodopa. Bromocriptine resulted in improvement in 25 of 66 patients (38%), while lergotrile resulted in improvement in 21 of 53 patients (39%). The drugs are effective against all of the major signs of the disease, and in the management of "on–off" phenomena. The efficacy of these drugs in patients with advanced PD and particularly in those with "on–off" phenomena is probably related to their properties as dopamine agonists (requiring no metabolic conversion to dopamine) and to their longer duration of action. "On–off" phenomena have been related both to the severity of PD and to treatment with levodopa (23). With increasingly severe PD, there is a decrease in the number of presynaptic dopaminergic nigrostriatal neurons. The remaining neurons partially compensate for their decreased number through an increased metabolism (by individual neurons) of exogenous levodopa to dopamine. As the principal means of inactivation of this dopamine, in the synaptic cleft, is through reuptake by the same presynaptic nerve terminals, a decrease in the number of these terminals may lead, at times, to excessive concentrations of dopamine at the receptor site. This may result in a depolarization block analagous to the cholinergic crisis of myasthenia gravis. In this scheme, "on" periods are visualized as resulting from activation of the receptors by a specific concentration of dopamine designated as an "adequate" or "sufficient" concentration. "Off" periods are visualized as resulting from failure of the receptors to be activated. One of two mechanisms may be responsible for this failure,

TABLE 5. *Results of treatment in 24 patients able to tolerate at least 25 mg of bromocriptine and at least 20 mg of lergotrile*

	Rigidity	Tremor	Bradykinesia	Gait	Total	Stage	IMs
Bromocriptine							
before	25.2 ± 5.2	7.4 ± 2.3	39.8 ± 4.3	36.3 ± 6.6	30.1 ± 3.8	2.9 ± .23	20.7 ± 3.9
after	18.3 ± 4.2	3.5 ± 0.9	26.8 ± 4.3	31.9 ± 5.9	23.6 ± 3.4	2.3 ± .24	35.1 ± 7.0
change	−27%	−53%	−33%	−12%	−22%	−21%	+70%
	$p < 0.01$		$p < 0.01$		$p < 0.01$	$p < 0.01$	$p < 0.01$
Lergotrile							
before	27.5 ± 5.0	9.8 ± 3.0	39.8 ± 3.9	31.5 ± 6.2	27.3 ± 2.9	2.8 ± .22	27.3 ± 5.4
after	20.8 ± 4.5	5.1 ± 1.7	30.3 ± 4.1	29.7 ± 6.6	19.9 ± 2.5	2.2 ± .24	28.5 ± 5.6
change	−24%	−48%	−24%	−6%	−27%	−21%	+4%
	$p < 0.01$		$p < 0.01$		$p < 0.01$	$p < 0.01$	

All values are mean ± SEM.

TABLE 6. *Adverse effects necessitating withdrawal of ergot alkaloid (no. of patients)*

	Total no. of patients entering study	Total no. patients discontinued	Mental changes	Orthostatic hypotension	IMs	Hepato-toxicity	Other
Bromocriptine	66	29	14	4	9	1	1
Percentage of total		44%	21%	6%	14%	1.5%	1.5%
Lergotrile	53	33	12	8	1	11	1
Percentage of total		62%	23%	15%	2%	21%	2%

Structure of lergotrile mesylate.

Structure of bromocriptine

and these mechanisms may alternate with each other in an unpredictable manner. In one mechanism, failure of receptor activation occurs because of "inadequate" or "insufficient" dopamine concentrations in the synaptic cleft. In the second mechanism, failure of receptor activation occurs because of "excessive" dopamine concentrations in the synaptic cleft, resulting in depolarization blockade. Such a scheme could explain the two major types of "off" phenomena encountered clinically. In the first, an "off" period occurs several hours after the last dose of levodopa and is not accompanied by IMs; it is usually benefited by the next dose of levodopa. This type of "off" period is related to decreased plasma concentrations of DOPA (and presumably to decreased concentrations of DOPA in the synaptic cleft) and has been variously called "end of dose deterioration" (30), "wearing off" (7), or type 1–3 diurnal fluctuations (1). The second type of "off" period occurs in no fixed relationship to the last dose of levodopa. This type of "off" period has been, at times, related to increased plasma DOPA concentrations and may result from depolarization blockade. Additionally, it must be noted that "on–off" periods may be precipitated by emotional upsets and positional changes. The abruptness of these changes suggests that factors other than the dopamine concentration in the synaptic cleft are important. Bromocriptine and lergotrile decrease those "off" periods related to "end of dose deterioration" and to a lesser extent other types of "off" periods as well.

Best results were obtained when bromocriptine or lergotrile was combined with levodopa, and for individual patients there was usually an optimal ratio of bromocriptine or lergotrile to levodopa (38). This follows observations in animal models of PD where the effect of the ergot alkaloids could be enhanced by pretreating with levodopa or diminished by blocking the synthesis of dopamine (11,12,32). This suggests that although the dopamine receptor stimulating property of these drugs is important, presynaptic mechanisms involving dopamine synthesis are also important.

The difference in involuntary movements between lergotrile and bromocriptine was anticipated by the preclinical studies (11,12,33). Both drugs behave like mixed pre- and postsynaptic dopamine agonists and antagonists, with lergotrile a more potent agonist and bromocriptine a more potent antagonist. These differences in agonist–antagonist properties may explain the observed difference in involuntary movements.

The effectiveness of both drugs in patients with advanced PD is encouraging and suggests that with some modifications even more effective agents may be developed.

SUMMARY

Bromocriptine and lergotrile were administered at different times to 81 patients with advanced PD and increasing disability, despite optimal treatment with levodopa. Sixty-six patients were treated with bromocriptine, and 45 of them tolerated at least 25 mg/day (adequately treated); 53 patients were treated with lergotrile, and 39 of them tolerated at least 20 mg/day (adequately treated). Both adequately treated groups had significantly decreased rigidity, tremor, bradykinesia, gait disturbance, total score, and stage upon addition of bromocriptine or lergotrile to levodopa. Twenty-five patients improved at least one stage on bromocriptine, and 21 improved at least one stage on lergotrile. Nineteen of 27 patients with "on–off" effects improved on bromocriptine, while 13 of 21 patients with "on–off" effects improved on lergotrile. The mean dose of bromocriptine in adequately treated patients was 47 mg, and the mean dose of lergotrile was 49 mg, permitting a 10% reduction in levodopa. Bromocriptine was discontinued in 29 of 66 patients because of adverse effects, including mental changes (14 patients) and IMs (nine patients). Lergotrile was discontinued in 33 of 53 patients because of adverse effects including hepatotoxicity (11 patients), mental changes (12 patients), and orthostatic hypotension (eight patients). While the results of treatment with bromocriptine or lergotrile were comparable, there were differences among individual patients with some improving more on bromocriptine and others more on lergotrile. Both drugs were useful in the management of patients with advanced disease, and suggest that even more effective agents may be developed.

ACKNOWLEDGMENTS

The authors wish to thank Drs. E. Estey and G. Gopinathan for their assistance in evaluating the patients; Dr. P. Berczeller (Dept. of Medicine), Dr. M. Leibowitz (Dept. of Medicine, Div. of Cardiology), Dr. H. Tobias (Dept. of Medicine, Div. of Hepatology), Dr. H. Plasse (Dept. of Otorhinolaryngology), Drs. B. Angrist, M. Serby, and B. Shopsin (Dept. of Psychiatry), E. Boyd, R.N., C. Strohsahl, R.N., and the staff of 10 East for their detailed observations; Drs. H. Langrall, P. Arcese, and R. Elton of Sandoz, East Hanover, New Jersey, for their kindness and cooperation; Drs. L. Lemberger, R. Burt, R. Shulman and Mr. W. Flamme of Eli Lilly, Indianapolis, Indiana, for their kindness and cooperation; Dr. C. T. Randt for his sound counsel; and Ms. K. Faridazar for her help in preparation of the manuscript.

REFERENCES

1. Barbeau, A. (1973): Treatment of Parkinson's disease with L-DOPA and RO44602: Past and present status. *Adv. Neurol.,* 2:173–198.
2. Bernheimer, H., Birkmayer, W., and Hornykiewicz, O. (1973): Brain dopamine and the syndromes of Parkinson and Huntington. *J. Neurol. Sci.,* 20:415–455.
3. Calne, D. B., Teychenne, P. F., and Claveria, L. E. (1974): Bromocriptine in parkinsonism. *Br. Med. J.,* 4:442–444.
4. Calne, D. B., Williams, A. C., and Neophytides, A. (1978): Long-term treatment of parkinsonism with bromocriptine. *Lancet,* 1:735–738.
5. Celesia, G. C., and Barr, A. N. (1970): Psychosis and other psychiatric manifestations of levodopa therapy. *Arch. Neurol.,* 23:193–200.
6. Davidson, L., Lloyd, K., Dankova, J., et al. (1971): L-DOPA treatment in Parkinson's disease: Effect on dopamine and related substances in discrete brain regions. *Experientia,* 27:1048–1049.
7. Fahn, S. (1974): "On-off" phenomenon with levodopa therapy in parkinsonism. *Neurology,* 24:431–441.
8. Fahn, S., Libsch, R., and Cutler, R. W. (1971): Monoamines in the human neostriatum: Topographic distribution in normals and in Parkinson's disease and their role in akinesia, rigidity, chorea and tremor. *J. Neurol. Sci.,* 14:427–455.
9. Godwin-Austen, R. B., and Smith, N. J. (1977): Comparison of the effects of bromocriptine and levodopa in Parkinson's disease. *J. Neurol. Neurosurg. Psychiatry,* 40:479–482.
10. Goldstein, M., Anagnoste, B., and Battista, A. F. (1969): Studies of amines in the striatum in monkeys with nigral lesions. The disposition, biosynthesis and metabolites of (^{3}H)dopamine and (^{14}C)serotonin in the striatum. *J. Neurochem.,* 16:645–653.
11. Goldstein, M., Battista, A. F., and Matsumoto, W. (1976): Pre and postsynaptic effects of dopamine agonists: Anti-parkinsonian efficacy and effects on dopamine synthesis. *Advances in Parkinsonism,* edited by W. Birkmayer and O. Hornykiewicz, pp. 236–243. Roche, Basle.
12. Goldstein, M., Lew, K. Y., Hata, F., and Lieberman, A. N. (1977): Binding interactions of ergot alkaloids with monoaminergic receptors in the brain. *Gerontology (Suppl.),* 24:76–85.
13. Hoehn, M. M., and Yahr, M. D. (1967): Parkinsonism: Onset, progression and mortality. *Neurology (Minneap.),* 17:427–442.
14. Hunter, K. R., Shaw, K. M., and Lawrence, D. R. (1973): Sustained levodopa therapy in parkinsonism. *Lancet,* 2:929–931.
15. Kartzinel, R., and Calne, D. B. (1976): Studies with bromocriptine. Part 1. "On-off" phenomena. *Neurology,* 26:508–510.

16. Kartzinel, R., Perlow, M., Teychenne, P. F., et al. (1976): Bromocriptine and levodopa (with or without carbidopa) in parkinsonism. *Lancet,* 2:272–275.
17. Langrall, H. M., and Joseph, C. (1972): Evaluation of safety and efficacy of levodopa in Parkinson's disease and syndrome. *Neurology (Minneap.) (Suppl.),* 22:3–16.
18. Lees, A. J., Shaw, K. M., and Stern, C. M. (1975): Bromocriptine in parkinsonism. *Lancet,* 2:709–710.
19. Lieberman, A. N., Estey, E., and Gopinathan, G. (1978): Bromocriptine and lergotrile in Parkinson's disease. Presented at the Fourth International Catecholamine Symposium, Pacific Grove, California.
20. Lieberman, A. N., Estey, E., and Kupersmith, M. (1977): Treatment of Parkinson's disease with lergotrile mesylate. *J.A.M.A.,* 238:2380–2382.
21. Lieberman, A. N., Gopinathan, G., and Estey, E. (1979): Lergotrile in Parkinson's disease: Further studies. *Neurology,* 29:267–270.
22. Lieberman, A. N., Kupersmith, M., Estey, E., and Goldstein, M. (1976): Treatment of Parkinson's disease with bromocriptine. *N. Engl. J. Med.,* 295:1400–1404.
23. Lieberman, A. N., Kupersmith, M., and Gopinathan, G. (1978): Modification of the "on-off" effect with bromocriptine and lergotrile. Presented at the International Symposium on Dopaminergic Ergot Derivatives and Motor Function, Stockholm, Sweden.
24. Lieberman, A. N., Kupersmith, M., and Gopinathan, G. (1979): Bromocriptine in Parkinson's disease: Further studies. *Neurology,* 29:363–369.
25. Lieberman, A. N., Miyamoto, T., and Battista, A. F. (1975): Studies on the anti-parkinsonian efficacy of lergotrile. *Neurology,* 25:459–462.
26. Lieberman, A. N., Zolfaghari, M., and Boal, D. (1976): The antiparkinsonian efficacy of bromocriptine. *Neurology,* 26:405–409.
27. Ludin, H. P., and Bass-Verrey, F. (1976): Study of deterioration in long-term treatment of parkinsonism with L-DOPA plus decarboxylase inhibitor. *J. Neural Transmiss.,* 38:249–258.
28. Lloyd, K. G., Davidson, L., and Hornykiewicz, O. (1973): Metabolism of levodopa in the human brain. *Adv. Neurol.,* 3:173–188.
29. Lloyd, K. G., and Hornykiewicz, O. (1970): Parkinson's disease: Activity of L-DOPA decarboxylase in discrete brain regions. *Science,* 170:1212–1213.
30. Marsden, C. D., and Parkes, J. D. (1976): "On-off" effect in patients with Parkinson's disease on chronic levodopa therapy. *Lancet,* 1:292–296.
31. Parkes, J. D., DeBono, A. G., and Marsden, C. D. (1976): Bromocriptine in parkinsonism: Long-term treatment dose response and comparison with levodopa. *J. Neurol. Neurosurg. Psychiatry,* 39:1101–1108.
32. Poirier, L. J., Singh, P., and Sourkes, T. L. (1967): Effect on amine precursors on the concentration of striatal dopamine and serotonin in cats with an without unilateral brain stem lesions. *Brain Res.,* 6:654–666.
33. Poirier, L. J., and Sourkes, T. L. (1965): Influence of the substantia nigra on the catecholamine content of the striatum. *Brain,* 88:181–192.
34. Selby, G.: Long-term treatment of Parkinson's disease with L-DOPA: A clinical study of 148 patients. *Brain Res.,* 6:473–482.
35. Serby, M., Angrist, B., and Lieberman, A. N. (1979): Mental disturbances during the treatment of Parkinson's disease with bromocriptine and lergotrile: Determinants of response pattern. *Am. J. of Psychiatry,* 135:1227–1229.
36. Sweet, R. D., McDowell, F. H., and Feigenson, J. (1976): Mental symptoms in Parkinson's disease during chronic treatment with levodopa. *Neurology (Minneap.),* 26:305–310.
37. Teychenne, P. F., Leigh, P. N., and Reid, J. L. (1975): Idiopathic parkinsonism treated with bromocriptine. *Lancet,* 2:473–476.
38. Teychenne, P. F., Pfeiffer, R. F., and Bern, S. M. (1978): Comparison between lergotrile and bromocriptine in parkinsonism. *Ann. Neurol.,* 3:319–324.
39. Yahr, M. D. (1976): Evaluation of long-term therapy in Parkinson's disease, Mortality and therapeutic efficacy. *Advances in Parkinsonism,* edited by W. Birkmayer and O. Hornykiewicz, pp. 435–443. Roche, Basel.

Advances in Neurology, Vol. 24, edited by
L. J. Poirier, T. L. Sourkes, and P. J. Bédard.
Raven Press, New York © 1979.

Long-Term Study and the Effect of Human Growth Hormone in Parkinsonian Patients Treated with Levodopa

Part 1. Ten-Year Follow-up Study of Levodopa-Treated Patients with Parkinson's Disease/ *(F. H. McDowell and R. Sweet)*
Part 2. Stability of Response to Levodopa Treatment *(P. Papavasiliou and F. H. McDowell)*
Part 3. Effect of Human Growth Hormone on Levodopa Treatment of Parkinson's Disease *(P. Papavasiliou)*

F. H. McDowell, P. Papavasiliou, and R. Sweet

Department of Neurology, Cornell University, Medical College, Ithaca, New York 10021

PART 1. TEN-YEAR FOLLOW-UP STUDY OF LEVODOPA-TREATED PATIENTS WITH PARKINSON'S DISEASE

We began treating patients at the Cornell University, New York Hospital Medical Center, during the first part of 1968. By the fall of 1968, we had accumulated our first 100 patients, and these patients have been periodically reviewed to try to understand the long-range efficacy of levodopa on Parkinson's disease, its complications, and hopefully something of the natural history of levodopa-treated Parkinson's disease. The latest complete review of the status of the patients in this original group was completed this summer. The analysis revealed that as of 1978, of the 100 patients who began treatment in 1968, 56 are dead, 41 are living, one was misdiagnosed and did not have Parkinson's disease, and two have been lost to follow-up. Among the 41 living patients, 31 patients are followed by regular contact in clinic or by home visit. Ten patients are confined to nursing homes and are totally immobilized but are followed by frequent telephone and letter contact with either the institution in which the patient is living or by contact with family members. All of the patients are still taking regularly either levodopa or levodopa/carbidopa (Sinemet®); over 90% are receiving Sinemet. None of them are being treated regularly with any other dopaminergic-like agents such as piribedil, bromocriptine, or apomorphine derivatives, although many of them have taken part in treatment trials with some of these agents in the past.

The mean total score for all of the original 100 patients was 118 and for those followed 10 years 102 (Table 1); both scores represent a significant degree of physical impairment, i.e., total incapacity is indicated by a score of around 230. After 2 years of treatment, the average score had fallen to 66, but it has gradually risen over the ensuing 8 years, so that by the end of 10 years of treatment, the mean score for the group of patients now alive is 100.7. This score is not statistically different than the initial average score of the living patients from the original group of patients who started in 1968, but it is statistically different than the score for the entire group. This suggests that despite the initial alleviation of symptoms of Parkinson's disease among the treated patients, the condition has progressed steadily over the ensuing 10 years, with most of the patients having almost as much disability now as they had at the beginning of treatment. The reasons for the current disability may not be the same as the original reasons, because some of the complications of treatment, such as the "on–off" response, the development of postural instability, and the increasing frequency of dementia, have increased and weighted these scores. In general, the improvement in motility with a decrease in bradykinesia, rigidity, and tremor has continued.

The percentage of patients who are remarkably improved has steadily declined over the 10 years of follow-up (Table 2). At 2 years of treatment, 49% of our patients were improved 51% or more, but after 10 years of treatment only 12% are improved 51% or more. The number of patients who were improved 25 to 50% initially has dropped from 33 to 18%. The percentage of those who were unchanged by treatment, i.e., an improvement of ±25%, has risen from 18 to 52%. Some of the patients have worsened considerably, so that now 10% of our patients are much worse than they were when they first began treatment. Among the 41 survivors, 8 patients need nearly total care, and only

TABLE 1. *Mean disability scores for all patients and for those followed for 10 years*

	Total score						
	Pretreatment						
	All patients	10-year patients	2 years	4 years	6 years	8 years	10 years
Mean	118.7[a]	102.4[b]	66.0	72.9	78.7	88.9	100.7[a,b]
SEM	3.8	4.9	4.6	4.8	4.9	6.1	7.4
No. of patients	99	41	75	52	41	45	41

[a]All patients at 0 years vs. 10 years significant at $p < 0.05$.
[b]10-year patients at 0 years vs. 10 years not significant.

TABLE 2. *Degree of improvement from levodopa therapy at 2, 5, and 10 years of follow-up*

Change from pretreatment score	Percentage of patients at		
	2 years	5 years	10 years
Improved 51% +	49	19	12
Improved 26–50%	33	34	18
Unchanged (± 25%)	18	30	52
Worsened 26–50%	—	9	7
Worsened 51% +	—	8	10

18 are able to care for themselves, despite complications, and lead relatively normal lives. These changes reflect the progression of the disease and the increase in the occurrence of serious disabling symptoms which have not been altered by the administration of levodopa or Sinemet.

We have investigated our data to see if the changes in patients observed over 10 years are related to any obvious factors, such as severity of the disease at onset of treatment, and age or sex of the patient.

Table 3 shows that at the time we began treatment, most of our patients were moderately or severely afflicted by Parkinson's disease, with the largest percentage of them being moderately impaired. At 10 years, the percentage of those patients with mild, moderate, or severe Parkinson's disease has changed considerably. One-quarter of the patients doing well and still being followed at 10 years had mild Parkinson's disease in 1968, and half of the patients who are still followed had moderate Parkinson's disease. The number of patients who had severe Parkinson's disease at the start of treatment and who have been followed for 10 years has declined from 33 to 24%.

In Table 4 it can be seen that those patients who died during the 10 years of follow-up were generally those who were older at the time of beginning treatment and who had more severe Parkinson's disease. Twenty-six percent of those who died during the 10 years of follow-up were aged 60 to 69 at the onset of treatment and 22% were 70 to 79. Thirty-four of the 56 patients who

TABLE 3. *Number of patients with a particular level of severity of Parkinson's disease pretreatment and at 5 and 10 years of follow-up*

Severity of Parkinson's disease (score)	Percentage of patients		
	Pre-treatment	5 years	10 years
Mild (0–50)	5	34	25
Moderate (61–135)	62	51	51
Severe (136+)	33	15	24

TABLE 4. *Severity of Parkinson's disease at the start of levodopa treatment related to age at the start of treatment and mortality*

	Severity of Parkinson's disease before L-DOPA			
Age in 1968	Mild	Moderate	Severe	Total
50–59	1	5	2	8
60–69	—	16	10	26
70–79	1	7	14	22
Total	2	18	16	56

died had moderate to severe Parkinson's disease. The patients in the older age groups with the more severe disease at the onset of treatment are the ones most likely to do less well and to die, while those in the younger age groups with mild to moderate disease have survived and done better overall.

The problem of adverse effects continued and has involved an increasingly larger percentage of the patients. In Table 5, it can be seen that the percentage of patients who have developed the "on–off" effect has risen from 11% at the end of 2 years to 54% at the end of 10 years of treatment. In some patients, this problem is as disturbing as the original Parkinson's disease and is almost as disabling.

A particular problem is the number of patients who have shown evidence of mental or intellectual decline and dementia. Among the individuals who have survived 10 years, only 9% had evidence of dementia at the time treatment began, but the percentage of those surviving 10 years who are now frankly demented has risen to 49% at the end of 10 years. Many of the patients who died in the interim had severe dementia. Dementia has become a major problem for a large segment of our patient population and is frequently a much more troublesome problem than the motility disturbances associated with Parkinson's disease.

The problem of postural instability is a growing one. At the time treatment began, 87% of our patients had postural abnormalities. Initially, postural abnormalities were grouped and included not only postural instability but postural deformity, such as stooped posture. Postural abnormality of some sort is ex-

TABLE 5. *Percentage of patients with adverse effects of treatment before treatment and at 2, 4, 6, 8, and 10 years of follow-up*

Adverse effect	Pre-treatment	2	4	6	8	10
"On–off" effect	0	11	37	49	51	54
Mental	9	24	33	44	42	49
Postural instability	87	69	—	—	71	71

TABLE 6. *Expected and observed mortality rates for patients with Parkinson's disease treated with levodopa*

	Mortality–10 years	
Age in 1968	Expected deaths	Observed deaths
30–34	0.02	0
35–39	0	0
40–44	0.16	0
45–49	0.21	0
50–54	0.59	1
55–59	2.50	7
60–64	5.89	7
65–69	8.45	19
70–74	9.82	14
75–79	8.84	8
Total	36.46	56

tremely common in patients with Parkinson's disease. After 10 years' follow-up, 71% of the patients who are still alive have major problems with postural instability, not just postural deformity. These patients are quite unsteady on their feet, fall down frequently, and have a high incidence of fractures. They are the patients with start–hesitation and festinating gait and are the patients who are in increasing jeopardy of injuring themselves by falling. Medication has offered them very little in the way of relief.

The mortality in this group of 100 patients can be seen in Table 6. The number of deaths in the group each year during the 10 years of follow-up shows that mortality is related to age of the patient at the time of treatment in 1968. This clearly indicates that the patients who were older at the time of beginning treatment had a markedly increased "observed" mortality compared to the "expected."

The excess mortality observed compared to the expected mortality for the whole group is 1.54, which is slightly lower than was reported earlier for our total group (Fig. 1).

This analysis of 100 patients after 10 years of follow-up reveals a sizeable mortality among the group (1.54 in excess of the expected mortality) and a steady increase in disability from Parkinson's disease, despite continued treatment. There has been a steady decline in the number of patients who have been strikingly improved by the treatment, a steady rise in serious side-effects

EXCESS MORTALITY

FIG. 1.

$$\frac{\text{OBSERVED DEATHS}}{\text{EXPECTED DEATHS}} = \frac{56}{36.46} = 1.54$$

of treatment such as "on–off" phenomenon, mental deterioration, dementia, and postural instability. All of this points to a steady progression of Parkinson's disease, despite treatment. However, the overall impression is that this group of patients is better off and functions better in general than patients did before the availability of levodopa treatment.

Among those who have survived are individuals with very stable responses to treatment whose conditions have remained stable or even improved, without major side-effects, over the past 10 years. This group makes up <5% of the total, but they are important examples. It is not clear if the response of these patients represents variations in the natural course of Parkinson's disease or if it is the result of levodopa treatment.

PART 2. STABILITY OF RESPONSE TO LEVODOPA TREATMENT

In order to understand these patients better, we have studied the relation of therapeutic effect to the plasma content of levodopa. From our patient population, nine patients who had had a stable response to levodopa of carbidopa over a number of years were identified and compared to a group of 10 patients who had an unstable response to levodopa or carbidopa with an "on–off" response. The "off" effects occurred at either unpredictable intervals or at the end of a dose, alternating with periods of good motility. In all patients levodopa alone, or Sinemet were given in multiple daily doses. Many of the patients in the unstable group were given smaller doses more frequently in an effort to alleviate symptom fluctuation. Three out of the 19 patients also received anticholinergic medication.

The patients were studied on a research ward during an overnight admission to the hospital or during a full-day in the clinic. Studies were carried out in the stable group with all patients in a nonfasting state. Four patients in the unstable group were nonfasting, and six patients were fasting during the study to investigate the effects of eating on the stability of response.

A patient's response to medication was rated clinically by scoring, using our disability rating scale which analyzes the patient for the presence of tremor, rigidity, hypokinesia, changes in facial expression, performance of rapid alternating movements, difficulties with speech, sialorrhea, and the performance of a number of tasks. The scores were obtained by blind observers, every 15 or 30 min during the observation period. Blood was drawn for the determination of plasma DOPA content prior to scoring and then hourly for the next 5 to 7 hr.

The data obtained were analyzed by calculating the deviations from the mean for the clinical Parkinson scores and deviations from the mean for plasma DOPA levels. Because of the variability of the Parkinson dyskinesia scores and plasma DOPA levels, log transformation was applied to stabilize variances and to render the distributions more symmetric. An analysis of variance was used to compare variability between patients and variability of a particular patient's response and to compare individual patient variability in the two groups.

Figure 2 shows the deviations from the mean for the clinical scores. In the upper portion of the figure, the clinical deviations of those patients who were deemed to have a stable response to levodopa are shown. There is a rather narrow fluctuation around the mean as compared to that seen in the lower portion of the figure, which illustrates the clinical fluctuations of those patients believed on clinical grounds to have an unstable response to levodopa or Sinemet. There is a striking difference between the two groups.

In Fig. 3, the deviations from the mean for plasma DOPA are illustrated. The top portion of the figure shows the deviations of plasma DOPA for the group found to be stable clinically. At the bottom of the graph are the variations of plasma DOPA for those patients who were found to be unstable clinically. The patients in the stable group had lower mean plasma DOPA levels and showed significantly less fluctuation of plasma DOPA levels than those in the unstable group. Higher means and median plasma DOPA levels were found in the unstable group, whether a patient was fasting or nonfasting. The lower

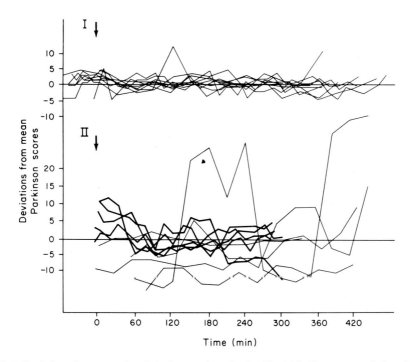

FIG. 2. Deviations from mean for clinical scores in patients with stable (I) responses to levodopa and in patients with unstable (II) responses to levodopa and Sinemet.

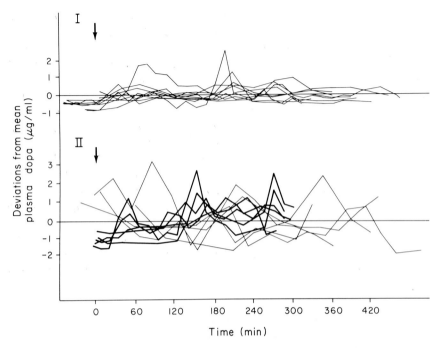

FIG. 3. Variations of plasmadopa in patients with stable (I) and unstable (II) responses to treatment.

mean plasma DOPA levels in the group who were stable clinically could not be attributed to differences in dosages as the percentage difference in dose was much smaller than the difference in plasma DOPA levels. The differences in the two groups were not related to whether the patient took Sinemet or levodopa. The dosages of Sinemet received by patients in the unstable and stable groups were similar, but there were wide differences in the plasma DOPA levels, and these differences were present with or without carbidopa, suggesting that at least gastrointestinal decarboxylation of DOPA was not involved.

There was no consistent correlation between the magnitude and timing of a clinical response and the isolated peaks and valleys of the plasma DOPA levels in the unstable patients. The peaks of plasma DOPA were also not consistently related to the time that medication was given, and often a particular dosage was not accompanied by an increase in plasma DOPA. In neither the stable nor the unstable group of patients was there a correlation between dose and plasma DOPA level. There was a correlation between periods of dyskinesia and the higher plasma DOPA levels.

Patients with unstable symptomatic control showed fluctuations of their plasma DOPA levels throughout the day, but patients with stable motor performance showed relatively stable and lower mean and median plasma DOPA levels. Since the daily dose was similar in the two groups and the more frequent drug administration to unstable subjects failed to stabilize plasma DOPA, these findings indicate that stable and unstable clinical responses may be reflected in plasma DOPA levels and suggest that there are different mechanisms of peripheral DOPA metabolism operant in patients with unstable and stable symptomatic control. The apparent metabolic defect in the unstable group may be due to erratic absorption, varying peripheral catabolism of levodopa, or both. To date, the extent to which central and peripheral metabolic defects directly influence the cerebral effects of levodopa has not been determined. The data presented suggest that peripheral metabolism of DOPA may strongly influence the clinical response and may be in part responsible for the problem of "on–off" effect.

PART 3. EFFECT OF HUMAN GROWTH HORMONE ON LEVODOPA TREATMENT OF PARKINSON'S DISEASE

In the search for a common metabolic factor that might explain the side-effects of chronic levodopa therapy in parkinsonism and on the basis of animal data, it has been suggested that one factor might be the episodic release of growth hormone (GH) during levodopa therapy. No correlation between the pattern of the cumulative secretion of plasma GH and the patients' diurnal symptomatic control while on levodopa has been found. The episodic release of GH has not been shown in any consistent way to influence the therapeutic results or side-effects of levodopa therapy. To clarify the questions arising from the different protocols applied in these experiments, and to conclusively demonstrate whether sufficiently raised and maintained plasma GH levels might influence the cerebral effects of levodopa, exogenous human GH was administered in doses sufficient to achieve and maintain high hormone levels.

Four patients with long-standing dyskinesia were selected; two of them had pronounced fluctuation of symptom control, mainly end-of-dose akinesia, and the other two had fairly stable performance (Table 7). They were studied according to a double-blind protocol while receiving optimum daily doses of levodopa or Sinemet, given in multiple doses. Following 1 week of evaluation, either saline or 5 IU of human growth hormone (hGH) was injected i.m. at 9 A.M.

TABLE 7. *Patient clinical characteristics*

Case no.	Sex	Age	Illness duration (years)	Treatment (years)	Daily dose (mg)
A	F	65	10	8	L/C = 115/1150
B	M	74	9	5	L/C = 120/1200
C	F	72	10	9	L/C = 187.5/1875
D	F	64	16	8	L = 3800

L/C, levodopa/carbidopa; L, levodopa.

TABLE 8. *Effect of human growth hormone (hGH) on neurologic scores, plasma dopa, and GH levels*

Case no.	Parkinson scores		Dyskinesia scores		Plasma dopa µg/ml		Plasma GH ng/ml	
	Placebo	hGH	Placebo	hGH	Placebo	hGH	Placebo	hGH
A	31.2 ± 6.3	33.1 ± 9.8	13.8 ± 2.3	21.7 ± 3.0[a]	2.56 ± 0.3	3.2 ± 0.4	4.4 ± 0.9	129.0 ± 20.3[c]
B	18.3 ± 1.2	19.9 ± 0.8	3.2 ± 0.3	1.7 ± 0.5	1.39 ± 0.2	1.9 ± 0.3	2.5 ± 0.6	22.3 ± 2.7[c]
C	22.8 ± 5.7	16.1 ± 3.6	12.1 ± 3.0	18.2 ± 2.9	2.70 ± 0.3	6.8 ± 0.9[b]	11.6 ± 1.1	370.1 ± 70.2[c]
D	28.7 ± 5.2	23.5 ± 3.3	0.2 ± 0.2	0.3 ± 0.2	1.50 ± 0.4	1.8 ± 0.3	3.1 ± 0.5	80.0 ± 16.4[c]

Data obtained during fourth injection of hGH. Values represent means ± standard errors.
[a] $p < 0.05$; [b] $p < 0.01$; [c] $p < 0.0005$.

TABLE 9. *Parkinson and dyskinesia scores before and during hGH administration*

Case no.	Parkinson scores			Dyskinesia scores		
	Placebo	hGH		Placebo	hGH	
	Mean ± SE	Mean ± SE	p Value	Mean ± SE	Mean ± SE	p Value
A	25.9 ± 6.9	21.1 ± 3.5	NS	19.8 ± 3.4	24.9 ± 1.7	NS
B	21.8 ± 1.2	17.7 ± 0.9	NS	3.2 ± 0.2	2.3 ± 0.2	<0.01
C	22.2 ± 3.6	21.3 ± 3.2	NS	14.2 ± 2.7	14.7 ± 2.2	NS
D	33.1 ± 3.9	36.7 ± 3.6	NS	0.0 ± 0.0	0.2 ± 0.1	NS

Means ± SE of parkinson and dyskinesia scores obtained during first three injections of hGH. The differences in scores were statistically insignificant (NS), with the exception of the dyskinesia scores of patient B ($p < 0.01$).

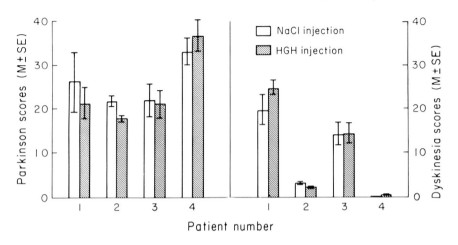

FIG. 4. Parkinson and dyskinesia scores before and during hGH administration.

every other day for a total of four injections. Cholesterol, fat, and protein content of breakfast and luncheon were kept constant throughout the experimental periods. During the period of the first three injections, the patient's motor performance was scored four times a day and at 30-min intervals for 6 hr during the day of the fourth injection. Blood samples were drawn every 30 min, just prior to each clinical evaluation, for the determination of plasma GH and DOPA. All data obtained during administration of hGH were compared to those obtained during saline injections (Tables 7–9).

Figure 4 shows the means and standard errors of parkinson and dyskinesia scores obtained after the first three injections of either saline (clear bars) or hGH (shaded bars). With the possible exception of case 2, there were no statistically significant differences in either symptom control or dyskinesia with hGH or saline administration (Table 9).

Figure 5 shows the lack of significant changes in these parameters when individual scores obtained every 30 min on the fourth injection of GH were compared to those after placebo injection. In this figure, motility is illustrated by the horizontal bars, the clear portion representing motility and the shaded, akinesia. These were not materially different between saline injection (left side of graph) and GH (right side). Scores for dyskinesia, depicted by the graded vertical blocks representing degree of severity, were not materially different between placebo and GH. Failure of GH to affect the levodopa's cerebral effects were noted in patients tested during akinetic episodes (point at shaded areas of A, B, C) and while their plasma GH levels were markedly elevated.

The absence of change in the clinical response to levodopa after hGH, was, however, accompanied by marked elevation of plasma GH. Plasma GH rose soon after GH injection reached a peak, within 120–180 min, and remained above basal levels 3 hr later. Plasma GH elevations after hGH administration

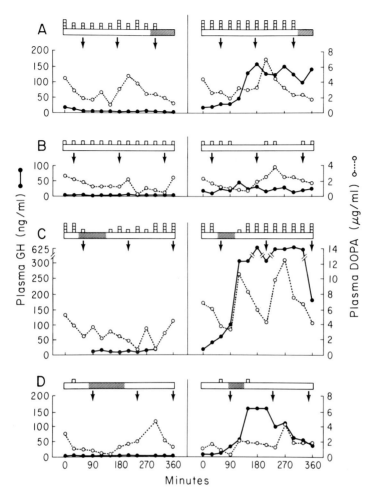

FIG. 5. Plasma GH and DOPA levels during fourth injection of hGH. hGH was injected just after first blood sample was drawn. *Arrows* indicate times at which levodopa/carbidopa (cases A, B, and C), or levodopa (case D) were administered. ▭, "on" periods; ▨, "off" periods; ▭, mild dyskinesia; ▤, moderate dyskinesia; ▤, pronounced dyskinesia.

differed from one subject to the next, and the highest levels were not always associated with changes in performance or dyskinesia. One of the patients (case B) had less dyskinesia after GH than after saline administration. The differences in GH levels were not correlated with age, weight, the dose of DOPA, or plasma DOPA levels. They may be related to different hepatic clearance for GH.

No subjective or other objective changes were observed during or after the periods of plasma GH elevation.

Plasma DOPA levels were determined concomitantly with GH, to find if the marked elevations of GH affect the transfer of DOPA from this extracellular compartment. With the exception of case D, no striking changes in plasma DOPA patterns were observed, suggesting that this hormone does not influence the transport of DOPA, as is the case for other members of this amino acid group.

These and earlier findings showed that the earlier speculations for a role of GH in the beneficial results and side-effects of levodopa therapy could not be substantiated since neither quantitative nor temporal correlations can be shown, whether correlations were sought between endogenous GH secretion under levodopa therapy or plasma elevation following exogenous GH and clinical responses to levodopa. They further show that exogenous GH does not modify the cerebral effects of the levodopa in either an immediate or delayed fashion, regardless of whether dopaminergic effects are present or not. This indicates that the GH release in response to levodopa treatment in patients with parkinsonism occurs independently of its cerebral effects and probably is the result of dopamine repletion of the hypothalamus, the dopaminergic output of which participates in the regulation of GH secretion by the pituitary.

Neither the endogenous GH release nor high doses of exogenous GH alter in any consistent way the therapeutic results or side-effects of chronic levodopa therapy.

Advances in Neurology, Vol. 24, edited by
L. J. Poirier, T. L. Sourkes, and P. J. Bédard.
Raven Press, New York © 1979.

Mortality of Parkinson Patients Treated with Sinemet

Shirley G. Diamond and Charles H. Markham

*Reed Neurological Research Center, UCLA School of Medicine,
Los Angeles, California 90024*

The advent of levodopa therapy in 1970 marked a dramatic advance in the treatment of Parkinson's disease. Efficacy of this drug in controlling symptoms of the disease has been well documented (3,4,11,13). The related question of life expectancy has also been examined. In pre-levodopa days, the death rate of persons with Parkinson's disease was three times the rate of the general population (4,7). After levodopa had been used for a number of years, two studies examining Parkinson patients treated with levodopa (without DOPA decarboxylase inhibitors added) demonstrated a distinct increase in longevity (4,8). Other investigators have examined groups of patients, some of whom were receiving levodopa alone and some levodopa plus a DOPA decarboxylase inhibitor, and these studies also reported an increase in longevity (10,12,14). Although these various reports have differed with respect to methodology, most have concluded that life expectancy of persons with Parkinson's disease has increased in the last decade.

From 1972 to 1974, Merck Sharp & Dohme sponsored clinical trials in the United States of a compound containing ten parts levodopa to one part carbidopa, a peripherally acting DOPA decarboxylase inhibitor. This preparation, since marketed as Sinemet®, has proven to be a highly effective treatment for Parkinson's disease. The addition of the inhibitor enabled the dosage of levodopa to be reduced 80% with concomitant decrease of such peripheral side-effects as nausea and vomiting (9). At the same time, patients switched from plain levodopa to Sinemet (levodopa/carbidopa) or to Madopa®, (a Hoffmann-La-Roche levodopa preparation containing the peripherally acting inhibitor benserazide) generally showed further improvement in the signs and symptoms of parkinsonism (6). The patients who began Sinemet during the early clinical trials have now received this drug for approximately 5 years, and provide a large body of data for examining mortality rates in a Parkinson population treated with this agent.

METHODS

Twenty-five neurologists across the United States participated in clinical trials of Sinemet during the years 1972 to 1974. Criteria for patient inclusion into these studies are listed elsewhere (9). The names and addresses of the investigators, and the Merck numbers identifying the patients enrolled in each study were kindly made available to us by Merck Sharp & Dohme. There were a total of 1564 patients enrolled in the entire series, a mean of 62.6 patients per investigator. Four investigators had fewer than 20 patients, but most had many more. We randomly selected 20 patients from each investigator by the Merck identifying numbers, or took the entire group of patients from those investigators with 20 or fewer enrolled. We then asked the investigators for data on these persons.

Information requested was date of birth; sex; date beginning Sinemet; if the patient was still taking Sinemet as of December 31, 1977, and if not, when Sinemet therapy had terminated; if the patient was still alive as of December 31, 1977, and if not, date of death. If the patient was lost to follow-up, we asked for the date he was last seen and if he was taking Sinemet at that time. These dates enabled calculation of each patient's age at entry into the study and age at termination, which was defined as the first-occurring of the following: the December 31, 1977, conclusion date, discontinuation of Sinemet therapy, last visit before loss to follow-up, or death. The interval between age at entry and age at termination represented the period of time each individual was observed. Using the method described in a previous study (4), the probability of death during the period of observation was computed for each individual, using the U.S. Life Table 1, 1969 to 1971. Briefly, this method uses the sum of individual probabilities to derive a ratio of observed number of deaths in a particular group to the expected number of deaths in an age-matched group drawn from the general population observed over the same period of time.

RESULTS

Of the 25 neurologists contacted, 19 responded with the data we requested. These investigators and their geographic locations are listed in Appendix 1. They had been asked for information on 356 patients, and usable data were received on 327. Unusable data from 29 patients consisted of 15 who had been on Sinemet too short a time for a probability of death to be computed, namely less than 6 months. Another 6 patients never actually entered the study, although a Merck number had been assigned to them during prestudy tests. Finally, eight were lacking various bits of information that prevented computation, e.g., date of birth; and one patient did not have Parkinson's disease. The usable data from the 327 patients represented 1,162 person-years of observation, a mean of 3.56 years per patient. There were 193 men and 134 women. Mean age at entry into the study was 62.4 years for all patients; mean ages in the

19 groups ranged from 57.6 to 67.0 years. Forty-five deaths were observed. Mean age at death was 70.8 years. The data are summarized in Table 1, where it may be seen that in a group of this age composition drawn from the general population and observed over the same intervals, 31.6611 deaths would be expected. The ratio of observed deaths to expected deaths was 1.4213 to 1. This may also be expressed as mortality 42% in excess of normal, and is a statistically significant difference ($p < 0.05$, two-tailed binomial test).

DISCUSSION

The ratio of observed to expected deaths found in the 19 individual groups comprising this study ranged from 5.1813 (3 deaths observed to 0.5790 expected) to 0 (no deaths observed in two studies where there were 1.9255 and 2.0419 deaths expected). See the last column in Table 1. This large variability in the ratios is not surprising in view of the fact that fractional deaths occur in probability tables, while only whole deaths are observed in the real world. Dealing with the small number of patients contained in each of the 19 studies, this mathematical phenomenon will sometimes produce the extreme ratios noted above. Clearly, small numbers of patients are insufficient to provide data for reliable mortality studies, and this was one reason we prevailed upon the investigators whose cooperation made this study possible. (Another reason was to get a wide geographic representation.) Ideally, we would have liked information on all patients from all investigators, but as some investigators had as many as 144 patients enrolled in the study, we did not feel we could impose on them the considerable effort of assembling information on so large a number. Asking for data on a maximum of 20 patients specified by us seemed a realistic compromise and provided us with a reasonable total of 327 patients observed over 1165 person-years.

The wide variability of the individual ratios seen in this study may explain why in earlier studies Diamond et al. (5) found a ratio of 0.97 in 93 patients and 1.03 in 1087 patients while Sweet and McDowell (12) obtained a ratio of 1.9 in 100 patients, all three groups being subsets of 1625 patients in a Hoffmann-LaRoche collaborative study which showed an unadjusted (see below) ratio of 1.03 (8). Those findings are analogous in the present study to Investigator 19 showing a ratio close to that of the whole group while Investigator 2 has a ratio approximately twice as great.

The Sweet and McDowell (12) study found a ratio of 1.5 in the patients who continued in (or died during) their study. Carefully pursuing the persons who were considered lost to follow-up, they determined that these drop-outs had a considerably higher death rate than those patients who remained in the study. Consequently, these investigators adjusted their ratio to 1.9 (or 29% higher) to compensate for those deaths.

Diamond et al. *(unpublished data),* tracing those lost to follow-up in their study, found the death rate of the drop-outs was no different than the patients

TABLE 1. Summary of mortality data on 327 Parkinson patients treated with levodopa/carbidopa (Sinemet®)

Investigator[a]	No. of patients	Person-years	Mean age	Deaths observed	Deaths expected	Ratio
1	17	60	59.8	2	1.2990	1.5396
2	20	68	63.7	5	1.8593	2.6892
3	5	11	63.7	1	0.5077	1.9697
4	20	71	64.7	5	2.1462	2.3207
5	11	28	62.9	3	0.5790	5.1813
6	19	72	59.6	3	1.6037	1.8707
7	20	49	64.2	2	1.5627	1.2798
8	18	53	63.6	2	1.6751	1.1940
9	19	51	61.9	1	1.3195	0.7579
10	18	90	58.6	0	1.9255	0
11	18	61	62.9	3	1.9816	1.5139
12	19	71	61.4	3	1.7742	1.6909
13	19	49	65.3	3	1.5963	1.8793
14	16	66	65.3	2	2.1946	0.9113
15	16	71	64.2	1	2.2970	0.4354
16	16	55	57.6	1	1.1455	0.8737
17	20	77	62.6	0	2.0419	0
18	16	56	67.0	5	1.9203	2.6038
19	20	95	59.7	3	2.2330	1.3435
	327	1162		45	31.6611	

$$\text{ratio} \frac{\text{observed}}{\text{expected}} = \frac{45}{31.6611} = 1.4213$$

[a]Number assigned in order data were received.

followed for the whole duration of the study. In their study, Joseph et al. (8), researchers at Hoffmann-LaRoche, Inc., a major marketer of levodopa, took the conservative action of adjusting the ratio of 1.03 derived from the actual person-years of observation upward by 29% in the Sweet and McDowell manner to 1.33, and thereby avoided presenting results possibly biased in favor of levodopa.

The present study is based solely on the actual person-years of observation. Deaths occurring after discontinuation of Sinemet were not included. Patients lost to follow-up were counted as "observed" only during the time they were followed, and no assumptions were made regarding their fate after that time.

In examining the observed to expected ratios found in the various mortality studies summarized in Table 2, it may be seen that up until the present time no mortality study has examined only patients receiving Sinemet. Four studies examined patients on plain levodopa, and two looked at groups containing some patients on plain levodopa and some on Sinemet or Madopar (levodopa/benserazide). If Barbeau's (1) study of severely akinetic patients is excluded, the plain levodopa studies show a mortality rate substantially the same as that seen in the general population. The mixed studies (some patients receiving plain levodopa, others levodopa plus a peripherally acting decarboxylase inhibitor) show ratios approximately twice normal. The death rates of the levodopa-only and the levodopa-plus-inhibitor patients in these studies are not presented separately, and therefore no conclusions can be drawn. However, one can compare the levodopa-only studies with the present study and note that although both represent a distinct improvement over the prelevodopa 2.9 ratio, greater longevity seems to have been demonstrated on plain levodopa.

The reasons for apparently greater longevity on plain levodopa than on Sinemet are unclear. There are several possible explanations for the findings of the present investigators, who used the same method of mortality analysis on their plain levodopa and on their Sinemet studies. First, the populations studied may have differed in some respects, e.g., extent of disability or duration of disease. (Age is not relevant, as the technique of analysis is age-adjusted, i.e., an older group would have greater numbers of observed and expected deaths, but the ratio would be unaffected.) Data collected from the 19 Sinemet investigators did not include disability measures, so comparison of the whole Sinemet group with a large number of plain levodopa patients is not possible. However, a comparison of the UCLA levodopa and Sinemet groups can be made (Table 3). From these data it would appear that if the UCLA groups differed, it was in the direction of less severe disease in the Sinemet group. It is unknown if the UCLA Sinemet group was typical of the other Sinemet groups, but the UCLA levodopa group was typical in the one comparison the Joseph et al. (8) levodopa study permits: Mean stage of disease of the 1589 patients of Joseph et al. was 3.2 compared to the UCLA mean of 3.1. Criteria of inclusion into the levodopa and Sinemet studies were similar: at least two major manifestations of Parkinson's disease or one major and two minor manifestations. Exclusions

TABLE 2. Ratio of observed to expected deaths in studies of Parkinson patients

Investigators	No. of patients	Levodopa only	Mixed	Levodopa/ carbidopa	Ratio
Diamond et al. (5)	93	x			.97
"	1087	x			1.03
Joseph et al. (8)	1625	x			1.03 (1.33[a])
Barbeau (1)	80[b]	x			2.4
Sweet and McDowell (12)	100		x[c]		1.5 (1.9[a])
Marttila et al. (10)	349		x[d]		1.85
Present study	327			x	1.42

[a] Adjusted ratio. See text for explanation.
[b] Severely akinetic.
[c] Levodopa/carbidopa given to 17 patients; remainder on plain levodopa. Mortality not reported separately.
[d] Levodopa only given to 194 patients; 150 patients on levodopa/benserazide; 5 on levodopa/carbidopa. Mortality not reported separately.

TABLE 3. *Comparison of the UCLA levodopa and Sinemet groups*

	UCLA levodopa	UCLA Sinemet
No. of patients	93	20
Mean age at entry	62	63.9
Duration of disease at entry (years)	10	8.6
Mean initial disability score	121	77
Mean initial stage of disease	3.1	1.6

in both were cancer; cardiac, pulmonary, renal, other neurologic or musculoskeletal disease; or infections.

One possible difference between the UCLA levodopa and Sinemet groups, unmeasured and subjective on the part of the investigators, was a certain persistence and drive in the levodopa group, a pioneer spirit which did not seem evident in the chronologically later Sinemet group. Levodopa was an entirely new form of drug therapy and Sinemet was a variation of an existing drug. Perhaps a psychologically (and/or physically) hardier person was attracted to the earlier study.

Another possibility is that compared to the carbidopa-containing compound, the much higher doses of plain levodopa may favor longevity. This would seem highly unlikely, yet Cotzias et al. (2) found increased longevity in rats fed large amounts of levodopa, with life spans increasing as dosage increased. Human application of this finding has not been shown, and the reasons for the apparently greater longevity of Parkinson patients on plain levodopa remain unknown.

SUMMARY

Nineteen neurologists across the United States who participated in clinical trials of levodopa/carbidopa (Sinemet®) in 1972 to 1974 provided data on 327 randomly specified Parkinson patients representing 1162 person-years of observation. The group studied consisted of 193 men and 134 women, with a mean age of 62.4 years at entry into the Sinemet trials. According to U.S. Life Tables, a group of this age composition drawn from the general population would be expected to show 31.6611 deaths over this period of time. Deaths observed in these patients numbered 45, resulting in a ratio of observed to expected deaths of 1.4213, or 42% higher than normal. Death rates in Parkinson patients prior to levodopa therapy were approximately three times higher than normal, so longevity has greatly increased in recent years. However, studies of mortality in patients receiving plain levodopa apparently show lower ratios of observed to expected deaths than patients receiving 80% less levodopa plus carbidopa.

ACKNOWLEDGMENTS

The authors are grateful to Donald W. Nibbelink, M.D., Director of Clinical Research, Merck Sharp & Dohme, whose unfailing cooperation was essential to this study. We also wish to thank the 19 investigators listed in Appendix 1 who provided data from their own investigational groups.

This study was partially supported by the Scott Trust, the Roselynn Foundation, and the Research Society for Parkinson's Disease and Movement Disorders, Inc.

APPENDIX

Clinical Investigators Providing Data on Mortality Study of Sinemet[1]

Nicholas A. Bercel, M.D.
Beverly-Sunset Medical Center
Los Angeles, CA 90069

Stanley Fahn, M.D.
Neurological Institute of New York
New York, NY 10032

Melvin Greer, M.D.
University of Florida
Gainesville, FL 32610

Geraldine King, M.D.
University of Pennsylvania
Philadelphia, PA 19104

Myoung Chong Lee, M.D.
University of Minnesota
Minneapolis, MN 55455

Abraham Lieberman, M.D.
New York University Medical Center
New York, NY 10016

Charles H. Markham, M.D.
University of California
Los Angeles, CA 90024

Harold Mars, M.D.
Case-Western Reserve University
Cleveland, OH 44106

Fletcher McDowell, M.D.
Cornell Medical College
New York, NY 10021

Robert J. Mones, M.D.
New York, NY 10029

Manfred D. Muenter, M.D.
Mayo Clinic
Rochester, MN 55901

Larry A. Pearce, M.D.
Wake Forest University
Winston-Salem, NC 27103

Henry Peters, M.D.
University of Wisconsin
Madison, WI 53704

Thomas J. Preziosi, M.D.
The Johns Hopkins Hospital
Baltimore, MD 21205

Stanley Stellar, M.D.
St. Barnabas Medical Center
Livingston, NJ 07039

Richard A. Thompson, M.D.
Barrow Neurological Institute
Phoenix, AZ 85013

Alice H. Wilson, M.D.
Freeman Hospital
Joplin, MO 64801

Robert Young, M.D.
Massachusetts General Hospital
Boston, MA 02114

Arthur W. Yount, M.D.
Medical Arts Building
North Palm Beach, FL 33408

---

[1] Addresses in effect at time studies were initiated.

REFERENCES

1. Barbeau, A. (1976): Six years of high-level levodopa therapy in severely akinetic parkinsonian patients. *Arch. Neurol.,* 33:333–338.
2. Cotzias, G. C., Miller, S. T., Tang, L. C., Papavasiliou, P. S., and Wang, Y. Y. (1977): Levodopa, fertility, and longevity. *Science,* 196:549–550.
3. Cotzias, G. C., Papavasiliou, P. S., and Gellene, R. (1969): Modification of parkinsonism: Chronic treatment with L-dopa. *N. Engl. J. Med.,* 280:337–345.
4. Diamond, S. G., and Markham, C. H. (1976): Present mortality in Parkinson's disease: The ratio of observed to expected deaths with a method to calculate expected deaths. *J. Neural Transmiss.,* 38:259–269.
5. Diamond, S. G., Markham, C. H., and Treciokas, L. J. (1976): Long-term experience with L-dopa: Efficacy, progression and mortality. In: *Advances in Parkinsonism,* edited by W. Birkmayer and O. Hornykiewicz. Fifth International Symposium on Parkinson's Disease, Vienna, 1975. Editions Roche, Basel.
6. Diamond, S. G., Markham, C. H., and Treciokas, L. J. (1978): A double-blind comparison of levodopa, Madopa, and Sinemet in Parkinson's disease. *Ann. Neurol.,* 3:267–272.
7. Hoehn, N. M., and Yahr, M. K (1967): Parkinsonism: Onset, progression and mortality. *Neurology (Minneap.),* 17:427–442.
8. Joseph, C., Chassan, J. B., and Koch, M-L. (1978): Levodopa in Parkinson disease: A longterm appraisal of mortality. *Ann. Neurol.,* 3:116–118.
9. Markham, C. H., Diamond, S. G., and Treciokas, L. J. (1974): Carbidopa in Parkinson disease and in nausea and vomiting of levodopa. *Arch. Neurol.,* 31:128–133.
10. Marttila, R. J., Rinne, U. K., Siirtola, T., and Sonninen, V. (1977): Mortality of patients with Parkinson's disease treated with levodopa. *J. Neurol.,* 216:147–153.
11. McDowell, F., Lee, J. E., Swift, T., Sweet, R. D., Ogsbury, J. S., and Kessler, J. T. (1970): Treatment of Parkinson's syndrome with 1-dihydroxyphenylalanine (levodopa). *Ann. Intern. Med.,* 72:29–35.
12. Sweet, R. D., and McDowell, F. H. (1975): Five years' treatment of Parkinson's disease with levodopa: Therapeutic results and survival of 100 patients. *Ann. Intern. Med.,* 83:456–463.
13. Treciokas, L. J., Ansel, R. D., and Markham, C. H. (1971): One to two year treatment of Parkinson's disease with levodopa. *Calif. Med.,* 114:7–14.
14. Zumstein, H., and Siegfried, J. (1976): Mortality among Parkinson patients treated with L-dopa combined with a decarboxylase inhibitor. *Eur. Neurol.,* 14:321–327.

Advances in Neurology, Vol. 24, edited by
L. J. Poirier, T. L. Sourkes, and P. J. Bédard.
Raven Press, New York © 1979.

Neuropharmacological Principles and Problems of Combined L-DOPA Treatment in Parkinson's Disease

*W. Birkmayer, **P. Riederer, and **W. D. Rausch

*Evangelisches Krankenhaus, A-1090, Vienna, Austria; and **L. Boltzmann Institute of Clinical Neurobiology, Lainz-Hospital, A-1130, Vienna, Austria

Parkinson's disease is characterized by a degeneration of the dopamine-containing neurons of the striatum. In general, patients with this disease respond well to the therapeutic administration of the dopamine precursor L-DOPA. The efficiency of L-DOPA therapy is dependent on the availability of L-DOPA in the plasma and on its conversion to dopamine in the cerebral dopaminergic neurons (4). Plasma L-DOPA concentrations may be further increased by combining peripherally acting aromatic amino acid decarboxylase inhibitors with L-DOPA medication (7). Clinical experience has demonstrated that a high L-DOPA medication leads to a rapid progression of the degeneration of the nigrostriatal dopaminergic system, the consequence of which is an earlier appearance of side-effects (13).

Table 1 shows the percentage improvement in parkinsonian patients treated with the combined therapy (L-DOPA plus the peripherally acting decarboxylase inhibitor benserazide) and its dependence on the duration of combined treatment. Results were obtained over the past 15 years. The disability score was established according to rating scale of Birkmayer and Neumayer (9). It is remarkable that the percentage improvement has not changed since the first report (6). We find that 21.5% of the 1414 patients are nonresponders (≤20% improvement in disability), 61.0% have responded well (30–40% improvement), and 17.5% show a very good improvement (50–60% improvement).

Table 2 summarizes the various side-effects in these parkinsonian in patients during L-DOPA/benserazide (Madopar®) treatment. In agreement with other reports (1,9,13,14,16,18), abnormal involuntary movements (AIM), dyskinesias, "on–off" effects and toxic delirium are the most frequent side-effects. It is evident that AIM, which are suffered by 18.5% of patients, are more frequent in the early stage of the disease than in the advanced stage. A reduction of L-DOPA dosage is generally not sufficient to overcome AIM. To restore the balance between the dopaminergic and cholinergic systems, it would seem that stimulation of the cholinergic activity might be useful; however, treatment of such

TABLE 1. *Percentage improvement of disability in Parkinson's disease after long-term L-DOPA/ benserazide treatment*

Duration of medication (years)	1	3	5	7	9	11	13	15	Total
Number of cases per year	147	455	315	210	210	42	21	14	1414 (100%)
Percentage improvement of disability									
10%	3%	0.5%						0.5%	4.0%
20%	5%	6%	4.5%	1.5%				0.5%	17.5%
30%	2%	12.0%	6%	3%	3.5%	0.5%			27.0%
40%	0.5%	8%	6.5%	7.5%	9.0%	1.5%	1%		34.0%
50%		3.5%	3.5%	2.5%	2%	1%	0.5%		13.0%
60%		1.5%	2%	0.5%	0.5%				4.5%

Medication was between 125 mg and 250 mg L-DOPA/benserazide, three times daily.

The functional disability score (9) for each patient consisted of ten different parameters: gait, pushing, jumping, speed, writing, associative movements, posture, mimic, start and self-care. A complete disability in a particular function is given ten points and normal function is rated one point. A disability score of ten is equivalent to normal healthy subjects and a disability score of 100 is equivalent to the last stage of Parkinson's disease, when the patient is completely akinetic. This disability rating scale especially takes into consideration the "motor behavior" of the patients. Besides these ratings, the depressed phases, toxic delirium, and other mental side-effects, occasionally occurring during treatment have been registered according to neurological practice.

patients with infusions of the acetylcholine precursor choline (2 g) or with deanol (Deaner®, 3 × 100 mg/day) has not given satisfactory results. In another clinical trial, infusions of taurine were given, but this therapy was also unsuccessful. Although taurine induces motor sedation, it sometimes produces orthostatic hypotension, which limits its application as a treatment for AIM. It is commonly observed that emotional stress induces AIM as well as sustained tremor. Treatment with propranolol (Trasicor®, 3 × 20 mg/day), a blocker of norepinephrergic receptors, leads to a decrease in tremor but not in AIM, thus indicating a relationship between the occurrence of tremor and the norepinephrergic system. Abnormal involuntary movements seem not to be related to norepinephrergic activity.

Another side-effect (19.0% of patients) is the occurrence of toxic delirium. After the initial symptoms of sleeplessness, vivid dreams, nightmares, and anxiety, there appear confusion, hallucinations, and delusions. In the latter stage, an increase of 5-hydroxyindol-3-acetic acid could be observed in the CSF and in postmortem brains (5). Depletion of serotonin by dopamine being synthesized in excess in serotoninergic neurons seems to be responsible for this result (2,20). Administration of L-tryptophan (3 × 500 mg/day) (8) has improved the condition of these patients, presumably by restoring the biochemical balance between the serotoninergic and dopaminergic systems, since a reduction of 5-HIAA could be observed in the CSF of these patients after recovery (15.5% of the patients recovered with L-tryptophan) (3). Competition between L-DOPA and L-trypto-

TABLE 2. *Occurrence of side-effects of L-DOPA benserazide therapy in the course of Parkinson's disease*

Duration of L-DOPA medication (years)	1	3	5	7	9	11	13	15	% Total
Number of cases per year	147	455	315	210	210	42	21	14	
Side effects (%)									
gastrointestinal		1.5			1				2.5
cardiac		2	2.0	1	1.0				6.0
orthostatic hypotension			3.0	3.0	1.0				7.0
dizziness	0.5	1	2	1	1	0.5			6
AIM		2.5	4	6.5	4.5	1			18.5
sleeplessness		1.5	2.5	1.5	2	1			8.5
depression	2.0	7.5	3		3.0	0.5			16.0
toxic delirium recovery by L-tryptophan		4	5.5	3.5	2		0.5		15.5
nonresponders		1	1.5	0.5	0.5				3.5
"on–off" phenomena		1	2.5	4	1				8.5
cramps		1	2.0	2.0	2.0	1.0			8.0

phan at the blood-brain barrier as well as at the level of neuronal membranes is assumed to be responsible for the observed effects (2,20–22).

Clinical experience demonstrates that there are two different syndromes of confusion as a component of toxic delirium:

1. Agitated confusion: This type is associated with an increase in motor behavior. L-Tryptophan (3 × 500 mg/day) or 5-hydroxytryptophan (50 mg i.v.) are able to overcome this side-effect in a high percentage (82%) of the cases.

2. Retarded confusion: Patients are quiet, but disoriented. In senile dementia we find this type frequently. In such patients, L-tryptophan does not improve behavior.

Toxic delirium resulting from L-DOPA therapy responds to a high degree to L-tryptophan therapy; 15.5% of the group of our patients with agitated confusion recovered, while only 3.5% of the group with retarded confusion did not respond. In the latter patients, L-DOPA treatment had to be discontinued. It should be mentioned that L-DOPA treatment was continued in patients who responded to L-tryptophan.

Depression (15% of our patients) is another side-effect encountered during L-DOPA therapy. There is good agreement that reduced activity of the serotoninergic system is one component of the unipolar depression syndrome, as shown by postmortem brain analysis (10,23, review ref. 14). However, it could be demonstrated that in such patients, dopamine also drops to about 20 to 30%

in the striatal regions, the red nucleus, and nucleus accumbens. Concentrations of norepinephrine were not significantly different from those in normal controls, except in the red nucleus. Free 3-methoxy-4-hydroxyphenylglycol (MHPG), the presumed main metabolite of brain norepinephrine, showed a different pattern in the brain areas where it was determined; i.e., MHPG was normal in the striatum, thalamus, nucleus ruber, nucleus amygdalae, gyrus cinguli and gyrus dentatus, but decreased in the globus pallidus, hypothalamus, corpus mamillare, substantia nigra, raphe, and nucleus accumbens (25).

L-DOPA treatment seems to be responsible for this imbalance of neurotransmitter systems in parkinsonian patients (28). As the nigrostriatal dopaminergic system degenerates and the storage capacity for dopamine is progressively lost in the course of the disease, it may be that extrastriatal areas are involved in the depressed phases. The administration of antidepressive drugs is efficient in nearly all such cases. Therefore, about 80% of the parkinsonian patients are administered antidepressant drugs prophylactically. In addition, some of these drugs, such as nomifensine, improve the therapeutic action of L-DOPA by well-known pharmacological mechanisms (see review ref. 12).

A major problem in the long-term treatment of Parkinson's disease is the occurrence of the "on–off" phenomena, which correspond to fluctuations in response to L-DOPA. They occur every few hours.

Common experience has demonstrated that in Parkinson's disease the improvement in the disability score after L-DOPA, Madopar® (L-DOPA/benserazide) or L-DOPA/carbidopa (Sinemet®) treatment decreases as the disease progresses (1,13,14,16,18). Moreover, in the course of a recent study (W. Birkmayer, P. Riederer, and M. B. H. Youdim, *in preparation*) a distinction between a benign and malignant type of Morbus Parkinson could be disclosed. It could be shown (Table 3) that in malignant patients, akinetic crises, "off" phases, and toxic delirium occur more frequently during a combined treatment with L-DOPA and a peripherally acting decarboxylase inhibitor than in the benign patients. High dosage of L-DOPA induced "off" phases in some patients. In addition, this side-effect occurs sooner after the onset of the disease (10a). However, hyperkinesia was significantly reduced in the malignant group. There seems to be a correlation between the onset of the above-mentioned side-effects and the progression of the disease, as the duration of Parkinson's disease was also significantly reduced in the malignant group.

In early stages of the disease, the addition of L-deprenyl (Jumex®) (5 to 10 mg/day) to L-DOPA therapy (i.v., alone, or orally, combined with a peripherally acting decarboxylase inhibitor, benserazide or carbidopa) is generally efficient and prevents "off" phases (see review 11). In terminal patients, the best therapy is to discontinue L-DOPA medication. Bromocriptine (3 × 2 mg/day) or 1-amino-adamantane sulfate (AS) infusions (PK Merz, 1 × 500 ml/day = 0.2 g AS) occasionally improves the kinetic behavior of such patients. Therefore, bromocriptine and AS are good adjuvant therapies in terminal stages of the disease.

TABLE 3. Clinical data characterizing different types of idiopathic parkinsonism and the occurrence of side-effects in parkinsonians after the start of L-DOPA/benserazide treatment (years)

Clinical parameter	I Benign type (39)	% of group	II Benign type (10)	% of group	Malignant type (20)	% of group
age (years)	63.85 ± 1.38		77.7 ± 1.22		71.4 ± 1.19[a]	
sex	17F, 22M		5F, 5M		12F, 8M	
age at onset of parkinsonism	56.7 ± 1.25		67.0 ± 1.63		68.0 ± 1.11[b]	
duration of parkinsonism (years)	12.51 ± 0.44		12.7 ± 0.45		4.0 ± 0.28[b,c]	
Side effects						
akinetic crises	5.5 ± 0.51 (14)	36%	10 ± 1.0 (3)	30%	3.20 ± 0.28 (14)[d]	70%
"off" phases	5.3 ± 0.56 (17)	44%	9.6 ± 0.74 (5)	50%	2.70 ± 0.20 (11)[d]	55%
hyperkinesia	4.1 ± 0.30 (22)	56%	10.6 ± 0.87 (5)	50%	2.50 ± 0.5 (2)[d]	10%
toxic delirium (L-DOPA-psychosis)	4.4 ± 0.70 (8)	21%	5.3 ± 0.6 (3)	30%	2.60 ± 0.37 (13)[d]	65%

Number of patients in parenthesis.
Means = SEM; Student's t-test.
Treatment with L-DOPA/benserazide (3 × 250 mg daily): benign type, 12.51 ± 0.44 years (group I) and 11.6 ± 0.6 years (group II); malignant group, 4.0 ± 0.28 years.
Rating of disability according to (9) and Table 1. Data are taken from (1).

[a] $p < 0.01$ when compared to I.
[b] $p < 0.001$ when compared to I.
[c] $p < 0.001$ when compared to II.
[d] $p < 0.01$ when compared to both groups of benign cases.

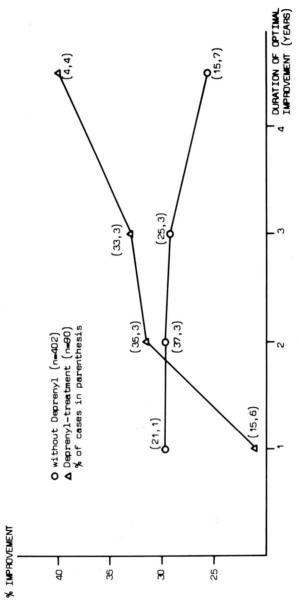

FIG. 1. Duration of optimal improvement of disability in Parkinson's disease with Madopar® plus L-deprenyl treatment. Daily oral Madopar® dosage: 3 × 250 mg. Daily oral dosage of Madopa® plus L-deprenyl: 3 × 250 mg Madopar® plus 1 × 10 mg L-deprenyl.

"Off" phases, which are generally reported by outpatients and last for about 1 to 3 hr, are characterized by an akinetic phase followed by a very rapid recovery, with even an increased ability to move. This effect can also be observed in the absence of any effect of the drugs. Therefore, enzymatic exhaustion (of tyrosine hydroxylase and/or aromatic amino acid decarboxylase) or insensitivity of dopaminergic receptors appears to be responsible for this time-dependent akinetic phase. As mentioned above, "off" phases can generally be prevented by administering L-deprenyl (see review 11).

Figure 1 shows that the addition of L-deprenyl to Madopar® treatment leads to a gradual improvement of the patient's disability, whereas L-DOPA/benserazide treatment alone is less efficient with time. It is shown (Fig. 2) that Madopar® treatment alone improves patient disability in the order of 33% within the first 8 years after onset of the disease. However, when the same patients were given in addition L-deprenyl for the next 3 years, the average improvement increased to 42%. Combined therapy with L-deprenyl permits the use of a lower dosage of Madopar® with the same or even better effect than with Madopar® alone. In our opinion, it is very important to be able to decrease L-DOPA dosage during the long-term treatment, as an increase of L-DOPA supply (together with the degeneration of the nigrostriatal system) causes side-effects such as toxic delirium or AIM. Clinical experience shows that the earlier the side-effects ("on–off" effects, toxic delirium) are observed, the more malignant is the progress of the disease (10a).

The fluctuation in patients' disability, as indicated by AIM, hyperkinesia, "on–off" effect, or akinetic crisis, as well as the occurrence of toxic delirium or depressed phases are triggered by the imbalanced neurotransmission due to the degenerative process (9,11). Therefore, it was of some interest to look at the activity of the key enzymes tyrosine hydroxylase (TH) and adenylate cyclase (AC), as well as at the dopamine-induced stimulation of the latter system.

Tyrosine hydroxylase and cyclic AMP have been determined in various regions of human postmortem brains according to standard methods (15,19). The brain dissection techniques have been reported elsewhere (28). Tyrosine hydroxylase activity has been shown to be decreased in the striatum of parkinsonian patients (17). However, evidence is lacking regarding the dopamine-sensitive AC. This system seems to be associated with the dopamine receptor (15). Cyclic AMP has been reported to be the mediator for the physiological effects of dopamine (DA). Therefore, TH and cyclic AMP have been determined in postmortem brains of parkinsonian patients, and the effect of drug treatment on these substances has been assessed. In addition, the determination of TH activity in the adrenal gland could provide evidence for a generally disturbed function and/or synthesis of TH in the disease.

The rate-limiting enzyme in the biochemical pathway, TH, is reduced by more than 80% in the nigrostriatal system, which reflects the degeneration of the presynaptic dopaminergic neurons (Table 4). In addition, it is shown for the first time that TH is decreased also in the adrenal gland, a finding that is

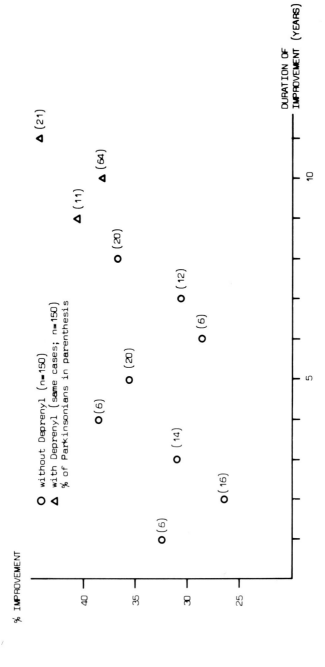

FIG. 2. Duration of optimal improvement of disability in Parkinson's disease after 8 years treatment with oral Madopar® (3 × 250 mg daily) and subsequent supplement with oral L-deprenyl (1 × 10 mg daily).

TABLE 4. *Tyrosine hydroxylase activity in postmortem human tissue. Tyrosine hydroxylase has been determined in various regions of human postmortem brains according to appropriate methods (9,19)*

	No. of subjects	Normal subjects	Parkinsonian patients			
			P1	P2	P3	P4
Brain areas						
caudate nucleus	15	27.8 ± 2.3	4.0	4.9	6.9	1.5
putamen	5	16.2 ± 5.9	0.6	2.4	1.2	NE
substantia nigra	4	19.4 ± 6.2	1.7	7.6	NE	NE
locus ceruleus	4	3.3 ± 0.1	NE	2.0	NE	NE
nucleus ruber	5	5.7 ± 1.9	0.8	4.9	NE	NE
raphe + reticular formation	2	0.4	1.0	1.8	2.4	0.8
hypothalamus	5	3.1 ± 1.0	1.1	2.4	NE	NE
corpus mamillare	5	0.6 ± 0.4	NE	0.5	NE	NE
nucleus accumbens	5	2.0 ± 0.7	0.9	ND	7.1	NE
Adrenal gland (medulla)	5	186.2 ± 5.5	31.8	86.3	41.6	39.2

Hours postmortem: Control subjects, 3.6 ± 0.4; parkinsonian subjects, 2.7 ± 0.3.
Values are given in nmoles DOPA/h.g
Age: Control subjects, 68.4 ± 2.8 years; parkinson subjects, 75.3 ± 2.3 years.
Mean ± SEM.
NE, not estimated; ND, not detectable.

consistent with the suggestion that a general disturbance of TH activity takes place in Parkinson's disease (24). Cyclic AMP was not changed in parkinsonian patients who died in the course of bronchopneumonia or heart failure (group A), but its level tended to be lower in patients who died following long-lasting akinetic crises (group B). Stimulation of cyclic AMP by 100 μM dopamine in group A showed a significant increase above basal levels, but this stimulation of cyclic AMP production was significantly less pronounced than in the controls. The AC system was not stimulated at all by 100 μM dopamine in parkinsonian patients with therapy-resistant akinetic crises (Fig. 3, Table 5). Long-term drug treatment failed to alter the ability of DA to stimulate cyclic AMP production. These findings indicate also a disturbance of the postsynaptic neuronal activity in Parkinson's disease. Evidence from the results in Fig. 3 indicates that in the final stage of Parkinson's disease, AC is stimulated only by very low doses of DA and is inhibited by higher doses. This effect seems to have clinical importance regarding the "off" phenomenon, which is exaggerated by high doses of L-DOPA or L-DOPA/benserazide.

Recent studies demonstrate the presence of a second dopaminergic receptor in the striatum, which seems to be unrelated to the AC system (28). In this case, it can be assumed that a complete loss in the DA stimulation of the cyclic-AMP-dependent dopaminergic receptor need not be accompanied by complete akinesia if the cyclic-AMP-independent dopaminergic receptor is intact. Unfortunately, clinical experience demonstrates that in the end stage of

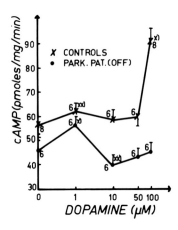

FIG. 3. Stimulation of adenylate cyclase by dopamine in the caudate nucleus. $^{a}p < 0.01$. $^{b}p < 0.05$ compared to basal level, means in pmoles/mg. protein/min $\pm$ S.E.M. number of experiments Brain material was taken from postmortem parkinsonian patients (group B, therapy-resistant akinetic crises; see legend to Table 5).

Parkinson's disease, the patient's disability cannot be changed by drug treatment, thus indicating a functional loss of sensitivity also in this axonic cyclic-AMP-independent dopaminergic receptor (26).

These results do not support the theory of denervation supersensitivity. However, denervation of the presynaptic dopaminergic system in the nigrostriatal tract may lead to a supersensitivity of the extrastriatal dopaminergic systems,

TABLE 5. *Stimulation of adenylate cyclase in the caudate nucleus by dopamine (DA) dependence on drug treatment*

	Cyclic AMP (pmoles/mg/min)	
	Basal level	Dopamine stimulated (100 μM)
Controls (7)	54.2 ± 7.3	90.3 ± 16.5 [a]
Liver cirrhosis (5)	65.1 ± 13.8	45.2 ± 8.9
Carcinoma (4)	47.9 ± 12.9	33.7 ± 11.6
Parkinson's disease		
group A: kinetic patients (4)	53.4 ± 5.3	73.6 ± 4.3 [a,b]
nomifensine (2)	54.2	65.3
group B: therapy-resistant		
akinetic crisis (8)	46.7 ± 11.9	44.3 ± 8.6 [c]
L-DOPA/benserazide (6)	79.9 ± 13.9	57.8 ± 10.9
(—)deprenyl (6)	61.7 ± 14.9	47.9 ± 9.2
2-bromoergocryptine (4)	76.6 ± 3.3	65.3 ± 10.6
1-aminoadamantane (5)	78.5 ± 10.6	61.4 ± 9.2
clomipramine (4)	69.3 ± 8.3	52.1 ± 8.9
anticholinergics (3)	47.2 ± 6.4	33.0 ± 9.9

No. of patients in parentheses.
[a] $p < 0.01$ comp. to basal levels.
[b] $p < 0.01$ comp. to controls (100 μM DA).
[c] $p < 0.01$ comp. to kinetic parkinsonian patients (100 μM DA).

and this effect could be related to the "L-DOPA psychosis" in which mesolimbic, limbic, and some brainstem areas seem to be involved.

ACKNOWLEDGMENTS

We are grateful to Österreichische Nationalbank for supporting our work by research grant project 1113.

Wolf-Dieter Rausch is the recipient of a HOECHST fellowship.

We thank Dr. G. P. Reynolds for his help during the preparation of this manuscript and Dr. Elisabeth Handerek for secretarial work.

REFERENCES

1. Barbeau, A. (1973): Treatment of Parkinson's disease with levodopa and Ro 4–4602: Review and present status. *Adv.' Neurol.,* 2:173–198.
2. Bartholini, G., Da Prada, M., and Pletscher, A. (1968): Decrease of cerebral 5-hydroxytryptamine by 3,4-dihydroxyphenylalanine after inhibition of extracerebral decarboxylase. *J. Pharm. Pharmacol.,* 20:228–229.
3. Birkmayer, W., Danielczyk, W., Neumayer, E., and Riederer, P. (1972): The biochemical aspects of behaviour. In: *Parkinson's Disease, Vol. 1,* edited by J. Siegfried, pp. 176–185. Hans Huber, Bern, Stuttgart, Wien.
4. Birkmayer, W., Danielczyk, W., Neumayer, E., and Riederer, P. 1973): L-Dopa level in plasma, Primary condition for the kinetic effect. *J. Neural Transm.,* 34:133–143.
5. Birkmayer, W., Danielczyk, W., Neumayer, E., and Riederer, P. (1974): Nucleus ruber and L-dopa psychosis, Biochemical post mortem findings. *J. Neural Transm.,* 35:93–116.
6. Birkmayer, W., and Hornykiewicz, W. (1961): Der L-Dioxyphenylalanin (L-Dopa) Effekt bei der Parkinson Akinese. *Wien. Klin. Wochenschr.,* 73:787–788.
7. Birkmayer, W., and Mentasti, M. (1967): Weitere experimentelle Untersuchungen über den Catecholaminstoffwechsel bei extrapyramidalen Erkrankungen. *Arch. Psychiatr. Nervenkr.,* 210:29–35.
8. Birkmayer, W., and Neumayer, E. (1972): Die Behandlung der Dopa-Psychosen mit L-Tryptophen. *Nervenarzt,* 43:76–78.
9. Birkmayer, W., and Neumayer, E. (1972): Die moderne medikamentöse Behandlung des Parkinsonismus. *Z. Neurol.,* 202:257–280.
10. Birkmayer, W., and Riederer, P. (1975): Biochemical post mortem findings in depressed patients. *J. Neural Transm.,* 37:95–109.
10a. Birkmayer, W., Riederer, P. and Youdim, M. B. H. (1979): *(in preparation).*
11. Birkmayer, W., and Yahr, M. (1978): Deprenyl, an inhibitor of MAO-Type B in the treatment of parkinsonism. *J. Neural Transm.,* 43:177–286.
12. Carlsson, A., and Lindquist, M. (1978): Effects of antidepressant agents on the synthesis of brain monoamines. *J. Neural Transm.,* 43:73–91.
13. Cotzias, G. C. (1971): Levodopa in the treatment of parkinsonism. *J.A.M.A.,* 218:1903–1908.
14. Diamond, S. G., Markham, C. H., and Treciokas, L. (1976): Long term experience with L-dopa: Efficacy, progression and mortality. In: *Advances in Parkinsonism,* edited by W. Birkmayer and O. Hornykiewicz, pp. 444–455. Editiones Roche, Basel.
15. Kebabian, J. W., Petzold, G. L., and Greengard, P. (1972): Dopamine sensitive adenylate cyclase in the caudate nucleus of rat brain and its similarity to the "dopamine receptor." *Proc. Natl. Acad. Sci. (USA),* 69:2145–2149.
16. Liebermann, A., Goodgold, A., Jonas, S., and Leibowitz, M. (1975): Comparison of dopa decarboxylase inhibitor (carbidopa) combined with levodopa and levodopa alone in Parkinson's disease. *Neurology (Minneap.),* 25:911–916.
17. Lloyd, K. G., Davidson, L., and Hornykiewicz, O. (1975): The neurochemistry of Parkinson's disease: Effect of L-dopa therapy. *J. Pharmacol. Exp. Ther.,* 195:453–464.
18. Ludin, H. P., and Bass-Vervey, F. (1976): Study of deterioration in long term treatment of parkinsonism with L-dopa plus decarboxylase inhibitor. *J. Neural Transm.,* 38:249–258.

19. McGeer, E. G., Gibson, S., and McGeer, P. L. (1967): Some characteristics of brain tyrosine-hydroxylase. *Can. J. Biochem.,* 45:1557–1563.
20. Ng, K. Y., Chase, T. N., Colburn, R. W., Kopin, I. J. (1970): L-Dopa-induced release of cerebral monoamines. *Science,* 170:76–77.
21. Riederer, P. (1978): Amino acid competition and ammonia detoxification by L-dopa and L-valine during oral and parenteral nutrition. *Nutr. Metab. (in press).*
22. Riederer, P. (1978): Regional brain studies on indoles and tyrosine in Mongolian gerbils during nutrition with artificial mixtures high in branched chain amino acids compared to a protein rich diet. *Z. Ernaehrungswiss. (in press).*
23. Riederer, P., Birkmayer, W., Neumayer, E., Ambrozi, L., and Linauer, W. (1974): The daily rhythm of HVA, VMA, (VA) and 5-HIAA in depression syndrome. *J. Neural Transm.,* 35:23–45.
24. Riederer, P., Birkmayer, W., Rausch, W. D., Jellinger, K., and Seemann, D. (1978): CNS modulation of adrenal tyrosine hydroxylase in Parkinson's disease and metabolic encephalopathies. *J. Neural Transm. (Suppl. 14),* 121–131.
25. Reiderer, P., Birkmayer, W., Seemann, D., and Wuketich, S. (1979): Brain noradrenaline turnover, as measured using MHPG in endogenous depressed patients. *Acta Psychiatr. Scand. (in press).*
26. Riederer, P., Rausch, W. D., Birkmayer, W., Jellinger, K., and Danielczyk, W. (1978): Dopamine-sensitive adenylate cyclase activity in the caudate nucleus and adrenal medulla in Parkinson's disease and in liver cirrhosis. *J. Neural Transm. (Suppl. 14):* 153–161.
27. Riederer, P., and Wuketich, S. (1976): Time course of nigrostriatal degeneration in Parkinson's disease. *J. Neural Transm.,* 38:277–301.
28. Rossum, J. M. van (1978): Two types of dopamine receptors in behavioral regulation. *Fed. Proc.,* 37:2415–2421.

Advances in Neurology, Vol. 24, edited by
L. J. Poirier, T. L. Sourkes, and P. J. Bédard.
Raven Press, New York © 1979.

Effect of Long-Term Treatment with L-DOPA on Dopamine Receptors in the Striatum and Pituitary

P. Rondot, J. L. Ribadeau Dumas, and M. Ziegler

Service de Neurologie, Centre Hospitalier Sainte-Anne, 75014 Paris, France

The long-term treatment of Parkinson's disease is complicated by two major secondary effects: disorder movements and efficiency fluctuations (1,13,16). Does the occurrence of these secondary effects involve phenomena related to important variations of exogenous L-DOPA? Certain authors have shown that there is a correlation between plasma levels and the time of appearance of the phenomena (5,6,11). Or does it concern modification in the response of dopamine receptors? It is more difficult to answer this question, since there is no way of testing receptor sensitivity. However, it is relatively easy to assess the influence of L-DOPA on infundibulum–hypothalamus receptors. It stimulates growth hormone (GH) and inhibits prolactin (PRL) release (2,3,7,15).

Since the dopamine receptors in the striatum seem to be related to the parkinsonian phenomena, it might be enlightening to compare the effects of L-DOPA on symptoms of this disease with the effect of L-DOPA on the secretion of PRL and GH. Both hormones are under catecholamine control: Tuberoinfundibular dopamine inhibits the former, norepinephrine seems to stimulate the latter. In both cases, the L-DOPA plasma levels are used to determine L-DOPA absorption by the blood.

METHODS

This study was carried out on 12 parkinsonians treated during an average period of 6 years (from 2 to 9 years). The average duration of the disease was 8 years.

Therapeutic and side-effects were observed each day, and included: (a) degree of improvement; and (b) occurrence of disorder movements, i.e., middle-of-dose disorder movements and biphasic or start- and end-of-dose disorder movements (8,10). Both types of disorders have been studied clinically and electrophysiologically. Therefore, the fluctuations of the phenomena can be very clearly individualized according to their relation to the time of administration of the drug (13 and Fig. 1).

akinesia

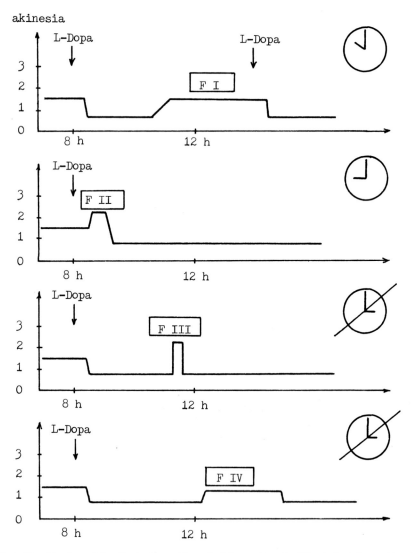

FIG. 1. Classification of the fluctuations. FI: end-of-dose akinesia; FII: start of dose akinesia; FIII: paroxystic akinesia; FIV: circadian akinesia.

Plasma L-DOPA was assayed according to the method of Sharpless et al. (14) modified (17). Blood samples were taken at regular intervals, every 30 min at the start, then hourly for 3 hr after administration of the drug (100 to 200 mg L-DOPA + 25 to 30 mg benserazide, a decarboxylase inhibitor). Growth hormone and PRL plasma levels were assessed in 7 patients by sampling every 30 min at the start, then hourly for the next 3 hr following L-DOPA administration. A radioimmunological assay was used for the determination of GH and PRL. Besides these systematic examinations, dopamine receptors were stimulated during periods where therapeutic efficiency was weak or absent. Stimulation was induced either by subcutaneous injection of 10 mg apomorphine or by slow i.v. injection of piribedil (1 ml = 0.03 g/ml).

RESULTS

Striatal Receptors

Nine of 12 patients showed a close relationship between the response of striatal receptors and the L-DOPA plasma levels (Fig. 2). Disorder movements showed the same clinical type, same localization, and same electrophysiological pattern (Rondot, Bathien, Thomas, *this volume*) in a given patient regardless of the time of appearance of the phenomena after L-DOPA. The appearance corresponded either to high plasma L-DOPA levels (2 cases), or to important variations in the L-DOPA level (7 cases). During the low-efficiency periods of treatment, disorder movements could be produced by stimulating the dopamine receptors. Both apomorphine and piribedil induced the movements without affecting the mode of appearance (middle-of-dose or biphasic disorder movements), but both shortened the time interval.

The results lead to the following comments. The striatal response to dopaminergic stimulation is remarkably steady in each patient whatever the dopaminergic agonist used (Fig. 3). Disorder movements are probably not due to a L-DOPA metabolite—for example 3-*O*-methyldopa—as they are identical whether they follow an L-DOPA injection or a drug directly stimulating the receptors. The variation of the level rather than the level itself seems to determine the time of appearance of disorder movements. These may be regarded as a consequence of plasma L-DOPA with respect to time (Fig. 4): Middle-of-dose disorder movements correspond to the first derivative of L-DOPA level biphasic disorder movements correspond to the second derivative, which suggests that the two phenomena are independent.

Are two types of receptors involved? Some might be sensitive to the amount of L-DOPA, resulting in the suppression of akinesia; others might be sensitive to the L-DOPA variation, causing movement disorders, especially when clinical and electrophysiological phenomena correspond.

Receptors Controlling GH and PRL Secretion

Several modes of reactions have been observed (Fig. 5): (a) Normal (or regular) response (2 cases). Prolactin release decreases, GH release increases, and in parallel the striatal response is satisfactory. (b) Paradoxical response (3 cases). While the striatal response is good, the PRL level is increased and the GH level decreases. (c) Dissociated response (1 case). Prolactin is inhibited as ex-

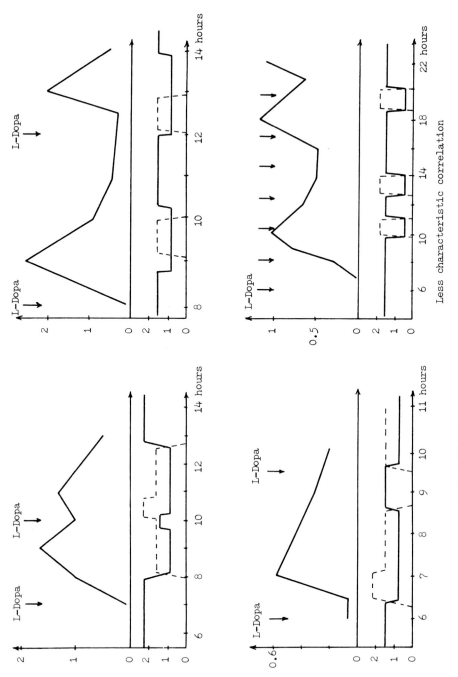

FIG. 2. Clinical responses and L-DOPA plasma level correlations.

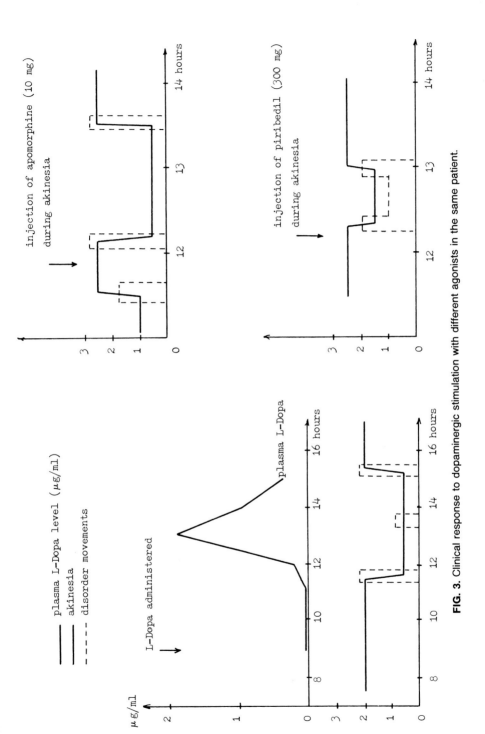

FIG. 3. Clinical response to dopaminergic stimulation with different agonists in the same patient.

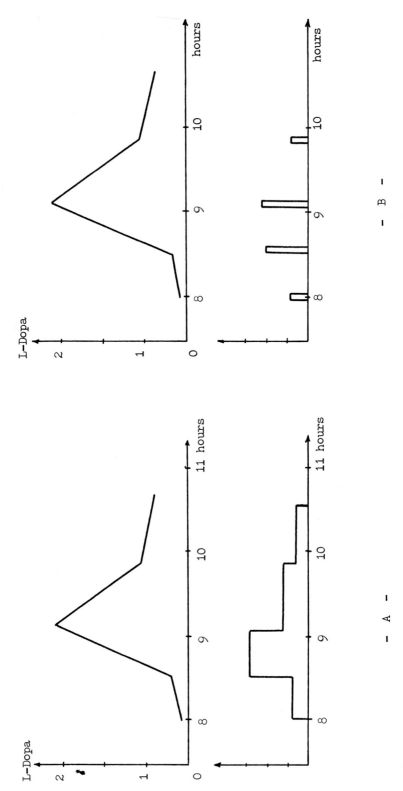

FIG. 4. Middle-of-dose and biphasic disorder movements correlated with ʟ-DOPA plasma levels. These movements may appear as a derived function of the plasma level of ʟ-DOPA varying with time. **A:** Primary derived function recalls the aspect of middle-of-dose disorder movements. **B:** Secondary derived function recalls the aspect of biphasic disorder movements.

PATIENTS	DISORDER MOVEMENTS	STRIATAL RESPONSE	PROLACTINE SECRETORY RESPONSE (ng/ml of plasma)	GROWTH HORMONE SECRETORY RESPONSE (ng/ml of plasma)	L-DOPA ABSORPTION	TOTAL RESPONSE
1	Middle-of-dose	Normal	45 → 8	4 → 50	Normal	Normal
2	—	Normal	17 → 2	3 → 60	Normal	Normal
3	Middle-of-dose	Normal	50 → 300	30 → 4	Normal	Paradoxical
4	Biphasic	Normal	2 → 65	20 → 3	Normal	Paradoxical
5	Middle-of-dose	Normal	100 → 65 → 270	2 → 9 → 2	Normal	Normal then paradoxical
6	—	Normal	12 → 1	30 → 3	Normal	Dissociated
7	Middle-of-dose	Normal	12 → 12	2 → 2	Normal	No response

FIG. 5. Responses of striatal receptors and receptors controlling the secretion of growth hormone and prolactin after L-DOPA administration.

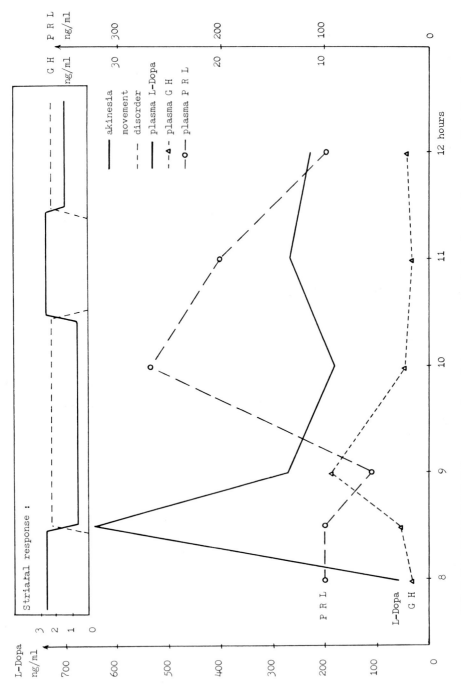

FIG. 6. Normal and paradoxical response of growth hormone and prolactin release in the same patient. Case 6.

pected, striatal response is satisfactory, but GH is decreased. (d) Absence of response (1 case). The striatal response is satisfactory, but the GH and PRL levels are not significantly modified.

The diversity of hypothalamus–infundibulary receptor (9,12) responses can be opposed to the normal but short response of striatal receptors during long-term treatment with L-DOPA. In one of the preceding cases where the striatal response was satisfactory, GH and PRL levels displayed important variations (case 6). Does this show that there is no correlation between GH and PRL levels and clinical responses? This absence of correlation has already been noted in respect to plasma and GH levels (4).

Apparent desensitizing of GH and PRL following administration of several doses of L-DOPA has been noted. A similar phenomenon is observed with striatal receptors, although to a lesser degree. Often the effect of the first morning dose of L-DOPA is greater than that of the following doses, as far as the intensity or duration of effects is concerned. Therefore it seems worthwhile to recommend avoiding too-frequent administration of L-DOPA during the day.

In certain patients (Fig. 6, case 5), the GH and PRL paradoxical response was preceded by a normal response, which might suggest that the receptors controlling GH and PRL secretion were inhibited as a consequence of too strong a dose of the drug. In this case, the striatal response remained satisfactory. In certain cases, however, especially in efficiency fluctuation of type II (start-of-dose akinesia), the striatal receptors could be involved.

Alternatively, we wonder whether in long-term treatment, the modification of the striatal response could represent hypersensitivity. This would explain a paradoxical effect of the treatment, since in a few patients, very low doses of L-DOPA induce abnormal movements. Some phenomena of sudden fluctuations might be related to alternative states of desensitizing and hypersensitivity. This is, indeed, one of the most important problems in long-term treatment with L-DOPA.

REFERENCES

1. Barbeau, A. (1975): Biphasic dyskinesia during levodopa therapy. *Lancet,* 29:756.
2. Boyd, A. E., Lebovitz, H. E., and Pfeiffer, J. B. (1970): Stimulation of human growth-hormone secretion by L-DOPA. *N. Engl. J. Med.,* 28:1425–1429.
3. Frantz, A. G. (1978): Prolactin. *N. Engl. J. Med.,* 298:201–207.
4. Galea-Debono, A., Jenner, P., Marsden, C. D., Parkes, J. D., Tarsy, D., and Walters, J. (1977): Plasma dopa levels and growth hormone response to levodopa in parkinsonism. *J. Neurol., Neurosurg. Psychiatry,* 40:162–167.
5. Granerus, A. K., Jagenburg, R., Rodjer, S., and Svanborg, A. (1974): Variations in L-dopa absorption. *Acta Med. Scand.,* 196:459–463.
6. Hare, T. A., Beasley, B. L., Chambers, R. A., Boehme, D. H., and Vogel, W. H. (1973): Dopa and amino acid levels in plasma and cerebrospinal fluid of patients with Parkinson's disease before and during treatment with L-dopa. *Clin. Chim. Acta,* 45:273–280.
7. Kostyo, J. L., and Reagan, C. R. (1976): The biology of growth hormone. *Pharm. Ther. B,* 2:591–604.
8. Lhermitte, F., Agid, Y., Signoret, J. L., and Studler, J. M. (1977): Des dyskinésies de début et de fin de dose provoquées par la L-dopa. *Rev. Neurol.,* 5:297–308.

9. Malarkey, W. B., Cyrus, J., and Paulson, G. W. (1974): Dissociation of growth hormone and prolactin secretion in Parkinson's disease following chronic L-dopa therapy. *J. Clin. Endocrinol. Metab.*, 39:229–233.
10. Muenter, M. D., Sharpless, N. S., Tyce, G. M., and Darley, F. L. (1977): Patterns of dystonia "IDI and DID" in response to L-dopa therapy for Parkinson's disease. *Mayo Clin. Proc.*, 52:163–174.
11. Muenter, M. D., and Tyce, G. M. (1971): L-Dopa therapy of Parkinson's disease: Plasma L-dopa concentration, therapeutic response and side-effects. *Mayo Clin. Proc.*, 46:231–239.
12. Pontiroli, A. E., Castegnaro, E., Vettaro, M. P., Barret, R. E., and Hoehn, M. M. (1976): Stimulatory effect of the dopa decarboxylase inhibitor Ro. 4–4602 on prolactin release; Inhibition by L-dopa, metergoline, methysergide and 2-Br- -ergocryptine. *Acta Endocrinol.*, 84:36–44.
13. Rondot, P., Ribadeau Dumas, J. L., and Cardon, P. (1975): Effets à court et moyen termes de l'association levodopa inhibiteur de la décarboxylase périphérique. *Thérapie*, 30:653–666.
14. Sharpless, N. S., Muenter, M. D., Tyce, G. M., and Owen, C. A. (1972): 3-O-Methyldopa in plasma during oral L-dopa therapy of patients with Parkinson's disease. *Clin. Chim. Acta*, 37:359–369.
15. Werder, K. V., Van Loon, G. R., Yatsu, F., and Forshan, P. H. (1970): Corticosteroid and growth hormone secretion in patients treated with L-dopa. *Klin. Wochenschr.*, 45:1454–1456.
16. Yahr, M. D., Duvoisin, R. C., Schear, M. J., Barret, R. E., and Hoehn, M. M. (1969): Treatment of parkinsonism with levodopa. *Arch. Neurol.*, 21:343–354.
17. Ziegler, M. (1978): Corrélations biologiques et cliniques au cours des mouvements anormaux induits par la L-dopa. (Thèse) Université Cochin-Port Royal, Paris.

Subject Index

A

Acetylcholine, 102, 103, 230, 293, 387-389, 391-392
  estrogen influence on, 417-418, 421
  opiate influence on release of, 233
  replacement therapy, 444-445
Acetylcholinesterase, 17-19, 22
  in pallidal complex, 1-10
  in substantia nigra, 15, 16-17
Acetylpromazine maleate, 145-147
Adenosine monophosphate, cyclic, 505, 507
Adenylate cyclase system, 204, 228-229, 285, 291
  DOPA dose and, 507, 508
  estrogen influence on, 416-418
Adipsia, 71-72, 81
Aging
  of brain, 32
  L-DOPA therapy and, 403
  essential tremor and, 373
  hydroxylase cofactor levels and, 306
  Parkinson syndrome and, 327, 329-334
  substantia nigra changes and, 231
Agonism, dopaminergic, 217, 218-224, 249-251
Akinesia, 278, 403-405, 442, 512
Alcohol, influence of on essential tremor of, 344, 348, 373, 374
Alpha-gamma coactivation, 178-179
Alpha motoneurons, 142, 143, 177-178
Alzheimer dementia, 333
Amantadine, 335
1-Amino-adamantane sulfate, 502
Amphetamine
  chronic abuse of, 217, 218-220
  dopamine release and, 192
  torticollis treatment with, 335
Anticholinergic agents, 335, 347

Antipsychotic drugs, 457
Antireticulin antibodies, 323
Aphagia, 71-72, 81
Apomorphine, 434-435
  action on dopamine receptors, 380, 383
  in treatment of torticollis, 335, 340, 344, 347
Aspiny neurons, 94-95, 97-99, 106
Autoimmunity, 321, 322-325
Axons, reserpine effects on development of, 26, 29-30

B

Basal ganglia
  acetylcholinesterase in, 19, 22
  estrogen influence on, 411, 414
  motor functions of, 131-139, 141, 155, 156-157
  in Parkinson's disease, 141, 155-157, 368
  somatotropic organization of, 136-137, 138
Basal nucleus of Meynert, 1, 5-6, 7, 9, 133-134
Benserazide, 433, 439, 499-507
Benztropine, 192, 335, 342-345, 346-347
Bradykinesia, 454-456
Bromocriptine
  adverse effects of, 467, 469, 471
  in Parkinson disease therapy, 247, 248, 251, 425-430, 438-439, 461, 463-471, 502
  plasma renin activity and, 314, 315, 317
  in tardive dyskinesia therapy, 380-381, 382, 383
  torticollis therapy with, 335
Butyrophenone, 379